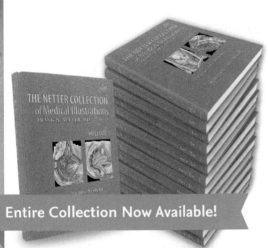
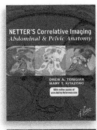
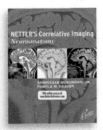
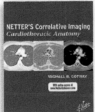
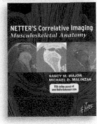

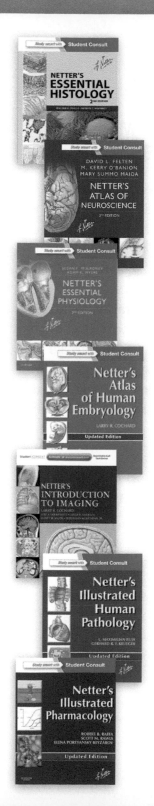

# NETTER'S ESSENTIAL BIOCHEMISTRY

**PETER RONNER, PhD**

Professor of Biochemistry and Molecular Biology
Professor of Pharmaceutical Sciences
Department of Biochemistry and Molecular Biology
Thomas Jefferson University
Philadelphia, Pennsylvania

*Illustrations by*
**Frank H. Netter, MD**

*Contributing Illustrators*
**Carlos A.G. Machado, MD**
**James A. Perkins, MS, MFA**
**Kip Carter, MS, CMI**
**Tiffany Davanzo, MA, CMI**

**ELSEVIER**

# ELSEVIER

1600 John F. Kennedy Blvd.
Ste 1800
Philadelphia, PA 19103-2899

**Library of Congress Cataloging-in-Publication Data**

Names: Ronner, Peter, 1951- author. | Netter, Frank H. (Frank Henry),
    1906-1991, illustrator. | Machado, Carlos A. G., illustrator. |
    Craig, John A., illustrator. | Perkins, James A., illustrator.
Title: Netter's biochemistry / Peter Ronner ; illustrations by
    Frank H. Netter ; contributing illustrators, Carlos A.G. Machado,
    John A. Craig, James A. Perkins.
Other titles: Biochemistry
Description: Philadelphia, PA : Elsevier, [2018] | Includes bibliographical
    references and index.
Identifiers: LCCN 2016024484 | ISBN 9781929007639 (pbk. : alk. paper)
Subjects: | MESH: Biochemical Phenomena | Biochemistry
Classification: LCC QP514.2 | NLM QU 34 | DDC 572–dc23 LC record available at
    https://lccn.loc.gov/2016024484

*Executive Content Strategist:* Elyse O'Grady
*Content Development Specialist:* Stacy Eastman
*Publishing Services Manager:* Patricia Tannian
*Senior Project Manager:* Carrie Stetz
*Design Direction:* Julia Dummitt

Working together
to grow libraries in
developing countries

www.elsevier.com • www.bookaid.org

Printed in the United States of America
Last digit is the print number:   9   8   7   6   5   4

*To Wanda and Lukas*

# About the Author

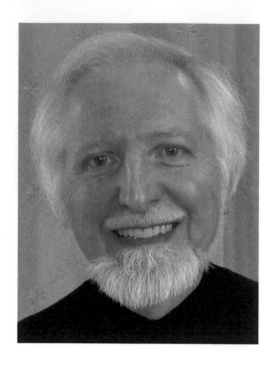

**Peter Ronner, PhD**, is Professor of Biochemistry and Molecular Biology at the Sidney Kimmel College of Medicine at Thomas Jefferson University in Philadelphia. He holds a secondary appointment as Professor of Pharmaceutical Sciences in the College of Pharmacy at Thomas Jefferson University. Dr. Ronner received his PhD in Biochemistry from the Swiss Federal Institute of Technology (ETH) in Zurich. His former laboratory research involved studies of pancreatic hormone secretion. Dr. Ronner has taught medical students for nearly 30 years and pharmacy students for almost 10 years. He is also a past chair of the Association of Biochemistry Course Directors (now Association of Biochemistry Educators). At Jefferson, he has received numerous awards for his teaching, including a Lindback Award and a portrait painting.

# Acknowledgments

Many people have helped me write this book, but Dr. John Thomas from New York University School of Medicine deserves a place of honor. He and I worked on this book together until we were forced to pause for a few years.

Years earlier, at the University of Pennsylvania, the late Dr. Annemarie Weber introduced me to teaching biochemistry to medical students. She was a tremendous role model. At Thomas Jefferson University, Dr. Darwin Prockop planted in my mind the idea of writing a biochemistry textbook. Many years later, Paul Kelly (then at Icon Learning Systems), approached me with the idea of using Dr. Netter's images for a biochemistry review book. This appealed to me because biochemistry is taught as a rather abstract science that students have difficulty linking to actual patients. The Netter images, I hoped, would provide the views of the practicing physician. Thanks to the support of my chairman, Dr. Jeffrey Benovic, this book project became part of my scholarly pursuits. I am thankful for the invaluable feedback the many students of medicine and pharmacy at Jefferson gave me over the years.

I would like to thank the team at Elsevier for their support, especially Elyse O'Grady (Senior Content Strategist), Stacy Eastman and Marybeth Thiel (Content Development Specialists), as well as Carrie Stetz (Senior Project Manager/Specialist).

Finally, I would like to thank my family and friends for their support while writing this book.

This book is dedicated to my wife Wanda and my son Lukas. Wanda has been a key influence on me, because she has continuously given me her perspective as a practicing physician and medical student educator. Lukas, a chemistry major and current medical student, has been my most trusted adviser on questions about young learners, chemistry, and artwork, and he has reviewed much of my writing.

## COAUTHORS AND CHAPTER REVIEWERS

I am deeply indebted to John Thomas for his contributions, which involved designing this book and writing drafts of several chapters: Clinical Tests Based on DNA or RNA; Basic Genetics for Biochemistry; Transcription and RNA Processing; Translation and Posttranslational Protein Processing; Pentose Phosphate Pathway, Oxidative Stress, and Glucose 6-Phosphate Dehydrogenase Deficiency; Oxidative Phosphorylation and Mitochondrial Diseases; Fatty Acids, Ketone Bodies, and Ketoacidosis; Triglycerides and Hypertriglyceridemia; Cholesterol Metabolism and Hypercholesterolemia; Steroid Hormones and Vitamin D; Eicosanoids; and Signaling.

**John Thomas, PhD**
Research Associate Professor (Retired)
Department of Biochemistry and Molecular Pharmacology
New York University School of Medicine
New York, New York

I am very thankful to Emine Ercikan Abali for coauthoring the chapters on Triglycerides and Hypertriglyceridemia and Cholesterol Metabolism and Hypercholesterolemia.

**Emine Ercikan Abali, PhD**
Associate Professor of Biochemistry and Molecular Biology
Rutgers Robert Wood Johnson Medical School
Piscataway, New Jersey

I am very grateful to the following persons for contributing their expertise and reviewing chapters:

**David Axelrod, MD**
Associate Professor of Medicine
Department of Medicine
Sidney Kimmel Medical College at Thomas Jefferson University
Philadelphia, Pennsylvania

**Samir K. Ballas, MD**
Emeritus Professor of Medicine and Pediatrics
Cardeza Foundation for Hematologic Research
Department of Medicine, Division of Hematology
Sidney Kimmel Medical College at Thomas Jefferson University
Philadelphia, Pennsylvania

**James C. Barton, MD**
Medical Director
Southern Iron Disorders Center;
Clinical Professor of Medicine
Department of Medicine
University of Alabama at Birmingham
Birmingham, Alabama

**Jeffrey L. Benovic, PhD**
Professor
Department of Biochemistry and Molecular Biology
Sidney Kimmel Medical College at Thomas Jefferson University
Philadelphia, Pennsylvania

**Bruno Calabretta, MD, PhD**
Professor
Department of Cancer Biology
Sidney Kimmel Medical College at Thomas Jefferson
    University
Philadelphia, Pennsylvania

**Gino Cingolani, PhD**
Professor
Department of Biochemistry and Molecular Biology
Sidney Kimmel Medical College at Thomas Jefferson
    University
Philadelphia, Pennsylvania

**Joe Deweese, PhD**
Associate Professor
Department of Pharmaceutical Sciences
Lipscomb University, College of Pharmacy and Health
    Sciences
Nashville, Tennessee

**Tina Bocker Edmonston, MD**
Associate Professor
Department of Pathology and Laboratory Medicine
Cooper University Health Care, Cooper Medical School at
    Rowan University
Camden, New Jersey

**Steven Ellis, PhD**
Professor
Department of Biochemistry
University of Louisville
Louisville, Kentucky

**Masumi Eto, PhD**
Associate Professor
Department of Molecular Physiology and Biophysics
Sidney Kimmel Medical College at Thomas Jefferson
    University
Philadelphia, Pennsylvania

**Andrzej Fertala, PhD**
Professor
Department of Orthopaedic Surgery
Sidney Kimmel Medical College at Thomas Jefferson
    University
Philadelphia, Pennsylvania

**Elizabeth Gilje, BS**
Medical Student
Sidney Kimmel Medical College at Thomas Jefferson
    University
Philadelphia, Pennsylvania

**Christopher Haines, MD**
Assistant Professor
Department of Family and Community Medicine
Sidney Kimmel Medical College at Thomas Jefferson
    University
Philadelphia, Pennsylvania

**Steven K. Herrine, MD**
Professor
Department of Medicine
Sidney Kimmel Medical College at Thomas Jefferson
    University
Philadelphia, Pennsylvania

**Jacqueline M. Hibbert, PhD**
Associate Professor
Department of Microbiology, Biochemistry and
    Immunology
Morehouse School of Medicine
Atlanta, Georgia

**Jan B. Hoek, PhD**
Professor
Department of Pathology, Anatomy, and Cell Biology
Sidney Kimmel Medical College at Thomas Jefferson
    University
Philadelphia, Pennsylvania

**Tanis Hogg, PhD**
Associate Professor
Department of Medical Education
Texas Tech University Health Sciences Center El Paso, Paul
    L. Foster School of Medicine
El Paso, Texas

**Ya-Ming Hou, PhD**
Professor
Department of Biochemistry and Molecular Biology
Sidney Kimmel Medical College at Thomas Jefferson
    University
Philadelphia, Pennsylvania

**Serge A. Jabbour, DM**
Professor
Department of Medicine
Sidney Kimmel Medical College at Thomas Jefferson
    University
Philadelphia, Pennsylvania

**Francis E. Jenney Jr, PhD**
Associate Professor
Department of Biomedical Sciences
Georgia Campus–PCOM
Suwanee, Georgia

**Erica Johnson, PhD**
Genomics Program Manager
Clinical Laboratories
Thomas Jefferson University Hospital
Philadelphia, Pennsylvania

**Leo C. Katz, MD**
Clinical Associate Professor
Department of Medicine, Division of Gastroenterology and
    Hepatology
Sidney Kimmel Medical College at Thomas Jefferson
    University
Philadelphia, Pennsylvania

**Janet Lindsley, PhD**
Associate Professor
Department of Biochemistry
University of Utah, School of Medicine
Salt Lake City, Utah

**Diane Merry, PhD**
Professor
Department of Biochemistry and Molecular Biology
Sidney Kimmel Medical College at Thomas Jefferson
    University
Philadelphia, Pennsylvania

**Michael Natter, BA**
Medical Student
Sidney Kimmel Medical College at Thomas Jefferson
    University
Philadelphia, Pennsylvania

**John M. Pascal, PhD**
Associate Professor
Department of Biochemistry and Molecular Medicine
University of Montreal
Montreal, Québec, Canada

**Puttur D. Prasad, PhD**
Professor
Department of Biochemistry and Molecular Biology
Medical College of Georgia at Augusta University
Augusta, Georgia

**Lawrence Prochaska, PhD**
Professor
Department of Biochemistry and Molecular Biology
Wright State University, Boonshoft School of Medicine
Dayton, Ohio

**Lucy C. Robinson, PhD**
Associate Professor
Department of Biochemistry and Molecular Biology
Louisiana State University Health Sciences Center
Shreveport, Louisiana

**Lukas Ronner, BS**
Medical Student
Icahn School of Medicine at Mount Sinai
New York, New York

**Wanda Ronner, MD**
Professor of Clinical Obstetrics and Gynecology
Department of Obstetrics and Gynecology
Perelman School of Medicine of the University of
    Pennsylvania
Philadelphia, Pennsylvania

**Richard Sabina, PhD**
Professor (Retired)
Department of Biomedical Sciences
Oakland University William Beaumont School of Medicine
Rochester, Minnesota

**John Sands, PhD**
Professor
Department of Biochemistry
Ross University, School of Medicine
Picard, Dominica

**Charles Scott, PhD**
Director, Jefferson Discovery Core
Department of Biochemistry and Molecular Biology
Sidney Kimmel Medical College at Thomas Jefferson
    University
Philadelphia, Pennsylvania

**Philip Wedegaertner, PhD**
Professor
Department of Biochemistry and Molecular Biology
Sidney Kimmel Medical College at Thomas Jefferson
    University
Philadelphia, Pennsylvania

**Charlene Williams, PhD**
Professor
Department of Biomedical Sciences
Cooper Medical School of Rowan University
Camden, New Jersey

**Edward Winter, PhD**
Professor
Department of Biochemistry and Molecular Biology
Sidney Kimmel Medical College at Thomas Jefferson
    University
Philadelphia, Pennsylvania

**Takashi Yonetani, PhD**
Professor
Department of Biochemistry and Biophysics
Perelman School of Medicine of the University of
    Pennsylvania
Philadelphia, Pennsylvania

# About the Artist

## FRANK H. NETTER, MD

Frank H. Netter was born in 1906 in New York City. He studied art at the Art Student's League and the National Academy of Design before entering medical school at New York University, where he received his MD degree in 1931. During his student years, Dr. Netter's notebook sketches attracted the attention of the medical faculty and other physicians, allowing him to augment his income by illustrating articles and textbooks. He continued illustrating as a sideline after establishing a surgical practice in 1933, but he ultimately opted to give up his practice in favor of a full-time commitment to art. After service in the United States Army during World War II, Dr. Netter began his long collaboration with the CIBA Pharmaceutical Company (now Novartis Pharmaceuticals). This 45-year partnership resulted in the production of the extraordinary collection of medical art so familiar to physicians and other medical professionals worldwide.

In 2005, Elsevier, Inc. purchased the Netter Collection and all publications from Icon Learning Systems. There are now over 50 publications featuring the art of Dr. Netter available through Elsevier, Inc. (in the US: www.us.elsevierhealth.com/Netter and outside the US: www.elsevierhealth.com).

Dr. Netter's works are among the finest examples of the use of illustration in the teaching of medical concepts. The 13-book *Netter Collection of Medical Illustrations*, which includes the greater part of the more than 20,000 paintings created by Dr. Netter, became and remains one of the most famous medical works ever published. The Netter *Atlas of Human Anatomy*, first published in 1989, presents the anatomical paintings from the Netter Collection. Now translated into 16 languages, it is the anatomy atlas of choice among medical and health professions students the world over.

The Netter illustrations are appreciated not only for their aesthetic qualities, but, more important, for their intellectual content. As Dr. Netter wrote in 1949, ". . . clarification of a subject is the aim and goal of illustration. No matter how beautifully painted, how delicately and subtly rendered a subject may be, it is of little value as a *medical illustration* if it does not serve to make clear some medical point." Dr. Netter's planning, conception, point of view, and approach are what inform his paintings and what make them so intellectually valuable.

Frank H. Netter, MD, physician and artist, died in 1991.

Learn more about the physician-artist whose work has inspired the Netter Reference collection: http://www.netterimages.com/artist/netter.htm.

# Preface

This book provides an introduction to and review of biochemistry as it pertains to the competencies required for graduation as a doctor of medicine or pharmacy. Increasingly, the basic sciences are taught alongside clinical science, often organ by organ. This book can help students in such integrated curricula gain a discipline-specific understanding of biochemistry, particularly metabolism. The book is structured so that it is useful for both the novice and the student who needs a quick review in preparation for licensure exams. The chapters are extensively cross-referenced so the material can be used in almost any chapter sequence. Descriptions of disease states are a regular part of the book rather than an addendum in the margin. Students often find it challenging to use their knowledge of basic science to solve clinical problems. Hopefully, Dr. Netter's images ("Medicine's Michelangelo"), as well as the text and other diagrams in this book, will help students build mental bridges between basic science and clinical practice.

The chapters have a structure that makes it easy for the reader to decide what to read and review:

■ The Synopsis is an introductory overview of the content of the chapter that requires very little preexisting knowledge.
■ The Learning Objectives indicate what the reader should be able to do when mastering the material presented in the chapter.

■ Each section starts with a preview.
■ Selected terms are printed in bold to make it easier to find relevant text when starting from the index.
■ The diagrams contain only the most essential information.
■ The Summary provides a brief overview of the chapter material for the expert.
■ A Further Reading section provides the reader with a starting point to satisfy deeper interests.
■ Review Questions provide the reader with an opportunity to apply newly acquired knowledge. Answers to these questions are at the end of the book.

Writing this text and designing the accompanying graphs has been a wonderful and interesting journey for me. I have also enjoyed many years of teaching biochemistry to future physicians and pharmacists. I hope that you, the reader, will also be amazed by the processes that underlie human existence, both in health and in sickness.

**Peter Ronner**

*P.S.: Please feel free to email suggestions for improvements to peterronner1@gmail.com.*

# Contents

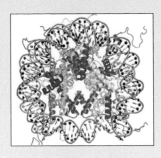

# Chapter 1

# Human Karyotype and the Structure of DNA

## SYNOPSIS

- Heritable information is encoded in deoxyribonucleic acid (DNA). DNA is a linear polymer of deoxyribonucleotides, and it is present in the nucleus and mitochondria of cells.
- The DNA of a cell comprises pairs of complementary molecules; each pair assumes a double-helical structure.
- DNA double helices in the nucleus are wound into higher-order structures. The simplest of such structures is the nucleosome; the most complex structures exist in the form of condensed chromosomes during cell division. Light microscopic examination of these chromosomes is part of karyotyping.
- Helicases and topoisomerases change the coiling of DNA for transcription, replication, and repair of DNA.
- Inhibitors of DNA topoisomerases can be used to destroy cancer cells or bacteria.

## LEARNING OBJECTIVES

*For mastery of this topic, you should be able to do the following:*
- Describe the components and architecture of a DNA double helix and explain where proteins bind to DNA helices.
- Provide an example of reporting a DNA sequence in the customarily abbreviated style.
- Describe the most basic unit for packaging DNA into the nucleus.
- Describe the normal human karyotype and list the number of DNA double helices that make up a single metaphase chromosome.
- Describe the function of DNA topoisomerases and explain the role of these enzymes in changing the topology of chromosomes.

## 1. CHEMICAL STRUCTURE OF DNA

*Mitochondria and the nucleus of each cell contain DNA that is a polymer of four basic types of nucleotides. DNA stores heritable information by way of its nucleotide sequence.*

DNA is a linear polymer of the **deoxyribonucleotides** deoxyadenosine monophosphate (dAMP), deoxyguanosine monophosphate (dGMP), deoxycytidine monophosphate (dCMP), and thymidine monophosphate (dTMP, TMP; Fig. 1.1). Each deoxyribonucleotide consists of deoxyribosephosphate (derived from a pentose, a 5-carbon sugar) covalently linked to a base that is **adenine, guanine, cytosine** (or 5-methyl cytosine), or **thymine**. Adenine and guanine structurally resemble purine; hence, they are called **purine** nucleotides (synthesis, turnover, and degradation of these nucleotides are described in Chapter 38). Cytosine and thymine structurally resemble pyrimidine; hence, they are called **pyrimidine** nucleotides (synthesis of these nucleotides is described in Chapter 37).

As part of epigenetic regulation, ~4% of the cytidine nucleotides of DNA in the nucleus are **methylated to 5-methyl deoxycytidine** (see Fig. 1.1). The term *epigenetic regulation* refers to changes in the DNA or DNA-associated proteins that do not affect the sequence of the bases but affect gene expression. Some of these changes can be heritable and passed from one cell to its descendants (see imprinting in Chapter 5). Quite generally, methylation influences the higher-order packing and transcription of DNA (see Chapter 6). Methylation is required for the inactivation of the second X chromosome in females (see Chapters 5 and 21), the silencing of certain transposons (movable genetic elements), regulation of the expression of genes during development, and determining the expression of particular genes from only the mother or only the father.

Each DNA molecule has a **5′ end** and a **3′ end** (Fig. 1.2). To distinguish the atoms of the deoxyribose from those of the base, the deoxyribose carbon atoms are given a **prime** as a postfix (e.g., 3′). The dinucleotide shown in Fig. 1.2 has a phosphate group at the 5′ position of nucleotide 1 and a hydroxyl group at the 3′ position of nucleotide 2, which is typical of DNA. The nucleotides are linked by **phosphodiester bonds**. DNA is normally elongated at the 3′ end (see Section 1 in Chapter 3).

By convention, the **sequence** of a DNA is written as the sequence of the bases in the **5′→3′** direction, using **A** for adenine, **C** for cytosine, **G** for guanine, and **T** for thymine. If the sequence is instead written 3′→5′, this must be indicated. The sequence of bases in DNA contains heritable information. DNA is found in the nucleus (see Section 4) and in mitochondria (see Section 3 in Chapter 23).

## 2. HYDROGEN BONDING BETWEEN COMPLEMENTARY BASES

*In the fashion of a zipper, complementary DNA molecules associate by hydrogen bonding. A and T can be linked by two hydrogen bonds, C and G by three hydrogen bonds.*

In Watson-Crick base pairing, A and T are hydrogen bonded to each other, and so are C and G. Each base of a nucleotide contains one or more hydrogen donors (–OH and –NH₂) and one or more hydrogen acceptors (=O and =N–). A hydrogen acceptor can form a partial bond to a donor's hydrogen atom; such a bond is called a **hydrogen bond**. A and T each contain one hydrogen donor and one hydrogen acceptor in suitable positions, such that A and T can be linked by a total of two hydrogen bonds (Fig. 1.3). C has one hydrogen donor and two hydrogen acceptors, while G has two hydrogen donors

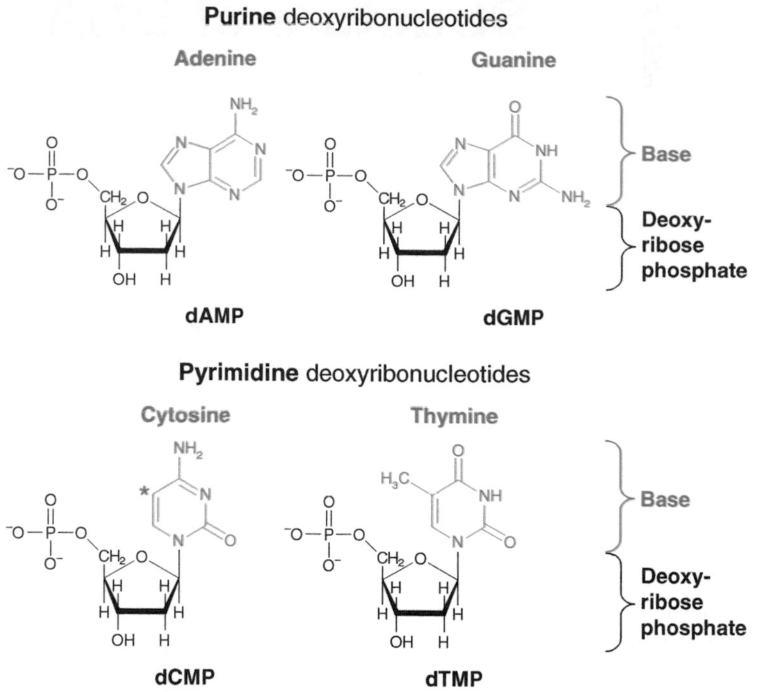

**Purine** deoxyribonucleotides

Adenine                     Guanine

} Base

} Deoxy-
  ribose
  phosphate

dAMP                        dGMP

**Pyrimidine** deoxyribonucleotides

Cytosine                    Thymine

} Base

} Deoxy-
  ribose
  phosphate

dCMP                        dTMP

**Fig. 1.1** **Structures of deoxyribonucleotides found in DNA.** The asterisk indicates the site of potential cytosine methylation.

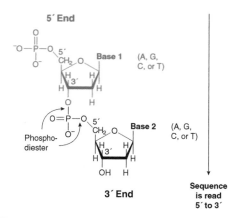

**Fig. 1.2** **The structure and polarity of a single strand of DNA.**

in complementary strands that, in vivo, usually assume a double-helical structure (Fig. 1.5). In mitochondria, each DNA strand consists of about 16,000 nucleotides; in the nucleus, each DNA strand consists of more than 45 million nucleotides.

When a DNA sequence is reported, the sequence of the complementary strand is usually omitted because it can easily be inferred.

According to the **Chargaff rule**, DNA contains equimolar amounts of A and T, as well as equimolar amounts of C and G. AT and CG base pairing are the basis of Chargaff's finding.

and one hydrogen acceptor in suitable positions so that C and G can be linked by a total of three hydrogen bonds. Since they form hydrogen bonds with each other, A and T are called **complementary bases**; likewise, C and G are complementary bases. CG base pairs are harder to separate than AT base pairs because they have more hydrogen bonds. (Non–Watson-Crick base pairing is observed predominantly in RNA, where it is common.)

In two complementary DNA molecules, all bases form hydrogen-bonded AT and GC base pairs, and the molecules are paired in an antiparallel fashion. For instance, the molecules 5′-AACGT-3′ and 3′-TTGCA-5′ are complementary (Fig. 1.4). The nucleotide at the 5′ end of one DNA strand is thus hydrogen bonded to the nucleotide at the 3′ end of its complementary DNA strand. All heritable human DNA exists

## 3. DNA DOUBLE HELIX

*Most human DNA assumes a double-helical structure. The double helix consists of two complementary strands that run in opposite directions.*

Complementary hydrogen-bonded DNA molecules normally assume the structure of a **DNA double helix** (see Fig. 1.5). In this structure, the hydrogen-bonded bases are close to the central long axis of the DNA helix. The covalently linked deoxyribose phosphates of the two DNA strands wind around the periphery of the helix cylinder, akin to the threads of an unusual screw (a typical screw has only one thread). As is evident from Fig. 1.3, the bonds between the bases and the deoxyribose moieties (i.e., the N-glycosidic bonds) do not point in exactly opposite directions. Hence, the two strands of linked deoxyribose phosphates are closer together on one side of the base pair than on the other side. Thus, the DNA double

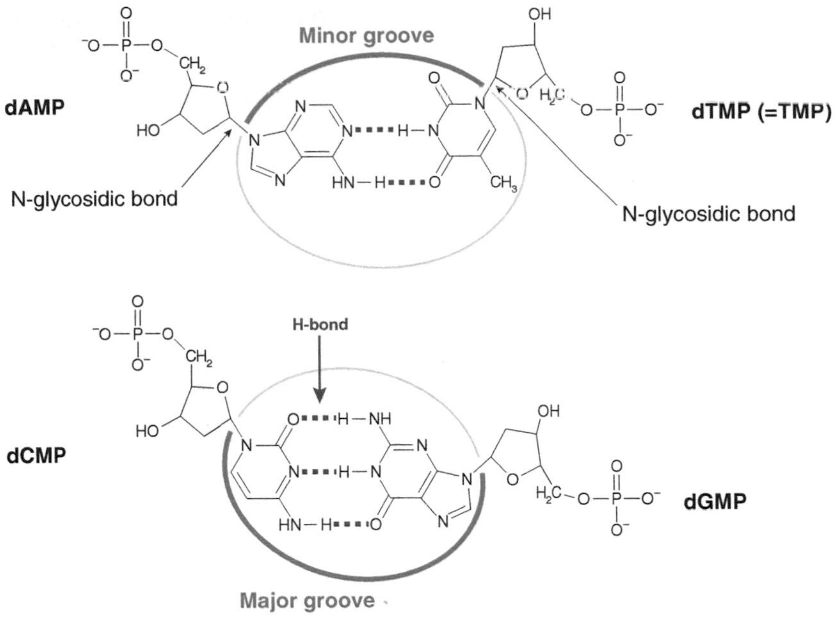

**Fig. 1.3** **Hydrogen bonding between complementary bases.**

helix has unequal grooves: a **minor groove** and a **major groove**.

There are several double-helical DNA structures that differ in handedness, diameter, and rise per turn. The most prominent of these structures are referred to as **A-DNA**, **B-DNA**, and **Z-DNA**. In cells, most DNA is in a double-helical form that resembles B-DNA.

**Transcription factors** that bind to DNA (see Chapter 6) bind to atoms at the surface of the major or minor groove and can thereby recognize a particular nucleotide sequence. Some transcription factors increase the contact with DNA further by bending or partially opening the double helix.

Certain positively charged side chains of **DNA-binding proteins**, as well as certain positively charged **stains** used in histochemistry (e.g., the basic dyes **hematoxylin**, **methylene blue**, and **toluidine blue**), bind to DNA by interacting with the negatively charged phosphate groups. These phosphate groups line the backbone of DNA and are exposed on the outside of the double helix (see Fig. 1.5). Among DNA-binding proteins, positive charges are found on some amino acid side chains of histones (see below) and of certain transcription factors (see Chapter 6). Complexes of DNA and the DNA-binding histone proteins are referred to as **chromatin**. The negative charges of the phosphate groups of DNA alone give rise to an overall negative charge of DNA that is taken advantage of in the **electrophoresis** of DNA (see Chapter 4).

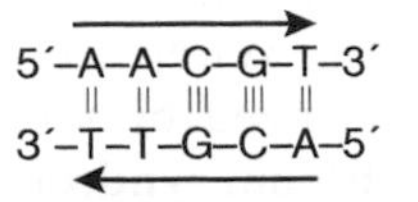

**Fig. 1.4** **Basic structure of double-stranded DNA.** Double-stranded DNA can form a double helix (see Fig. 1.5).

In vivo, hydrogen bonds between bases of complementary DNA strands are broken and reformed during replication, repair, or transcription of DNA (see Chapters 2, 3, and 6). In vitro, the separation and "rejoining" (hybridization) of complementary DNA strands are an important part of many diagnostic DNA-based procedures (see Chapter 4).

## 4. PACKING OF DNA DOUBLE HELICES INTO CHROMATIDS

*The length of human DNA molecules far exceeds the diameter of the cell nucleus. DNA is compacted into orderly structures ranging from nucleosomes to metaphase chromatids.*

In the nucleus, DNA is folded into nucleosomes, which in turn are part of increasingly higher orders of folding. The greatest degree of DNA compaction is needed for cell division. The longest human chromosome (chromosome 1) contains about 246 million base pairs and has a length ~15,000 times the diameter of a typical nucleus. The organization of DNA also affects the transcription of genes. The basic unit of folding is the **nucleosome**, of which several types exist. Nucleosomes contain a **core particle** that consists of eight histone proteins, a DNA helix of ~147 base pairs that encircles the **histones** ~1.7 times (Fig. 1.6), and **linker DNA** of ~40 base pairs to which histone H1 is often bound. N- and C-terminal **tails** of the histones protrude from nucleosome core particles. Certain amino acids in these histone tails can be modified (Table 1.1). The resulting structure of the histone tails affects the packing, **replication** (see Chapter 3), and **transcription** of DNA (see Chapter 6).

Nucleosomes can be organized into **30-nm** diameter **chromatin fibers**. Chromatin fibers, in turn, can be condensed into yet higher-order structures, and finally into

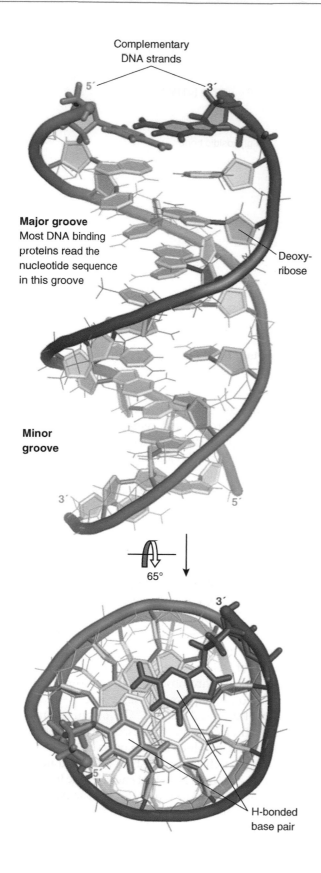

Complementary DNA strands

5′  3′

**Major groove**
Most DNA binding proteins read the nucleotide sequence in this groove

Deoxy-ribose

**Minor groove**

3′  5′

65°

3′

5′

H-bonded base pair

**Fig. 1.5** **The double-helical structure of DNA.** The structure of an 11-base-pair segment of the human N-ras gene is shown (the sequence of the purple strand is 5′-GGCAGGTGGTG; this sequence frequently undergoes mutation and then promotes the development of a tumor). The bases are in the center, and the riboses are located in the periphery of the helix. The blue and purple snaking cylinders are imaginary forms that connect the phosphorus atoms and show the progress of the helix. The bonds that connect phosphates and riboses and that form the true backbone of a DNA strand are generally situated just outside the calculated cylinders. The planes of the rings of deoxyriboses and bases are shown in light gray. The two DNA strands are antiparallel; the blue strand is winding downward (5′ to 3′), while the purple strand is winding its way up (5′ to 3′). The structure of this oligomer mostly resembles the structure of B-DNA. (Based on Protein Data Bank [www.rcsb.org] file 1AFZ from Zegar IS, Stone MP. Solution structure of an oligodeoxynucleotide containing the human N-ras codon 12 sequence refined from 1H NMR using molecular dynamics restrained by nuclear Overhauser effects. *Chem Res Toxicol.* 1996;9:114–125.)

chromatids. Chromatids are found only in dividing cells during mitosis.

## 5. CHANGES IN DNA TOPOLOGY

*The cellular processes of DNA repair, replication, and transcription (discussed in Chapters 2, 3, and 6) require, at times, the unwinding of DNA from its structures (e.g., the 30-nm chromatin fiber, the nucleosomes, and the double helix) followed by rewinding. Changes in the winding of DNA are catalyzed by helicases and topoisomerases.*

Topology is a field of mathematics that describes the deformation, twisting, and stretching of objects such as DNA. As outlined above, DNA of human chromosomes is organized into nucleosomes and higher-order structures. The chemical structure of DNA can accommodate only a limited amount of torsional strain, and the chromatin structure prevents the dispersion of strain over a large distance. (As an analogy, consider how winding affects the three-dimensional shape of a phone cord or garden hose.) Thus, the winding of DNA (the topological state of DNA) matters. Torsional strain can result from the partial opening of a DNA helix (e.g., during repair, replication, or transcription) or from a nonrotatable complex of enzymes that moves in between the two strands of a DNA double helix (Fig. 1.7). Replication and transcription, for example, cause overwinding, or positive supercoiling, within the chromosomes.

**Helicases** can use energy from ATP hydrolysis to separate the two strands of the double helix. The energy input from ATP is needed to pay the penalty for breaking hydrogen bonds between bases in DNA. Humans produce several different helicases. The physiological roles of these helicases are largely unknown. Mutations in a few helicases are known to cause disease: a deficiency in WRN causes **Werner syndrome** (predominantly characterized by premature aging); a deficiency in BLM causes **Bloom syndrome** (accompanied by an increased rate of tumorigenesis); and a deficiency in RECQ4 causes **Rothmund-Thomson syndrome** (associated with skin

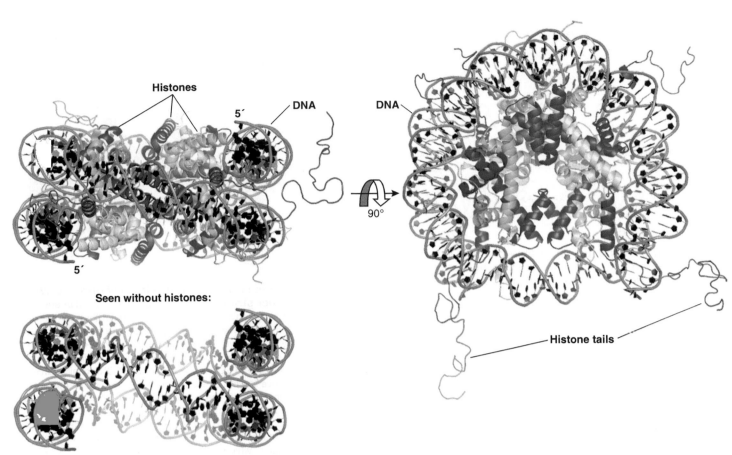

Histones

DNA

5′

5′

DNA

Seen without histones:

90°

Histone tails

**Fig. 1.6** **Packing of DNA into a nucleosome core particle in the nucleus.** Nucleotides are shown in black. An idealized cylinder through all phosphorus atoms is shown in light brown. DNA winds almost twice around a core of eight histone proteins. There are two copies each of histone H2A (gold), H2B (red), H3 (blue), and H4 (green). (Based on Protein Data Bank [www.rcsb.org] file 1KX5 from Davey CA, Sargent DF, Luger K, Maeder AW, Richmond TJ. Solvent mediated interactions in the structure of the nucleosome core particle at 1.9 Å resolution. *J Mol Biol.* 2002;319:1097–1113.)

**Table 1.1**    **Modifications of Histones**

| Amino Acid | Side Chain Modification |
|---|---|
| Lysine | Methylation (mono-, di- or tri-; CH₃– is a methyl group) Acetylation (CH₃–CO– is an acetyl group) Ubiquitylation (ubiquitin is a 76-residue protein) Sumoylation (SUMO = small ubiquitin-like modifier, a small group of ~100-residue proteins) ADP-ribosylation (conjugation with a ribose that in turn forms a phosphodiester with ADP) |
| Arginine | Methylation (mono- or di-; there are two possibilities for dimethylation) Deimination (exchange of =NH for =O, turning arginine into citrulline) |
| Glutamate | ADP-ribosylation |
| Serine | Phosphorylation |
| Threonine | Phosphorylation |
| Tyrosine | Phosphorylation |

*ADP*, adenosine diphosphate.

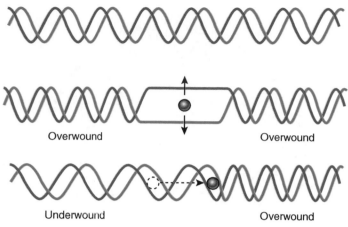

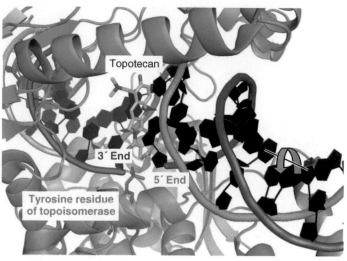

**Fig. 1.7** **Strain imposed on double-helical DNA when the helix is opened up partially, or when a nonrotatable object moves in between the two complementary strands.**

**Fig. 1.8** **Topoisomerase I cuts one strand of DNA and swivels around the other strand.** The riboses and bases of DNA are shown in black. An artificial, smoothed backbone is drawn through the phosphorus atoms in red, brown, or orange (there are three segments of DNA). The enzyme is shown in greenish blue. A tyrosine residue (magenta) is covalently linked to the 3′ end of the "red" DNA chain. The "brown" DNA chain, together with a portion of the "orange" DNA chain, can rotate and thereby relieve torsion stress. Normally, the 5′ end of the "brown" chain then reconnects with the 3′ end of the "red" chain. Here, the chemotherapeutic drug topotecan (shown as a stick model with C in grey, N in blue, and O in red) binds in between the 3′ base of the "red" chain and the 5′ base of the "brown" chain; topotecan thereby prevents religation of these chains, which leads to cell death. (Based on Protein Data Bank [www.rcsb.org] file 1K4T from Staker BL, Hjerrild K, Feese MD, Behnke CA, Burgin Jr. AB, Stewart L. The mechanism of topoisomerase I poisoning by a camptothecin analog. *Proc Natl Acad Sci.* 2002; 99:15387–15392.)

abnormalities). All of these disorders are rare and show autosomal recessive inheritance.

Once a part of two complementary DNA strands has been separated, **single-strand binding proteins** (e.g., replication protein A [RPA]) can prevent the pairing of bases.

**Topoisomerases** can relieve strain in DNA and thus alter the topology of DNA. **Supercoiled DNA** is DNA that has folded back on itself to accommodate under- or overwinding (negative or positive supercoiling, respectively) of the double helix. Topoisomerase I and topoisomerase II both relax supercoiled DNA during replication and transcription. Topoisomerase II also untangles (decatenates) DNA for chromosome segregation during mitosis. Type I topoisomerases cut one strand, whereas type II topoisomerases cut both strands of a double helix. In both cases, the enzyme forms a transient covalent link with either the 5′ or 3′ end of the broken DNA.

**Type I topoisomerases** (including topoisomerase I) relieve the torsional strain of DNA by cutting one strand of the double helix, swiveling around the intact strand or passing the intact strand through the break, and then ligating the cut strand again (Fig. 1.8).

Inhibitors of topoisomerase I offer a means of preferentially damaging tumor cells that divide more frequently than normal cells. Analogs of **camptothecin** prolong the lifetime of a covalent DNA–topoisomerase I complex that is formed as a normal reaction intermediate. As the genome is copied during replication (see Chapter 3), the obstructing DNA–topoisomerase I–camptothecin complex can result in permanent strand breaks, which the cell may attempt to repair. When the number of double-strand breaks exceeds a cell's capacity for repair (see homologous recombination repair in Chapter 2), the cell undergoes apoptosis (i.e., programmed cell death; see Chapters 2 and 8). Camptothecin analogs (e.g., **topotecan** and **irinotecan**) are used predominantly in the treatment of advanced malignancies (e.g., relapsing small-cell lung cancer or metastatic ovarian cancer).

**Type II topoisomerases** (topoisomerase II in humans, and DNA gyrase and topoisomerase IV in bacteria) cleave both

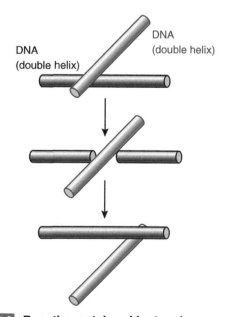

**Fig. 1.9** **Reaction catalyzed by topoisomerase II.**

strands of one double helix, use conformational changes in the enzyme subunits to pass a separate DNA segment between the break, and then ligate the cut strands (Figs. 1.9 and 1.10). This process requires ATP. Type II topoisomerases are involved in relaxing the supercoils that result from DNA replication or

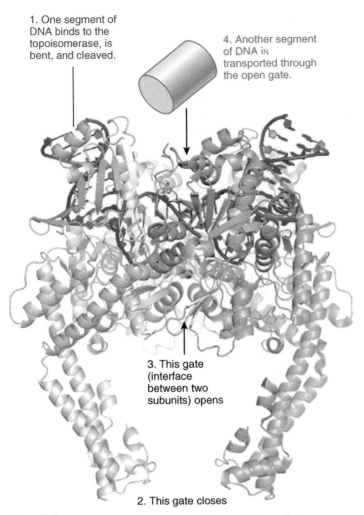

1. One segment of DNA binds to the topoisomerase, is bent, and cleaved.

4. Another segment of DNA is transported through the open gate.

3. This gate (interface between two subunits) opens

2. This gate closes

**Fig. 1.10** **Human topoisomerase IIα catalyzes the passage of one DNA strand through another DNA strand.** The enzyme functions as a dimer. The image shows the catalytic core domain, including the central gate and the lower, C-terminal gate; not shown is the ATPase domain, which is at the top of the structure. (Based on Protein Data Bank [www.rcsb.org] file 4FM9 from Wendorff TJ, Schmidt BH, Heslop P, Austin CA, Berger JM. The structure of DNA-bound human topoisomerase II alpha: conformational mechanisms for coordinating inter-subunit interactions with DNA cleavage. *J Mol Biol.* 2012;424: 109–124.)

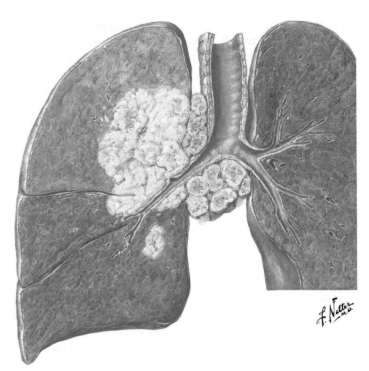

**Fig. 1.11** **Etoposide is an inhibitor of topoisomerase II and is often used in the treatment of extensive small-cell lung cancer.** These patients typically have disseminated disease. Etoposide is often combined with a platinum drug.

transcription. Sister chromatids become intertwined during DNA replication; this linking is called *catenation*. The essential function of type II topoisomerases, which cannot be performed by type I enzymes, is the separation (decatenation) of replicated chromosomes before compaction and cell division.

Inhibitors of topoisomerase II are useful as anticancer agents. Most of these inhibitors are part of a class called topoisomerase II poisons. Two drugs of this class that are widely used in chemotherapy are **doxorubicin** (an anthracycline) and **etoposide** (an epipodophyllotoxin; Fig. 1.11). In the presence of these drugs, topoisomerase II can cleave DNA but cannot ligate it. Therefore, DNA replication and transcription are both inhibited. As a consequence, DNA strand breaks accumulate and lead to apoptosis (programmed cell death). However, these drugs are also mildly mutagenic and thus increase a patient's risk of developing therapy-related leukemia. Aside from poisons, catalytic inhibitors of topoisomerase II inhibit other portions of the catalytic mechanism of the enzyme (e.g., ATP hydrolysis) and cause cell death without inducing DNA strand breaks.

Some polyphenols in our diet also poison topoisomerase II. Soybeans contain **genistein**, which binds to estrogen receptors and can help ameliorate symptoms of menopause. Genistein also poisons topoisomerase II. Genistein appears to have anticancer activity, but in pregnant mothers it also confers a higher risk of childhood leukemia in the offspring. Green tea contains the polyphenol **epigallocatechin gallate** (EGCG), which also poisons topoisomerase II. The biological impact of these poisons has not been fully established, and there is some evidence that these agents may be chemopreventive.

**Fluoroquinolone antibacterials** inhibit bacterial DNA gyrase (the name given to the positively supercoiling topoisomerase II in bacteria) and topoisomerase IV. Commonly used quinolones are the broad-spectrum antibiotics **ciprofloxacin**, levofloxacin, ofloxacin, and moxifloxacin.

## 6. HUMAN KARYOTYPE

*The human karyotype consists of 46 chromosomes. Stained metaphase chromosomes are used for karyotyping.*

Each normal human cell nucleus in the $G_0$ phase of the cell cycle (see Chapter 8) contains 46 chromosomes (i.e., 46 DNA double helices). In preparation for cell division, the 46 double helices are replicated to form 92 double helices (see

Chapter 3). Then, each one of these helices is greatly condensed into **chromatids** (see Section 4). Proteins join pairs of identical chromatids at their centromeres to form **metaphase chromosomes**.

With basophilic stains (e.g., **Giemsa stain**), metaphase chromosomes can be visualized under a light microscope (Fig. 1.12). Images of stained chromosomes are used to characterize the chromosomes of an individual (i.e., to describe an individual's **karyotype**). Stains used in karyotyping produce various diagnostically useful **banding patterns**, which depend on the staining procedure used, the degree of DNA compaction, and the presence of DNA-bound proteins.

Two of the 46 chromosomes are called **sex chromosomes**; the remaining 44 chromosomes are called **autosomes**. Humans typically inherit one sex chromosome and 22 autosomes from each parent. There are two types of sex chromosomes, X and Y. Each female with a normal karyotype has two X chromosomes (one of which gets inactivated by methylation; see Chapter 5). Each male with a normal karyotype has one X and one Y chromosome. The 22 autosomes are numbered from 1 to 22 in approximate order of decreasing size (see Fig. 1.12).

Segregation of chromosomes occurs during both cell division (mitosis) and gamete formation (meiosis). During **mitosis**, pairs of chromatids are pulled apart so that each daughter cell gets 46 chromatids (i.e., 46 DNA double helices). In nondividing cells, the term **chromosome** is used to designate a single chromatid (i.e., a single DNA double helix). Every cell in the $G_0$ phase of the cell cycle has 46 chromosomes (in this case, 46 DNA double helices). During **meiosis I**, homologous chromosomes form pairs that are then pulled to separate poles (yielding only 23 chromosomes per cell, whereby each chromosome contains two chromatids). During **meiosis II**, paired chromatids are pulled apart to yield cells that contain only 23 chromatids (i.e., 23 DNA double helices).

Cells contain more than 100 times more DNA in their nucleus than in their mitochondria. Although a cell's network of mitochondria contains thousands of copies of **mitochondrial DNA**, even the shortest of the 46 chromosomes contain more than 3000 times the number of base pairs in the mitochondrial genome.

## SUMMARY

- DNA is a polymer of dAMP, dCMP, dGMP, and dTMP. The bases of these nucleotides can hydrogen bond to form AT or GC base pairs. A and T are thus complementary bases, as are G and C.
- DNA is mostly present as double helices that consist of two complementary DNA strands. Complementary strands pair in a head-to-tail fashion (i.e., the 5′ end of one strand is paired with the 3′ end of its complementary strand). Unless indicated otherwise, DNA sequences are written in a 5′→3′ direction.
- DNA binding proteins can bind selectively to a specific DNA sequence by interacting with the atoms of bases that are at the surface of the DNA helix grooves.
- The length of nuclear DNA molecules far exceeds the diameter of the nucleus. Inside the nucleus, most of the DNA is condensed into nucleosomes; this, in turn, is condensed into higher-order structures. These structures play critical roles in the regulation of transcription and make the orderly separation of DNA molecules possible during cell division.
- Helicases separate complementary strands of DNA. Single-stranded DNA binding proteins prevent the pairing of separated strands. Topoisomerases cut one or both strands of double-helical DNA, relieve torsional strain (topoisomerases I and II) or untangle chromosomes in preparation for mitosis (topoisomerase II), and then religate the strands. Inhibitors of topoisomerases are used in chemotherapy for cancer.
- Human cells with a normal karyotype contain 46 chromosomes: 23 from the mother and 23 from the father. Of the chromosomes, 44 are autosomes and two are sex chromosomes.

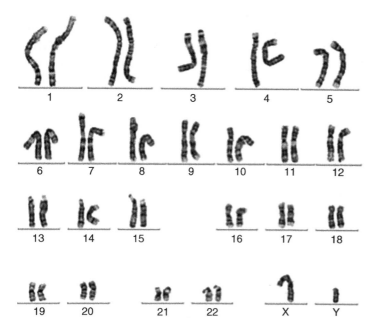

**Fig. 1.12** **Normal male karyogram.** For karyotyping, cultured cells are arrested in metaphase. This karyogram shows the light-microscopic images of stained chromosomes from a single cell. The chromosomes are sorted and analyzed according to their size and banding pattern. (Courtesy Dr. Barry L. Barnoski, Oncocytogenetics Laboratory, Cooper University Hospital, Camden, NJ.)

## FURTHER READING

- Deweese JE, Osheroff MA, Osheroff N. DNA Topology and topoisomerases: teaching a "knotty" subject. *Biochem Mol Biol Educ.* 2008;37:2-10.
- Ozer G, Luque A, Schlick T. The chromatin fiber: multiscale problems and approaches. *Curr Opin Struct Biol.* 2015;31:124-139.

■ Tessarz P, Kouzarides T. Histone core modifications regulating nucleosome structure and dynamics. *Nat Rev Mol Cell Biol.* 2014;15:703-708.

■ Vos SM, Tretter EM, Schmidt BH, Berger JM. All tangled up: how cells direct, manage and exploit topoisomerase function. *Nat Rev Mol Cell Biol.* 2011;12:827-841.

■ Wapner RJ, Martin CL, Levy B, et al. Chromosomal microarray versus karyotyping for prenatal diagnosis. *N Engl J Med.* 2012;367:2175-2184.

■ Zhu P, Li G. Structural insights of the nucleosome and the 30-nm chromatin fiber. *Curr Opin Struct Biol.* 2016; 36:106-115.

# Review Questions

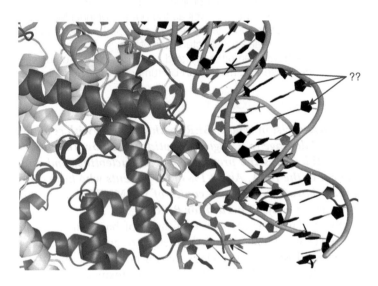

1. The figure above shows part of a nucleosome. The three pentagons identified by arrows represent which of the following?

   A. Deoxyriboses
   B. Phosphate groups
   C. Proline residues
   D. Pyrimidine bases

2. In the image shown in Question 1, the DNA binds to positively charged amino acid residues of histones via which of the following?

   A. Covalent bonds
   B. Electrostatic interactions
   C. Hydrogen bonds

3. A 69-year-old male patient with metastatic colon cancer receives treatment with a cocktail of chemotherapeutic drugs that contains irinotecan. This drug inhibits which one of the following processes?

   A. Modification of histone tails
   B. Pairing of complementary bases
   C. Reading of bases in the major groove
   D. Relaxation of supercoiled DNA

4. Many DNA-based diagnostic tests use a DNA polymerase from *Thermus aquaticus*, a bacterium that can survive high temperatures. Compared with the DNA of bacteria that grow at 25°C, the DNA of *T. aquaticus* is expected to have a higher fraction of which of the following nucleotides?

   A. A and C
   B. A and G
   C. A and T
   D. C and G
   E. C and T
   F. G and T

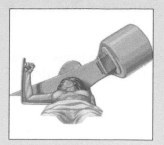

# Chapter 2

# DNA Repair and Therapy of Cancer

## SYNOPSIS

■ DNA damage may be due to the inherent properties of DNA or the damaging effects of ultraviolet light, radiation, drugs, or noxious agents in the environment. Damage may manifest as lesions to nucleotides, DNA adducts, crosslinks within or between DNA strands, or single- or double-strand breaks in the DNA. Diverse DNA repair mechanisms exist, ensuring near constancy of the genome.

■ Knowledge of DNA repair is important for understanding how inadequate DNA repair leads to tumorigenesis and how chemotherapy and radiotherapy of cancer can lead to overwhelming damage and death of tumor cells, as well as neoplasms among previously normal cells.

■ DNA repair has been studied extensively in bacteria and yeast. Although humans have more complex DNA repair pathways than these single-cell organisms, DNA repair proteins are highly evolutionarily conserved. Appropriately, many human DNA repair proteins are named after their counterparts in bacteria and yeast.

■ The base-excision repair pathway becomes active when a single nucleotide is altered. The faulty nucleotide is excised and replaced with a new one that fits the complementary DNA strand.

■ The mismatch repair pathway detects mismatches of base pairs and bulges due to missing or excess nucleotides that arise from faulty DNA replication. The most recently synthesized portion of DNA is removed, and new DNA is synthesized based on the complementary DNA strand.

■ The nucleotide-excision repair pathway repairs damage that grossly distorts DNA. Such damage may stem from exposure to the sun, cigarette smoke, or platinum chemotherapeutic drugs. A section of the damaged strand is cut out, and the DNA is then resynthesized.

■ Nonhomologous end-joining repairs double-strand breaks by joining the broken ends. The product is often different from the original DNA. Double-strand breaks can arise from DNA damage by x-rays or chemotherapeutic drugs.

■ The homologous recombination pathway repairs double-strand breaks by producing long, single-strand overhangs that invade a homologous DNA strand. The invaded strand then serves as a template for resynthesis of the lost DNA.

■ Hereditary and acquired defects in DNA repair favor tumorigenesis (e.g., in the colon, breast, ovaries, pancreas, and skin).

## LEARNING OBJECTIVES

*For mastery of this topic, you should be able to do the following:*
■ Summarize the major DNA repair pathways.
■ Describe how ultraviolet light and high-energy x-rays damage DNA, and how this damage is repaired.
■ Describe how polycyclic aromatic hydrocarbons in cigarette smoke damage DNA and how this damage is repaired.

■ Explain how platinum drugs and nitrogen mustards (e.g., cyclophosphamide) damage DNA and how this damage is repaired.
■ Describe and explain commonly used lab tests for DNA mismatch repair in biopsy tissues.
■ Explain the term microsatellite instability, describe a lab test for microsatellite instability, and link microsatellite instability to a deficiency in a DNA repair pathway.
■ List hereditary cancer syndromes and specify the associated defects in DNA repair, as well as the pattern of inheritance. List any modifications in chemotherapy or radiotherapy of tumors that must be made for affected patients.
■ Describe how chemotherapy and radiotherapy kill tumor cells and how these treatments can be tumorigenic in normal cells.

## 1. BASE-EXCISION REPAIR

*The base-excision repair (BER) pathway deals with common forms of damage to a single nucleotide. It removes an altered nucleotide, adds the proper deoxyribonucleotide, and seals the cut in the DNA. About 1% of all patients who have colon cancer have two defective copies of the MUTYH gene that encodes an enzyme needed for BER.*

Every day, in every cell, thousands of bases in DNA are altered (Fig. 2.1). Bases (mostly adenine or guanine) are spontaneously **lost** from the DNA deoxyribose backbone. Bases can be **deaminated**, especially 5-methylcytosine and cytosine, which thus give rise to thymine and uracil, respectively. **Hydroxyl radicals** can react with bases; this happens especially with guanine, forming **8-oxo-guanine** (also called **8-hydroxyguanine**). The physiological methyl-group donor S-adenosylmethionine can react with adenine to form **3-methyladenine**. **Ionizing radiation** (e.g., x-rays, γ-rays) can ionize water (thereby giving rise to a hydroxyl radical), oxidize a base, cleave a base from the deoxyribosephosphate backbone, or fragment a deoxyribose and thereby cut one of the complementary DNA strands.

In **the short-patch BER** pathway, enzymes recognize a damaged nucleotide and then replace it (Fig. 2.2). Humans produce many **DNA glycosylases** that slide along DNA, recognize deaminated, hydroxylated, or methylated bases, and remove them. This generates a substrate that is recognized by AP endonuclease 1, which cuts the DNA where the base is missing. Polynucleotide kinase/phosphatase (PNKP) then phosphorylates the free 5′ end and dephosphorylates the adjacent 3′ end. **Poly-ADP-ribose polymerase (PARP)** binds to the strand break and recruits the protein **XRCC1**, which serves as a platform for recruiting other repair proteins. Then, **DNA polymerase β** excises the abasic deoxyribose and replaces it with a proper new nucleotide. Finally, **DNA ligase**

**Deamination**

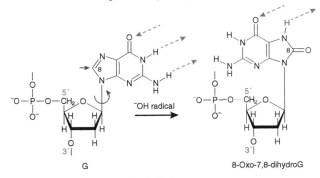

**Damage from hydroxyl radicals**

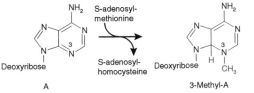

**Methylation**

**Loss of a base**

**Fig. 2.1** **Spontaneous alterations of DNA that are repaired by the base-excision repair pathway.**

IIIα seals the nick in the DNA strand to reestablish a contiguous DNA molecule.

A single defect also triggers the **long-patch BER pathway**, which replaces 2 to 10 consecutive nucleotides. Certain oxidation products of a **deoxyribose** must be removed via the long-patch pathway. In addition, this pathway completes some of the repairs that cannot be completed by single-patch BER.

If damage to a base is not repaired, DNA **replication** (see Chapter 3) may insert an incorrect nucleotide, or it may come to a halt until the damaged base is repaired. Replication stops when methyladenine (see Fig. 2.1) is present so that BER can replace methyladenine with adenine. When a base is missing, **translesion DNA synthesis** inserts a nucleotide into the newly synthesized DNA strand, but this nucleotide may be the wrong one. If replication inserts an inappropriate base opposite a

damaged one, the **mismatch repair (MMR)** pathway (see Section 2) often detects the error. For instance, it recognizes an A opposite a U (from deamination of C) or opposite an oxo-G (from the hydroxylation of guanine).

The enzyme **DNA MYH glycosylase**, encoded by the *MUTYH* gene, partners with the MMR pathway (see Section 2) to excise A opposite 8-oxo-guanine (see Fig. 2.1). The BER pathway then replaces the 8-oxo-G with G. MUTYH stands for MutY homolog (from bacteria).

About 1% of all patients who have **colorectal cancer** have **MUTYH-associated polyposis (MAP)**, a disease that is caused by deficient **DNA MYH glycosylase** activity. The disease shows autosomal recessive inheritance. In patients with MAP, G→T mutations accumulate (persistent A opposite 8-oxo-G yields a T in place of 8-oxo-G in the next round of replication). Interestingly, such G→T mutations are found in the same genes that are mutated or no longer transcribed in some patients who have *sporadic* colorectal cancer (i.e., in patients who do not have MAP). In patients with MAP, colon cancer typically occurs in the late forties. At this time, the colon often contains tens to hundreds of polyps.

**PARP inhibitors** are in clinical trials for patients who have tumors with defective homologous recombination (HR) repair (see Section 4) and therefore rely unusually heavily on PARP-dependent BER and nonhomologous end joining (NHEJ; see Section 4). PARP inhibitors inhibit BER and NHEJ because poly-ADP-ribose recruits DNA repair proteins (e.g., XRCC1) to damaged sites in the DNA. While PARP inhibitors are relatively innocuous to normal cells, they are especially toxic to tumor cells that are deficient in BRCA1 or BRCA2, proteins that play a role in HR repair.

## 2. MISMATCH REPAIR

*The mismatch repair (MMR) system handles improper base matches, as well as single-strand loops that stem from insertions or deletions during replication. Repair is directed to the most recently synthesized DNA strand. MMR is defective in ~10% to 20% of sporadic cancers of the colon, rectum, stomach, or endometrium. Hereditary mutations that affect MMR are the cause of Lynch syndrome, which most often causes colorectal or endometrial cancer.*

The MMR pathway detects noncomplementary base pairs and repairs them. Mismatches may stem from the following (Fig. 2.3): (1) spontaneous tautomerization of bases during DNA polymerization; (2) deamination of cytosine to uracil or of 5-methylcytosine to thymine; (3) DNA polymerase error of inserting a base that is not complementary to the DNA strand that is being copied; and (4) DNA polymerase slippage in nucleotide sequence repeats.

In MMR, **MSH** proteins recognize the damage and **MLH** proteins help initiate the excision of a stretch of the most recently synthesized DNA (Fig. 2.4). Heterodimeric MSH proteins (homologs of bacterial MutS proteins; Table 2.1) detect mispaired and unpaired bases. MLH proteins (homologs of bacterial MutL proteins) then attach to the MSH proteins. In

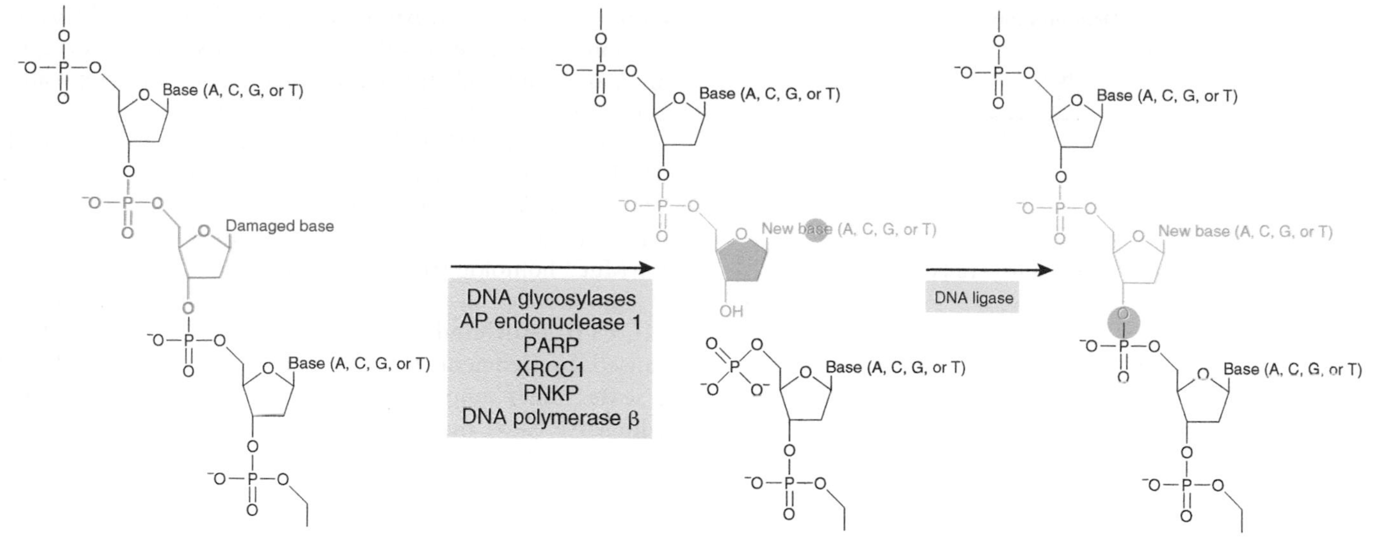

**Fig. 2.2** **The short-patch base-excision repair pathway.**

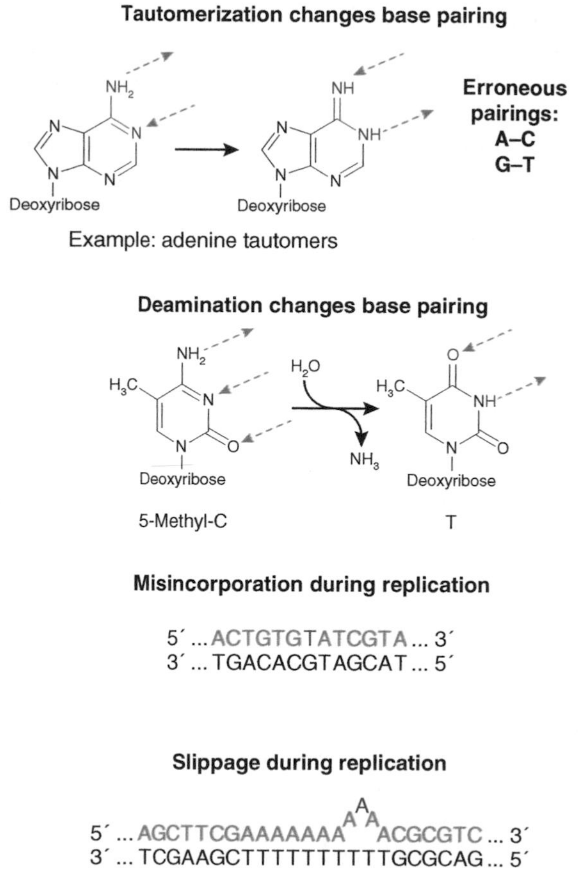

### Tautomerization changes base pairing

**Erroneous pairings:**
**A–C**
**G–T**

Example: adenine tautomers

### Deamination changes base pairing

5-Methyl-C        T

### Misincorporation during replication

5′ ... ACTGTGTATCGTA ... 3′
3′ ... TGACACGTAGCAT ... 5′

### Slippage during replication

5′ ... AGCTTCGAAAAAAA $^{A\,A}_{\,\,\,A}$ ACGCGTC ... 3′
3′ ... TCGAAGCTTTTTTTTTTGCGCAG ... 5′

**Fig. 2.3** **Causes of base mismatches that are repaired by the mismatch repair pathway.** *Blue arrows* indicate hydrogen bonding for base pairing.

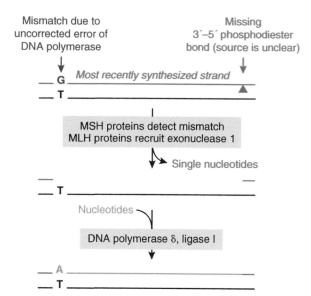

Mismatch due to uncorrected error of DNA polymerase

Missing 3′–5′ phosphodiester bond (source is unclear)

__ G    *Most recently synthesized strand*
__ T

MSH proteins detect mismatch
MLH proteins recruit exonuclease 1

Single nucleotides

__ T

Nucleotides

DNA polymerase δ, ligase I

__ A
__ T

**Fig. 2.4** **DNA mismatch repair.** Shown is the repair of a G–T mismatch.

the DNA strand, using the complementary strand as a template. Finally, **DNA ligase I** ligates the pieces of DNA.

Inactivation of the DNA MMR system leads to an increased susceptibility to cancer, especially **cancer** of the colon, stomach, or endometrium. Cells with impaired MMR accumulate mutations at a vastly increased pace. This leads to frameshift mutations that impair the production and function of tumor suppressors, prevent programmed cell death, or alter signaling, transcription, or immune surveillance.

The tumors from ~15% of patients who have **colon cancer** and ~20% each of patients who have **endometrial** or **gastric cancer** have defective MMR systems. In patients with a **sporadic** form of this cancer, the MMR deficiency is usually due to the **methylation** of the promoter of both copies of the **MLH1** gene. The methylation essentially abolishes the expression of the MLH1 protein.

addition, MLH proteins bind to an exonuclease. Tethered to MSH and MLH proteins, the **exonuclease 1** (Exo1) begins the degradation of the most recently synthesized DNA strand at a nearby cut in the DNA (it is unclear how this cut arises). **DNA polymerase δ** then resynthesizes the missing portion of

**Table 2.1** **Proteins That Are Involved in DNA Mismatch Repair in the Nucleus**

| Absolutely Required Protein | Possible Partners to Form a Heterodimer* | Heterodimer |
|---|---|---|
| **RECOGNITION OF MISMATCH** | | |
| MSH2[†] | MSH3 (for up to 15 extra or missing nucleotides in microsatellites) | MutSβ |
| | MSH6[†] (for mismatches and ≤2 extra or missing nucleotides in microsatellites) | MutSα |
| **INITIATION OF NUCLEOTIDE EXCISION** | | |
| MLH1[†] | PMS1 | MutLβ |
| | PMS2[†] (used in most mismatch repair processes) | MutLα |
| | MLH3 | MutLγ |

*One partner can partially make up for another.
[†]Most patients with Lynch syndrome inherited an inactivating mutation in MSH2, MSH6, MLH1, or PMS2.

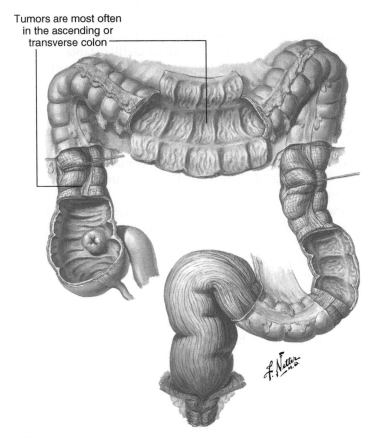

Tumors are most often in the ascending or transverse colon

**Fig. 2.5** **Patients with hereditary defects in mismatch repair have Lynch syndrome and are at a high risk of colon cancer.**

**Lynch syndrome** is a **hereditary** predisposition to cancer that is due to a germline mutation in a DNA MMR gene (Fig. 2.5). At least 1 in 1,000 individuals has Lynch syndrome, and about 3% of all patients who have colon cancer have Lynch syndrome. Most patients with Lynch syndrome inherited a mutation that inactivates MSH2, MSH6, MLH1, or PMS2 (see Table 2.1). The second copy of the gene or its associated promoter then undergoes mutation or epigenetic inactivation (via DNA methylation) in certain cells of the body, such that no functional protein is produced in these cells (e.g., in the colon). Patients who have Lynch syndrome have a ~70% lifetime risk for cancer of the colon, ~40% risk for cancer of the endometrium, and ~15% risk for cancer of the stomach or an ovary. These cancers occur at an unusually early age (e.g., colon cancer typically in the mid-40s). In contrast to patients who have a sporadic tumor with defective MMR mechanisms, patients who have Lynch syndrome also have a mutant MMR gene in blood lymphocytes. Since only one defective allele needs to be inherited, the disease shows autosomal dominant inheritance (see Chapter 5). This means that if only one parent is affected, each offspring has a 50% chance of inheriting the disease.

**Immunohistochemical detection** of MMR proteins in a tumor of the colon or endometrium is often part of the diagnosis of an MMR deficiency. The tissue is commonly stained for MLH1, MSH2, PMS2, and MSH6. Patients who have sporadic colon cancer or endometrial cancer due to hypermethylation of the promoter for the *MLH1* gene do not show immunoreactivity for MLH1. Similarly, patients who have Lynch syndrome, and therefore only a mutant version of a particular MMR protein, exhibit an absence or greatly reduced immunoreactivity for that protein. To complicate matters (see Table 2.1), a lack of MLH1 often leads to the degradation of the PMS2 protein, and a lack of MSH2 leads to the loss of the MSH6 protein (but not vice versa). Results of immunohistochemical assays can be used for guidance in DNA-based testing for mutations, hypermethylation, and microsatellite instability (see below).

Defective MMR can be detected as the **microsatellite instability (MSI)** of DNA. Microsatellites are 5- to 100-fold repeats of sequences that contain one to five nucleotides [e.g., $(A)_{16}$ or $(GT)_9$]. Microsatellites are also called **short tandem repeats**. When a patient is tested for MSI, DNA is obtained from the excised tumor and occasionally also from peripheral blood lymphocytes (the DNA in lymphocytes is assumed to be representative of the DNA in the germline). By using PCR (see Chapter 4), DNA that contains certain microsatellites (e.g., the mononucleotide repeats BAT25 and BAT26 and the dinucleotide repeats D2S123, D5S346, and D17S250) is amplified and analyzed for size. BAT26 is within the *MSH2* gene, but the remaining microsatellites are outside the genes that encode MMR proteins. In MMR-deficient tumor cells, these repeats usually become *shortened*, giving rise to a shorter piece of PCR-amplified DNA. Most tumors that have MSI show abnormal lengths of four or five of the five microsatellite sequences mentioned. A tumor is usually said to have **high MSI** instability if two or more of the five tested microsatellites show a change in length. If only one of the five microsatellites is unstable, there is **low MSI**. If all five microsatellites are stable, the tumor is said to be **microsatellite stable**.

In patients who have tumors that show MSI, pathogenic changes can occur in the lengths of the $A_{26}$ microsatellite BAT26 in the *MSH2* gene, in the $C_8$ microsatellite of the *MSH6* gene, in the $A_{10}$ microsatellite of the **tumor growth factor β receptor 2** gene, or in the $G_8$ tract of the gene for the cell-death-inducing protein **BAX**. Changes in the repeat lengths of the other four diagnostically measured microsatellites (BAT25, D2S123, D5S346, D17S250) are not known to be pathogenic.

Patients who have a colon tumor that demonstrates microsatellite instability do not derive any benefit from adjuvant chemotherapy with **5-fluorouracil** (the mechanism of action of fluorouracil is described in Chapter 37). In contrast, 5-fluorouracil is often part of adjuvant chemotherapy for microsatellite-*stable* colon tumors.

Persons who are **homozygous** or compound heterozygous for mutations in DNA MMR proteins not only develop gastrointestinal cancer but also have brain tumors and hematologic malignancies in childhood. This disorder is called **constitutional MMR deficiency syndrome** (CMMR-D).

## 3. NUCLEOTIDE-EXCISION REPAIR

*The nucleotide-excision repair (NER) pathway recognizes distortions of the DNA double helix that arise from environmental insults (e.g., sunlight or smoking) or chemotherapeutic agents (e.g., platinum drugs). In addition, it repairs lesions that lead to the stalling of transcription. A section of ~30 nucleotides of one DNA strand is removed in one piece and then resynthesized.*

NER can be divided into two subpathways: **global genome** (GG) repair and **transcription-coupled** (TC) repair. GG-NER occurs throughout the genome when helix-distorting lesions (e.g., interstrand crosslinks) are recognized. By contrast, TC-NER occurs when RNA polymerases, which negotiate helix-destabilizing lesions inefficiently, become stalled on the DNA. In TC-NER, the transcribed strand of the DNA is repaired more efficiently than the nontranscribed strand. A network of histone-modifying processes appears to assist access to histone-bound DNA. GG-NER and TC-NER activate the same set of NER enzymes to repair the DNA.

Distortions of DNA helices, recognized by GG-NER, are a hallmark of many types of DNA damage. GG-NER deals mostly with **intrastrand DNA adducts** and **crosslinks**. Common intrastrand DNA adducts include the following lesions: (1) TT-, TC-, CT-, and CC-**cyclobutane dimers** that are caused by **ultraviolet (UV) light** (either from the sun or tanning lights; Fig. 2.6); (2) adducts between adenine or guanine and **polycyclic aromatic hydrocarbons** (found in **cigarette smoke** and environmental contaminants; Fig. 2.7); and (3) adducts between GG or AG sequences and **platinum drugs** (e.g., **cisplatin**, **carboplatin**, or **oxaliplatin**, which are used in chemotherapy for solid tumors; Figs. 2.8 and 2.9).

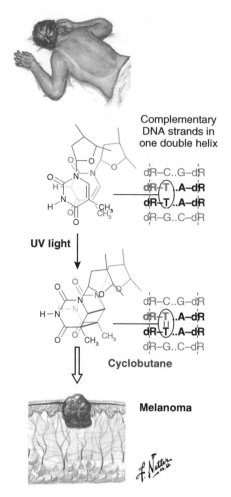

**Fig. 2.6** **UV light induces intrastrand crosslinking of pyrimidine bases into cyclobutane dimers.**

Once the damage is detected, helicases in **TFIIH** (a protein complex with roles in both GG-NER and TC-NER) unwind nearby DNA and verify the presence of damage (Fig. 2.10). RPA binds to single-stranded DNA and prevents the reformation of hydrogen bonds between base pairs. The **ERCC1**-XPF endonuclease complex cuts unwound DNA 5′ of the lesion. A section of ~30 nucleotides is removed and a **DNA polymerase** (e.g., δ, ε, or κ) resynthesizes the missing region. Finally, a **DNA ligase** (I or III) links the 3′ end of the newly synthesized region to the rest of the DNA strand.

Patients with deficient TC-NER mostly show impaired development, premature aging, and neurodegeneration; some also have increased sensitivity to UV light. If many transcription sites are halted and stopped for long periods, the cell undergoes programmed cell death (**apoptosis**; see Chapter 8).

Patients who have abnormalities specifically in GG-NER tend to have very early-onset cancer (in part induced by UV light) because error-prone translesion DNA polymerases (see Chapter 3) bypass the many unrepaired lesions during DNA replication.

The inadequate repair of intrastrand crosslinks promotes the formation of **tumors**. Inadequate repair of UV-induced DNA damage plays a role in the development of **basal cell**

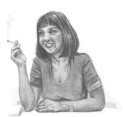

Dibenzo[*a*,*l*]pyrene:

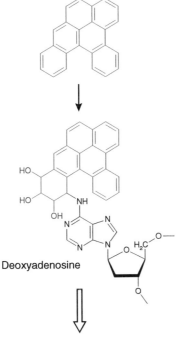

Deoxyadenosine

Bronchogenic carcinoma,
squamous cell type

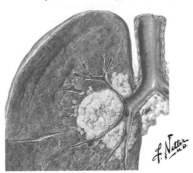

**Fig. 2.7** Adduct of the principal metabolite of the carcinogen dibenzo[*a*,*l*] pyrene with deoxyadenosine in DNA.

carcinomas, **squamous cell carcinomas**, and **melanomas** of the skin (see Fig. 2.6). Inadequate repair of *smoking*-induced damage plays a role in the development of **lung cancer** (see Fig. 2.7).

Debilitating heritable deficiencies in NER are seen in the rare autosomal recessively inherited diseases **xeroderma pigmentosum**, **Cockayne syndrome**, and a form of light-sensitive **trichothiodystrophy** (all occur in less than 1 in 100,000 people). All these diseases can, in turn, be subdivided into several types, depending on the protein that is mutated. Patients with xeroderma pigmentosum readily develop tumors

when exposed to UV light, and they also have an increased susceptibility to cancer that results from smoking or carcinogens in the diet. Cockayne syndrome is characterized by emaciation and short stature as well as neurological impairment, often also by photosensitivity. Trichothiodystrophy is characterized by brittle hair and sometimes also by photosensitivity. These disorders dramatically reveal the importance of components of the NER system.

Inadequate repair of drug-induced damage is taken advantage of in the treatment of **cancer.** Testicular cancer cells, for instance, have a low capacity for NER and thus readily undergo programmed cell death (see Section 5 and Chapter 8) when exposed to platinum drugs. This drug sensitivity is a major reason for the high cure rate of testicular cancer that is achieved with therapy that includes **cisplatin** (see Figs. 2.8 and 2.9).

The NER pathway works together with HR (see Section 4.2) to repair interstrand crosslinks, such as those generated by platinum compounds, nitrogen mustards, or psoralen.

## 4. REPAIR OF DOUBLE-STRAND BREAKS AND INTERSTRAND CROSSLINKS

*Nondividing cells repair double-strand breaks chiefly via NHEJ. Dividing cells repair double-strand breaks and interstrand crosslinks via a combination of NHEJ and HR repair. HR repair involves the copying of information from a nearby sister chromatid or homologous chromosome. Patients who have hereditary deficiencies of HR repair have a variety of cancer syndromes.*

### 4.1. Nonhomologous End Joining

**Ionizing radiation** (e.g., in the form of high-energy **x-rays**) can give rise to single- and **double-strand breaks**. Ionizing radiation damages DNA directly or indirectly by forming DNA-damaging free radicals (mostly hydroxyl radicals, OH$^\bullet$, from water). When ionizing radiation cuts both DNA strands within 10 to 20 base pairs of each other, the cuts generate a double-strand break. The ends of the breaks often contain an inappropriate phosphate group or a fragment of deoxyribose.

In nondividing cells, double-strand breaks are largely repaired by **NHEJ** (see Fig. 2.11). The proteins **Ku70** (also called **XRCC6**) and **Ku80** (also called **XRCC5**) bind to the broken ends of the DNA. The Ku proteins recruit the DNA-dependent protein kinase catalytic subunit and the **nuclease** Artemis, which processes the ends of the strands if needed. End processing may be accompanied by a loss of nucleotides. As needed, the **DNA polymerases** λ and μ then insert nucleotides with or without a template. A **DNA ligase** complex (consisting of XLF, XRCC4, and DNA ligase IV) then ligates the ends of the DNA; this ligase complex tolerates some gaps and mismatches. (In contrast to *double*-strand breaks, *single*-strand breaks are repaired by BER; see Section 1.)

NHEJ can introduce mutations and is therefore a potentially *tumorigenic* process. Nonetheless, these mutations are

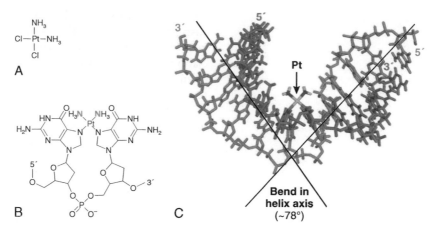

**Fig. 2.8** **Cisplatin-induced intrastrand crosslinking between two adjacent guanine bases.** **A,** Cisplatin. **B,** Cisplatin adduct with guanine bases in DNA. **C,** Solution structure of a cisplatin-DNA intra-strand crosslink. Platination causes partial unwinding of the double helix, an unusual angle of the planes of the guanine bases, and an overall bend in the long axis of the helix. Platinum drugs also generate *inter*strand crosslinks, which have to be repaired via homologous recombination repair (see Section 4.2). (Based on Protein Data Bank [www.rcsb.org] 1A84 from Gelasco A, Lippard SJ. NMR solution structure of a DNA dodecamer duplex containing a cis-diammineplatinum [II] d[GpG] intrastrand cross-link, the major adduct of the anticancer drug cisplatin. *Biochemistry.* 1998;37:9230–9239.)

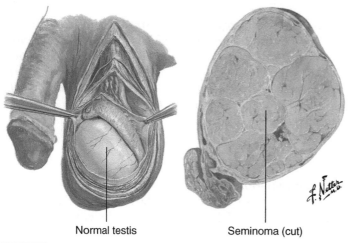

Normal testis        Seminoma (cut)

**Fig. 2.9** **Use of cisplatin in the treatment of testicular cancer.** Patients usually undergo orchidectomy and then often receive adjuvant chemotherapy with cisplatin. Treatment is successful in part largely because the tumor cells have a low capacity for nucleotide-excision repair and then undergo apoptosis.

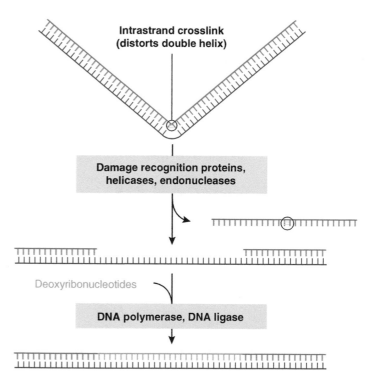

**Fig. 2.10** **Nucleotide-excision repair of intrastrand cross-links.** The crosslinks can be TT-, CT-, or CC-cyclobutane dimers (UV induced; see Fig. 2.6), single nucleotides linked to polycyclic aromatic compounds (as found in cigarette smoke; see Fig. 2.7), or platinum-linked purine nucleotides (e.g., cisplatin induced; see Fig. 2.8).

thought to be less damaging to cells than unrepaired DNA double-strand breaks because unprotected ends at the break-point would be degraded. Furthermore, some of the unre-paired DNA segments would lack centromeres or telomeres, which would be catastrophic for the genome of a cell. NHEJ can take various paths even with the same starting damage. Mutations caused by NHEJ often consist of one to 10 nucleo-tide **deletions** or three or fewer nucleotide **insertions**. When a nucleus contains numerous double-stranded DNA frag-ments, NHEJ even carries a risk of joining the wrong DNA fragments, which results in **translocation** (material from one chromosome is joined to another chromosome). This can cause a protein-coding segment of a gene to be controlled by a promoter that induces aberrant transcription and thus

pathogenic protein production. As described in Chapter 8, an increased rate of mutations paves the way for the development of a tumor.

Intense irradiation of cells with **ionizing radiation** pro-duces such extensive and persistent DNA damage that affected, heavily damaged cells undergo programmed cell death; this is the basis of **radiation therapy** of tumors. Radiation therapy aims not only to introduce double-strand breaks but also additional DNA lesions within the region of the break. Cells that have DNA with such **clustered lesions** are especially likely to die.

In the **adaptive immune system**, NHEJ is involved in recombining V, D, and J segments of antibodies and T-cell receptors. The inaccuracies of NHEJ help increase the diversity of antibodies and T-cell receptors. Patients who have a deficiency in NHEJ can also have a deficiency in their adaptive immune system.

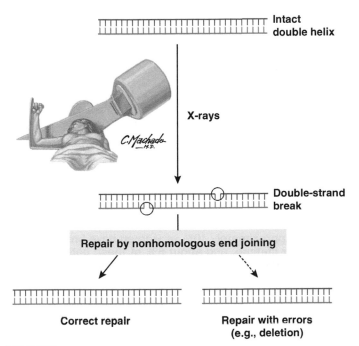

**Fig. 2.11** **Repair of radiation-induced double-strand breaks by nonhomologous end joining.** Some radiation is natural. Radiation is also a mainstay of cancer treatment.

## 4.2. Homologous Recombination Repair (Homology-Directed Repair)

HR repair, like NHEJ described above, repairs DNA double-strand breaks. HR most often uses a **sister chromatid** as a template for repair. In contrast to NHEJ, HR is generally accurate. In the S and G2 phases of the cell cycle, double-strand breaks can arise mostly from problems with DNA replication (see Chapter 3), such as unrepaired **single-strand breaks** or complexes of DNA with **poisoned topoisomerase**. It is estimated that a normal dividing cell under physiological circumstances needs to repair ~50 double-strand breaks per cell cycle, and most of these breaks are handled by HR.

**Interstrand crosslinks** are repaired by NER alone (GG-Ner and/or TC-NER; see Section 3) or by an obligatory combination of HR repair and NER. (*Intra*strand crosslinks are repaired by NER.) Interstrand crosslinks result from platinum drugs, nitrogen mustards, or psoralens. **Platinum drugs** (e.g., **cisplatin, carboplatin**) and **nitrogen mustards** (e.g., **cyclophosphamide**) are used in chemotherapy to kill tumor cells. **Psoralens** (e.g., **methoxypsoralen**) are used for the treatment of **psoriasis** and **vitiligo**. UV light induces psoralens to form cyclobutanes with staggered pyrimidine bases on the two strands of a DNA double helix. Psoriasis (Fig. 2.12) is a common skin disorder that is marked by the hyperproliferation of keratinocytes; treatment with a psoralen plus light reduces this hyperproliferation. Vitiligo (see Fig. 35.18) is a condition involving the patchy loss of skin pigmentation that affects 1% to 2% of the population. The loss of pigmentation is due to an absence of melanin pigment-producing cells, which in turn may be due to inflammation (see Chapter 35). Treatment with a psoralen plus light is effective and might work by diminishing inflammation. Although the psoralens kill some cells as intended, they also increase the rate of mutation in other cells, which explains the side effect of an increased rate of skin cancer.

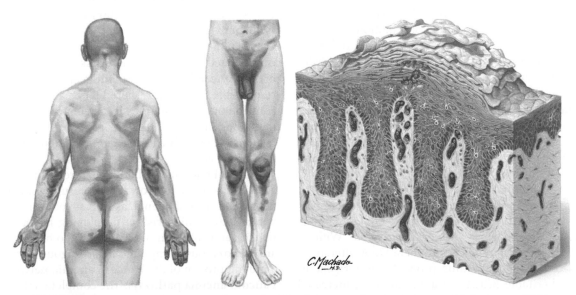

**Fig. 2.12** **Psoriasis is sometimes treated with photoreactive psoralens, which cause DNA intrastrand and interstrand crosslinks.**

After a double-strand break occurs, the **MRN complex** (consisting of Mre11, Rad50, and Nbs1) binds to the ends of the DNA and activates the signaling kinase **ATM** (ataxia telangiectasia mutated). ATM, in turn, phosphorylates numerous proteins, some of which halt the cell cycle, while others increase the DNA repair activity. The MRN complex cuts one DNA strand ~100 to 200 base pairs from the break and then resects this strand toward the break. Another protein complex resects the same strand in the opposite direction so that a single-strand overhang is generated that can be greater than 1000 bp long. One such overhang is generated in each piece of broken DNA. Meanwhile, MRN also tethers together the ends of the two pieces of DNA. The **BRCA1** protein (breast cancer 1) forms a dimer with the **PALB2** protein and recruits the **BRCA2** protein, which in turn helps load the recombinase RAD51. RAD51 then fosters the invasion of a sister chromatid or a homologous chromosome by a 3′ overhang. The invaded DNA strand serves as a template for an elongation of the 3′ overhang. Subsequently, helicases and nucleases resolve the entangled DNA strands.

The use of a homolog for HR repair leads to **gene conversion**, which can be the cause of a **loss of heterozygosity** (**LOH**). The homologous chromosomes, derived from the mother and father, contain similar but not identical sequences. Gene conversion refers to the finding that the sequence of one parental allele converts to the sequence of the other parental allele. Hence, a somatic cell with one functional and one nonfunctional copy of a gene may give rise to a cell with two nonfunctional copies. LOH can also be used to describe the deletion of the examined sequence. The term **uniparental disomy** is applied when there is a loss of a chromosome or chromosome segment (usually containing multiple genes) from one parent and a gain of the lost sequence from the other parental chromosome. In patients who are heterozygous for a deficiency of a tumor suppressor, HR repair may lead to the complete loss of tumor suppressor activity, which may be tumorigenic (see Chapter 8).

Impairment of the activity of the **MRN** complex or the **ATM** kinase leads to an increased rate of mutation, and to an increased sensitivity toward therapeutic ionizing radiation. **Ataxia-telangiectasia**, seen in about one per 300,000 births, is due to homozygosity or compound heterozygosity for inactivating mutations in the ATM gene. **Nijmegen breakage syndrome** and **ataxia-telangiectasia–like disease** are much rarer diseases that are due to homozygosity or compound heterozygosity for inactivating mutations that affect the MRN complex. Reduced amounts of the MRN complex are also observed in about 20% of **breast tumors.**

About 5% of women who have breast cancer (Fig. 2.13), or ~0.1% of all men and women, have inherited a mutation in the **BRCA1** or **BRCA2** genes. Over time, the remaining, normal *BRCA* allele becomes lost or inactivated. Without functional BRCA proteins, cells accumulate DNA alterations at an increased rate and are thus prone to tumorigenesis. Patients with a heritable *BRCA* mutation are at an increased risk for **breast cancer**, **ovarian cancer**, and other tumors. The propensity for tumor formation is inherited in **autosomal**

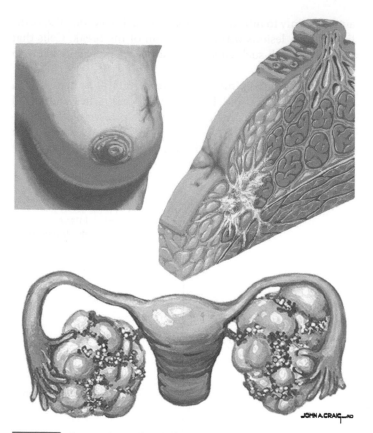

JOHN A.CRAIG—AD

**Fig. 2.13** **Approximately 10% of women have breast cancer during their lifetime, and about 5% of these patients inherited one mutant BRCA allele that encodes a protein with impaired function.** With time, the other, normal allele becomes nonfunctional, thereby impairing homologous recombination repair of DNA. Cells without functioning homologous recombination repair accumulate mutations at an increased rate and are more likely to give rise to a tumor. Patients can be tested for *BRCA* gene mutations.

**dominant** fashion (as in Lynch syndrome; see Section 2). Heterozygosity for a defective BRCA1 or BRCA2 allele is a frequent cause of the **hereditary breast and ovarian cancer syndrome** (**HBOCS**).

Germline heterozygosity for a mutation in the *PALB2* gene is associated with an increased risk of **pancreatic cancer** and **breast cancer**. Together, mutations in *PALB2* and *BRCA2* are responsible for much of hereditary pancreatic cancer (other contributors are mutations in a gene for a MMR protein and mutations in the *CDKN2A* gene). *PALB2* mutations are responsible for only a few percent of patients who have hereditary breast cancer.

**Fanconi anemia** is a heritable, rare syndrome that is characterized by bone marrow failure, resulting in anemia, leukopenia, and thrombopenia, as well as malformations. Affected persons are at high risk of developing hematological malignancies and solid tumors. Patients who have Fanconi anemia are homozygous, compound heterozygous, or hemizygous for a mutant protein of the **Fanconi anemia network** (also called **Fanconi anemia pathway**). The complete network consists of at least 16 proteins that play a role in DNA repair. PALB2 and BRCA2 are members of the Fanconi anemia network. Patients who have *two* mutant BRCA2 alleles have the D1-type of Fanconi anemia, and patients who have two mutant PALB2 alleles have the N-type. Protein complexes of the Fanconi anemia network coordinate some of the DNA excision, strand invasion, and resolution of HR. In the general population, several types of sporadic tumors are deficient in one of the proteins of the Fanconi anemia network, which bears on the susceptibility of these tumors to DNA crosslinking agents. Patients who have Fanconi anemia are hypersensitive to ionizing radiation and DNA crosslinking agents (e.g., cisplatin or cyclophosphamide).

HR not only plays a role in DNA repair but also in forming crossovers in **meiosis** for the purpose of identifying and pairing homologous chromosomes, thereby increasing genetic diversity among offspring.

## 5. DNA DAMAGE RESPONSE HALTS THE CELL CYCLE AND REGULATES APOPTOSIS

*As is outlined in Chapter 8, cancer is the result of damage to the genome such that cell growth and survival are no longer properly regulated. Inadequate DNA repair increases the rate of mutation and thus favors the formation of a tumor. Cells have means of assessing DNA damage and determining whether to survive or self-destruct.*

A cell's **DNA damage response** senses DNA damage, slows progression through the cell cycle, and coordinates this with DNA repair; when DNA damage is persistent, the response can also initiate apoptosis. Most DNA repair pathways are discussed in Sections 1 to 4. Translesion DNA synthesis is discussed in Section 2 of Chapter 3. Fig. 2.14 provides an overview of these repair pathways.

The DNA damage response is best studied in cells that contain double-strand breaks. Such breaks eventually lead to the activation of the kinases ATR and ATM, which in turn activate the checkpoint kinases Chk1 and Chk2. Through various means, the checkpoint kinases lead to a halt in the cell cycle by blocking the G1/S transition, S phase, the G2/M transition, or M phase (see Section 1 in Chapter 8). This allows DNA repair pathways, including translesion DNA synthesis, to repair DNA damage.

DNA repair pathways are often redundant: although a particular type of damage is typically repaired mostly by one pathway, it can often be repaired by an alternative pathway. If DNA damage is repaired, the signal blocking the cell cycle is eliminated, and progression through the cycle resumes. If the damage is not repaired, the DNA damage signal persists and can trigger apoptosis.

Some **chemotherapeutic drugs** kill cells by inducing DNA damage that is so overwhelming that the cells undergo apoptosis. The sensitivity of normal and abnormal cells to chemotherapy-induced DNA alterations depends on many variables, including drug uptake and efflux, the capacity for DNA repair, the ability of cells to sense and transduce the DNA damage response, and the likelihood that DNA damage leads to apoptosis. Many tumor cells have altered sensitivity to DNA damage-induced apoptosis. Cells that survive damage from chemotherapeutic drugs (e.g., because entry into apoptosis is misregulated or DNA damage-sensing mechanisms fail to detect the damage) may give rise to a new tumor or aggravate the behavior of the existing tumor.

Intense **ionizing radiation**, such as that used for radiation therapy of cancer, causes cell death not just by the sheer volume of damage to DNA, but also by clustering damage within one to two turns of the DNA helix. It is unclear why clustered damage is particularly lethal.

### SUMMARY

■ The base-excision repair (BER) pathway mends the damage from deamination, hydroxylation, methylation, the loss of a base, from the alteration of a deoxyribose, or from a single-strand break. Such damage is a result of the chemical

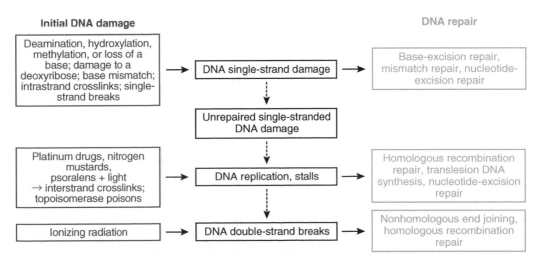

**Fig. 2.14** **Overview of DNA repair pathways.** DNA replication and translesion DNA synthesis are explained in Chapter 3.

properties of DNA, the destructive effects of other cellular constituents, or ionizing radiation. The short patch repair pathway replaces a single damaged nucleotide, while the long-patch repair pathway replaces a stretch of 2 to 10 consecutive nucleotides. The complementary DNA strand serves as a template for the insertion of nucleotides.

- MUTYH-associated polyposis (MAP) is caused by a homozygous or compound heterozygous deficiency of DNA MYH glycosylase, which plays a role in repairing 8-oxo-guanine (produced from guanine by a radical). The disease is associated with the formation of numerous polyps in the colon, as well as early colorectal cancer.

- DNA mismatch repair (MMR) processes tackle single-base DNA mismatches and DNA loops, which arise from errors in the synthesis of DNA, from the spontaneous deamination of C to U or methyl-C to T, or from homologous recombination (HR) repair. Enzymes of the DNA MMR pathway degrade and resynthesize a portion of a DNA strand, which is often the most recently synthesized strand.

- Lynch syndrome is due to an inherited MMR deficiency. Both inherited and acquired deficiencies in MMR can cause cancer, especially of the colon, uterus, and ovaries. An MMR deficiency in tumor cells can often be detected as deficient immunohistochemical staining of MMR proteins and by DNA microsatellite instability (MSI) (i.e., a shortening of the lengths of certain nucleotide repeats).

- Nucleotide-excision repair (NER) involves the removal and appropriate replacement of a contiguous stretch of ~24 to 32 nucleotides around a helix-distorting lesion on one strand of a DNA double helix. Such lesions commonly stem from the crosslinking of the pyrimidine bases (T or C) by exposure to UV light, from the reaction of metabolites of polycyclic aromatic hydrocarbons (found in smoke) with purine bases (A or G), or from the crosslinking of adjacent purine bases by platinum drugs (used in chemotherapy of tumors). A high rate of production of helix-distorting DNA lesions is associated with an increased risk of cancer (e.g., melanoma and lung cancer).

- After a double-strand break, HR involves resection of one strand to produce a long single-strand overhang, invasion of the homologous chromatid, copying of the information, and separation of the two chromatids.

- Ionizing radiation (e.g., high-energy x-rays) causes double-strand breaks that can be repaired by NHEJ or by HR.

- The therapeutically used platinum drugs, nitrogen mustards, and photoreactive psoralens produce interstrand crosslinks that can be repaired by HR repair. The BRCA1 and BRCA2 proteins participate in HR repair. Mutations in the *BRCA* genes can convey increased susceptibility to breast and ovarian cancer.

- DNA damage-sensing pathways can halt the cell cycle to allow time for DNA repair. Cells with excessive unrepaired DNA damage often undergo apoptosis. Some of the drugs used in the chemotherapy of cancer kill cells by causing DNA damage in excess of the cells' capacity for repair. These drugs are inherently mutagenic to all cells.

## FURTHER READING

- Brenerman BM, Illuzzi JL, Wilson III DM. Base excision repair capacity in informing healthspan. *Carcinogenesis.* 2014;35:2643-2652.
- Erie DA, Weninger KR. Single molecule studies of DNA mismatch repair. *DNA Repair (Amst).* 2014;20:71-81.
- Lafrance-Vanasse J, Williams GJ, Tainer JA. Envisioning the dynamics and flexibility of Mre11-Rad50-Nbs1 complex to decipher its roles in DNA replication and repair. *Prog Biophys Mol Biol.* 2015;117:182-193.
- Lindahl T. Instability and decay of the primary structure of DNA. *Nature.* 1993;362:709-715.
- Marteijn JA, Lans H, Vermeulen W, Hoeijmakers JH. Understanding nucleotide excision repair and its roles in cancer and ageing. *Nat Rev Mol Cell Biol.* 2014;15: 465-481.
- Mehta A, Haber JE. Sources of DNA double-strand breaks and models of recombinational DNA repair. *Cold Spring Harb Perspect Biol.* 2014;6(9):a016428.

# Review Questions

1. A 48-year-old woman has endometrial cancer and undergoes a hysterectomy. Immunohistochemistry of tumor tissue reveals the presence of MLH1 and PMS2, but an absence of MSH2 and MSH6. Based on this finding, the most likely diagnosis is which of the following?

   A. Cockayne syndrome
   B. Hereditary breast and ovarian cancer syndrome
   C. Lynch syndrome
   D. MUTYH-associated polyposis

2. Some nitrofurans form adducts with bases in DNA that cannot be repaired via the base-excision repair pathway. The adduct leads to distortion of the DNA double helix. The lesion is most likely repaired by which one of the following DNA repair pathways?

   A. Homologous recombination repair
   B. Mismatch repair
   C. Nonhomologous end joining
   D. Nucleotide-excision repair

3. On a colonoscopy, a 45-year-old patient with a family history of colon cancer is found to have about 90 polyps. A genetic workup revealed homozygosity for a common mutation in the *MUTYH* gene. This patient most likely developed adenomas in the colon due to a deficiency in which one of the following DNA repair pathways?

   A. Base-excision repair
   B. Homologous recombination repair
   C. Mismatch repair
   D. Nonhomologous end joining
   E. Nucleotide-excision repair

4. Aflatoxin is a polycyclic aromatic hydrocarbon that is produced by *Aspergillus* species, which often grow on cereals, peanuts, and nuts. The liver converts ingested aflatoxin to a compound that reacts with guanine in DNA. A stable adduct of guanine and the aflatoxin derivative is predominantly repaired by which one of the following DNA repair pathways?

   **A.** Base-excision repair
   **B.** Homologous recombination repair
   **C.** Mismatch repair
   **D.** Nonhomologous end joining
   **E.** Nucleotide-excision repair

5. Loss of heterozygosity (LOH) is frequently observed in tumor tissue. Thereby, the allele from one parent is lost. Which one of the following DNA damage (1) and repair (2) pathways most readily gives rise to LOH?

   **A.** (1) Deamination of C to U and (2) mismatch repair
   **B.** (1) Double-strand break and (2) homologous recombination repair
   **C.** (1) Formation of TT cyclobutane dimer and (2) nucleotide-excision repair
   **D.** (1) Opening of deoxyribose ring and (2) base-excision repair

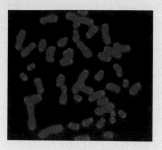

# Chapter 3

# DNA Replication

## SYNOPSIS

- During DNA replication, each DNA strand serves as a template for the synthesis of a new, complementary DNA strand. Replication starts at many sites on each chromosome. As double-stranded DNA is opened up for replication, each strand can be copied continuously in one direction, but it must be copied in many small segments in the opposite direction.
- Translesion DNA polymerases help DNA replication continue through unrepaired DNA lesions.
- Telomeres, the ends of chromosomes, shorten with each round of replication. This shortening plays a role in senescence. Cells of the germline and stem cells use telomerase to keep the length of their telomeres constant.

## LEARNING OBJECTIVES

*For mastery of this topic, you should be able to do the following:*
- Outline the replication of DNA.
- Describe the factors that contribute to the fidelity of DNA replication.
- Describe the structure of telomeres, explain how replication leads to shortening of telomeres, and describe how select cells maintain an adequate length of their telomeres.

## 1. DNA REPLICATION

*During replication, each strand of a DNA double helix serves as a template for the synthesis of a new complementary DNA strand. Topoisomerase I releases the superhelical strain and helicases catalyze the separation of complementary DNA strands. Replication of a section of DNA starts with the synthesis of an RNA primer. Then, DNA polymerase catalyzes the addition of deoxyribonucleotides. Finally, the RNA primer is replaced by deoxyribonucleotides.*

The packing of nuclear DNA into nucleosomes, 30-nm chromatin fibers, and higher-order structures is described in Chapter 1. In preparation for **DNA replication** (i.e., the copying of the genome), higher-order DNA structures are dismantled by **chromatin remodeling factors**. Such factors include enzymes that modify proteins in chromatin (e.g., acetylases and deacetylases, methylases and demethylases, kinases, and phosphatases) and proteins that replace existing proteins in chromatin.

Nuclear DNA is replicated during **S phase** of the cell cycle (see Chapter 8), which usually takes a few hours. Mitochondrial DNA is replicated on demand, which can occur independently of the replication of nuclear DNA. The following is an account of DNA replication in the nucleus.

Replication of a DNA double helix is **semiconservative**: each strand of an existing DNA double helix serves as a template for the synthesis of a new complementary strand. At the end of this process, each of the two double helices contains one of the old DNA strands and one of the newly synthesized DNA strands (Fig. 3.1).

During replication, DNA synthesis proceeds in a 5′ to 3′ direction (Fig. 3.2). The 3′ hydroxyl group at the end of a growing DNA strand performs a nucleophilic attack on the phosphorus atom of the incoming deoxyribonucleoside triphosphate that is closest to the sugar (i.e., the α-phosphate of the incoming dNTP). If the nucleotide at the 3′ end of a DNA strand lacks the 3′ hydroxyl group, the DNA strand cannot be elongated.

Replication can start at thousands of predetermined regions, the **origins of replication** (ORIs). ORIs are spaced ~50,000 to 300,000 base pairs apart. The use of these origins is regulated. There are early- and late-replicating origins. Furthermore, most origins are never used under normal circumstances (i.e., they are dormant). Dormant origins can become active when replication stalls.

The following processes ensure that the DNA around each ORI is replicated only once per cell cycle: During the $G_1$ phase of the cell cycle, just before S phase (see Chapter 8), multiprotein **origin-recognition complexes** assemble on the ORIs in a process termed licensing. This happens only in the presence of loading factors, which in turn are present only during this $G_1$ phase. In the $G_1$-to-S-phase transition and during S phase (when loading factors are no longer present), an ATP-driven helicase in the assembled complex is activated, and the complex departs from the ORI. The activity of cyclin-dependent kinases (CDKs; see Chapter 8) is high as cells exit from $G_1$ and enter S phase, and it remains high until chromosome segregation takes place during M phase. This high CDK activity inhibits licensing during the S and M phases, thus preventing rereplication.

Starting at an ORI, separation of the complementary DNA strands gives rise to two **replication forks** (see Fig. 3.3). As ATP-driven helicases separate double-helical DNA into single strands, **single-strand–binding proteins** such as **RPA (replication protein A)** partially wrap around the single-stranded DNA and prevent the hybridization of bases within the same strand or with the complementary DNA strand. **Topoisomerase I** removes the superhelical stress from the DNA (see Chapter 1). Each strand of the DNA double helix is read in a 3′→5′ direction, giving rise to new, complementary DNA strands that are called **leading strands** (see Figs. 3.3 and 3.5).

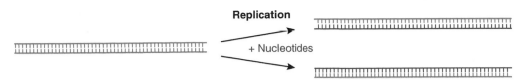

**Fig. 3.1** **DNA replication is semiconservative.**

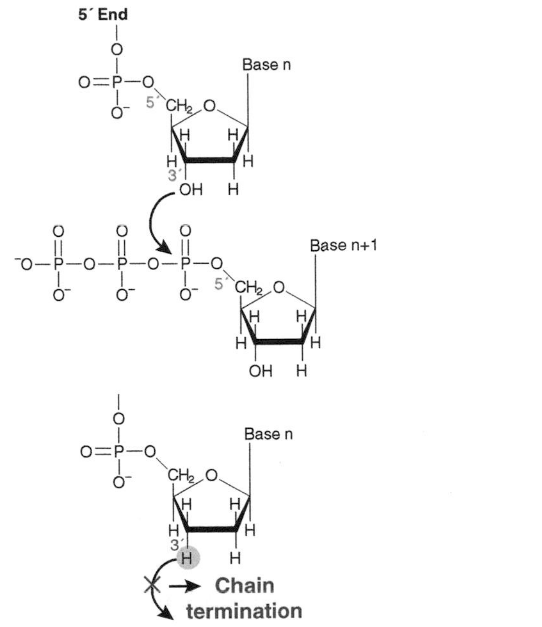

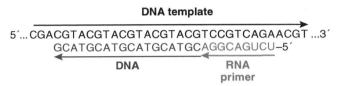

**Fig. 3.4** **Primer synthesis during DNA replication.**

**Fig. 3.2** **DNA replication occurs 5′ to 3′ and is stopped by incorporated synthetic dideoxyribonucleotides that lack the 3′ hydroxyl group.** Dideoxyribonucleotides are used clinically to treat cancer and in the laboratory for DNA sequencing and various DNA-based tests.

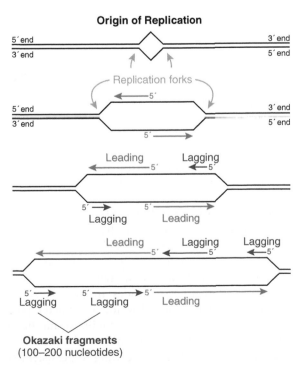

**Okazaki fragments**
(100–200 nucleotides)

**Fig. 3.3** **Replication forks during DNA replication.**

As replication proceeds, an increasing length of DNA on the 3′ side of the ORI remains uncopied, because the template can be read only in the 3′→5′ direction. Once approximately 100 to 200 uncopied bases are exposed, a DNA polymerase works on these strands as well, producing 100 to 200 nucleotide-long pieces of DNA that are called **Okazaki fragments** (see Figs. 3.3 and 3.5). The Okazaki fragments are eventually ligated, and this strand is called the **lagging strand**. Thus, synthesis of the leading strand is continuous, while synthesis of the lagging strand is discontinuous.

**DNA polymerase α** is a multisubunit enzyme complex that contains a DNA polymerase and an RNA polymerase. It uses ribonucleoside triphosphates (i.e., ATP, CTP, GTP, UTP) to synthesize a complementary **RNA primer** that is ~7 to 12 nucleotides long (Figs. 3.4, 3.5). The DNA polymerase then extends the RNA primer by ~20 nucleotides. All RNA and DNA is synthesized by the addition of a nucleoside 5′-triphosphate to the 3′-hydroxyl group of the preceding nucleotide (i.e., the newly synthesized strand grows in a 5′→3′ direction). Neither the RNA polymerase or the DNA polymerase in the DNA polymerase α complex can carry out proofreading; the complex therefore incorporates noncomplementary nucleotides at a higher frequency than DNA polymerase δ (see below).

**DNA polymerase δ** (the DNA polymerase responsible for the bulk of nucleotide incorporation) and **DNA polymerase ε** (which plays a minor role not shown in Fig. 3.5) elongate the strand synthesized by DNA polymerase α. Each polymerase has a proofreading function; if the bases of the growing DNA strand do not match the template, the enzyme stalls, excises the mismatched nucleotide, and then continues polymerization.

When DNA polymerase δ reaches an RNA primer on the lagging strand, the primer and up to ~30 deoxyribonucleotides that follow it are displaced and excised. DNA polymerase δ inserts the missing complementary nucleotides, and the **DNA ligase** joins the 3′ end of the most recently synthesized piece of DNA with the appropriate 5′-end of the previously synthesized piece of DNA.

DNA replication has a very high **fidelity**. On average, each replication of the human genome (involving ~3 billion base pairs) introduces only about three base changes. The high accuracy is in large part due to the substrate specificity

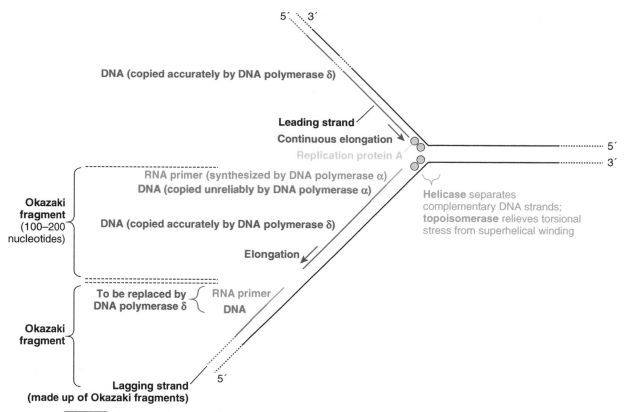

**Fig. 3.5** DNA replication, showing the leading and lagging strand at a replication fork.

and proofreading function of DNA polymerase δ, as well as the efficiency of postreplication DNA mismatch repair (see Section 2 in Chapter 2).

Following replication, DNA is assembled into nucleosomes and higher-order chromatin structures using chromatin assembly factors, including existing and newly synthesized histones.

**DNA polymerases** and **DNA ligases** from a variety of organisms are used for in vitro DNA diagnostic methods (see Chapter 4).

**Dideoxyribonucleotides** that interfere with DNA replication are used in cancer chemotherapy, as antiviral drugs, in DNA diagnostics, and in Sanger-type DNA sequencing (see Chapter 4). Nucleotides without a 3′-hydroxyl group (e.g., **ddATP, ddGTP, ddCTP,** and **ddTTP**), can be incorporated into the DNA, but because they lack a 3′-hydroxyl group, they are chain terminators (see Fig. 3.2).

**Zidovudine** and **lamivudine** (Fig. 3.6) both inhibit viral reverse transcriptases (enzymes that copy viral RNA into DNA) but have only a minor effect on human DNA polymerases. Both drugs are used against infections with **retroviruses** (i.e., viruses that contain an RNA genome). Zidovudine is an analog of thymidine. Enzymes in the cell convert zidovudine to the triphosphate form, and reverse transcriptase subsequently incorporates it into growing DNA strands. These DNA strands cannot be elongated because zidovudine lacks a 3′-hydroxyl group. Lamivudine likewise is phosphorylated inside cells and then markedly inhibits viral reverse transcriptases but not human DNA polymerases. Like zidovudine,

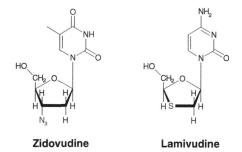

**Zidovudine**          **Lamivudine**

**Fig. 3.6** **Drugs that preferentially inhibit DNA synthesis in retroviruses.** Zidovudine is an analog of thymidine, and lamivudine is an analog of deoxycytidine. Residues that differ from the physiological nucleoside are shown in red.

lamivudine also acts as a chain terminator. Lamivudine is used in the treatment of hepatitis B and human immunodeficiency virus-1.

**Arabinosylcytosine** and **fludarabine** (Fig. 3.7) interfere with DNA replication, and both drugs are used for the treatment of acute **leukemias.** Inside cells, these drugs are phosphorylated. DNA polymerase incorporates arabinosylcytosine triphosphate and fludarabine triphosphate into DNA. However, these synthetic nucleotides are poor substrates for excision and replacement, as well as for continued replication. The decrease in replication leads to double-strand breaks. In addition, fludarabine at the 3′ terminus of a piece of DNA prevents ligation by DNA ligase, leading to persistent single-strand breaks (i.e., nicked DNA). Once a cell has incorporated

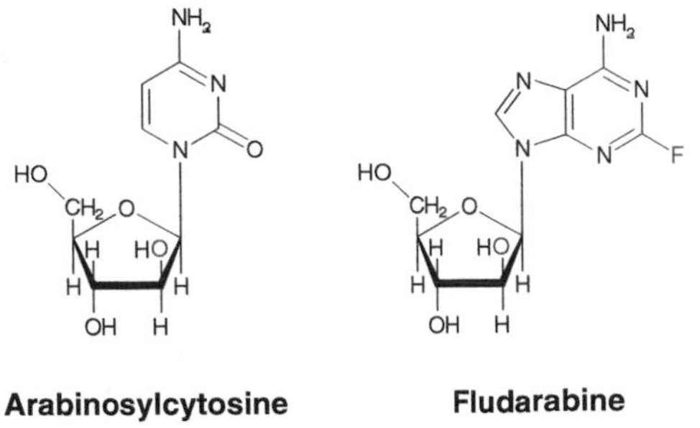

**Arabinosylcytosine**          **Fluradabine**

**Fig. 3.7** **Drugs that inhibit DNA replication.** Arabinosylcytosine is an analog of cytidine, and fludarabine is an analog of adenosine. Residues that differ from the physiological nucleoside are shown in red.

about 100,000 molecules of fludarabine into its DNA, it undergoes apoptosis.

## 2. TRANSLESION DNA SYNTHESIS

*Translesion DNA synthesis is carried out during DNA replication by polymerases that recognize damaged nucleotides that escape DNA repair mechanisms. These DNA polymerases usually incorporate the correct nucleotide opposite a damaged one, but the damaged DNA template strand is not repaired.*

During DNA replication, **bypass DNA polymerases** (**translesion DNA polymerases**) are recruited to DNA lesions that escape repair by the pathways of base excision, mismatch repair, and nucleotide excision (see Chapter 2). The major replicative DNA polymerases α and δ generally cannot copy damaged nucleotides. In contrast, bypass DNA polymerases copy a wide spectrum of DNA damage, but they also have lower copy fidelity than DNA polymerase δ. Bypass polymerases are much more active with damaged DNA as a template than with intact DNA; this characteristic prevents translesion DNA polymerases from inaccurate copying of appreciable stretches of undamaged DNA. Bypass DNA polymerases do not repair the damage to nucleotides in the template DNA.

Humans have several types of bypass DNA polymerases: η (eta), ι (iota), κ (kappa), and others. Collectively, these polymerases can insert A, T, C, or G opposite an abasic site, insert G opposite U (U derives from the deamination of C), or insert C opposite 8-oxoguanine, for lesions that should have been repaired by the base excision repair pathway (see Chapter 2). Bypass DNA polymerases can also insert an AA opposite the cyclobutane TT dimers, T opposite adducts of polycyclic aromatic hydrocarbons with A, C opposite adducts of polycyclic aromatic hydrocarbons with G, or CC opposite cisplatin GG intrastrand crosslinks, for lesions that should have been repaired by the nucleotide excision repair pathway (see Chapter 2).

The physiological importance of translesion DNA synthesis is apparent from a variant form of **xeroderma pigmentosum** that is due to a deficiency in DNA polymerase η (eta). This DNA polymerase inserts an AA opposite cyclobutane TT dimers (it catalyzes DNA synthesis opposite other damaged

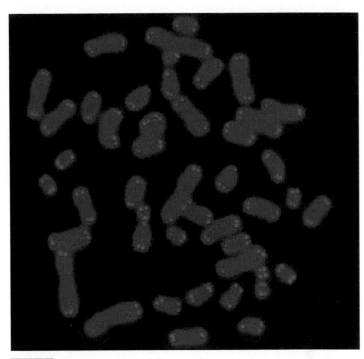

**Fig. 3.8** **Metaphase chromosomes with telomeres.** A metaphase chromosome consists of two sister chromatids (see Section 5 in Chapter 1). Each chromatid has two ends and thus two telomeres. The chromosomes were stained with a telomere-specific, pink fluorescent peptide nucleic acid probe and the chromosomes with the blue fluorescent DNA-binding molecule DAPI (4′,6-diamidino-2-phenylindole). (From Olaussen KA, Dubrana K, Domont J, Spano JP, Sabatier L, Soria JC. Telomeres and telomerase as targets for anticancer drug development. *Crit Rev Oncol Hematol.* 2006;57:191–214.)

nucleotides as well). Affected patients are extremely sensitive to sunlight and have an elevated risk of cancer.

## 3. REPLICATION OF THE ENDS OF CHROMOSOMES (TELOMERES)

*The ends of the chromosomes are called telomeres; they consist largely of repeats of the sequence TTAGGG. So that DNA repair complexes do not mistake telomeres for the ends of damaged DNA, the ends of the DNA strands are folded over, and the telomeric repeats are covered by proteins. In most somatic cells, upon replication, each DNA strand loses telomeric DNA until, eventually, short telomeres induce cell senescence. By contrast, telomerase maintains the lengths of the telomeres in germ cells, some stem cells, and most tumor cells.*

The ends of the chromosomes are called **telomeres** (Fig. 3.8), and they play an important role in aging and cancer. Telomeres prevent DNA repair mechanisms from attacking the ends of the chromosomes, provide a means to limit the number of times a cell can divide, and can prevent the irreversible loss of genetic information from the ends of the chromosomes during DNA replication. Immortal cancer cells circumvent the telomere-limitation of cell division.

A telomeric nucleoprotein structure shields the telomeres from recognition by DNA repair complexes (Fig. 3.9).

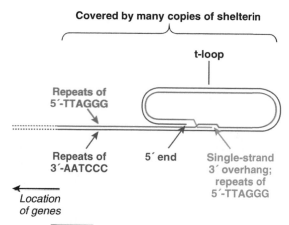

**Covered by many copies of shelterin**

t-loop

Repeats of
5′-TTAGGG

Repeats of
3′-AATCCC

5′ end

Single-strand
3′ overhang;
repeats of
5′-TTAGGG

Location
of genes

**Fig. 3.9** **Structure of a telomere.**

Telomeres are about 4,000 to 15,000 bases long and consist mostly of repeats of the sequence **TTAGGG** (5′-CCCTAA on the complementary strand). The last 20 to 35 TTAGGG repeats at the 3′ end of each DNA strand have no partners in the complementary strand (i.e., they form a single-strand 3′ overhang). A double-strand portion of the telomere loops back, and the single-strand 3′ overhang invades a double-strand portion of the telomere, forming a **t-loop**. Telomeric DNA is covered by **shelterin** protein complexes that specifically bind to telomeric DNA repeats and protects telomeres from being recognized by DNA repair proteins, thereby preventing fusion of chromosomes.

In most somatic cells, the **telomeres shorten** with each cell division (Fig. 3.10). Therefore, telomere length provides the cells with a potential mechanism to count and limit the number of cell divisions. Since the DNA polymerases that are involved in DNA replication require template DNA 3′ to their catalytic site, the normal replication machinery described in

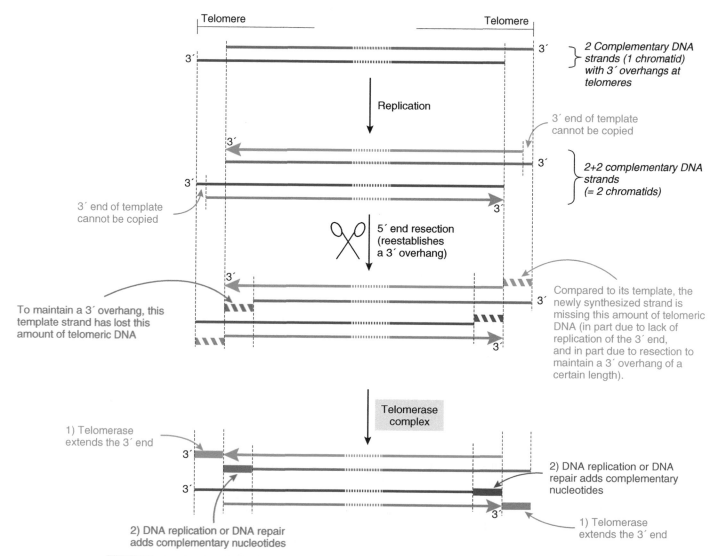

**Fig. 3.10** **Telomere shortening and lengthening.** Telomere shortening occurs during replication of the genome. Cells that express telomerase can rebuild the telomere length.

Section 1 cannot replicate the 3′ end of the DNA strand. In addition, an exonuclease degrades a portion of each 5′ end to maintain the length of the 3′ overhang. In vitro measurements show that **fibroblasts** on *average* lose 40 to 120 bp per telomere with each cycle of replication. Fibroblasts that have a relatively small number of TTAGGG repeats no longer divide (i.e., they enter replicative **senescence**) and stay in the $G_0$ phase of the cell cycle (see Chapter 8).

The **telomerase** protein complex can maintain telomere length by adding telomeric DNA repeats, nucleotide by nucleotide, using an RNA template (**telomerase RNA component, TERC**) that is stably bound to the protein complex. Thus, telomerase has reverse transcriptase activity that can repeatedly copy the sequence 3′-CAAUCCCAAUC-5′ contained within the long TERC RNA to produce the 5′-TTAGGG-3′ telomeric DNA repeats. Numerous proteins regulate the placement of telomerase on single-strand telomeric DNA. Once telomerase is displaced from the telomere, DNA replication or repair processes add complementary nucleotides (deoxy-C, T, and deoxy-A) to the 5′ end of the complementary DNA strand.

Cells with a high or unlimited potential for replication, such as embryonic stem cells, germ cells, stem cells in the bone marrow or the villi of the intestine, activated lymphocytes, and tumor cells express telomerase. Otherwise, normal somatic cells typically have little or no telomerase activity.

For unknown reasons, despite the presence of telomerase in precursor cells, the telomeres of many cells (e.g., circulating white blood cells, muscle, skin, and adipose tissue) become shorter by ~25 bp per year of age. Factors such as smoking, psychological stress, asthma, and chronic obstructive pulmonary disease (COPD) hasten the shortening.

Short telomeres are associated with high mortality, while long repeats are associated with an increased risk for a select number of neoplasms.

The **heritable telomeropathies (inherited telomere syndromes)** known to date are caused by mutations in a subunit of telomerase or in a protein that binds to telomeres. Most pathogenic mutations are accompanied by haploinsufficiency, and telomeropathies therefore usually show autosomal dominant inheritance. Impaired telomere maintenance causes a spectrum of symptoms that may include leukoplakia (white patches on the mucosa of the mouth), skin hyperpigmentation, nail dystrophy, fibrosis of the lungs, bone marrow failure, and liver cirrhosis.

**Tumor cells** have the means to avoid replicative senescence and apoptosis due to telomere shortening. Tumor precursor cells may avoid senescence by inactivating a cell cycle checkpoint (see Chapter 8). As telomeres continue to shorten as a result of DNA replication, the cells reach a crisis point, at which the telomeres no longer protect the genetic information and apoptosis normally ensues; only cells that can establish protective telomeres survive. Indeed, most immortal tumor cells have active **telomerase** that helps them maintain telomeres, although these telomeres are relatively short. Telomerase is thus a potential target for antitumor drugs. In a minority of tumors, telomeres are maintained by the recombination of chromosome ends or short pieces of circular DNA that contain telomeric repeats; this is called the **alternative lengthening of telomeres (ALT)** pathway. Telomeres that are maintained by the ALT pathway are unusually long and differ greatly in length. The ALT pathway is found most frequently in sarcomas.

## SUMMARY

- Most nuclear DNA is replicated during the S-phase of the cell cycle. Replication starts at the origins of replication (ORIs). Helicases separate complementary DNA strands, while topoisomerases relieve torsional superhelical strain. DNA polymerase α, which shows low fidelity, synthesizes an RNA primer and then extends it with deoxyribonucleotides. DNA polymerase δ and ε extend the growing DNA strand with high fidelity and also replace the RNA primer and the inaccurately copied DNA region with an accurate copy of DNA. DNA ligase joins contiguous pieces of the newly synthesized DNA.

- As a DNA double helix is opened and replicated at an ORI, each parental strand is read continuously on one strand and discontinuously on the other strand. Discontinuous replication of DNA gives rise to Okazaki fragments that are subsequently ligated.

- Nucleotides without a 3′-hydroxyl group can inhibit DNA replication.

- During replication, the translesion DNA polymerases ε (eta), ι (iota), and κ (kappa) read damaged nucleotides on the template DNA that escaped the repair processes. These damaged nucleotides include 8-oxoguanine, cyclobutane thymine dimers, cisplatin intrastrand crosslinks, and adducts of polycyclic hydrocarbons with a base. These polymerases insert a nucleotide in the growing DNA strand, but they do not repair the damaged nucleotides in the template strand.

- The ends of the chromosomes are capped by telomeres. Telomeres consist of 700 to 2,500 TTAGGG repeats, the end portion of which forms a t-loop. Shelterin covers the repeats. In most somatic cells, the telomeres shorten with each cycle of replication, and short telomeres induce replicative senescence. Telomerase lengthens telomeres by adding TTAGGG repeats based on its own internal RNA template. Germline cells and some stem cells use telomerase to maintain their telomeres. Tumor cells use telomerase or a recombination-based pathway (termed alternative lengthening of telomeres) to maintain telomeres. Abnormal function of the telomerase complex can lead to premature aging of a number of tissues (e.g., bone marrow, lungs, and liver).

## FURTHER READING

- Fragkos M, Ganier O, Coulombe P, Méchali M. DNA replication origin activation in space and time. *Nat Rev Mol Cell Biol.* 2015;16:360-374.

■ Holohan B, Wright WE, Shay JW. Cell biology of disease: telomeropathies: an emerging spectrum disorder. *J Cell Biol.* 2014;205:289-299.

■ Yang K, Weinacht CP, Zhuang Z. Regulatory role of ubiquitin in eukaryotic DNA translesion synthesis. *Biochemistry.* 2013;52:3217-3228.

# Review Questions

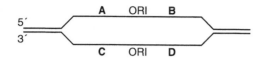

1. The figure above represents DNA undergoing replication. Lagging strand synthesis occurs in which of the following areas?

    A. A and B
    B. A and C
    C. A and D
    D. B and C
    E. B and D

2. Translesion DNA synthesis accomplishes which of the following?

    A. Extends DNA strands that end in a dideoxyribonucleotide
    B. Inserts nucleotides opposite the damaged nucleotides
    C. Joins the lagging strands
    D. Refills deletions of DNA nucleotides
    E. Replicates the DNA of adjoining Okazaki fragments

3. Which of the following is true about telomeres?

    A. A metaphase chromosome contains two telomeres and consists of two chromatids.
    B. Telomere length positively correlates with mortality rate.
    C. Telomeres shorten during DNA replication.
    D. The shelterin complex elongates telomeres.

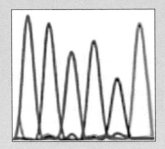

## SYNOPSIS

- DNA- and RNA-based tests are widely used in the clinic, for instance prenatal diagnosis, diagnosis of hereditary diseases, screening for infectious agents, and optimization of cancer treatment.
- For traditional cytogenetic determination of the karyotype (the set of chromosomes), cells from biopsy material are grown in vitro and arrested in mitosis. The chromosomes are then stained and analyzed under a light microscope.
- In fluorescence in situ hybridization (FISH), fluorescently labeled DNA probes are hybridized with chromosomes. The main application of FISH is detecting chromosome alterations.
- In the polymerase chain reaction (PCR), synthetic DNA primers are used to define a segment of DNA that is then amplified, sometimes by a factor of more than $10^9$.
- DNA microarrays consist of an inert surface onto which numerous known DNA sequences are deposited in known locations. Hybridization of test DNA or of test DNA plus competing control DNA, followed by detection, allows analysis of the test DNA for deletions, duplications, and, in special cases, even sequence. There is great variation in the resolving power of DNA microarray–based tests.
- Sanger sequencing is the traditional method for sequencing nucleic acids. More recently, massive parallel sequencing has revolutionized molecular diagnostics; it is used, for example, to detect inherited mutations and analyze mutations in a tumor.
- DNA from the placenta circulates in the pregnant mother's blood and can be analyzed by massive parallel sequencing to estimate the chromosome complement of the fetus.

## LEARNING OBJECTIVES

*For mastery of this topic, you should be able to do the following:*
- Describe the sample requirements for a traditional cytogenetic analysis and the level of detail one can expect to find in the final karyotype report.
- Describe FISH and explain the results one can expect to obtain.
- Explain how PCR can amplify one or more specific DNA fragments. Describe quantitative (real-time) PCR. Explain how the threshold cycle is used for quantification of test DNA.
- Explain how restriction enzymes and capillary electrophoresis can be used to determine the presence or absence of a mutation.
- Explain how DNA melting curve analysis can be used to determine the presence or absence of a mutation.
- Describe the type of result one can expect from aCGH (array comparative genomic hybridization) and from DNA SNP (single nucleotide polymorphism) microarrays.
- Compare and contrast Sanger sequencing and massive parallel sequencing.
- Explain how DNA from a pregnant woman's blood can be used to estimate the karyotype of her fetus.

## 1. CONVENTIONAL CYTOGENETICS AND FLUORESCENCE IN SITU HYBRIDIZATION

*In conventional cytogenetics, viable cells from biopsied tissue, blood, or bone marrow are grown in vitro and arrested in metaphase, when the chromosomes are maximally condensed and clearly separated from each other. The results of analyzing stained chromosomes are summarized in a karyotype report. For FISH, one or more fluorescently labeled nucleic acid probes for genetic loci of interest are allowed to hybridize with nucleic acids that have been made single stranded. Then, fluorescent spots are then assessed for rearrangements.*

For a traditional cytogenetic analysis and determination of karyotype, viable cells from a fetus or a patient are grown in vitro, arrested at metaphase (when chromosomes are condensed), dropped onto a glass slide, stained, and analyzed for abnormalities based on the unique banding pattern of each type of chromosome (Fig. 4.1; also see Fig. 1.12). Cells used for cytogenetic analyses must therefore be able to divide and be free of infection. The most commonly used chromosome stain is Giemsa in a technique called **G-banding,** or Giemsa banding. The two most common indications for determining a karyotype are cancer and prenatal diagnosis.

**Aneuploidy** is the presence of a number of chromosomes that is not an exact multiple of 23, such as 45 chromosomes instead of the 46 present in a normal diploid karyotype (see Fig. 4.1).

To be visible in a cytogenetic karyotype analysis, a deletion or insertion must be at least approximately 5 million base pairs (bp) long.

For **FISH,** metaphase or interphase chromosomes of cells from a patient are hybridized with a DNA segment that is specific for the genetic locus of interest and conjugated with a fluorescent molecule (Fig. 4.2). FISH on metaphase chromosome spreads allows determination of the chromosome location of the signal. FISH on interphase chromosomes is performed on nondividing cells and can therefore be used on histology tissue sections, so that the FISH signal can be correlated with histologic features. In cells that have a normal karyotype, two signals (fluorescent spots) per nucleus are seen, one for each gene in the two autosomes. If there is partial or complete duplication of a chromosome, or if the genetic locus under study is amplified, more than two signals are seen. Conversely, the deletion of the gene under study leads to a reduction in the number of signals. FISH detects deletions larger than approximately 150,000 bp. Accordingly, FISH can detect **microdeletions** and **microduplications,** which have a size of approximately 1 million to 3 million bases and cannot

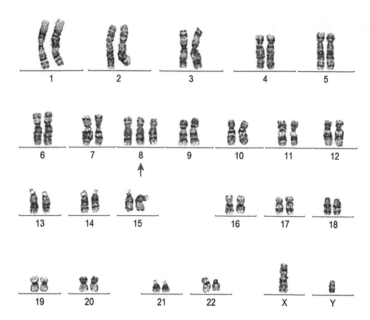

**Fig. 4.1** **Abnormal karyogram of a bone marrow cell from a patient with acute myeloid leukemia.** Cells in the bone marrow acquired a third copy of chromosome 8 *(arrow)*. (Courtesy Dr. Barry L. Barnoski, Oncocytogenetics Laboratory, Cooper University Hospital, Camden, NJ.)

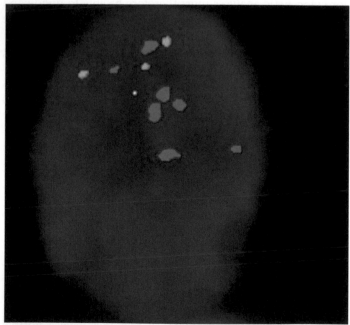

**Fig. 4.2** **Example of fluorescence in situ hybridization to interphase chromosomes.** Breast cancer cells were tested for epidermal growth factor 2 (*HER2*) status. The red fluorescent probe binds to *HER2*, and the green fluorescent probe binds to the centromere of chromosome 17. In a normal cell, two red and two green signals are present. In tumors that meet criteria for *HER2* amplification, the number of red signals is ≥6/cell, or the number of red signals is ≥4/cell and the ratio of red to green signals is ≥2. The image shows a single-cell nucleus *(blue)*. *HER2* is amplified. (Data from Pu X, Shi J, Li Z, Feng A, Ye Q. Comparison of the 2007 and 2013 ASCO/CAP evaluation systems for HER2 amplification in breast cancer. *Pathol Res Pract.* 2015;211:421-425.)

be detected with G-banding of metaphase chromosomes. FISH is not sensitive enough to detect point mutations or small deletions. It provides data on single cells.

FISH can also be used to detect **rearrangements** within and between chromosomes (e.g., translocations). The rearrangement may lead to **separation** or **fusion** of two differently colored FISH probes for two different genetic loci.

## 2. DNA AMPLIFICATION BY POLYMERASE CHAIN REACTION

*PCR is used to amplify select DNA segments in a DNA sample. Primers determine the start and end of a sequence to be amplified. In clinical lab tests, PCR is often used to determine the amount of a particular DNA in a sample, but the technique also has other applications (see Sections 3 and 4).*

PCR is a frequently used template amplification technique in RNA- or DNA-based clinical tests. PCR produces multiple copies of a segment of DNA that is bounded by two specifically chosen oligonucleotide sequences called **primers** (Fig. 4.3). The oligonucleotide primers (in vitro synthesized single-stranded DNA approximately 15 to 20 nucleotides long) are needed for **DNA polymerase** to be active. As shown in Chapter 1, complementary DNA strands are by convention presented with the 5′-end of the coding strand in the top left. In such a representation, the two primers are sometimes referred to as the **forward primer** and the **reverse primer**.

A **PCR cycle** involves heat denaturation to separate complementary DNA strands, cooling to allow hybridization (annealing) of primers to the complementary sequences of the template, and moderate heating to increase the activity of DNA polymerase, which extends the primers, using the hybridized DNA strand as a template (Fig. 4.4). To simplify DNA amplification, a heat-tolerant DNA polymerase is chosen (typically from an organism that lives in a hot spring). A full PCR cycle typically takes approximately 1 to 2 minutes.

After 20 and 30 PCR cycles, the template DNA molecule has been copied approximately 1 million ($2^{20}$) to 1 billion ($2^{30}$) times, respectively. At this point, the nonamplified DNA (the

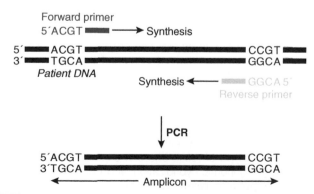

**Fig. 4.3** **Primer-directed in vitro DNA synthesis.** The forward primer uses the bottom strand as a template and thereby synthesizes a new top strand. The reverse primer uses the top strand as a template and thereby synthesizes a new bottom strand.

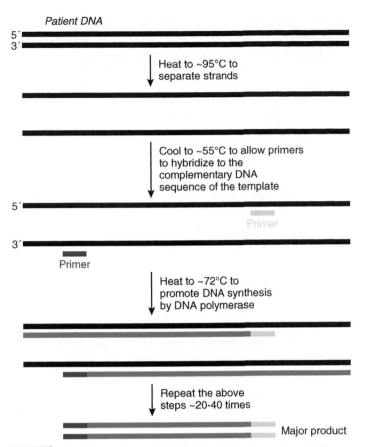

**Fig. 4.4** **Principle of the PCR amplification of a DNA sequence.** PCR requires two different primers so that both strands can be amplified with a defined start and end sequence. The DNA polymerase stems from an organism that is adapted to high temperature.

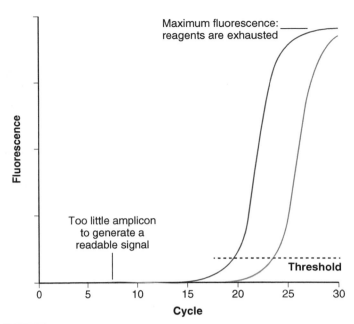

**Fig. 4.5** **Quantitative PCR amplification.** The amount of DNA in the sample increases exponentially and is followed with a fluorescent dye during each cycle. The cycle at which the amount of DNA crosses the predetermined threshold is a measure of the amount of DNA in the initial sample.

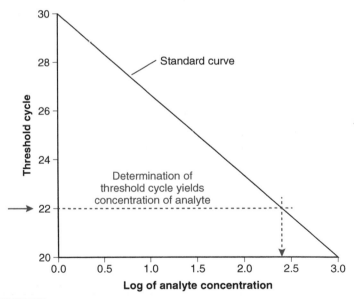

**Fig. 4.6** **Standard curve for real-time PCR that relates analyte concentration to threshold cycle.** Fig. 4.5 explains the threshold cycle. The higher the threshold cycle number for a sample, the lower the concentration of the analyte.

DNA that is not of interest) has faded into nonsignificant background abundance.

In **reverse transcription PCR (RT-PCR)**, an **RNA** template is reverse transcribed into complementary DNA (**cDNA**), which is then amplified as in regular PCR.

**Multiplex PCR** refers to a procedure during which more than two primers are present so that more than one DNA (or cDNA) sequence can be amplified simultaneously. Multiplex PCR can be used to analyze several regions of interest at the same time (one of these regions may be used for quality control).

After PCR amplification, the amplified DNA segment (**amplicon**) is analyzed further, often by one of the methods described in Sections 3 and 4.

The handling of amplicons for further analysis poses a risk of **contamination** because of the very high concentration of amplicon compared with the DNA segment of interest in patient samples. Many labs perform preamplification and postamplification steps in separate areas.

For **real-time PCR**, fluorescently labeled probes that are specific for the sequence of interest are added to the reaction, and fluorescence is measured at each PCR cycle (Fig. 4.5). This technology is often used for quantification and is sometimes called **quantitative PCR (qPCR)**. A threshold fluorescence is set, and a calibration curve (Fig. 4.6) is established that relates the threshold cycle (i.e., the cycle at which the fluorescence crosses the threshold) to the amount of template DNA. This permits quantification of template DNA in patient samples. Since real-time PCR provides the results directly during the run, no post-PCR handling of the amplicons is necessary, which significantly reduces the risk of contamination.

## 3. ELECTROPHORESIS AND MELTING CURVE ANALYSIS OF DNA

*Electrophoresis allows determination of the size of a nucleic acid fragment. Restriction enzyme digestion permits probing of a small part of the sequence of a DNA segment. Melting curves allow the detection of a difference between DNA sequences that match a probe perfectly and ones that match imperfectly. All of these tests are commonly performed on PCR-amplified DNA.*

**Electrophoresis** is commonly used for size separation of nucleic acid fragments. An electrical field pulls the negatively charged molecules through a matrix, such as an agarose or polyacrylamide gel or a polymer-filled capillary. Small DNA molecules migrate the fastest because they experience the least amount of drag in the matrix; conversely, large DNA molecules migrate the slowest.

**Capillary electrophoresis** is used in modern Sanger sequencing (see Fig. 4.10) and to determine the fragment length after PCR or digestion with a restriction enzyme (see below).

Digestion of PCR-amplified DNA with **restriction enzymes** (**restriction endonucleases**) allows one to gain limited sequence information (Fig. 4.7). Hundreds of restriction enzymes are available that cut only at specific sequences (these are mostly palindromic; i.e., they read the same on both DNA strands) and in a specific manner. It is likely that a restriction enzyme can be found that cuts either only the normal or the known mutant sequence. After the reaction has gone to completion, the size of the products is determined by electrophoresis.

Instead of digestion with a restriction enzyme, **melting curve analysis** by real-time PCR (Fig. 4.8) can be used to identify small known sequence variations. The real-time PCR is performed with the usual primers and also with two labeled, sequence-specific nucleic acid probes. At low temperature, one of the two probes anneals with the segment where the known mutation is located, regardless of the presence or absence of the mutation. The probe that anneals closer to the 5′ end of the amplified DNA segment has a **donor** chromophore at its 3′ end, and the second probe (which hybridizes directly to the first probe) has an **acceptor chromophore** at its 5′ end. When the two probes bind next to each other on an amplified DNA, and when they are illuminated with the light that the donor chromophore absorbs efficiently, **Förster resonance energy transfer** to the acceptor chromophore takes place. The acceptor chromophore then fluoresces at its specific wavelength, which is measured by the real-time PCR instrument. At the end of the amplification cycles, the probes are annealed and the fluorescence intensity is high. The sample is then heated gradually, causing the probes to melt off the amplified DNA. If the probe does not perfectly match the patient's DNA, it dissociates at a relatively low temperature, thereby causing a loss in fluorescence. By contrast, the probe that perfectly hybridizes to the patient's DNA dissociates at a relatively high temperature. For interpretation, the melting curve for the test DNA is compared to a standard.

## 4. DNA MICROARRAY–BASED TECHNOLOGIES

*DNA microarrays contain known DNA sequences at known locations and can be used to probe test DNA for deletions, duplications, and—at a limited number of chosen locations—sequence.*

A **DNA microarray** (sometimes called a **chip**) consists of a treated flat surface (often glass) approximately $25 \times 25$ mm$^2$ in size that has been densely printed with several copies each of thousands to more than 1 million different segments of DNA (often called **probes**). The sequence of each probe is known, as is its location in the array. Sample DNA (and sometimes control DNA) is allowed to hybridize with the probes. The extent of hybridization is then measured.

Depending on the length, diversity, and design of the probes in a DNA microarray, different resolutions and goals are achieved. The longer probes bind DNA fragments regardless of a minor sequence variation. This is used to scan the entire genome for **copy number variations** (CNVs; i.e.,

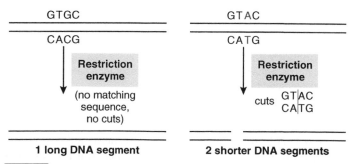

**Fig. 4.7** **Digestion of PCR–amplified DNA with a restriction enzyme.** After digestion with the restriction enzyme, DNA fragment length is determined by electrophoresis. The procedure can be used, for example, to test for the C282Y mutation in the *HFE* gene of patients suspected of having *HFE* hemochromatosis (see Section 9.2 in Chapter 15).

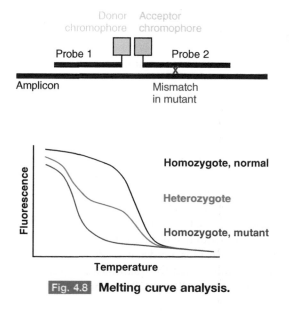

**Fig. 4.8** Melting curve analysis.

deletions or amplifications; see array comparative genomic hybridization below). Balanced translocations are not detectable because DNA is fragmented before analysis. The shorter probes can be designed to differentiate between short sequences that differ by a single nucleotide (see single nucleotide polymorphism microarrays below).

In one of the most common clinical applications, **array comparative genomic hybridization (aCGH)**, microarrays are exposed simultaneously to fragments of control DNA labeled with one particular fluorophore and fragments of test DNA labeled with a different fluorophore (Fig. 4.9). The test and the control DNA fragments compete for hybridization with complementary probes on the microarray. The fluorescence of each fluorophore is determined for every printed array location. At each location, the ratio of the fluorescence of the two fluorophores is indicative of the ratio of test DNA to control DNA.

DNA **single nucleotide polymorphism (SNP) microarrays** are designed to determine the identity of single nucleotides at thousands of specific loci in the genome. A SNP (pronounced "snip") is a locus in the genome at which a different single base (A, C, G, or T) is commonly found in the

population. SNPs are so polymorphic (diverse) in the population that people likely inherit two different versions of the SNP from their parents. The array includes probes for both DNA strands and for all relevant SNPs. Fluorescently labeled DNA of a patient is hybridized to the SNP array and binds mostly to perfectly complementary probes on the array.

SNP arrays can be used to identify sequence variations at SNPs, to compare the SNP distribution of related individuals and perform linkage analysis, and to determine sites of **loss of heterozygosity**. DNA segments that are involved in loss of heterozygosity contain numerous SNPs. If there is loss of heterozygosity (see Section 4.2 in Chapter 2), stretches of neighboring SNPs lose their natural diversity (because of uncompensated loss of a DNA segment or homologous recombination repair of DNA).

In clinical practice aCGH and SNP arrays are often combined.

## 5. DNA SEQUENCING

*Sanger sequencing is a highly accurate but slow and expensive way of sequencing DNA with chain-terminating nucleotides. Massive parallel sequencing is used extensively in molecular diagnostics. It involves attaching DNA fragments to a surface, multiplying them locally, and then sequencing them at their known location; with algorithms, the sequence data are assembled into a genome (akin to a puzzle).*

### 5.1. Sanger Sequencing

Sanger sequencing is built on the principle that DNA-synthesizing DNA polymerase can incorporate a **dideoxynucleotide**, which causes **chain termination** (dideoxynucleotides lack a 3′-hydroxyl group that could form a phosphodiester with an incoming nucleotide; see Fig. 3.2). If a mixture contains approximately 99% normal deoxynucleotides and approximately 1% chain-terminating dideoxynucleotides, a chain ends whenever a dideoxynucleotide is incorporated. Typically, the four different chain-terminating dideoxynucleotides (A, T, C, G) are labeled with four different fluorescent dyes. This generates DNA fragments that fluoresce with the color that befits the nucleotide at the 3′-end of the chain. Separating the resulting chains with one base resolution (now generally done with capillary electrophoresis; see Section 3) and detecting the four different fluorescence colors allow determination of the nucleotide sequence (Fig. 4.10).

### 5.2. Massive Parallel Sequencing

Massive parallel sequencing (**second-generation sequencing**, **next-generation sequencing**, or **deep sequencing**) refers to the simultaneous sequencing of multiple DNA segments. This is now often achieved by fragmenting DNA, enriching the DNA for regions of interest, creating a DNA library attached to a solid support, and then sequencing the attached DNA fragments at their specific location step by step while

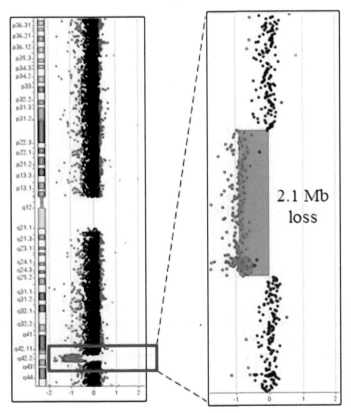

**Fig. 4.9 Microarray analysis of chromosome 1.** The leftmost part of the figure shows a schematic of chromosome 1. Each dot in the graph represents the reading of one oligonucleotide probe. In the area that is free of dots (approximately the centromere and q12 to q21.1), no oligonucleotide probes were present. The numbers on the horizontal axis refer to the numbers of DNA segments lost or gained relative to control DNA. The data relate to a newborn with brain malformation. (From Peters DG, Yatsenko SA, Surti U, Rajkovic A. Recent advances of genomic testing in perinatal medicine. *Semin Perinatol.* 2015;39:44-54.)

2.1 Mb loss

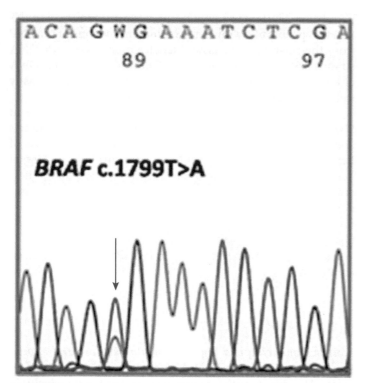

Fig. 4.10 **Sample result of Sanger sequencing of a lung nodule.** The nodule contained some cells that had a normal *BRAF* sequence with the expected red peak, signifying a T (fifth base shown, *red arrow*), and cells that contained a T→A mutation, seen as a smaller green peak at the same location. (From Yousem SA, Dacic S, Nikiforov YE, Nikiforova M. Pulmonary Langerhans cell histiocytosis: profiling of multifocal tumors using next-generation sequencing identifies concordant occurrence of BRAF V600E mutations. *Chest*. 2013;143: 1679-1684.)

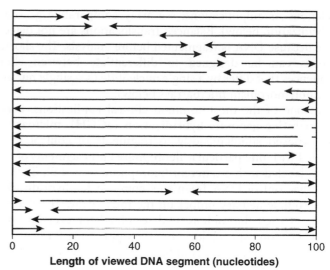

**Length of viewed DNA segment (nucleotides)**

Fig. 4.11 **Processed results of massive parallel sequencing.** Arrows indicate the direction of the sequenced strands (DNA has two antiparallel, complementary strands). Fragments with arrows that point to the very left or right end of the graph extend beyond the viewed frame. The maximum read depth for the depicted 100-base segment is 24.

following the reaction with imaging. Multiple competing technologies are available.

After massive parallel sequencing, the obtained sequences (**read**s) are assembled into whole chromosomes using computer-based algorithms (Fig. 4.11). The algorithms take advantage of overlapping sequences and knowledge of the human genome. For genetic testing (when all tested cells are expected to be genetically identical), there should be 30 or more reads. When searching for somatic mutations in tumors, the sequencing depth can be as high as 1000 reads; this permits the detection of a mutation in as little as approximately 5% of all cells.

In search of a genetic alteration, next-generation sequencing can cover the entire genome (**whole-genome sequencing**) or be limited to all exons (**exome sequencing**). The exome makes up only ~2% of the genome, yet it contains ~85% of disease-causing mutations. The cost of sequencing ~95% of the exome is currently ~10% of the cost of sequencing ~98% of the whole genome.

For sequencing, hotspot mutation panels are available that cover up to several hundred DNA segments in which mutations are known to occur. These panels can be used to determine the spectrum of significant mutations in a tumor or elucidate the genetic basis of a patient's heritable disorder.

At present, the challenge is not so much the generation of sequencing data at an affordable price and with reasonable speed, but the curation and interpretation of the highly complex data. For instance, exome sequencing of a single patient's DNA yields approximately 25,000 variants, and genome sequencing of the same DNA yields approximately 3 million variants. It is challenging to separate variants of clinical significance from **variants of unknown significance (VUS)**. Furthermore, it is difficult to determine which data should be disclosed and how the complex information should be explained to individual patients.

## 6. SELECTED CLINICAL APPLICATIONS OF DNA-BASED TESTING

*DNA-based testing is extensively used in prenatal diagnosis, in determining the cause of infections, in diagnosing certain hereditary disorders, and in assessing tumors for genetic alterations relevant to diagnosis, prognosis, or treatment.*

### 6.1. Prenatal Diagnosis

Several approaches are used for prenatal testing: proteins in the mother's serum (triple screen, quad screen, penta screen; see Section 2.3 in Chapter 31), ultrasound examination of the fetus, and analysis of DNA from the fetus.

About 1% to 2% of fetuses are **aneuploid**, and about another 3% to 4% have a **microdeletion** or **microduplication**. The major aneuploidies include trisomy 13 (**Patau** syndrome), trisomy 18 (**Edwards** syndrome), trisomy 21 (**Down** syndrome), **Turner** syndrome (only 1 X chromosome), and **Klinefelter** syndrome (XXY). Fetuses with most other aneuploidies are not viable. The major microdeletion syndromes are a microdeletion in the long arm of chromosome 7 causing **Williams** syndrome, a microdeletion or imprinting error of a region in the long arm of chromosome 15 near the centrosome causing either **Prader-Willi** or **Angelman** syndrome, and a microdeletion in the long arm of chromosome 22, near the centrosome (causing **DiGeorge** syndrome in its most severe manifestation).

DNA made by the fetus can be obtained by withdrawing **amniotic fluid** (**amniocentesis**), taking a biopsy of **chorionic villi** (**chorionic villus sampling**), or using a sample of the mother's **blood**. The invasive procedures of amniotic fluid sampling and chorionic villus sampling carry up to ~1% risk of pregnancy loss. Taking a blood sample of a pregnant woman for analyzing cell-free DNA carries no such risk, but the analysis of this DNA is far less sensitive and more complicated.

Fetal cells obtained from amniotic fluid or chorionic villus sampling can be cultured, arrested in metaphase, stained, and analyzed by **G-banding** (see Section 1). G-banding readily identifies aneuploidies but not microdeletions. **FISH** probes can detect the most common aneuploidies, and they are also used to find or confirm microdeletions and microduplications. A combination of **aCGH** and **SNP DNA microarray** of fetal DNA uncovers the same aneuploidies and unbalanced chromosome alterations as G-banding, but it cannot detect balanced translocations or triploidy (see also Section 4). However, this combined microarray technology reveals uniparental disomy (see Section 4.2 in Chapter 2), and it uncovers small chromosome changes that are below the level of resolution of G-banding. A sizable fraction of these small alterations are currently of unknown clinical significance.

Fragments of **fetal DNA** less than 200 bp in length circulate briefly in the pregnant mother's blood. These fetal DNA fragments are also referred to as **fetal cell-free DNA**. The DNA originates from the placenta. The peak size of fetal cell-free DNA is approximately 140 bp and that of maternal cell-free DNA is approximately 160 bp. The maternal DNA pieces correspond to the DNA in a nucleosome plus a linker, while the fetal DNA lacks the linker sequence (it must have been clipped). At 10 to 20 weeks of gestation, the serum of the mother contains approximately 10 times more DNA from the mother than from her fetus. After delivery, the concentration of fetal DNA in the mother's plasma drops rapidly because the half-life of fetal DNA is only about 15 minutes.

By using serum from the pregnant mother, there are various ways of determining abnormalities of fetal DNA in the sea of maternal DNA. In one approach, all DNA from the mother's blood is sequenced by **massive parallel sequencing**. The DNA fragments are then assembled into whole chromosomes with computer-based algorithms. If the fetus has a trisomy (e.g., trisomy 21, which gives rise to Down syndrome and occurs in approximately 1 in 750 pregnancies), a greater number of chromosomes 21 is apparent relative to the other chromosomes. Massive parallel sequencing is often limited to the clinically most relevant chromosomes. Other approaches include sequencing of the father's genome.

Sequencing of the cell-free DNA in the plasma of the mother is currently best established for detecting **aneuploidies**.

One or more of the aforementioned techniques are often used to determine the complement of **sex chromosomes** of the fetus. This is of special importance in families who are affected by X-linked disorders (e.g., Lesch-Nyhan syndrome; see Section 2.4 in Chapter 38) or by congenital adrenal hyperplasia (see Section 4.2 in Chapter 31).

Cell-free DNA can also readily be used to test for **rhesus D** positivity in the fetus in a rhesus D–negative mother. The condition requires treating the mother with anti-rhesus D immunoglobulin.

## 6.2. Other Common Nucleic Acid–Based Tests

To guide **cancer** treatment, some companies offer a combination of bioinformatics and **massive parallel sequencing** of known genetic alterations in tumor cells. Examples of such tests are FoundationOne, FoundationOne Heme, and Caris Molecular Intelligence.

**Massive parallel sequencing** of select DNA segments is also available for **hereditary diseases** that can be caused by a mutation in one of multiple genes, such as hereditary breast cancer (Section 4.2 in Chapter 2), Lynch syndrome (a form of hereditary colon cancer; see Section 2 in Chapter 2), or neonatal diabetes (see Sections 1 and 3 in Chapter 39).

The diagnosis of many **infectious agents** relies on **real-time PCR**. DNA- or RNA-based identification of infectious agents is much faster than tests that involve culture. Furthermore, not all infectious agents can be cultured. A short turn-around time is especially important in patients who are in critical care and have life-threatening infections. Rapid molecular testing for pathogens can be performed in 1 to 2 hours. Viral load testing is important in monitoring the effectiveness of human immunodeficiency virus, hepatitis C virus, and other viral infections. In the practice of gynecology, there are commonly used molecular tests for RNA from *Chlamydia trachomatis*, *Neisseria gonorrhoeae*, and *Trichomonas vaginalis*, as well as DNA from herpes simplex virus. Detection of DNA or mRNA from human papillomavirus plays an important role in determining which patients are at an increased risk of cancer of the cervix.

Leukemias and lymphomas are increasingly classified by their genetic alterations to guide diagnosis and treatment. For instance, chronic myelogenous leukemia and some forms of acute lymphoid leukemia are caused by a reciprocal translocation between chromosome 9 and chromosome 22, leading to the synthesis of a pathogenic BCR-ABL1 fusion protein. Therapy is available that blocks the kinase activity of the fusion protein. After initiating treatment, the amount of BCR-ABL1 mRNA is determined with **RT-PCR** (see Section 2) every few months to monitor the effectiveness of the treatment.

## SUMMARY

- Traditional cytogenetic testing requires sterile cells that grow in vitro. Cytogenetic testing can detect all alterations in chromosome number, as well as deletions, duplications, inversions, and translocations that are larger than approximately 5 million bp.
- Fluorescence in situ hybridization (FISH) is ideal for detecting deletions and amplifications of DNA segments of more than approximately 150,000 bp, such as *HER2* gene amplification in breast cancer. FISH is also used for rapid identification of translocations and inversions.
- In the polymerase chain reaction (PCR), the forward and reverse primers determine the 5′ end and the 3′ end of the amplicon. With every temperature cycle, DNA melts, primers anneal, and the heat-stable DNA polymerase extends the primers. In quantitative PCR (qPCR), quantitative information is derived from the threshold cycle number relative to a calibration curve. In multiplex PCR, multiple forward and reverse primers exist. In reverse transcription (RT)-PCR, RNA is first reverse transcribed into DNA and then amplified by PCR.
- Capillary electrophoresis is used extensively in clinical tests to determine the size of DNA fragments.
- Melting curve analysis provides information on sequence mismatches compared with a chosen probe. Restriction enzyme digestion is another way to test for the presence of a pathogenic point mutation in an amplicon.
- Array comparative genomic hybridization (aCGH) and single nucleotide polymorphism (SNP) DNA microarrays printed with oligonucleotides can provide detailed information on aneuploidies, microdeletions, microduplications, and uniparental disomy but not about balanced translocations.
- Sanger sequencing is based on dideoxynucleotide-induced chain termination, followed by electrophoresis (usually capillary electrophoresis).
- Massive parallel sequencing depends on attaching DNA fragments of the genome to a solid support and then following the sequencing reaction on the surface of the support. The DNA sequence fragments are assembled by computer-based algorithms.
- Cells obtained from amniocentesis of chorionic villus sampling can be analyzed by G-banding, FISH, aCGH, DNA SNP microarray, or massive parallel sequencing.
- By massive parallel sequencing, short fetal DNA segments in a pregnant woman's blood can be discerned from the cell-free DNA of the mother and used to uncover an aneuploidy of the fetus, as well as determine the sex chromosome complement of the fetus.
- Massive parallel sequencing of selected DNA segments is available to characterize genetic alterations in tumors.
- Infectious agents are often quantified by molecular methods, sometimes after reverse transcribing RNA into cDNA.

## FURTHER READING

- Moorthie S, Mattocks CJ, Wright CF. Review of massively parallel DNA sequencing technologies. *Hugo J.* 2011;5: 1-12.
- Peters DG, Yatsenko SA, Surti U, Rajkovic A. Recent advances of genomic testing in perinatal medicine. *Semin Perinatol.* 2015;39:44-54.
- Szuhai K, Vermeer M. Microarray techniques to analyze copy-number alterations in genomic DNA: array comparative genomic hybridization and single-nucleotide polymorphism array. *J Invest Dermatol.* 2015;135:e37.
- Wong AI, Lo YM. Noninvasive fetal genomic, methylomic, and transcriptomic analyses using maternal plasma and clinical implications. *Trends Mol Med.* 2015;21: 98-108.

# Review Questions

1. DNA-based diagnosis of a known point mutation that causes iron overload is best accomplished with which one of the following techniques?

   A. aCGH
   B. FISH
   C. Karyotype by G-banding
   D. PCR, then melting curve analysis

2. A part of the sequence of a section of a double-stranded DNA segment is as follows (only one strand is shown): 5′-..**GCTAT**…**ACTAC**..-3′. Which one of the following sets of primers can be used to amplify the DNA sequence that is bounded by the nucleotides that are in bold? (Only the 5′ ends of the primers are shown.)

   A. 5′-AAGCT.., 5′-TCAGC..
   B. 5′-CGATA.., 5′-CATCA..
   C. 5′-GCGAA.., 5′-AGTTC..
   D. 5′-GCTAT.., 5′-GTAGT..
   E. 5′-GCTAT.., 5′-AGTCG..

3. A 20,000,000-bp balanced translocation from one chromosome to another is most readily detected with which one of the following techniques?

   A. aCGH
   B. Karyotype by G-banding
   C. Massive parallel sequencing
   D. PCR, then melting curve analysis

4. A 500,000-bp inversion in chromosome 7 is most easily detected with which one of the following techniques?

   A. aCGH
   B. FISH
   C. G-banding
   D. Massive parallel sequencing

5. Patients who are homozygous for a mutant aldolase B have hereditary fructose intolerance. Asymptomatic carrier parents requested genetic testing of their newborn daughter for this condition. A defined portion of the aldolase B gene in the DNA of the newborn and her parents was amplified with PCR. The product was exposed to the restriction enzyme *Aha*II, which cuts the amplified DNA of a common pathogenic allele into 185 bp and 125 bp fragments; *Aha*II does not cut the amplified DNA of the normal allele. The digest was subjected to electrophoresis, and DNA fragments of the following number of base pairs were found:

Father: 310, 185, and 125
Mother: 310, 185, and 125
Daughter: 185 and 125

These results show which of the following?

A. The amplicons should have been exposed to more AhaII and for a longer time.
B. The daughter has hereditary fructose intolerance.
C. Each parent has three copies of the aldolase B gene.
D. The PCR tubes with the parents' DNA were contaminated.

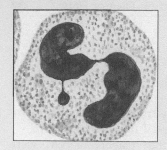

# Chapter 5

# Basic Genetics for Biochemistry

## SYNOPSIS

- This chapter explains some basic terms in genetics that are used throughout this book. It covers relevant and recurring essentials only and is not intended to provide an introduction to genetics.
- Normal nucleated human cells have 46 chromosomes, half of which are inherited from the mother and half from the father. In each parent, during meiosis, these chromosomes are newly assembled from existing chromosomes through a process of multiple crossing-over events.
- A person who is homozygous for a particular DNA sequence (e.g., a gene) has two exact copies of the sequence, while a person who is heterozygous has two different copies.
- X-linked diseases typically occur with greater frequency in males than in females. Early in female development, each cell randomly chooses one X chromosome for inactivation. Each cell then gives rise to daughter cells that maintain the inactivation of the same X chromosome. As a result, females are mosaics in terms of the X chromosomes they express.
- A small set of genes is imprinted in each oocyte and another small set in each sperm, such that these maternal and paternal copies of genes are not expressed in the offspring.
- An analysis of the association between disease and small sequence differences in known locations of the genome is often performed in the hope of elucidating the genetic basis of a disease.

## LEARNING OBJECTIVES

*For mastery of this topic, you should be able to do the following:*
- Describe the normal human karyotype and define the meaning of aneuploidy.
- Explain the terms allele, homozygosity, heterozygosity, and compound heterozygosity.
- Compare and contrast penetrance and variable expressivity.
- Compare and contrast dominant and recessive inheritance. Explain the meaning of the terms haploinsufficiency, gain-of-function mutation, loss-of-function mutation, and dominant negative effect, thereby relating these terms to dominant and recessive inheritance. Give an example for each of these terms.
- Compare and contrast the expected phenotypes of X-linked disorders in males and females.
- Compare and contrast Mendelian inheritance and non-Mendelian inheritance due to imprinting.
- Describe the pattern of inheritance of DNA in the mitochondria.
- Explain the terms germline and somatic cells.
- List common types of mutations.
- Describe the use of polymorphic markers in linkage analysis.

## 1. CHROMOSOMES AND ALLELES

*Except for the sex chromosomes, healthy humans have two copies of each chromosome. The mitochondria of a typical cell contain 1,000 or more copies of their own genome. A person who is homozygous for a piece of nuclear DNA has two identical copies of the piece, and a person who is heterozygous or compound heterozygous has two different copies.*

A normal nucleus in a human cell contains **46 chromosomes** (i.e., two copies each of **22 autosomes** and **two sex chromosomes**) (XX or XY; see Chapter 1). Half of these chromosomes stem from the mother and half from the father.

Since a typical, normal human cell has two copies of every chromosome (except possibly the sex chromosomes) it is said to be **diploid** (or 2n). By contrast, a normal egg and sperm are **haploid** (or 1n) (i.e., they have only 23 chromosomes [22 autosomes and 1 sex chromosome]). A cell that is **aneuploid** has more or less than 46 chromosomes.

The **karyotype** of cells is a description of the chromosome composition. The normal human karyotypes are 46,XX and 46,XY (number of chromosomes, followed by a description of the sex chromosomes). Fig. 1.12 shows an image of a normal karyotype.

**Aneuploidy** is typically pathogenic. Examples include Down syndrome (three copies of chromosome 21; karyotype: 47,XX,+21 or 47,XY,+21), Turner syndrome (45,X), and Klinefelter syndrome (47,XXY). Many tumor cells are aneuploid.

**Homologous chromosomes** have a similar architecture yet stem from different parents. For instance, chromosome 1 from the mother is homologous to chromosome 1 from the father.

Most human cells contain mitochondria, which have their own genome in the form of **mitochondrial DNA** (**mtDNA**; see Chapter 23). A typical cell contains 1,000 or more copies of mtDNA within its network of mitochondria (i.e., a "mitochondrion" has multiple copies of mtDNA). mtDNA is inherited exclusively from the mother. The inheritance of mtDNA and associated diseases is complex because mitochondria can contain mixtures of different mtDNAs that are passed on in a chance distribution (see Section 3 in Chapter 23).

Each chromosome contains many **genes**. A gene is often defined as a region of DNA that is transcribed into RNA. To the extent that we have two copies of every chromosome, we also have two copies of every gene; these two copies are referred to as **alleles**. We typically have one allele from the mother and one allele from the father.

A person who is **homozygous** has two similar copies of a gene; these can be two normal copies or two pathogenic copies. A person who is **heterozygous** has two different copies of the same gene, for example, one normal and one pathogenic copy. A person who is **compound heterozygous** has two different abnormal copies of the same gene. For example, a person who makes only a normal phenylalanine hydroxylase is homozygous for normal phenylalanine hydroxylase. A person who is a carrier for phenylketonuria has one normal and one abnormal allele for phenylalanine hydroxylase. A person who has two identical pathogenic mutant copies of the enzyme is homozygous for phenylalanine hydroxylase deficiency. A person who has two different mutant alleles for phenylalanine hydroxylase (of which there are many different mutants in the population) is compound heterozygous for a mutant phenylalanine hydroxylase.

Females have two X chromosomes, and males have one X and one Y chromosome. An XY male is **hemizygous** for all alleles on the X chromosome.

## 2. IMPRINTING AND PATTERNS OF INHERITANCE

*Traits encoded by chromosomes in the nucleus show dominant or recessive patterns of inheritance, whereby the type of inheritance depends on both the definition of the phenotype and the behavior of the relevant molecules. A small fraction of genes is expressed only when inherited from the mother or only from the father because of imprinting (DNA methylation). Traits encoded by mtDNA are inherited only via the mother.*

The **phenotype** describes the attributes of a person; this may include, for instance, physical characteristics, behavior, laboratory measurements, or the risk of neoplasms.

**Penetrance** refers to the frequency with which a particular disease-causing genotype leads to disease. Penetrance generally increases with age. Hemochromatosis (see Chapter 15), for example, has incomplete penetrance in that only a subset of persons who have an *HFE* gene with the C282Y mutation develops an iron overload (e.g., older men who abuse alcohol and are infected with hepatitis C virus show very high penetrance).

**Variable expressivity** refers to symptoms seen with a particular mutation. For instance, Marfan syndrome (see Chapter 13) is due to a mutation in fibrillin-1. Among family members who all have the same mutation, penetrance may be 100% (i.e., all clearly having Marfan syndrome), but there can be a large variation in phenotype. Some members, for instance, may have a normal chest while others have a sunken chest that needs to be corrected surgically.

In **autosomal dominant** inheritance, the phenotype is determined by the dominant allele. In osteogenesis imperfecta, one allele encodes a mutant type I collagen that impairs the assembly of type I collagens into fibrils (see Section 2.2 in Chapter 13). This allele is dominant (it causes disease on its own) and on an autosome. Hence, osteogenesis due to this particular allele is inherited in autosomal dominant fashion.

Autosomal dominant inheritance can be due to the following (examples are provided in Table 5.1):

- **Haploinsufficiency**: A single functional copy of a gene is not sufficient for normal function.
- **Gain-of-function mutation**: A protein acquires a new and pathogenic function (e.g., uncontrolled activity, aggregation, or the catalysis of a new reaction); it is also possible that extra copies of a gene are made and inserted into a chromosome (a process called gene duplication or gene amplification), or that a gene is transcribed at a greater rate.
- **Dominant negative effect**: An abnormal protein destroys the function of the normal protein. This is often seen in proteins that are active as dimers, trimers, tetramers, and so forth.

In **autosomal recessive** inheritance, the phenotype is present when there are two recessive alleles. This is commonly seen in deficiencies of enzymes that function as monomers.

**Table 5.1** **Examples of Mutation Types That Exhibit Autosomal Dominant Inheritance**

| Type of Mutation | Example 1 | Example 2 | Example 3 |
|---|---|---|---|
| Haploinsufficiency | Mutant glucokinase in maturity-onset diabetes of the young (MODY) type 2 (Chapter 39) | 16/heme, mutant porphobilinogen deaminase in acute intermittent porphyria (Chapter 14) | Mutant LDL receptor in heterozygous familial hypercholesterolemia (Chapter 29) |
| Gain of function | Mutant subunit of succinate dehydrogenase in hereditary pheochromocytoma and paraganglioma (Chapter 22) | Mutant fumarase in hereditary leiomyomatosis and renal cell cancer (Chapter 22) | Mutant PCSK9 in a type of congenital hypercholesterolemia (Chapter 29) |
| Dominant negative | Variant low-activity aldehyde dehydrogenase in East Asians that leads to flushing after the consumption of ethanol (Chapter 30) | Mutant type I collagen (which assembles into fibrils) in osteogenesis imperfecta (Chapter 12) | Mutant fibrillin-1 (which assembles into fibrils) in Marfan syndrome (Chapter 13) |

LDL, low-density lipoprotein.

Half the normal activity is often sufficient, but an activity of less than 10% of normal may be pathogenic. **Consanguinity** of parents frequently gives rise to an otherwise rare autosomal recessive disorder among offspring. In genetics, consanguinity refers to a close genetic relationship between two individuals. Two first-degree relatives (e.g., a parent and a child, or two siblings) have a coefficient of relationship of 0.5. Two second-degree relatives (e.g., a child and an aunt or grandmother) have a coefficient of relationship of 0.25. Two third-degree relatives (e.g., two first cousins) have a coefficient of relationship of 0.125.

Keep in mind that the type of inheritance (dominant or recessive) depends on both the definition of the phenotype or trait and the characteristics of the molecules that play a role in generating the phenotype. While a particular disease is inherited in a recessive fashion 99% of the time, 1% of all affected patients may carry a less common mutation in the same gene that shows dominant inheritance. Hence, there are always exceptions to statements such as "The disease shows autosomal recessive inheritance."

**Loss-of-function mutations** (**inactivating mutations**) are the norm in traits that show autosomal recessive inheritance.

In disorders that show **X-linked** inheritance, **males** are always affected. Female heterozygotes are clearly affected in **X-linked dominant** inheritance but may be unaffected in **X-linked recessive** inheritance.

As suggested in 1961 by Mary Lyon (the Lyon hypothesis), females **inactivate** all but one **X chromosome** per cell in the embryo in a patchwise fashion, a process referred to as **dosage compensation**. One cell inactivates the X chromosome from the father. A neighboring cell may inactivate the same X chromosome or the X chromosome from the mother in a process that is determined entirely by chance. These early cells give rise to progeny that maintain the same patterns of X inactivation. Hence, women are mosaics for X chromosome expression.

Statistically, it is most likely that a female expresses the maternal X chromosome in 50% of her cells and the paternal in the other 50%. It is least likely that a female expresses the X chromosomes from only one parent in all of her cells. Everything in between these two extremes is possible. If the inactivation is unequal, it is called **skewed X inactivation**. For this reason, an X-linked recessive disorder can produce very different phenotypes in heterozygous women.

Examples of X-linked disorders are glucose 6-phosphate dehydrogenase deficiency (see Chapter 21), ornithine carbamoyltransferase deficiency (see Chapter 35), and Lesch-Nyhan disease (see Chapter 38).

X chromosome inactivation in females occurs through DNA methylation. The inactivated X chromosome is condensed throughout the cell cycle and may be visible in the nucleus as the **Barr body** (Fig. 5.1).

A person is a genetic **mosaic** if some cells have a recognizably different genome from other cells. Mosaicism is typically a result of mutations that take place during development. Mosaicism can affect the germline or the somatic cells.

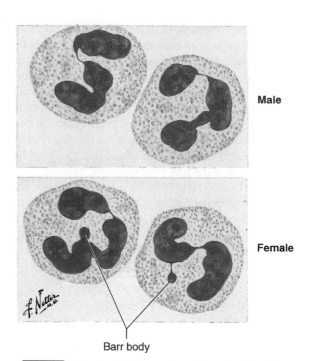

Barr body

**Fig. 5.1**  **Barr body in neutrophils of a female.**

The term **Mendelian inheritance** refers to inheritance patterns that are dominant or recessive, X linked or autosome linked, whereby it does not matter whether an allele is derived from the mother or father.

About 100 genes encoded on chromosomes in the nucleus show **non-Mendelian inheritance** due to **imprinting**. Imprinting disables the expression of small regions of chromosomes via the **methylation** of certain CpG dinucleotides. Maternally imprinted genes cannot be expressed in the mother's offspring, but that offspring can pass on these genes to the next generation. The same applies to paternally imprinted genes.

Existing imprinting is erased after fertilization in the cells that give rise to primordial germ cells, and it is reestablished later such that all oocytes have one customary set of genes imprinted, and all sperm have another customary set imprinted. For instance, the daughter of two parents cannot express the maternally imprinted genes; she will therefore express only the homologous paternal alleles. The reverse is true for paternally imprinted genes. This daughter's oocytes will imprint a predetermined set of genes; half of the alleles for these genes stem from her mother and half from her father.

## 3. MUTATIONS AND MARKERS

*Mutations are often classified by their effect on transcription and translation. Markers are known sequences in known locations of the genome. They are useful in linking a disease to a DNA location.*

The term **germline** refers to the cells in the gonads that give rise to the eggs and sperm. All other cells are called **somatic cells**. Germline mutations are heritable but somatic mutations are not. Most neoplasms occur in somatic cells.

A mutation is called a **de novo mutation** if it is seen in offspring but not in the peripheral blood or normal tissues of the parents. The mutation most likely occurred in the germline of a parent and is therefore heritable. It is also possible that only a part of a parent's germline carries the de novo mutation. Mutations in somatic cells occur frequently and may give rise to neoplasms; these mutations are simply called "mutations," not "de novo mutations."

Mutations are often subclassified into the following types:

- A **coding region** mutation occurs in a region of a gene that is transcribed and becomes part of mRNA that is translated into protein.
- A **frame-shift mutation** shifts the reading frame for codons.
- A **missense mutation** converts an amino acid codon to a different amino acid codon.
- A **nonsense mutation** converts an amino acid codon to a stop codon.
- A **promoter mutation may** alter the binding of transcription factors and thereby alter the amount of mRNA that is synthesized.
- A **silent substitution (synonymous substitution)** does not change the amino acid sequence of the encoded protein because the genetic code is degenerate (see Chapter 7).
- A **splice site mutation** may affect splicing efficiency and hence, alter the amount of normally spliced mRNA that is produced. In addition, abnormally spliced mRNA is usually degraded by nonsense-mediated decay.
- A **3′ end-processing mutation** may affect the efficiency of mRNA 3′ end processing and thereby alter the amount of mRNA that is produced.

**Trinucleotide repeats** are repeats of the same sequence of three nucleotides (e.g., CAG). Some trinucleotide repeats are unstable, expand, and give rise to disease once they are too long.

A **polymorphism** usually refers to a sequence variation that is less common but still occurs with some frequency (e.g., in more than ~1% of all persons).

A **single-nucleotide polymorphism (SNP)** is a polymorphism that affects only a single nucleotide.

**Polymorphic markers** are DNA sequences at known locations that show some sequence variation in the population. Notably, they allow a geneticist to determine whether a person inherited a particular sequence from the mother or the father and whether the sequence is associated with a disorder.

**Linkage analysis** refers to linking a DNA region to a phenotype. Linkage analysis is based on knowledge of marker sequences throughout the human genome and also on the fact that two DNA sequences that are close to each other on a chromosome are more likely to be inherited together than two DNA sequences that are far apart on a chromosome or even on different chromosomes. Crossing over during meiosis is the reason that two DNA sequences that are far apart on a chromosome are not necessarily inherited together.

Many diseases show **genetic heterogeneity** because a certain phenotype can be the result of a mutation in one of several different genes. Often, these genes play a role in the same pathway of metabolism or signaling pathway.

## SUMMARY

- 46,XX and 46,XY are the normal human karyotypes. Aneuploidy is an abnormal complement of chromosomes. It occurs, for instance, in Turner syndrome (45,X), Klinefelter syndrome (47,XXY), and Down syndrome (47,XY,+21).
- A compound heterozygous individual typically has two different disease-causing alleles.
- Penetrance refers to the frequency with which a pathogenic genotype gives rise to a defined phenotype. Variable expressivity refers to interindividual variability in the phenotype of the same pathogenic genotype.
- Haploinsufficiency indicates that a single normal copy of a gene is insufficient to maintain a normal phenotype. A gain-of-function mutation gives rise to a new or increased activity of a protein. A dominant-negative effect is often caused by a mutant molecule forming dimers and multimers with normal molecules that greatly impair the function of the resulting complex.
- Maternal and paternal imprinting of a small set of genes, which takes place in developing oocytes and sperm, leads to non-Mendelian inheritance.
- Linkage analysis uses polymorphic markers to elucidate a link between DNA and disease.

# Review Question

1. Within a family, individuals who have the same telomeropathy-causing mutation present with different abnormal phenotypes. The diversity of phenotypes is best referred to as which of the following?

   A. Dominant-negative effect
   B. Gain-of-function mutation
   C. Haploinsufficiency
   D. Incomplete penetrance
   E. Variable expressivity

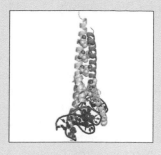

## Chapter 6

# Transcription and RNA Processing

## SYNOPSIS

- Transcription is the process of synthesizing an RNA based on a DNA template.
- DNA can be packaged into nucleosomes and compacted further into heterochromatin so that it is inaccessible to the transcription machinery.
- Upstream of a gene is a promoter region that contains binding sites for DNA-binding regulatory proteins called transcription factors. The availability of these transcription factors depends on development, cell type, and various environmental cues.
- Transcription also requires general transcription factors and RNA polymerase.
- During transcription, a protein complex recognizes the 5′-end of the RNA and adds a methyl guanosine cap, while another complex recognizes a polyadenylation site further downstream on the growing RNA chain, cleaves the RNA, and adds a poly(A) tail.
- Spliceosomes remove large segments (introns) from pre-mRNA and connect the remaining sequences (exons).
- Alternate transcription start sites, alternative polyadenylation sites, alternative splicing, alternative translation start sites, and alternate posttranslational protein modifications each contribute to protein diversity that far exceeds the diversity of genes.

## LEARNING OBJECTIVES

*For mastery of this topic, you should be able to do the following:*

- Describe the effect of chromatin structure on transcription, taking into account DNA methylation, histone methylation, and histone acetylation.
- Explain the meaning of the terms CpG dinucleotide and CpG island.
- Describe the basis of epigenetic inheritance.
- Describe the relationships of coding strands, noncoding strands, and template strands to each other and to an entire chromosome.
- Compare and contrast promoter elements, enhancers, activators, repressors, and silencers.
- Outline the assembly of a transcription initiation complex, paying special attention to steps that can be regulated by metabolites or hormones (particularly steroids).
- Interpret a graph of the structure of a promoter and a gene.
- Describe the modifications of precursor mRNA (pre-mRNA) at the 5′- and at the 3′-end and explain the purpose of these modifications.
- Describe the splicing of pre-mRNA and provide an example of alternative splicing.
- Compare and contrast exons and introns and relate these to a gene, as well as the final product of translation.
- Explain how a point mutation can alter splicing and hence the amino acid sequence of a protein.
- Explain the term *cryptic splice site* and provide an example.

## 1. DNA METHYLATION AND PACKING IMPEDE TRANSCRIPTION

*Methylation of DNA and histones generally leads to packing of methylated DNA into heterochromatin, which is not transcribed. The pattern of DNA methylation can be passed from cell to cell in a process called epigenetic inheritance. This is a normal part of development and cell differentiation. Methylation is abnormal in many neoplasms and also in most cases of Rett syndrome, which is associated with impaired development of the nervous system. Acetylation generally has the opposite effect of methylation in that it makes chromatin available for transcription.*

The term transcription refers to the synthesis of an RNA based on a DNA template.

Transcription is controlled at several levels: the compaction of DNA into nontranscribable heterochromatin, the formation of nucleosomes, the methylation of promoter regions, and the availability and activity of factors that are part of the transcription machinery.

In cells, DNA together with **histones** and other proteins forms **chromatin**. Light microscopy and electron microscopy reveal two forms of chromatin: **euchromatin** and **heterochromatin** (Fig. 6.1). Cells typically have more euchromatin than heterochromatin. Heterochromatin is somewhat concentrated near the periphery of the nucleus, and it is more densely packed than euchromatin. The physical structure of heterochromatin is not known, but it likely involves packing nucleosomes into a 30-nm chromatin fiber that is then folded into an even more compact form (see Fig. 1.6 and Section 4 in Chapter 1).

The nucleus is surrounded by an **inner** and an **outer membrane** that contains nuclear **pores**. The two membranes represent a layer of endoplasmic reticulum that envelops the nucleus. The membranes are stabilized by the **nuclear lamina**, which contains lamins, a type of protein that forms so-called intermediate filaments. Other proteins bind heterochromatin to the nuclear lamina.

Genes in **euchromatin** can be transcribed but those in **heterochromatin** cannot. In heterochromatin, nucleosomes are compacted into higher-order structures that prevent the access of proteins that are needed for transcription. DNA in euchromatin is also packaged in nucleosomes, but various mechanisms exist for modifying and moving nucleosomes to enable transcription.

Heterochromatin forms in a tissue-specific manner. During development and differentiation, perhaps one-third of the genome moves from euchromatin to heterochromatin or vice versa. Other parts of the genome, such as telomeres,

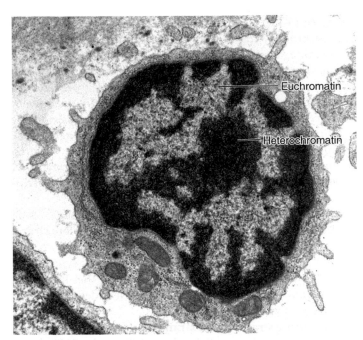

**Fig. 6.1** **Euchromatin and heterochromatin in the nucleus of a lymphocyte as seen by transmission electron microscopy.** The nucleus fills almost the entire lymphocyte.

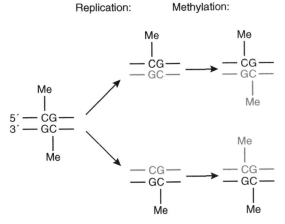

**Fig. 6.2** **Maintenance of CpG methylation, an epigenetic modification.** Methylation occurs only where a CpG on the complementary strand is already methylated. Me, methyl group.

centromeres, the long arm of the Y chromosome, and large segments of chromosomes 1, 9, and 16, are always condensed into heterochromatin. Since the DNA in these regions is not transcribed, even large DNA insertions and deletions have no known effect on a person's phenotype. Indeed, cytogenetics reports often mention an unusual size of one of these heterochromatic regions as being a normal polymorphism.

**Methylation** of cytosine bases by a **DNA methyltransferase** favors the incorporation of DNA into heterochromatin. DNA methylation occurs principally on the C of a 5′-CG-3′ sequence (often called a CpG dinucleotide, where p refers to the phosphate that forms a phosphodiester; see Fig. 1.2). For every 5′-CG on one DNA strand, a 5′-CG exists on the complementary DNA strand (Fig. 6.2). The Cs on both strands are typically methylated.

**CpG islands** are segments of DNA that contain a relatively high fraction of CG dinucleotides. Methylcytosine is mutagenic because occasional spontaneous deamination gives rise to thymine. Fittingly, the genome contains fewer CG dinucleotides than would be expected on the basis of statistics. By contrast, CpG islands contain almost the expected fraction of CG dinucleotides. Although ~70% of CG dinucleotides are methylated in the entire genome, CGs in CpG islands are mostly unmethylated. A typical CpG island is ~1000 bp long.

The pattern of CG methylation differs between cell types, and it can also change over time.

Methylation of C on DNA is passed on during cell division and thus gives rise to **epigenetic inheritance** (see Fig. 6.2). A cell therefore inherits not only the DNA of the parent cell (genetic inheritance) but also the pattern of chromatin packaging of the parent cell (epigenetic inheritance). Epigenetic events play a role, for instance in imprinting, development, cell differentiation, and X-inactivation in females (see Chapter 5). During DNA replication, a **DNA methyltransferase** methylates C of a CpG dinucleotide, but only if the C on the complementary strand is already methylated. In this way, methylated sequences remain methylated, and unmethylated sequences remain unmethylated. DNA methyltransferases use **S-adenosyl methionine** (see Fig. 36.6 and Section 4 in Chapter 36) as a methyl group donor.

The formation of blood cells (see Fig. 16.3 and Section 1.2 in Chapter 16) provides an example of epigenetic inheritance. Hematopoietic stem cells in the bone marrow give rise to red blood cells and various types of white blood cells. Each of these developing cell types possesses a different pattern of chromatin condensation. Erythroblasts (precursors to red blood cells) package the genes for immunoglobulins into heterochromatin, whereas white blood cells package the hemoglobin genes into heterochromatin.

A deficiency of the **methyl CpG-binding protein 2 (MECP2)** causes **Rett syndrome**, a progressive neurologic disorder that is the most common cause of a low IQ in females. MECP2 is widely expressed but especially abundant in mature neurons. The function of MECP2 is poorly understood. It binds to methylated Cs and nucleosomes, competes with a histone, bends DNA, and represses or activates transcription. Rett syndrome is inherited in X-linked dominant fashion and has a prevalence of ~1 in 12,000 births. In males, the disease is often lethal in utero. Females who have Rett syndrome start to regress at age 1 to 4 years.

In many **neoplasms**, CpG islands are methylated, which leads to suppression of transcription of the associated genes, typically **tumor suppressors** (see Chapter 8).

Compaction of DNA into heterochromatin is largely driven by the state of some of the **histone modifications** listed in Table 1.1. The packing of DNA and histones into nucleosomes is described in Fig. 1.6 and Section 4 in Chapter 1. Histone modifications (e.g., methylation and acetylation) occur on the tails of histones, which protrude from the nucleosomes. Compaction of nucleosomes into 30 nm fibers and then further into heterochromatin starts largely at the sites of repetitive or highly methylated DNA sequences, spreads, and is stopped by certain DNA elements and RNAs.

Methylated DNA can attract **histone methyltransferases** that methylate histones, and methylated histones can attract proteins that contain a **chromodomain** (chromatin organization modifier domain) and favor the formation of heterochromatin. Histone methyltransferases (like DNA methyltransferases) use S-adenosyl methionine (see Fig. 36.6 and Section 4 in Chapter 36) as a methyl group donor. Histone methyltransferases can methylate histone H3 at lysine residue 9 (shorthand H3K9). Proteins that contain a chromo domain can bind to the methylated histone H3 (H3K9me). By contrast, increased methylation of lysine-4 of the same histone H3 (H3K4me) favors the formation of euchromatin.

**Lysine acetyltransferases** in the nucleus and cytosol can use acetyl-coenzyme A (acetyl-CoA) to add an acetyl group to the amino group of the side chain of a lysine residue. The **acetyl-CoA** for this reaction stems from citrate that has been exported from mitochondria into the cytosol as described in Fig. 27.3 and Section 2 in Chapter 27.

Acetylation of histone lysine side chains leads to a more relaxed structure of chromatin. Lysine acetylation is read by proteins that contain an acetyl-lysine reader domain, such as a **bromodomain**.

**Histone deacetylases** (HDACs) can remove an acetyl group from a lysine side chain of a histone. Deacetylation of histones favors formation of heterochromatin. Humans produce 18 different HDACs.

Drugs in current use that are HDAC inhibitors include the following:

- **Vorinostat** and **romidepsin** are used in the treatment of cutaneous T-cell lymphoma, a disorder in which malignant T cells form tumors in the skin.
- **Belinostat** and romidepsin are used in the treatment of peripheral T-cell lymphoma, a disease in which malignant T cells are found in a variety of tissues, such as lymph nodes, liver, and bone marrow.
- **Panobinostat** is used together with bortezomib (a proteasome inhibitor) and dexamethasone (a glucocorticoid) in the treatment of multiple myeloma, a form of lymphoma caused by abnormal B cells.
- **Valproic acid** is used in patients who have seizures; some of its effects may be due to inhibition of HDACs.

Conjugation of lysine residue 120 of histone H2B with a single 76–amino acid protein **ubiquitin** by a ubiquitin ligase complex favors the transition from heterochromatin to euchromatin. Ubiquitin is a small protein and therefore much larger than a methyl or an acetyl group. Deubiquitinases remove ubiquitin from histones and thereby facilitate the incorporation of nucleosomes into heterochromatin.

## 2. THE PROCESS OF TRANSCRIPTION

*During transcription, one strand of the DNA is used as a template to synthesize an RNA. The RNA sequence is comple-mentary to the DNA template strand and identical to the coding strand, except that the RNA contains uracil in place of thymine. Upstream of a gene is a promoter region that contains multiple elements to which transcription factors bind. Formation of these protein-DNA complexes is essential to specific and regulated transcription of individual genes. The activity of some transcription factors depends on the binding of ligands, such as steroid hormones. Through the use of different promoter elements and transcription start sites, a single gene can give rise to several different proteins. A number of drugs in clinical use affect the activity of transcription factors.*

During transcription, RNA is synthesized in a $5' \rightarrow 3'$ direction based on the sequence of the DNA **template strand** (the DNA template strand is read in a $3' \rightarrow 5'$ direction). The $5' \rightarrow 3'$ synthesis of RNA resembles the $5' \rightarrow 3'$ synthesis of DNA during replication (see Fig. 3.4), except that RNA contains **ribonucleotides** (not deoxyribonucleotides) and **uracil** in place of thymine.

The **coding strand** (**sense strand**) has the same directionality and sequence (except T in place of U) as the RNA that is made from the template strand. The sequence of both the coding strand and the RNA is complementary to the sequence of the template strand. Sometimes, the template strand is called the **noncoding strand** or the **antisense strand**.

A **gene** is often defined as a segment of DNA that is transcribed into RNA.

By convention, the direction of a chromosome is from the end of the short arm toward the end of the long arm, and the direction of a gene is the direction of the coding strand ($5' \rightarrow 3'$; Fig. 6.3). A gene that has the same direction as the chromosome is said to be in **forward orientation**; if the directions are opposite, the gene is in **reverse orientation**. Each chromosome contains many genes that are in forward orientation and many that are in reverse orientation.

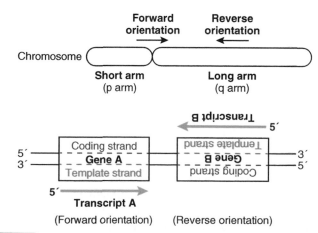

**Fig. 6.3 Genes in a chromosome can be oriented in two ways.** By convention, the orientation refers to the coding strand. The forward orientation is from the short-arm end of the chromosome toward the long-arm end of the chromosome. RNA is elongated at its 3′-hydroxyl group. The direction of transcription is the same as the direction of the green transcript arrow.

The genes on **mitochondrial DNA** (see Fig. 23.7) are likewise distributed between the two DNA strands (called heavy and light strand).

Transcription is often divided into initiation, elongation, and termination. Initiation refers to the highly regulated assembly of a complex of transcription factors and coactivators to which RNA polymerase then binds. Elongation refers to the synthesis of an RNA by RNA polymerase. Termination refers to the process that halts RNA polymerase and removes it from the DNA.

Upstream (5′) of a gene is a **promoter** region that consists of many **promoter elements (cis-acting regulatory elements**, Fig. 6.4), which affect the rate of transcription as detailed further in the chapter.

All **transcription factors** have a DNA-binding domain and bind to promoter elements, enhancers, or silencers (see below) on DNA. The promoter elements are often ~5 to 15 nucleotides long. Note that the term *transcription factor* excludes the general transcription factors (GTFs) introduced below.

Transcription factors are either transcription **activators** or transcription **repressors**; the binding of transcription factors to regulatory elements on DNA determines how often a gene is transcribed. Figs. 6.5 and 6.6 show examples of a part of a transcription factor bound to a segment of DNA.

Transcription factors bind to the periphery of a DNA double helix; that is, to the grooves in the helix (see Figs. 6.5 and 6.6); this most often involves both the coding strand and the template strand. The binding site of a transcription factor is usually only reported as the 5′ → 3′ sequence because the complementary sequence can easily be inferred.

Many transcription factors bind to DNA as homodimers or heterodimers and therefore contain a **dimerization domain**. A **leucine zipper** (see Fig. 6.6) is a common motif among some of these transcription factors. Apposition of leucine side chains generates a hydrophobic effect that holds the monomers together in a reversible fashion.

Some transcription factors contain a **ligand binding domain** (see Fig. 6.5). Among these transcription factors is the family of **nuclear hormone receptors**, which contains 48 members, including receptors for steroids, vitamin D, retinoic acid, and thyroid hormone, among many others.

The **steroid hormone receptors** encompass the receptors for glucocorticoids, mineralocorticoids, estrogen, progesterone, and dihydrotestosterone. The steroids are membrane permeable, and the steroid receptors that affect transcription are either in the cytosol or in the nucleus. A description of glucocorticoid receptors serves as an example of the complexity of steroid hormone receptor function.

In the absence of a glucocorticoid, **glucocorticoid receptors** reside mostly in the cytosol, where they are bound to a chaperone complex that includes heat shock protein 90 (HSP90; see also Section 4.1 in Chapter 7). When cortisol (the major glucocorticoid) binds to the glucocorticoid receptor, the receptor dissociates from HSP90 and moves to the nucleus thanks to its nuclear localization sequence. In the nucleus, the activated receptor can bind to a glucocorticoid response element (GRE). A typical GRE sequence is nGnACAnnnnGTnC (n = variable nucleotide). The GRE can be close to the promoter or far away from it (up to >100,000 nucleotides). The glucocorticoid receptor can directly bind to DNA and recruit coactivators and corepressors; alternatively, it can be tethered to DNA by binding to other transcription factors. There are also negative GREs (nGREs); when a GR binds to an nGRE, transcription is repressed. The nGREs have a different consensus sequence than the GREs.

Glucocorticoid action is complex and can vary from tissue to tissue as a result of receptor isoforms and epigenetic effects. Only one gene exists for the glucocorticoid receptor. **Alternative splicing** of RNA (see Section 3.4 and Fig. 6.14) yields

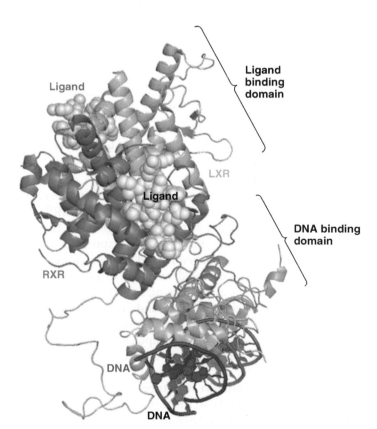

**Fig. 6.5 Structure of the liver X receptor–retinoid X receptor transcription factor bound to DNA.** The transcription factor binds to two AGGTCA sequences that are four nucleotides apart. The ligand binding domains bind oxysterols (e.g., 27-hydroxycholesterol) and retinoic acid, respectively (see Section 4.1 in Chapter 29). (Based on Protein Data Bank file 4NQA from Lou X, Toresson G, Benod C, et al. Structure of the retinoid X receptor α-liver X receptor β [RXRα-LXRβ] heterodimer on DNA. *Nat Struct Mol Biol.* 2014;21:277-281.)

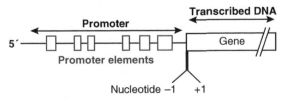

**Fig. 6.4 Promoter upstream of a gene.** By convention, the first nucleotide that is transcribed is +1, and the nucleotide 5′ to it is −1. All promoter elements are made up of nucleotides that carry negative numbers.

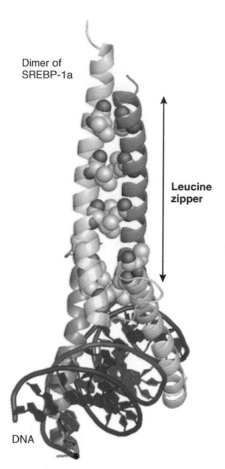

Dimer of
SREBP-1a

Leucine
zipper

DNA

**Fig. 6.6** **SREBP-1a as an example of a transcription factor that uses a leucine zipper to dimerize.** Leucine atoms are shown as spheres (O, red; N, blue; C, gray). (Based on Protein Data Bank file 1AM9 from Párraga A, Bellsolell L, Ferré-D'Amaré AR, Burley SK. Co-crystal structure of sterol regulatory element binding protein 1a at 2.3 A resolution. *Structure*. 1998;6:661-672.)

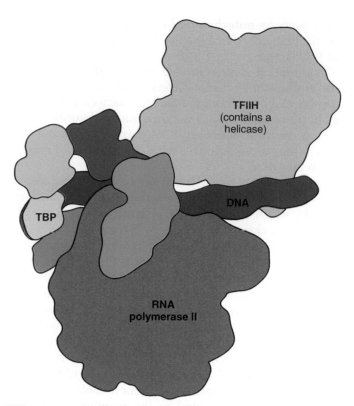

**Fig. 6.7** **Model of general transcription factors (GTFs) that are part of a preinitiation complex.** The complex contains GTFs and RNA polymerase II. Transcription factors and coactivators are not shown. (Data from Murakami K, Tsai KL, Kalisman N, Bushnell DA, Asturias FJ, Kornberg RD. Structure of an RNA polymerase II preinitiation complex. *Proc Natl Acad Sci U S A*. 2015;112:13543-13548.)

several isoforms. GRα is usually the predominant glucocorticoid receptor that responds to glucocorticoids. GRβ is an isoform that does not activate transcription and can therefore antagonize GRα. Indeed, the increased expression of GRβ observed in **asthma** and in **rheumatoid arthritis**, for example, is accompanied by a decreased response to glucocorticoids. Other GR isoforms can also antagonize GRα. Variations in the use of the **translation start site** and in **posttranslational modification** (e.g., phosphorylation and acetylation) can yield further isoforms (see also Chapter 7). Although a GRE is a prerequisite for the binding of GR, great variation is seen from cell to cell in the GREs that are available to bind GR due to a cell-specific **chromatin structure**.

Transcription depends on the formation of a **preinitiation complex** by transcription activators, transcription coactivators, GTFs (general transcription factors), and RNA polymerase in the promoter region of a gene (Fig. 6.7).

For transcription, transcription factors bind to **promoter elements (DNA response elements)**. Typically, a promoter contains many and diverse promoter elements (see Fig. 6.4).

Some transcription factors contain a **transactivation domain** through which they can bind **transcription coregu-**

lators. Transcription coregulators can either be **transcription coactivators** or **transcription corepressors**. Transcription coregulators bind to transcription factors but not to DNA. Some transcription coactivators facilitate formation of the preinitiation complex, others favor the binding of enzymes that modify histones and thus make DNA available for transcription, and yet other coactivators remove proteins from the DNA that would impede transcription.

The transcription of some genes is markedly enhanced when transcription factors bind to **enhancer sequences** in DNA. Enhancers can be part of the promoter, they can be thousands of nucleotides upstream or downstream of the promoter, and they can even be found inside genes. Enhancers increase transcription only when transcription activators are bound to promoter elements. Enhancers are equally active in both orientations relative to the transcription start site. For a transcription factor bound to an enhancer to increase the formation of a preinitiation complex, the DNA containing the enhancer may loop back. Chromatin is organized such that certain enhancers are physically close to their target promoter regions; this increases the specificity of transcription enhancement.

**Repressors** (proteins) bind to **silencer elements** on DNA and thus reduce the rate of transcription. Like enhancers, silencers may be in the promoter region, gene, or thousands of nucleotides from the promoter region, and they are equally active in both orientations relative to the transcription start site.

Transcription factors bound to promoter elements recruit **GTFs** (**TFII** proteins) that bind to the **core promoter**. In contrast to other transcription factors, the GTFs are used for the transcription of most genes. The core promoter is part of the promoter region and is close to the start site of the transcription. Some core promoters contain a **TATA box** (consensus sequence TATAAA) at about nucleotide −30; others contain an **initiator motif** at the transcription start site and a **downstream promoter element** (DPE) at about nucleotide +30 (i.e., downstream of the transcription start site). Transcription factors bound to DNA favor the binding of the GTF **TFIID** to the core promoter. The TFIID complex has a variable composition and contains **TATA-binding protein** (TBP), which binds to the TATA box. Subsequently, the GTFs TFIIA, TFIIB, TFIIC, TFIIE, TFIIF, TFIIG, and TFIIH bind to TFIID, thereby forming the **preinitiation complex**. TFIIB binds to the B recognition element (BRE) in the core promoter at approximately nucleotide −35 (immediately upstream of the TATA box, if there is one).

Once the initiation complex is assembled, the **helicase** of a GTF (see Fig. 6.7) unwinds the DNA helix so that a single strand can enter the active site of the **RNA polymerase**. RNA polymerase can then start transcribing the gene.

The **transcription start site** is determined by the location of promoter elements, including the TATA box (if present), by the local DNA conformation (a result of nucleotide composition), by the position of nucleosomes near the start site, and by the histone composition of nucleosomes (Table 6.1). The transcription start sites of some genes are limited to a single nucleotide, whereas those of others can extend over 30 to 100 nucleotides. Some genes contain a transcription start site that is in or near a particularly labile nucleosome (because of a special histone composition).

When alternate transcription start sites are used, multiple different RNA transcripts and proteins can be made from a single gene.

Eukaryotes contain three RNA polymerases. Under most circumstances, the activities of RNA polymerases I and III account for most of the transcription activity in a cell. We know most about transcription performed by RNA polymerase II.

RNA polymerase II transcripts encompass **messenger RNA** (**mRNA**), some of the **small nuclear RNAs** (**snRNAs**) that are used for splicing (see Section 3.3), and the **micro RNAs** (**miRNAs**) that can alter mRNA stability and translation (see Section 3 in Chapter 7). RNA polymerase uses the template DNA strand to synthesize a complementary RNA, inserting U in places where DNA polymerase would place T. The RNA itself is synthesized in a $5' \rightarrow 3'$ direction (like DNA synthesis). Consequently, the DNA template strand is read in a $3' \rightarrow 5'$ direction (like the DNA template strand during DNA replication). RNA polymerase II transcribes ~60 nucleotides per second.

The **3′ end of mRNAs** is not formed by termination of transcription but by **cleavage** of the RNA downstream of a polyadenylation signal. RNA polymerase II then terminates anywhere from a few to a few thousand base pairs downstream from the cleavage site via mechanisms that are still under investigation. As long as a preinitiation complex is present, RNA polymerase can start a new round of transcription.

Together, complexes of GTFs and **RNA polymerases I** and **III** accomplish transcription of genes that encode **ribosomal RNAs** (**rRNAs**; see Section 3 in Chapter 7), **transfer RNAs** (**tRNAs**; see Section 2 in Chapter 7), and some of the **snRNAs** that are part of the spliceosome (see Section 3.3). The abundance of these RNAs influences growth and cell replication.

**Mitochondria** contain a simpler transcription system compared with the nucleus. In its simplest form, the mitochondrial system requires **mitochondrial transcription factor A**, **mitochondrial transcription factor B2**, and **mitochondrial RNA polymerase**. The mitochondrial DNA encodes only two rRNAs, 22 tRNAs, and 13 proteins that play a role in oxidative phosphorylation (see Fig. 23.3 and Section 3 in Chapter 23). Hence, the entire transcription machinery is encoded in the nucleus, synthesized in the cytosol, and then imported into mitochondria. Mitochondrial DNA contains three promoters and generates various transcripts that give rise to multiple RNAs.

Some clinically used **drugs** and over-the-counter **supplements** influence transcription. **Glucocorticoids** are used widely for immunosuppression (see Section 3 in Chapter 31). In women, various **estrogens** and **progestins** are used for contraception, to treat infertility, and to reduce symptoms of menopause (see Section 2.4 in Chapter 31). **Fibrates** are used to reduce hypertriglyceridemia by activating peroxisome proliferator–activated receptor (PPAR)-α transcription factors (see Section 4 in Chapter 27 and Section 8.1 in Chapter 28). **Thiazolidinediones** are sometimes used to lower blood glucose by activating PPAR-γ transcription factors (see Section 5.3 in Chapter 39). **All-trans retinoic acid** is used in treating acne and acts at least in part by inducing activation of retinoic acid receptors and retinoid X receptors (RXR; see Section 7 in

**Table 6.1** **Characteristics of Transcription Start Sites**

| Transcription Start Site | Type of Transcription | Promoter Region | Nucleosomes |
|---|---|---|---|
| One specific nucleotide | Tissue-specific or highly regulated | Has TATA box | Positioning is flexible |
| ~30 to 100 nucleotides | Always transcribed (housekeeping) | Has CpG island (no TATA box) | Nucleosome-free DNA segment near the promoter and start site |

Chapter 28, Section 4.1 in Chapter 29, and Section 5 in Chapter 31). **Vitamin D**, which acts via heterodimeric transcription factors consisting of a vitamin D receptor and an RXR, regulates calcium and phosphate homeostasis (see Fig. 31.22 and Section 5 in Chapter 31).

# 3. PROCESSING OF RNA DURING AND AFTER TRANSCRIPTION

*During transcription, the 5′ end of the growing RNA chain is capped with methylguanosine triphosphate. In response to a polyadenylation signal, the 3′ end of the growing RNA chain is cut and a poly(A) tail is added. Alternate polyadenylation sites can influence mRNA stability and even protein sequence. The RNA contains long segments (introns) that are removed and shorter segments (exons) that are retained and spliced together during and after transcription. Most RNAs can be spliced in multiple alternate ways by including or excluding whole exons or parts of exons, thus giving rise to diverse proteins. Mature mRNA is exported from the nucleus into the cytosol.*

## 3.1. Capping of Pre-mRNA

During transcription, the 5′ end of the growing RNA chain is capped with 7-methyl guanosine triphosphate (Fig. 6.8). The methyl guanosine is added in "reverse" orientation, as it is joined to the RNA in a 5′ to 5′ fashion (not the usual 5′ to 3′). Furthermore, a triphosphate group is present between the 7-methyl guanosine and the 5′-end of the RNA. The cap structure is often abbreviated as $m^7GpppN$ (by analogy, the remainder of the RNA would be described as pNpNpN…).

For capping, a phosphate group is first removed from the triphosphate group at the 5′ end of the newly synthesized RNA, then guanosine monophosphate is attached, and then the guanine base is methylated at $N^7$. The enzymes that catalyze capping bind to RNA polymerase transiently. Capping is complete by the time the RNA polymerase has produced a ~30-nucleotide transcript.

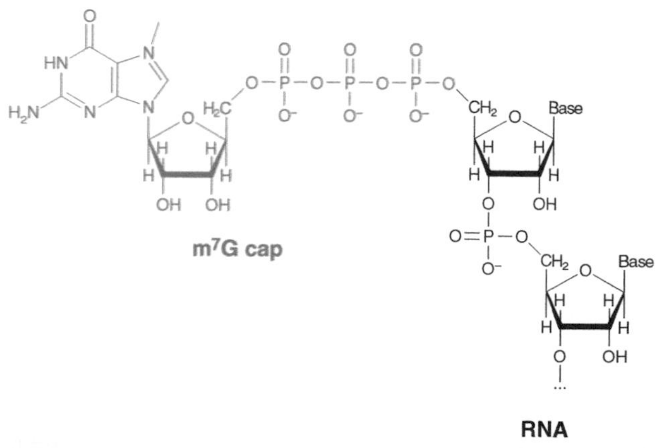

The cap is essential for the export of mRNA from the nucleus (see Section 3.5) and for translation (see Section 3 in Chapter 7).

## 3.2. Polyadenylation of Pre-mRNA

Most precursor mRNAs (pre-mRNAs) are polyadenylated; that is, their 3′-end is extended with a ~50- to 100-nucleotide **poly(A) tail**. During transcription, a large protein complex recognizes the sequence AAUAAA (or a similar sequence) on pre-mRNA as a **polyadenylation signal** and then cuts the pre-mRNA between the polyadenylation signal and a U- or GU-rich **downstream sequence element** (DSE). A poly(A) polymerase then generates a poly(A) tail without using a DNA template (Fig. 6.9). The actual site of polyadenylation is ~10 to 35 nucleotides downstream of the polyadenylation signal.

Polyadenylation stabilizes an mRNA against degradation, and it also favors export from the nucleus into the cytosol.

The use of alternate polyadenylation sites can alter mRNA stability (Fig. 6.10) and protein amino acid sequence (Fig. 6.11). Through the use of alternate polyadenylation signals, transcription of most genes gives rise to multiple pre-mRNAs. The choice of signal site used depends on the exact nucleotide sequence of the signal, other elements of the pre-mRNA, and proteins that bind to pre-mRNA.

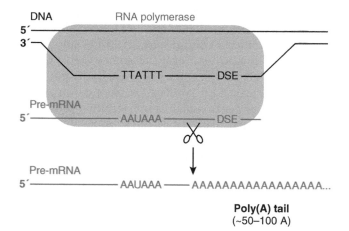

**Fig. 6.9** **Polyadenylation of RNA.** DSE, downstream sequence element.

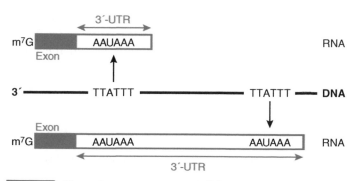

**Fig. 6.10** **Use of an upstream poly(A) site leads to termination of transcription and a shortened 3′-untranslated region (UTR).** The longer 3′-UTR may contain sequences that regulate mRNA half-life. Exons are explained in Section 1.3.

![Capping of RNA structure diagram with m7G cap and RNA]

**Fig. 6.8** **Capping of RNA with methylated guanosine triphosphate.**

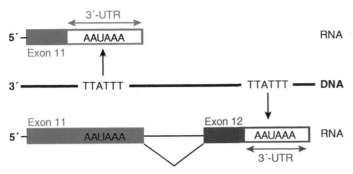

**Use of upstream poly(A) site leads to termination of transcription and a reduced number of exons, altering protein structure.** Filled boxes indicate protein-coding regions. A similar result is obtained if the upstream poly(A) site lies within an intron. Exons and introns are explained in Section 3.3.

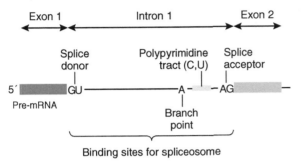

**Basic requirements for splicing of pre-mRNA.** The figure shows the 5′ part of a pre-mRNA.

## 3.3. Splicing of Pre-mRNA

Splicing is part of the processing of pre-mRNA that gives rise to mature mRNA. Spliceosomes remove **introns** and join the remaining **exons**. A typical human pre-mRNA contains approximately 25 exons of ~150 nucleotides each as well as 24 introns of ~2,000 nucleotides each (total length ~50,000 nucleotides).

Splicing of pre-mRNA starts during transcription. Some splicing proteins can bind to RNA polymerase, but much of the splicing takes place after the RNA polymerase has disengaged from the DNA.

Splicing is determined by the following elements of the pre-mRNA (Fig. 6.12): splice site donor (5′), splice site acceptor (3′), polypyrimidine tract upstream of the splice acceptor, splicing branch point, splicing enhancers, and splicing silencers.

The consensus **splice donor** sequence is **GU**, and the consensus **splice acceptor** sequence is **AG**. Nucleotides flanking these sequences affect the choice of splice site.

The core spliceosome, which performs almost all RNA splicing, consists of a dynamic complex that, over the course of splicing, involves five **snRNAs** and more than 300 proteins. Since the snRNAs of the spliceosome catalyze the actual splicing, the spliceosome (like the ribosome) is a **ribozyme**.

In addition to splice donors, splice acceptors, and spliceosomes, splicing is directed by sequences called exonic and intronic **splicing enhancers**, as well as exonic and intronic **splicing silencers**, respectively. SR proteins recognize and bind to splicing enhancers and favor splicing. Conversely, hnRNPs (RNA-protein complexes) bind to splicing silencers and block splicing.

Exons are spliced together only in the sequence in which they occur in pre-mRNA, though it is possible to skip one or more exons. During splicing, the ends of exons are always bound to the spliceosome; that is, they are never free.

During splicing, a multiprotein **exon junction complex (EJC)** is deposited on the spliced mRNA upstream of each splice junction. EJCs are required for the export of mRNA from the nucleus. In the cytosol, EJCs are removed during the first round of translation, but if a stop codon is close to an EJC, the mRNA enters nonsense-mediated RNA decay (see Section 3 in Chapter 7).

Acquired mutations in splicing factors (proteins) occur especially frequently in **myelodysplastic syndrome (MDS)**. MDS is characterized by impaired production of blood cells and an increased risk of development of acute leukemia.

**Mutations** of splice donor or splice acceptor sites can abolish correct splicing and may also induce splicing at **cryptic splice sites**, which are splice sites that are normally not used. Furthermore, a mutation may create a new splice site.

Mutations frequently cause only a partial shift in splicing, thereby generating two or more mRNAs. An example of a partial shift to use a new splice acceptor site is a form of **β-thalassemia** that originated in the Mediterranean basin (see Fig. 17.3).

## 3.4. Alternative Splicing of Pre-mRNA

Most RNAs that contain two or more exons undergo alternative splicing, which greatly increases the diversity of proteins that can be synthesized. Through alternative splicing, parts of a protein can be exchanged, added, or deleted.

Four essential types of alternative splicing are available: use of an alternative 5′ splice site, use of an alternative 3′ splice site, cassette exon inclusion/skipping, and intron retention (Fig. 6.13).

The splicing of the RNA transcript from the gene for glucocorticoid receptors is an example of the use of an alternative splice acceptor (Fig. 6.14). In this case, alternative splicing leads to receptors that do or do not bind to a glucocorticoid.

In summary, a gene is a segment of DNA that is transcribed into RNA, and after transcription, introns are removed from the RNA, while exons are retained (Fig. 6.15). As explained in Chapter 7, an mRNA is translated into protein, but the 5′ end, 3′ end, and poly(A) tail are not translated. The untranslated ends are called the **5′-untranslated region (5′-UTR)** and the **3′-untranslated region (3′-UTR)**.

A single gene can give rise to diverse proteins thanks to alternative transcription start sites and polyadenylation sites, alternative splicing (see Sections 2 and 3), translation initiation, and posttranslational modifications (see Sections 3 and 4 in Chapter 7).

**Alternative splice donor:**

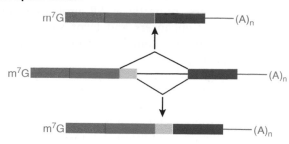

**Alternative splice acceptor:**

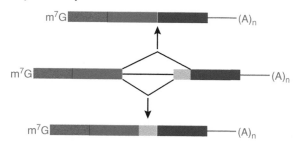

**Exon inclusion or skipping (cassette exon):**

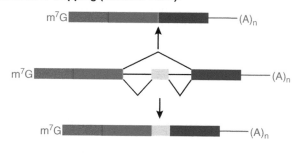

**Intron splicing or retention:**

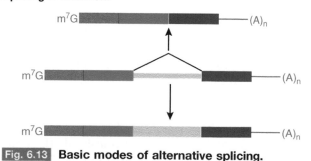

**Fig. 6.13** Basic modes of alternative splicing.

## 3.5. Export of mRNA Into the Cytosol

**Messenger ribonucleoprotein particles** (complexes of mRNA and proteins) are exported from the nucleus through **nuclear pore complexes** (NPCs), which dot a layer of endoplasmic

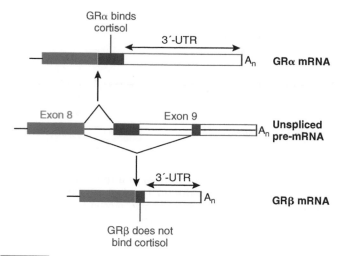

**Fig. 6.14** **Alternative splicing of glucocorticoid receptor pre-mRNA.** Filled boxes indicate translated sequences. Exon 9 encodes the glucocorticoid binding domain. Exons 1–7 are not shown. (There is an additional form of GRα mRNA with a shorter 3′-untranslated region due to use of an upstream alternative polyadenylation site that is not shown.)

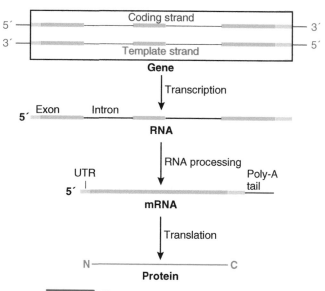

**Fig. 6.15** From gene to RNA to protein.

reticulum around the nucleus (Fig. 6.16). For export through the NPCs, RNA **export factors** need to be bound to the complex of mRNA and its associated proteins (e.g., the cap-binding complex, poly(A)-binding protein, and EJCs).

## 3.6. Degradation of mRNA

The quality of pre-mRNA and mRNA is controlled extensively. RNAs that do not meet requirements are degraded, and there is ongoing turnover of all mRNAs. In the cytosol, the 5′ cap and 3′ poly(A) tail, bound to proteins, allow mRNA to survive. mRNA is degraded first by shortening of the poly(A) tail by deadenylases, producing adenosine monophosphate. The resulting RNA can then be degraded in a 3′→5′ direction by the **exosome**, a large protein complex, until only the m7GpppN

*Nucleus*

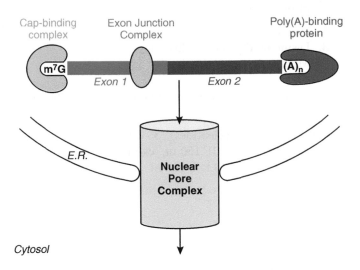

**Export of messenger ribonucleoprotein particle (mRNP) complexes from the nucleus.** Additional proteins are needed to shepherd the mRNP complex through the nuclear pore complex.

cap remains, which is degraded by a dedicated enzyme. Alternatively, after the removal of the poly(A) tail, the RNA can be degraded first by 5′ **decapping** and then by a **5′→3′ exonuclease** (Xrn1). Both pathways of RNA degradation are under the control of many proteins that activate or inhibit.

## SUMMARY

- DNA in heterochromatin is tightly packed and is not transcribed. DNA in euchromatin can be transcribed.
- Methylation of DNA on C's of CpGs, recognition of methylated CpGs, and methylation of histones favor the formation of heterochromatin. DNA methylation is the basis of epigenetic inheritance. CpGs are methylated as part of development, differentiation, and inactivation of X chromosomes when two or more X chromosomes are present. DNA segments that contain a relatively high fraction of CpGs are called CpG islands. Most CpG islands are unmethylated.
- In tumor cells, excessive DNA methylation is often responsible for decreased transcription of genes that encode tumor suppressors.
- Acetylation of histones, catalyzed by lysine acetyltransferases, makes DNA more amenable to transcription. A similar effect is achieved clinically with inhibitors of histone deacetylases (HDACs). Among these inhibitors, valproic acid is used to treat seizures, while vorinostat, romidepsin, belinostat, and panabinostat are used to treat certain forms of lymphoma.
- A gene is commonly defined as a segment of DNA that is transcribed. The template strand of DNA is transcribed in a 3′→5′ direction so that RNA is synthesized in a 5′→3′ direction. The resulting RNA has the same sequence as the coding strand, except for U in place of T.

- Neighboring genes can be oriented in opposite directions. Of the two complementary DNA strands that make up a chromosome, one DNA strand is the coding strand of only the genes that are oriented in one particular direction, while the other strand contains the coding strands for genes that are oriented in the opposite direction.
- Upstream of the gene is a promoter region that contains a core promoter. For transcription to take place, transcription factors need to bind to promoter elements in the promoter region, and general transcription factors (GTFs) must bind to the core promoter. Some transcription factors are active only when bound to a ligand, such as a steroid. Once the initiation complex is assembled, RNA polymerase synthesizes RNA from the DNA template.
- Some drugs that are in clinical use, such as glucocorticoids, estrogens, progestins, fibrates, and retinoic acid, activate transcription factors.
- During transcription, transcribed RNA receives a 7-methylguanosine triphosphate cap and a 50- to 100-nucleotide poly(A) tail.
- Both during and after transcription, spliceosomes remove introns and link exons. The first exon contains the 5′-UTR and the last exon contains the 3′-UTR. Alternative splicing is due to the use of an alternate splice donor or acceptor, exon skipping, or intron retention. A cryptic splice site is a site that is not normally used for splicing but is used under special conditions, such as when a new mutation is present.
- Mature mRNA with cap, cap-binding complex, exon junction complexes (EJCs), poly(A) tail, and poly(A)-binding protein binds additional proteins and is then exported into the cytosol via the nuclear pore complex (NPC).

## FURTHER READING

- de Klerk E, 't Hoen PA. Alternative mRNA transcription, processing, and translation: insights from RNA sequencing. *Trends Genet.* 2015;31:128-139.
- Houseley J, Tollervey D. The many pathways of RNA degradation. *Cell.* 2009;136:763-776.
- Matera AG, Wang Z. A day in the life of the spliceosome. *Nat Rev Mol Cell Biol.* 2014;15:108-121.
- Meijsing SH. Mechanisms of glucocorticoid-regulated gene transcription. *Adv Exp Med Biol.* 2015;872:59-81.
- Wickramasinghe VO, Laskey RA. Control of mammalian gene expression by selective mRNA export. *Nat Rev Mol Cell Biol.* 2015;16:431-442.

# Review Questions

1. For a particular protein, the template strand contains the sequence 5′-ACCGT. After transcription into RNA, the RNA contains which one of the following sequences?

   **A.** 5′-ACCGU
   **B.** 5′-ACGGU
   **C.** 5′-UGCCA
   **D.** 5′-UGGCA

2. A couple had a son who had β-thalassemia (i.e., the child made only a small amount of β-globin). The couple sought genetic counseling. The father was found to have one normal and one mutant β-globin allele. The mutant allele contained an A→G mutation at position −30 of the β-globin promoter. The A nucleotide is most likely in which of the following?

   A. Downstream promoter element
   B. Enhancer
   C. Initiator motif
   D. Nuclear receptor
   E. TATA box

3. Rett syndrome in a 4-year-old girl is caused by a hereditary deficiency in which one of the following processes?

   A. DNA methyltransferase
   B. Histone acetyltransferase
   C. Histone methyltransferase
   D. Methyl CpG-binding protein

4. Most nuclear receptors bind to which of the following?

   A. Both the template and the coding strand
   B. Coding strand only
   C. Template strand only

5. Which one of the following processes generally favors transcription of a gene?

   A. Lysine acetylation of histones
   B. Lysine methylation of histones
   C. Methylation of CpG islands

6. Given the following data, what is the length of the mature mRNA?

   5′-UTR: 20 nt (nucleotides), 3′-UTR: 50 nt without the poly(A) tail, exon 1: 150 nt, exon 2: 150 nt, intron 1: 2000 nt, and poly(A) tail: 100 nt

   A. 231 nt
   B. 331 nt
   C. 401 nt
   D. 471 nt
   E. 2301 nt
   F. 2401 nt

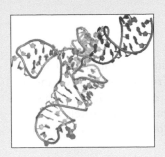

# Chapter 7

# Translation and Posttranslational Protein Processing

## SYNOPSIS

- As detailed in Chapter 6, the nucleotide sequence of DNA gives rise to an mRNA of essentially complementary sequence.
- In translation, ribosomes synthesize proteins according to the rules of the genetic code and the genetic information contained in mRNA. The mRNA sequence is read in units of three nucleotides, called codons. Each codon specifies either a particular amino acid or a signal to terminate the synthesis of the protein.
- Aminoacyl-tRNA synthetases charge each tRNA with an appropriate amino acid, thus generating aminoacyl-tRNAs.
- Ribosomes scan mRNA for a start codon to initiate protein synthesis. At each codon, the translating ribosome matches the codon sequence with a specific aminoacyl-tRNA and catalyzes peptide bond formation.
- In humans, if a newly synthesized peptide contains a signal sequence, ribosomes dock to the endoplasmic reticulum (ER) and feed the growing peptide chain into the ER through a peptide channel. As soon as certain asparagine side chains reach the lumen of the ER, they are glycosylated. Glycosylation can influence protein folding and later also protein sorting. Bacteria do not have an ER.
- Proteins fold mostly in the ER. Chaperones detect misfolded proteins, refold them, or direct them to degradation.
- Proteins travel from the ER in vesicles to the Golgi. In the Golgi, proteins can be extensively modified and are further sorted for transport inside vesicles to specific parts of the cell.
- Many commonly used antibiotics selectively impair translation in bacteria.

## LEARNING OBJECTIVES

*For mastery of this topic, you should be able to do the following:*
- Describe the factors that determine the start, continuation, and end of translation.
- Explain why some DNA mutations in the coding sequence do not result in a mutant protein.
- Explain why a one-base or two-base insertion or deletion is usually a loss-of-function mutation and why no mutant protein accumulates in the tissue.
- List factors that set the gross rate of protein synthesis.
- List antibiotics that interfere with protein synthesis and describe their mechanism of action.
- Describe the synthesis of membrane proteins.
- Describe the factors that influence sorting of newly synthesized proteins and their transport to different subcellular compartments.
- Describe common posttranslational modifications.
- Discuss how cells control the quality of newly synthesized proteins and degrade these proteins if needed.

## 1. CODONS AND THE GENETIC CODE

*The amino acid sequence of a protein is encoded in messenger RNA (mRNA) in the form of a sequence of codons. Each codon consists of three nucleotides and encodes one amino acid or a signal to stop translation. The genetic code describes the correlation between codons and amino acids; it allows one to predict the effects of some mutations on the amino acid sequence of a protein.*

**Translation** is the process of synthesizing proteins in ribosomes according to the nucleotide sequence of mRNA.

There are 20 different amino acids that are incorporated into proteins, and their sequence is encoded in mRNA as **codons** that consist of three nucleotides. Since there are four different bases, 3-nucleotide codons can have a total of $4^3 = 64$ different sequences, enough to encode 20 amino acids (2-nucleotide codons would offer only $4^2 = 16$ options).

The **genetic code** is a list of codon sequences and the corresponding amino acids that are used in translation (Table 7.1). The AUG codon codes for Met and signals the **start** of translation. The codons UAA, UAG, and UGA are **stop codons** (**nonsense codons**, **termination codons**) and usually end translation.

Since all possible codon sequences are used, multiple different codons may code for the same amino acid; that is, the genetic code is **degenerate**.

The **coding strand** of DNA has the same sequence as the mRNA that is generated from the template strand, except that it contains T in place of U. Both the coding strand and the mRNA are complementary to the template strand (see Section 2 in Chapter 6).

**Silent mutations** (**synonymous substitutions**) are mutations that do not lead to a change in amino acid sequence because the genetic code is degenerate. However, silent mutations can affect mRNA splicing or mRNA stability and may therefore be pathogenic.

**Nonsense mutations** are mutations that lead to the formation of a stop codon. Only a small amount of the altered protein may be produced because the premature stop codon causes destruction of the mRNA by **nonsense-mediated mRNA decay** (see Section 3).

**Missense mutations** are mutations that lead to the substitution of an amino acid with another amino acid. Substitutions of amino acids with very different properties (nonconservative substitutions; e.g., substitution of a hydrophobic amino acid with a charged amino acid) have more severe effects than substitutions of amino acids with similar properties (conservative substitutions).

**Table 7.1**  **Genetic Code for Information Stored in Chromosomes**

| First Base | Second Base | | | | Third Base |
|---|---|---|---|---|---|
| | U | C | A | G | |
| U | Phe | Ser | Tyr | Cys | U |
| U | Phe | Ser | Tyr | Cys | C |
| U | Leu | Ser | Stop | Stop | A |
| U | Leu | Ser | Stop | Trp | G |
| C | Leu | Pro | His | Arg | U |
| C | Leu | Pro | His | Arg | C |
| C | Leu | Pro | Gln | Arg | A |
| C | Leu | Pro | Gln | Arg | G |
| A | Ile | Thr | Asn | Ser | U |
| A | Ile | Thr | Asn | Ser | C |
| A | Ile | Thr | Lys | Arg | A |
| A | Met | Thr | Lys | Arg | G |
| G | Val | Ala | Asp | Gly | U |
| G | Val | Ala | Asp | Gly | C |
| G | Val | Ala | Glu | Gly | A |
| G | Val | Ala | Glu | Gly | G |

To decode the coding strand of DNA, replace U with T. The genetic code for mitochondria differs in that AGA and AGG are additional stop codons, UGA codes for Trp, and both AUU and AUA code for Met.

Since each codon contains three nucleotides, there are theoretically three different **reading frames** for mRNA. The actual reading frame is usually determined by the first occurrence of the nucleotide sequence AUG (encoding Met) in a particular sequence context (see Section 3). The alternate reading frames usually contain relatively frequent stop codons (statistically, ~1:20 random codons is a stop codon). Since the physiologically used reading frame has fewer stop codons than the other two reading frames, it is sometimes called the **open reading frame**.

**Frame-shift mutations** are nucleotide insertions or deletions that are not divisible by 3 and thus change the reading frame for part of the mRNA. Because the alternate reading frames have frequent stop codons, a frameshift mutation generally leads to protein truncation and to degradation of the mRNA by **nonsense-mediated mRNA decay** (see Section 3).

With the exception of **mitochondria**, which have their own translation machinery and employ a modified form of the genetic code (see Table 7.1), all organisms use the same genetic code (i.e., the code is universal). Hence, genetically modified

bacteria, for instance, can be used in a straightforward manner to manufacture human proteins (**recombinant proteins**) for use as biologicals (e.g., insulin, erythropoietin). However, posttranslational processing of eukaryotic proteins in prokaryotes may be incomplete or incorrect and may thus require further manipulation.

## 2. TRANSFER RNAs

*In preparation for protein synthesis, aminoacyl-tRNA (transfer RNA) synthetases charge their cognate tRNAs with the cognate amino acids to form aminoacyl-tRNAs. Each tRNA contains an anticodon that will read the corresponding codon of an mRNA. The anticodon of each tRNA must match the first two nucleotides of a codon according to the common (Watson-Crick) base pairing rule; however, there is flexibility in matching the third nucleotide because of wobble base pairing.*

**tRNAs** are bifunctional molecules that read selected codons and carry a matching amino acid. While there are 20 different amino acids that are incorporated into proteins and 61 codons that code for these amino acids, there are more than 500 different tRNAs.

tRNAs consist of ~80 nucleotides, and they all fold into an L-shaped tertiary structure (Fig. 7.1). The sequence of each tRNA is encoded in chromosomes and in mitochondrial DNA (see Fig. 23.8). Each tRNA is synthesized by transcription of a gene and then processed. The 3′ end of all tRNAs is extended with the sequence CCA-3′. Nucleotides of tRNAs are extensively modified, most often by methylation. A few adenosines can be edited by deamination to give rise to inosines. In the L-shaped tRNA, one end contains three nucleotides that are complementary to the three nucleotides in the codon; this region is called the **anticodon**.

Each tRNA anticodon can often read multiple different codons due to **wobble base pairing**. An anticodon has to match the first two nucleotides of each mRNA codon according to Watson-Crick base-pairing rules (A-U, C-G), but there is flexibility with the third nucleotide. The third nucleotide of a codon can be A, C, or U and still bind sufficiently well to inosine (I, an edited A; see above) in the anticodon; furthermore, G and U can form a wobble base pair. As an example of wobble base pairing, the anticodon of the glycine-tRNA has the sequence 5′-ICC, which can pair with three codons: GGA, GGC, and GGU.

tRNAs are named for the amino acid they are charged with and the codons that are assigned to this amino acid. For instance, tRNA$^{Cys}$ is charged with cysteine and recognizes the cysteine codons. The initiator tRNA$_i^{Met}$ is used selectively for the initiation of protein synthesis, and the elongator tRNA$^{Met}$ is used during chain elongation. Although there are usually multiple tRNAs that code for the same amino acid, these tRNAs are not further distinguished in this book.

**Aminoacyl-tRNA synthetases** use ATP to couple the CCA-3′ end of a tRNA to the appropriate amino acid. For each amino acid, there is one aminoacyl-tRNA synthetase. The

The 3′ end contains 4 more
nucleotides (not shown),
and the amino acid is added
to the last nucleotide

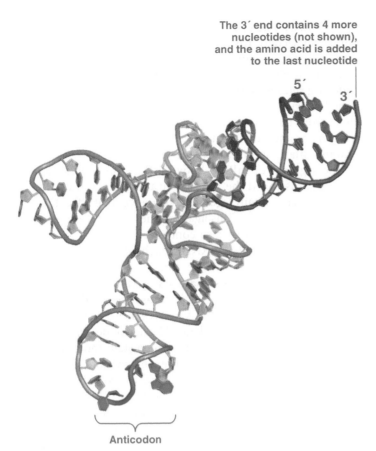

**Anticodon**

**Fig. 7.1** **Structure of human tRNA^Sec.** (Based on Protein Data Bank file 3A3A from Itoh Y, Chiba S, Sekine SI, Yokoyama S. Crystal structure of human selenocysteine tRNA. *Nucleic Acids Res.* 2009; 37:6259-6268.)

aminoacyl-tRNA synthetases recognize tRNAs in varied ways but mostly via the nucleotide sequence in the amino acid acceptor stem (colored red in Fig. 7.1) and in the anticodon region.

For some amino acids, such as Leu, multiple tRNAs are needed to read all Leu codons. In such circumstances, the aminoacyl-tRNA synthetase (in this case, leucyl-tRNA synthetase) accepts multiple tRNAs^Leu as substrates. These isoacceptor tRNAs differ in nucleotides in the anticodon and in other regions of the L-shaped structure.

The aminoacyl-tRNA synthetases for leucine, isoleucine, valine, threonine, alanine, and phenylalanine contain an **editing** (**proofreading**) function. These synthetases can acylate their tRNA with the wrong amino acid. To compensate, these enzymes use a second catalytic site to remove incorrect amino acids.

**Selenocysteine** (see Fig. 9.2), an amino acid contained in a few proteins, is synthesized on tRNA^Sec (Sec = selenocysteine). First, seryl-tRNA synthetase aminoacylates tRNA^Sec with serine. An enzyme then phosphorylates the serine. A second enzyme exchanges the phosphate for a selenol (–SeH) group to yield selenocysteinyl-tRNA^Sec. tRNA^Sec is unique in that it carries the anticodon 5′-UCA-3′, which is complementary to the UGA stop codon. Selenocysteine is encoded in mRNA via

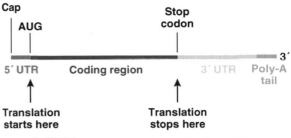

**Fig. 7.2** **Structure of a typical mRNA.**

a combination of a UGA stop codon and a downstream selenocysteine insertion sequence (SECIS).

The antibiotic **pseudomonic acid** (**mupirocin**) inhibits protein synthesis by inhibiting isoleucyl-tRNA synthetase in bacteria. It is often used to treat methicillin-resistant *Staphylococcus aureus*.

## 3. RIBOSOMES TRANSLATE mRNA INTO PROTEIN

*Ribosomes are large RNA-protein complexes that bind the mRNA, read the mRNA, accept tRNAs that match the codons of the mRNA, and catalyze peptide bond formation between amino acids attached to tRNAs. The first amino acid of a protein is usually methionine; however, it is typically removed soon after translation. Proteins that contain a signal sequence are transferred into the ER during synthesis. Nonsense-mediated RNA decay ensures that mRNAs that contain premature stop codons are not translated. Micro RNAs interfere with translation. Protein synthesis increases after a mixed meal and decreases during times of stress, viral infection, or nutrient deprivation. Several antibiotics used in clinical practice block translation in bacteria but not appreciably in humans.*

The production of mRNA, its 5′ cap structure, and its poly-A tail are described in Sections 2 and 3 in Chapter 6. The features of mRNA that are important to translation are shown in Fig. 7.2.

Each human ribosome is made up of four **ribosomal RNA**s (**rRNA**s) and ~80 proteins. The largest rRNA is a **ribozyme** that catalyzes peptide bond formation. A ribosome consists of a small subunit and a large subunit.

In the cytosol, a complex of translation **initiation factors**, Met-tRNA$_i^{Met}$ (methionine initiator tRNA acylated with methionine), and the small subunit of a ribosome binds to the **5′ cap** of an mRNA, checks for a poly-A **tail**, scans the mRNA from the 5′-cap, finds the **start codon** (almost always **AUG**), and starts translation. This AUG is often flanked by ACC on the 5′ side and by G on the 3′ side. If the flanking nucleotides of the AUG do not match sufficiently well, translation starts at a suitable AUG that is further away from the cap. **Insulin** and other **growth factors** increase protein synthesis in part by leading to increased binding of an initiation factor to the 5′ cap of mRNA.

The sequence between the 5′ cap and the start codon of the mRNA is called the **5′ untranslated region** (**5′ UTR**; see

Fig. 7.2). Occasionally, the 5′ UTR contains a regulatory element, such as an iron response element (see Section 3 in Chapter 15).

Once the start codon has been found, the large ribosome subunit binds to the mRNA. An **elongation factor** (eIF5A) brings an aminoacylated **tRNA** to the codon that follows the start codon. If the codon and anticodon match, guanosine triphosphate (GTP) is hydrolyzed and the aminoacylated tRNA undergoes a conformational change called accommodation. This change in structure moves the amino acid on the tRNA into the peptidyl transferase catalytic site of the ribosome and aligns it with the Met on the initiator tRNA. A new peptide bond forms via a nucleophilic attack of the amino group of the incoming amino acid on the carbonyl group of methionine on the initiator tRNA (Fig. 7.3). The new peptide bond forms such that Met is now linked to the amino acid on the newly added tRNA.

Next, a different **elongation factor** (EF-G) binds to the ribosome, GTP is hydrolyzed, and the ribosome moves on the mRNA by one codon in the 5′→3′ direction. The tRNA that now carries a dipeptide also moves in the ribosome. A new matching aminoacylated tRNA binds to the ribosome, and the deacylated ("empty") initiator tRNA leaves the ribosome. Repetition of the aforementioned processes leads to further elongation of the peptide chain according to the coding information

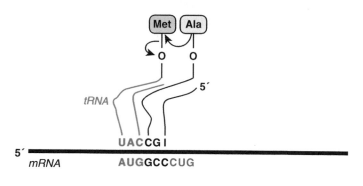

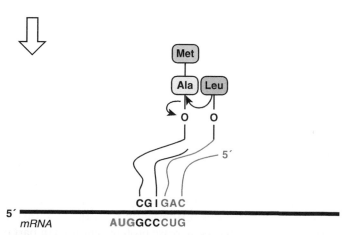

**Fig. 7.3** **Peptide synthesis in ribosomes.** The hydroxyl group at the 3′ end of the incoming tRNA is esterified with the carboxyl group of its cognate amino acid. The free amino group of this amino acid mounts a nucleophilic attack on the carboxyl group of the preceding amino acid of the growing peptide chain.

in the mRNA. Each ribosome forms about one to two peptide bonds per second. **Insulin** favors protein synthesis in part by increasing the activity of the elongation factor.

Once the ribosome encounters a **stop** codon (**termination** codon), a **release factor** (a protein) recognizes the stop codon. Together with another release factor, it releases the peptide chain from the ribosome. With the help of a ribosome recycling factor and other proteins, the ribosome then dissociates into the small subunit and the large subunit.

The segment of mRNA between the stop codon and the poly-A tail is called the **3′ UTR**. Just like the 5′ UTR, the 3′ UTR also may contain regulatory sequences that affect the rate of mRNA translation. This again applies to iron response elements. The 3′ UTR may also contain a sequence that leads to rapid degradation of the mRNA, which allows cells to express certain proteins for only a brief time.

mRNAs that contain **premature stop** (termination) codons may be degraded by the classic **nonsense-mediated decay** (**NMD**) pathway. When mRNA first reaches the cytosol, every exon-exon splice site is marked ~22 nucleotides upstream by exon junction complexes. If a ribosome stalls more than ~50 nucleotides upstream of an exon-exon junction, the mRNA enters NMD. In NMD, the 5′ cap and the 3′ poly-A tail are removed, and exonucleases degrade the mRNA from both ends. By contrast, if a ribosome moves smoothly along the mRNA without stalling, the exon junction complexes are removed, and the mRNA is now a bona fide template for translation. There are several other pathways that recognize abnormal mRNAs that are not discussed here. For the synthesis of many proteins, loss of abnormal mRNA, which may lead to haploinsufficiency, is the lesser evil compared to production of a truncated protein, which may have a dominant-negative effect (see Chapter 5). It is estimated that despite the degradation of mRNAs with premature stop codons, ~10% of all heritable diseases are caused by nonsense mutations.

Two different **methionine aminopeptidases** remove the N-terminal **Met** from most nascent proteins as they emerge from the ribosome (i.e., before the proteins fold). For these aminopeptidases to cleave the Met residue, the second amino acid of the nascent protein must not be bulky. Proteins start folding into secondary structures during translation. α-Helices are small enough to start forming in the exit tunnel of ribosomes. However, proteins can acquire a tertiary structure (see Chapter 9) only after leaving the ribosomes.

A single mRNA often contains many ribosomes that travel on it. Furthermore, the 5′ cap and the 3′ poly-A tail of an mRNA are held together by initiation factors. This facilitates recognition of the two mRNA ends and reassembly of ribosomes on the mRNA.

**Micro RNAs (miRNAs)** are RNAs that are ~22 nucleotides long, favor degradation of mRNA, and inhibit translation. miRNAs bind to complementary segments of mRNA. Humans produce more than 1000 different miRNAs. Each miRNA can bind to several different mRNAs, in part because a miRNA does not have to match exactly the sequence of the mRNA. About half of all mRNAs are subject to regulation by a miRNA.

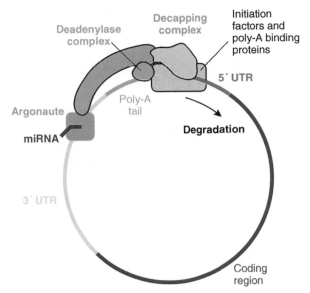

**Fig. 7.4** **miRNA-induced degradation of mRNA.**

miRNAs combine with the protein **Argonaute** to form the core of a **miRNA-induced silencing complex** miRISC (Fig. 7.4). miRNAs reduce protein synthesis mainly by favoring degradation of mRNA. miRNA and Argonaute first bind to the 3′ UTR of an mRNA and then recruit a scaffold protein, which in turn binds enzymes that remove the poly-A tail and the 5′ cap from the mRNA. Subsequently, a 5′ exonuclease in the cytosol degrades the decapped and deadenylated mRNA. Direct inhibition of translation might occur by interference with initiation factors.

Protein synthesis slows dramatically in response to conditions of **nutrient deprivation** (especially of amino acids and glucose), viral **infection**, and various forms of cellular **stress**. These conditions slow translation by lowering the concentration of aminoacyl-tRNAs available to ribosomes. The following three examples illustrate how this regulation works:

■ Cells that are starved for a single **amino acid** stop protein synthesis.

■ Red blood cell precursors that are actively synthesizing hemoglobin (see Chapter 16) devote almost all of their protein synthesis to the production of **globins**. If **heme** (the prosthetic group of globins) becomes scarce (e.g., due to iron deficiency), the rate of protein synthesis decreases and becomes limited by heme production.

■ Many **viruses** that infect human cells produce large quantities of double-stranded **RNA**. Most human cells contain a kinase that recognizes double-stranded RNA and inactivates an initiation factor for protein synthesis. Thus translation is shut down in a virus-infected cell. This prevents the synthesis of viral proteins. Type I **interferons**, which are proteins produced endogenously in response to virus infection or given as a drug, can stimulate the same double-stranded RNA-dependent kinase. Some viruses, including influenza, herpes simplex, and human immunodeficiency virus, have evolved mechanisms for antagonizing the kinase-directed shutdown of protein synthesis.

Some mRNAs contain **CUG** codons for **Leu,** which are used to initiate protein synthesis when translation initiation via AUG codons for Met is shut down due to stress or infection. This applies to mRNAs for major histocompatibility complex class I proteins, which present short peptides, including peptides of pathogens, to cytotoxic T-cells.

Proteins synthesized on ribosomes in the **cytosol** can be relocated to various subcellular compartments based on specific peptide sequences. For example, the presence of a **nuclear localization sequence** facilitates translocation of the protein into the nucleus; a **mitochondrial localization sequence** facilitates translocation of the protein into the mitochondria; and a **peroxisome-targeting sequence** sends the protein into peroxisomes.

The protein-transporting **translocase of the outer membrane** (TOM) and **translocase of the inner membrane** (TIM) complexes control the import of more than 1000 proteins into mitochondria across the outer and inner membrane. The electrochemical protein gradient of mitochondria (see Section 1.2 in Chapter 23) provides the energy for protein translocation.

About one-third of all proteins contain a **signal sequence** (leader sequence, preprosequence) and are therefore synthesized by transfer of the growing peptide chain into the **ER** (Fig. 7.5). This group encompasses proteins that end up in the plasma membrane, in the lysosomes, or in secretory vesicles. Examples include the following: G protein–coupled receptors in the plasma membrane (see Chapter 33), acid maltase in lysosomes (see Chapter 24), and insulin in secretory vesicles (see Chapter 26).

When a growing peptide chain emerges from the ribosome and contains a signal sequence, a **signal recognition particle** (**SRP**) binds to it (Fig. 7.6). The SRP consists of one RNA and six proteins. A part of the SRP reaches into the ribosome at the elongation factor binding site, pairs with rRNA, and temporarily halts translation. The SRP (with the ribosome bound to it) then binds to the **SRP receptor** on the surface of the ER. This facilitates binding of the ribosome to a channel (**translocon**) that allows the growing peptide chain to be transferred into the ER once translation resumes due to departure of the SRP.

Proteins that are synthesized via transfer of the growing peptide chain into the ER can be transferred entirely into the ER or partially inserted into the ER membrane. Proteins destined for secretion are entirely transferred into the ER, and the signal peptide is generally cleaved by **signal peptidase**. Because of the presence of internal start-transfer and stop-transfer sequences, multiple transmembrane sequences of a membrane protein can be inserted into the ER membrane. For example, G protein–coupled receptors cross the plasma membrane seven times (see Chapter 33). (In the ER membrane, the signal peptide is degraded by signal peptide peptidase.)

Ribosomes in **mitochondria** (**mitoribosomes**) differ appreciably from ribosomes in the cytosol (and also from those in bacteria). Mitoribosomes translate only the 13 mRNAs that are encoded by mitochondrial DNA (mtDNA; see Fig. 23.8). Mitoribosomes contain only two rRNAs (both encoded by mtDNA). Although all ~80 proteins of mitoribosomes are

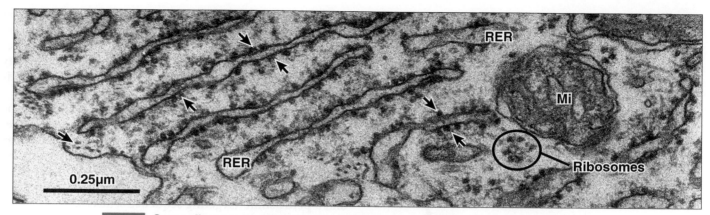

Fig. 7.5 **Some ribosomes attach to the endoplasmic reticulum.** Transmission electron microscopic view of part of a fibroblast. *Arrows* show ribosomes that are attached to the ER membrane. *Mi*, mitochondrion; *RER*, rough endoplasmic reticulum. The *circle* denotes free ribosomes. (Courtesy Dr. B.J. Crawford.)

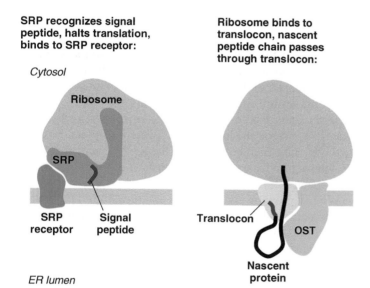

**SRP recognizes signal peptide, halts translation, binds to SRP receptor:**

*Cytosol*

Ribosome

SRP

SRP receptor    Signal peptide

*ER lumen*

**Ribosome binds to translocon, nascent peptide chain passes through translocon:**

Translocon    OST

Nascent protein

Fig. 7.6 **Transfer of a growing peptide chain into the endoplasmic reticulum.** *ER*, endoplasmic reticulum; *OST*, oligosaccharyltransferase; *SRP*, signal recognition particle, which adds a glycan (see Section 4.2).

dria), and the formyl group is then removed while the first methionine residue is left in place. The initiation factors, proteins in the ribosome, elongation factors, and release factors differ between prokaryotes and humans.

A number of important classes of **antibiotics** inhibit translation by bacteria but not by human cells:

- **Aminoglycosides**, such as **streptomycin**, **gentamycin**, **tobramycin**, and **amikacin**, interfere with the decoding of mRNA and the accommodation of incoming tRNA. As a result, erroneous amino acids are inserted, and elongation of the peptide chain is inhibited. Aminoglycosides have toxic side effects on tubule function in the kidneys and also on hearing and equilibrium.
- **Chloramphenicol** inhibits protein chain elongation by interfering with the peptidyl transferase activity of ribosomes.
- **Macrolides** such as **erythromycin**, **telithromycin**, **azithromycin**, and **clarithromycin** interfere with peptide synthesis by blocking the exit tunnel of the nascent peptide chain from the ribosome.

encoded in the nucleus, synthesized in the cytosol, and then imported into mitochondria, only about half of these proteins are the same as in ribosomes in the cytosol.

Mitoribosomes use a **genetic code** that differs somewhat from the one cytosolic ribosomes use (see Table 7.1). Mitochondrial mRNAs contain no 5′ cap and essentially no 5′ UTR. The start codon is AUG for 9 of the 13 proteins.

In mitochondria, membrane proteins can also be inserted into the inner membrane during translation. Few details are known about this process.

Translation of mRNA in **prokaryotes** differs from translation in the cytosol of humans in important ways. In prokaryotes, the small subunit of a ribosome binds to a conserved Shine-Dalgarno sequence, which is 5′ to the AUG start codon. The methionine on the initiation tRNA is formylated (a formyl group, –CHO, is added; this also occurs in human mitochon-

## 4. POSTTRANSLATIONAL MODIFICATION

*During and after synthesis, proteins fold and undergo processing. Protein folding is sometimes aided by chaperones. Proteins can be modified by proteolysis, by attachment of carbohydrates, lipids, or isoprenes, or by redox reactions. Misfolded or mutant proteins may be recognized and refolded or degraded. This quality control plays a major role in a variety of heritable diseases.*

### 4.1. General Comments

In the ER, as proteins fold, **protein disulfide isomerase** catalyzes the formation of **disulfide bonds** between cysteine residues.

**Peptidylprolyl isomerase** isomerizes cis and trans peptide bonds that involve **proline** (see Fig. 9.3).

**Chaperones** are proteins that help fold other proteins. They are found in the nucleus, cytosol, ER, mitochondria, cell surface, and extracellular space. Most chaperones are **heat shock proteins**, which were originally discovered as being expressed in increased amounts when cells are exposed to heat.

Most chaperones use ATP to facilitate folding and bind to misfolded proteins to prevent aggregation, as well as unfold and refold misfolded proteins. Chaperones often receive assistance from multiple cochaperones. Many tumors overexpress chaperones, thus favoring tumor progression and metastasis.

Chaperones recognize their targets by various means, including certain short peptide consensus sequences and surface hydrophobicity (hydrophobic residues are supposed to be buried; see Chapter 9).

Glycosylation (see below) can guide protein folding by preventing access to certain conformations.

## 4.2. Glycosylation

**N-linked glycosylation** occurs inside the ER on select asparagine residues of nascent proteins during translation. Oligosaccharyltransferase (**dolichyl-diphosphooligosaccharide-protein glycotransferase**) transfers a 14-residue preformed glycan to the nitrogen on the side chain of an **asparagine** in a consensus sequence (Fig. 7.7). The oligosacharyltransferase complex is bound to the translocon that transfers a nascent protein into the ER. For some proteins, the addition of a bulky, hydrophilic glycan influences protein folding.

The synthesis of the 14-residue glycan for N-linked glycosylation starts on the cytosolic side and ends on the luminal side of the ER (Fig. 7.8). On the outer surface of the ER, two N-acetyl glucosamine residues (activated by UDP) and five mannose residues (activated by GDP) are attached to dolichol phosphate. Dolichol is a lipid that stems from the same isoprene-producing pathway as farnesyl-PP, geranylgeranyl-PP, ubiquinone, and cholesterol (see Fig. 29.4). The resulting glycan is flipped to the luminal side of the ER membrane. There, four more mannose and three glucose residues (all activated by dolichol-P) are attached to generate the 14-residue glycan that contains three branches (all at mannose residues).

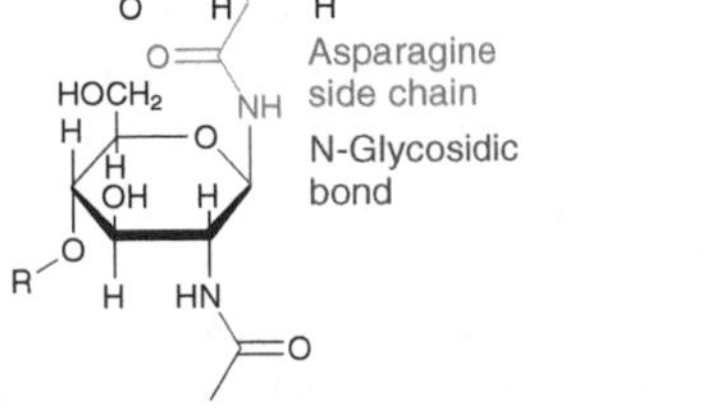

In the **Golgi**, protein-linked glycans are extensively modified by a combination of trimming of glucose and mannose residues; phosphorylation, sulfation, and acetylation of existing sugar residues; and addition of new sugar residues such as N-acetylglucosamine, galactose, fructose, and neuraminic acid. The trimming of residues depends on a proper protein conformation as sensed by chaperones.

One example of a secreted protein that must be glycosylated is **erythropoietin**, which stimulates red blood cell synthesis (see Chapter 16). For the production of **recombinant** human erythropoietin (**epoetin alfa**), mammalian cells are typically engineered to both produce human erythropoietin protein and glycosylate this protein so that a pharmacologically useful half-life can be attained. **Darbepoietin** is an engineered analog of erythropoietin that contains five instead of three N-linked glycans and has a threefold longer half-life than recombinant human erythropoietin when given intravenously.

Abnormal N-linked glycosylation is observed in certain **congenital disorders of glycosylation** (CDG). A CDG may be due to reduced glycosylation in the ER or abnormal

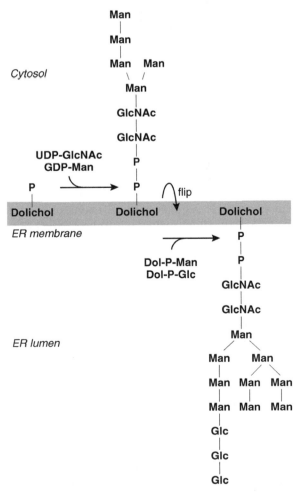

**Fig. 7.7** **N-glycosylation of the asparagine side chain of a protein.**

**Fig. 7.8** **Synthesis of a 14-residue glycan for N-linked glycosylation in the endoplasmic reticulum.** *Dol*, dolichol; *Glc*, glucose; *GlcNAc*, N-acetyl-glucosamine, *Man*, mannose; *P*, phosphate.

processing in the Golgi. CDGs cause a wide variety of clinical symptoms.

At a prevalence of ~1 in 20,000, **PMM2-CDG** (formerly **CDG-Ia**) is the most prevalent CDG. It is due to homozygosity or compound heterozygosity for a defective *PMM2* allele. The *PMM2* gene encodes **phosphomannomutase 2**, which catalyzes the following reaction:

$$\text{Mannose 6-phosphate} \leftrightarrow \text{mannose 1-phosphate}$$

Mannose 1-phosphate is normally activated with GDP and then added to the growing dolichol-PP-glycan toward the production of a 14-residue glycan in the lumen of the ER. Affected patients show a wide spectrum of disease and age of onset. The patients generally have some intellectual disability, impaired vision, peripheral neuropathy, and cerebellar ataxia that make it difficult for them to walk independently. Diagnosis is often based on finding abnormal glycosylation of transferrin by isoelectric focusing (transferrin is a protein that carries iron in blood; see Section 4 in Chapter 15). If positive, this test is followed with a measurement of the phosphomannomutase activity in leukocytes or fibroblasts.

The only CDG for which there is currently effective treatment is **MPI-CDG** (formerly **CDG-Ib**), which is treated with supplements of mannose. MPI-CDG is due to a deficiency of mannose 6-phosphate isomerase, which catalyzes the following reaction:

$$\text{Fructose 6-phosphate} \leftrightarrow \text{mannose 6-phosphate}$$

This reaction is a prerequisite for the synthesis of GDP-mannose.

The most commonly performed laboratory test for a type I CDG (which affects N-glycosylation) is a test of the glycosylation of **transferrin**.

Known CDGs are caused by mutations in more than 50 different genes, and sequences of all exons of thousands of persons (~20% of whom turned out to be carriers of a CDG) suggest that the overall prevalence of autosomal recessively inherited CDGs is perhaps ~1 in 1,000. This number implies that most affected patients are currently not diagnosed as having a CDG; because the field is young and some affected fetuses may not be viable, this seems possible.

**O-linked glycosylation** occurs in the Golgi apparatus on the –OH groups of **Ser** and **Thr** and starts with the addition of **N-acetyl-galactosamine** (**GalNAc**), which can be extended with N-acetyl-glucosamine, N-acetyl-neuraminic acid, or galactose, and subsequently with these and other sugars.

Proteoglycans and mucins are examples of proteins that undergo O-linked glycosylation. **Proteoglycans** are abundant in the extracellular matrix, where they absorb and distribute compressive forces, store growth factors, and bind to coagulation factors (see Section 2 in Chapter 13). **Mucins**, which are produced by many types of epithelial cells and are often secreted to give rise to mucus (e.g., in the digestive tract and in the airways), contain an abundance of Ser and Thr residues that can undergo O-linked glycosylation.

O-linked glycosylation is much less common than N-linked glycosylation, and the components of O-linked glycosylation have greater redundancy than the components of N-linked glycosylation. Accordingly, disorders of O-linked glycosylation are less common than disorders of N-linked glycosylation.

Disorders of O-linked glycosylation are typically tissue or organ specific. An example of such a disorder is **paroxysmal nocturnal hemoglobinuria** (see Section 1.5 in Chapter 11).

## 4.3. Acylation With Fatty Acids and Prenylation

The addition of a fatty acid to a protein can influence the association of the protein with a membrane or other protein and thus frequently plays a role in signaling. Fatty acylation of the –SH group of cysteine is reversible, whereas fatty acylation of the $-NH_3^+$ group of an N-terminal amino acid is irreversible.

A protein acylated with a single fatty acid has an increased affinity for membranes, but it resides in a membrane for only minutes. A second interaction in the form of an additional fatty acid, a prenyl group (see below), positively charged amino acids, or hydrophobic amino acids is generally needed to increase the residence time in membranes to a time scale of hours.

**Palmitoylation**, the addition of a 16-carbon fatty acid, occurs mostly on the –SH group of the side chain of cysteine, forming a thioester bond that can be cleaved again. Addition of palmitate by more than 20 different palmitoyltransferases occurs predominantly in the Golgi, whereas removal of palmitate by acyl protein thioesterases occurs throughout a cell, thereby affecting membrane association and traffic between membranes. Several palmitoyltransferases in the ER and Golgi as well as several acyl protein thioesterases at the plasma membrane can catalyze the addition and removal of palmitate to hundreds of different proteins.

**Myristoylation**, the addition of a 14-carbon fatty acid, occurs mostly on N-terminal glycine and is therefore irreversible. Whereas almost all newly synthesized proteins contain an N-terminal methionine, a methionine aminopeptidase commonly removes this residue, such that a glycine in second position may now be the N-terminal amino acid. Because of the substrate specificity of the myristoyl-CoA:protein N-myristoyl transferases, only some of the proteins that have an N-terminal Gly are myristoylated. During apoptosis, caspases (which are proteases) cleave proteins and thereby generate a fragment that often contains an N-terminal Gly residue, which may then be myristoylated.

On the cytosolic face of the ER, proteins can be irreversibly prenylated with **farnesyl pyrophosphate** or **geranylgeranyl pyrophosphate**. The synthesis of farnesyl pyrophosphate and geranylgeranyl-phosphate is shown in Fig. 29.4. Prenyl anchors are shown in Fig. 11.9. Prenylation occurs on the side chain of a cysteine residue within a consensus sequence near the C-terminus of a protein. The particular amino acid sequence determines whether farnesylation or geranylgeranylation occurs. Some proteins have a consensus sequence that specifies geranylgeranylation on two closely spaced cysteine side chains. After prenylation, the C-terminal amino acids are removed, such that the prenylated cysteine residue forms the new C-terminus. This C-terminus is then methylated, which renders it less hydrophilic. Prenylation makes a protein more hydrophobic, but for stable association with a membrane, a prenylated protein also needs to acquire a fatty-acid anchor (see above) or contain a series of positively charged amino acids that bind to the negative surface charge of a phospholipid-containing membrane. Prenylation favors a membrane-based interaction of proteins, such as in Ras protein signaling in the mitogen-activated protein kinase pathway (see Chapter 33).

## 4.4. Phosphorylation, Sulfation, and Nitrosylation

**Protein phosphorylation**, the addition of a phosphate group to the side chain of serine, threonine, or tyrosine, is a widespread means of regulating protein function. Humans have more than 500 kinases that catalyze phosphorylation and well over 100 phosphatases that dephosphorylate proteins.

For **sulfation**, protein-tyrosine sulfotransferase in the trans-Golgi network (TGN) uses 3′-phosphoadenosine-5′-phosphosulfate (PAPS; for synthesis see Fig. 36.16) to sulfate a tyrosine residue on some secreted proteins and some transmembrane proteins.

S-**Nitrosylation** by nitric oxide (NO) of cysteine residues in proteins gives rise to SNO-proteins (S-nitrosylated proteins). NO is formed by NO synthases and serves as a signaling molecule. Nitrosylation can be reversed by reduced glutathione (see Fig. 21.5) such that the original cysteine –SH group is restored.

## 4.5. Ubiquitylation and SUMOylation

**Ubiquitylation**, the conjugation of a protein with ubiquitin, a 76-amino acid polypeptide, is reversible, occurs in many different fashions, and serves a variety of roles. Humans have more than 100 deubiquitylases that can remove ubiquitin from ubiquitylated proteins. **Monoubiquitylation** plays a role in signaling, such as in the coordination of DNA repair or in silencing gene expression through histone modification. **Polyubiquitylation** via Lys-48 of ubiquitin is a signal for degradation of a protein in proteasomes (see Fig. 35.1 and Section 1.2 in Chapter 35). E3 ubiquitin-protein ligases (of which there are more than 600) play a crucial role in binding to proteins and initiating ubiquitylation. Misfolded proteins may be polyubiquitylated because they display excessive hydrophobicity or a normally hidden sequence that is recognized as a signal for degradation. Parkin is an E3 enzyme that plays a major role in protein quality control in mitochondria, as well as in the removal of mitochondria by autophagy. Mutant parkin gives rise to a form of **hereditary Parkinson disease** (see Section 8.5 in Chapter 9).

Conjugation of proteins with small ubiquitin-like modifier (**SUMO**) proteins plays a role in signaling (but not in protein degradation). Humans make three (possibly four) physiologically relevant SUMO proteins. At ~100 amino acids, SUMO proteins are slightly larger than ubiquitin. The set of enzyme activities required for SUMOylation resembles the set required for ubiquitylation. However, there are many fewer enzymes that play a role in selecting proteins for SUMOylation than those for ubiquitylation, in part because SUMOylation occurs on lysine side chains in a consensus sequence.

SUMO plays a role in chromatin organization, transcription, DNA repair, and the production of ribosomes. SUMOylation can prevent the formation of dimers or multimers by steric hindrance, or it can promote complex formation, whereby it is usually helped by proteins that contain a SUMO-interacting motif. There are many SUMO-specific hydrolases that can deSUMOylate a protein.

## 5. PROTEIN SORTING AND QUALITY CONTROL

*About one-third of all proteins are translated into the ER and end up in the membrane or lumen of the ER. Chaperone proteins recognize abnormally folded proteins foster refolding and guide defective proteins to degradation. Coated vesicles transport proteins from the ER to the Golgi. At the trans end of the Golgi, proteins are sorted according to destination, such as lysosomes, secretory vesicles, or plasma membrane.*

Generally, vesicles coated with clathrin, coat protein I (COPI), or coat protein II (COPII) transport proteins (and lipids) between subcellular compartments (Fig. 7.9). Coat proteins, along with cargo adaptor proteins, bind to the cytosolic face of a membrane, bend the membrane, bind cargo, and give rise to a vesicle (Fig. 7.10). After budding off, the vesicle is uncoated; that is, the coat proteins and the cargo adaptor proteins are removed (they are reused). Depending on the particular cargo adaptor proteins on the surface of vesicles (or cytosolic proteins that bind to cargo adaptors), the uncoated vesicles fuse with a target membrane with the help of SNARE complexes (see Fig. 9.7).

In the ER, newly synthesized, folded proteins enter budding coated vesicles at specific ER exit sites. Most proteins leave the ER in COPII-coated vesicles and then enter the Golgi at its cis face, where they start their migration through the Golgi.

Protein sorting takes place in the trans-Golgi network (TGN). About one-third of all newly synthesized proteins pass through the TGN. On the cytosolic side of the TGN, cargo adapters recognize amino acid sequences of transmembrane proteins. Such cargo adapters also recognize cargo receptors,

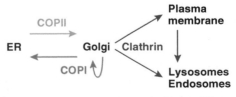

**Fig. 7.9** **Transport of proteins among intracellular compartments by coated vesicles.** *COP,* coat protein; *ER,* endoplasmic reticulum.

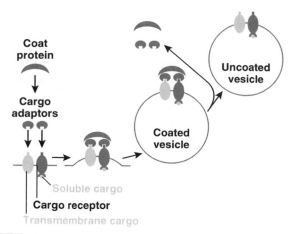

**Fig. 7.10** **Basic principle of vesicle formation and protein sorting in the endoplasmic reticulum and Golgi.**

which are proteins that in turn bind soluble proteins inside the TGN.

At the TGN, proteins can be sorted to end up in endosomes, lysosomes, secretory granules, or in the plasma membrane (in polarized epithelial cells, some proteins can be sorted so that they selectively end up in the apical or basolateral plasma membrane). Cargo adaptor proteins bind to transmembrane proteins that contain a matching localization sequence. At their destination, vesicles fuse with the new membrane and empty their soluble contents into the target compartment.

The cargo adaptor proteins can also bind cargo receptor proteins that in turn bind soluble cargo, such as **mannose 6-phosphate**–labeled enzymes destined for **lysosomes**. In the ER, most nascent hydrolases destined for lysosomes are conjugated with a 14-residue glycan. In the Golgi, some mannose residues in the 14-residue glycan are phosphorylated to form mannose 6-phosphate (this particular enzyme is missing in the very rare disease **I-cell disease**). Uncovering enzyme (N-acetylglucosamine-1-phosphodiester α-N-acetylglucosaminidase) removes terminal sugar residues to expose mannose 6-phosphate. In the TGN membrane, the mannose 6-phosphate receptor, a cargo receptor, binds an enzyme destined for lysosomes by virtue of its mannose 6-phosphate. On the cytosolic face of the TGN membrane, a cargo adapter binds to this mannose 6-phosphate receptor, resulting in the transport of the enzyme to lysosomes.

**Posttranslational quality control** takes place at several levels. In the ER, where protein folding predominantly takes place, chaperones are the main sensors of inappropriate protein folding, and they are involved in directing proteins toward refolding or degradation. For degradation, proteins are exported to the cytosol. There, protein monomers can be conjugated with ubiquitin and degraded inside proteasomes (see Fig. 35.1 and Section 1.2 in Chapter 35), or they can be recognized by a chaperone by virtue of their KFERQ motif (the sequence Lys-Phe-Glu-Arg-Gln, which is present in ~30% of all proteins in the cytosol) and be delivered to a lysosome for degradation. Protein aggregates in the cytosol are collected in

a central location and can enter macroautophagy, a process by which the aggregates are enveloped by an autophagosome that then fuses with a lysosome for protein degradation (macroautophagy also envelopes defective organelles).

Improperly folded, damaged, or defective proteins in the Golgi and in the plasma membrane are preferentially delivered to lysosomes for degradation.

## SUMMARY

- tRNAs can read multiple codons thanks to wobble base pairing at the third position of a codon.
- Silent mutations change the codon but not the amino acid residue, nonsense mutations create a stop codon, and missense mutations encode a different amino acid.
- Frameshift mutations change the reading frame of part of an mRNA.
- The most common start codon is AUG in an appropriate sequence context. AUG codes for Met, which is removed soon after protein synthesis.
- During the first round of translation, mRNAs with premature stop codons are degraded by nonsense-mediated decay (NMD).
- Translation in mitochondria differs from translation in the cytosol with regard to ribosome composition, tRNAs, and genetic code.
- There are more than 500 tRNAs that are encoded in the DNA of the nucleus. During processing, the tRNAs are extended by CCA, and many nucleotides are modified. Aminoacyl-tRNA synthetases charge these tRNAs with their cognate amino acid.
- Pseudomonic acid (mupirocin), which is used to treat methicillin-resistant *Staphylococcus aureus*, inhibits isoleucyl-tRNA synthetase in bacteria.
- miRNAs bind to mRNAs and thereby impair translation directly or induce mRNA degradation.
- Stress, infection, and nutrient deprivation inhibit translation and may lead to use of alternate start codons.
- Aminoglycosides, chloramphenicol, and macrolides are used clinically to impair translation in bacteria.
- Proteins that are destined for the cytosol, nucleus, mitochondria, or peroxisomes are synthesized by ribosomes in the cytosol. If needed, these proteins contain organelle-specific localization sequences.
- Proteins that are destined for the endoplasmic reticulum (ER), Golgi, secretory vesicles, plasma membrane, or lysosomes have a signal sequence. Signal recognition particles (SRPs) recognize the signal sequence on a nascent protein, bind to the SRP receptor, and set up the ribosome on the translocon to move the growing peptide chain into the ER.
- In the ER, some nascent proteins are glycosylated with a 14-residue glycan at the amino group of the side chain of an asparagine. Subsequently, in the Golgi, the glycan is often greatly modified. The Golgi can also glycosylate proteins on serine and threonine residues. Congenital disorders of glycosylation (CDGs) are a class of disorders that

can be due to a lack of a glycan addition in the ER or faulty processing in the Golgi.

- Chaperones can help fold proteins, bind to aggregated proteins, unfold and refold misfolded proteins, and direct proteins to degradation in proteasomes or lysosomes.
- Acylation with palmitate or myristate, or prenylation with a farnesyl or geranylgeranyl group increases the likelihood that a protein resides in a membrane. Long-term association with a membrane requires two or more such modifications or additional positively charged or hydrophobic amino acid sequences.
- Ubiquitylation of proteins can lead to protein degradation or play a role in a variety of processes, such as DNA repair and signaling. SUMOylation plays a role in signaling, often by creating steric hindrance or by inducing binding to proteins that contain SUMO-interacting motifs.
- Coated vesicles transport proteins between the ER, Golgi, plasma membrane, and lysosomes.

## FURTHER READING

- Barone R, Fiumara A, Jaeken J. Congenital disorders of glycosylation with emphasis on cerebellar involvement. *Semin Neurol.* 2014;34:357-366.
- Jonas S, Izaurralde E. Towards a molecular understanding of microRNA-mediated gene silencing. *Nat Rev Genet.* 2015;16:421-433.
- Khatter H, Myasnikov AG, Natchiar SK, Klaholz BP. Structure of the human 80S ribosome. *Nature.* 2015;520:640-645.
- Miller JN, Pearce DA. Nonsense-mediated decay in genetic disease: friend or foe? *Mutat Res Rev Mutat Res.* 2014;762:52-64.
- Neupert W. A Perspective on transport of proteins into mitochondria: a myriad of open questions. *J Mol Biol.* 2015;427:1135-1158.
- Ott M, Amunts A, Brown A. Organization and regulation of mitochondrial protein synthesis. *Annu Rev Biochem.* 2016;85:77-101.
- Palsuledesai CC, Distefano MD. Protein prenylation: enzymes, therapeutics, and biotechnology applications. *ACS Chem Biol.* 2015;10:51-62.
- Stroynowska-Czerwinska A, Fiszer A, Krzyzosiak WJ. The panorama of miRNA-mediated mechanisms in mammalian cells. *Cell Mol Life Sci.* 2014;71:2253-2270.
- Torres AG, Batlle E, Ribas de Pouplana L. Role of tRNA modifications in human diseases. *Trends Mol Med.* 2014;20:306-314.

# Review Questions

1. Which of the following most likely occurs when a ribosome encounters a UAG codon of an mRNA that derives from a normal, nonpathogenic allele?

   A. Eukaryotic release factor (a protein) binds to UAG
   B. Met is incorporated into the nascent peptide
   C. The ribosome binds to the SRP
   D. The ribosome stalls and the mRNA is degraded by NMD

2. The coding strand of a particular gene contains a codon that reads 5′-CAT. Based on the genetic code shown in Table 7.1, which amino acid is added to the nascent protein chain as a consequence of the aforementioned sequence?

   A. Gln
   B. His
   C. Met
   D. Tyr
   E. Val

3. The unprocessed transcript of a gene contains the following number of nucleotides:

   3′-UTR: 45
   5′-UTR: 15
   Exon 1: 120
   Exon 2: 120
   Intron 1: 240

   How many amino acid residues will the protein product of translation have?

   A. 60
   B. 80
   C. 100
   D. 180
   E. 300

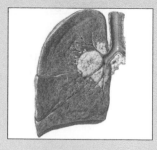

# Chapter 8

# Cell Cycle and Cancer

## SYNOPSIS

- The activity of cyclin-dependent kinases (CDKs) is a key regulator of the cell cycle. Cyclins increase CDK activity, whereas CDK inhibitor proteins decrease it.
- From a quiescent state, cells enter the cell cycle in response to growth factors. Growth factor stimulation activates CDKs, which in turn inhibit the activity of a protein called retinoblastoma (RB). RB then no longer binds to E2F transcription factors. Free E2Fs alter the expression of proteins to favor progress in the cell cycle.
- In the presence of DNA damage, the p53 pathway halts the cell cycle before the DNA is replicated.
- In tumor cells, the RB protein, which prevents cell cycle progression in normal cells, and the p53 protein, which arrests the cell cycle in response to DNA damage, are often nonfunctional.
- The WNT/β-catenin pathway plays a role in development and activates transcription of certain genes, such as the gene for cyclin D and MYC, a transcription factor. In tumors, this pathway is often overly active.
- Over time, all cells acquire mutations. A small fraction of these mutations is tumorigenic.
- Old age, a long history of smoking, obesity, and excessive alcohol consumption are major risk factors for cancer.
- Genes that drive the formation of tumors are divided into oncogenes and tumor suppressor genes. A single allele of an oncogene is sufficient to drive tumorigenesis, but both alleles of a tumor suppressor gene need to be nonfunctional to permit tumorigenesis. A typical tumor cell contains one oncogene and has lost the function of several tumor suppressors.
- Patients with an inherited cancer syndrome are at an increased risk of neoplasia at an unusually early age. Hereditary cancer syndromes are typically due to heterozygosity for a pathogenic tumor suppressor allele. Some somatic cells then acquire a genetic alteration that abolishes the function of the remaining, previously normal allele.
- About half of the cases of familial breast and ovarian cancer syndromes are due to inheritance of a mutation in the *BRCA* gene, which encodes a protein that plays a role in DNA repair. Similarly, about half of the cases of familial melanoma are due to an inherited mutation in the *CDKN2A* gene, which encodes an inhibitor of the cell cycle. Most cases of hereditary colon cancer are due to Lynch syndrome, which is caused by a DNA mismatch repair deficiency. A small fraction of hereditary colon cancer is due to familial adenomatous polyposis (FAP), which is caused by a mutation in the *APC* gene.
- Pharmacological treatment of metastatic cancer often involves drugs that induce DNA crosslinks, as well as drugs that inhibit deoxythymidine monophosphate synthesis, topoisomerases, or the rearrangement of microtubules before cell division.
- For the treatment of certain forms of breast cancer, lung cancer, colorectal cancer, and melanoma, there are several inhibitors of kinases in growth-promoting signaling pathways.
- Patients with prostate cancer are generally given androgen deprivation therapy, regardless of the genetic makeup of tumor cells.
- Tumor cells use considerably more glucose than normal cells. This makes it possible to locate metastases after radioactive fluorodeoxyglucose has been infused into a patient.

## LEARNING OBJECTIVES

*For mastery of this topic, you should be able to do the following:*
- Compare and contrast the RB and p53 pathways.
- Explain how DNA damage in the G1 phase normally leads to cell cycle arrest and possibly apoptosis.
- Compare and contrast an oncoprotein and a tumor suppressor.
- Describe the genetic makeup of a typical tumor.
- Describe lifestyle choices that can help patients minimize their cancer risk.
- Compare and contrast the major genetic causes of the hereditary breast and ovarian cancer syndrome, FAP, Lynch syndrome, and familial melanoma.
- Use patient history, clinical findings, and lab tests to determine whether a patient with colorectal cancer has sporadic cancer, FAP, or Lynch syndrome.
- Given an abnormality in a growth-promoting signaling pathway in a breast carcinoma, lung carcinoma, colorectal cancer, or melanoma, list drugs that target these signaling pathways and can potentially be used for treatment.

## 1. CELL CYCLE AND ITS REGULATION

*The cell cycle consists of phases G1, S (for DNA synthesis), G2, and M (for mitosis). Cyclin activation of cyclin-dependent kinases (CDKs) is essential to moving cells through the cell cycle. When growth factors stimulate quiescent cells to enter the G1 phase, cyclin-activated CDKs phosphorylate the retinoblastoma (RB) protein, which then no longer binds to E2F transcription factors. E2Fs alter transcription in cells to fit the needs of the cell cycle—for instance, the needs of DNA replication. If the protein p53 receives information about DNA damage, it prevents entry of the cell into S phase, and it may even induce apoptosis (self-destruction of the cell). In apoptosis, DNA and many cellular proteins are degraded in a regulated fashion.*

### 1.1. Cell Cycle and the Retinoblastoma Pathway

The cell cycle is commonly divided into the following **phases**: **G0** (quiescence), **G1** (gap 1), **S** (DNA synthesis), **G2** (gap 2), and **M** (mitosis). In adults, most cells are in a quiescent state (Fig. 8.1).

During the G0 phase, **RB** binds to **E2F** transcription factors (Fig. 8.2). E2Fs bind to promoter elements upstream of

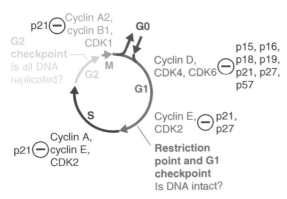

**Fig. 8.1** Cell cycle and its phase-specific kinase activities.

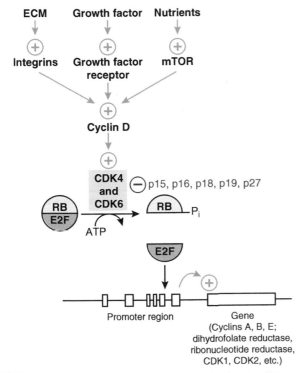

**Fig. 8.2** Phosphorylation of the retinoblastoma (RB) protein by cyclin-dependent kinases (CDKs) releases the transcription factor E2F.

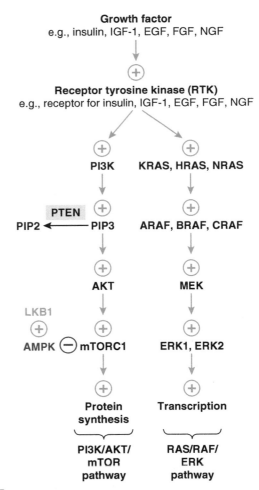

**Fig. 8.3** **Growth factor signaling.** IGF-1, insulin-like growth factor 1; EGF, epidermal growth factor; FGF, fibroblast growth factor; NGF, nerve growth factor.

genes (see Chapter 6). Binding of E2Fs to RB prevents the transcription of genes, the products of which play a role in cell proliferation.

To leave the G0 phase and enter into the G1 phase, cells need to sense a sufficiently high concentration of extracellular **growth factors** (Fig. 8.3); epithelial cells also need to sense **adhesion** to the extracellular matrix (see Fig. 8.2). Examples of growth factors are insulin, insulin-like growth factor 1, epidermal growth factor (EGF), fibroblast growth factor, transforming growth factors α and β (see Chapter 13), and erythropoietin (see Section 1.3 in Chapter 16). The receptors of these growth factors signal to the cytosol and the nucleus of cells (see Fig. 8.3). **Integrins** are membrane proteins that participate in linking actin filaments and intermediate filaments (part of the cytoskeleton) inside cells to the

extracellular matrix. Integrins can accomplish this link in response to intracellular signals, and they can also signal to the inside of a cell that attachment to the extracellular matrix has taken place.

Growth factor receptors that are tyrosine kinases signal via both the **PI3K/AKT/mTOR pathway** and via the **RAS/RAF/ERK pathway** (**MAPK pathway**). In the PI3K/AKT/mTOR pathway, phosphatidylinositol (3,4,5)-trisphosphate (PIP3) is a phospholipid in the plasma membrane that activates the kinase AKT. The phosphatase **PTEN** dephosphorylates PIP3 to PIP2, thereby inhibiting signaling in the PI3K/AKT/mTOR pathway.

An acquired loss of one or two alleles of PTEN is frequently seen in sporadic tumors, and an inherited loss of one allele for PTEN gives rise to **Cowden** syndrome, a heritable cancer syndrome associated with an increased likelihood of neoplasms in the thyroid gland, breast, endometrium, kidneys, colon, and rectum.

Adenosine monophosphate–activated protein kinase (AMPK) phosphorylates and thereby inhibits mTORC1 when energy production is impaired (see Fig. 8.3). LKB1 (encoded by the *STK11* gene) is a protein kinase that activates AMPK.

**Peutz-Jeghers syndrome** is most often caused by loss-of-function mutations in *STK11*, the gene that encodes LKB1 (see Fig. 8.3). Affected persons are at an increased risk of a variety of tumors, such as in the gastrointestinal system and breasts.

Progression through the cell cycle is promoted by **CDKs**, which in turn are activated by **cyclins** (see Figs. 8.1 and 8.2). The cyclins are present only during certain parts of the cell cycle, whereas the amount of CDK protein is much less variable. The major CDKs are CDK1, CDK2, CDK4, and CDK6. The major cyclins are A, B, D, and E. Cyclins are often overexpressed in tumor cells.

Stimuli from growth factors and cell adhesion lead to an increased production of **cyclin D**, which activates **CDK4** and **CDK6** (see Figs. 8.1 to 8.3). CDK4 and CDK6 in turn phosphorylate the **RB protein**, which then releases **E2F** transcription factors. Some E2Fs bound to promoter elements increase transcription, whereas others decrease it. As a result, the cell's transcription program is modified to fit the needs of the cell cycle. E2F leads to an increased transcription of the genes that encode CDK2, cyclins A and E, dihydrofolate reductase, and ribonucleotide reductase (all needed for the S phase), as well as CDK1 and cyclin B (needed for mitosis). Cyclin E–activated CDK2 further increases the phosphorylation of RB. Dihydrofolate reductase is needed for the synthesis of thymidine triphosphate (see Fig. 37.6), and ribonucleotide reductase is needed for the reduction of ribonucleotides to deoxyribonucleotides (see Fig. 37.5), which are needed for DNA replication (see Chapter 3).

**CDK inhibitor proteins** (**CKIs**) bind to CDKs and inhibit them. CKIs inhibit the binding of cyclins to CDKs and also impair catalysis in preformed cyclin/CDK complexes. The **Ink4** inhibitors (inhibitors of CDK4) inhibit only CDK4 and CDK6. The Ink4 family consists of **p15$^{Ink4b}$**, **p16$^{Ink4a}$**, **p18$^{Ink4c}$**, and **p19$^{Ink4d}$** (in short: p15, p16, p18, and p19; see Figs. 8.1 and 8.2).

The RB pathway is important for cells to enter the G1 phase; this pathway is abnormally active in most tumor cells (discussed later in this chapter). Common tumorigenic events include overexpression of cyclin D, loss of RB function, and loss of p16$^{Ink4a}$ function.

Children who inherited only one functional copy of the *RB1* gene develop **retinoblastoma**, often bilaterally and before 2 years of age. These children have an ~30% risk of developing bone cancer in their teenage years or a soft tissue sarcoma or skin melanoma at ~30 years of age.

After reaching the **restriction point** (see Fig. 8.1), a cell goes through the cell cycle independent of growth factors. This is achieved by phosphorylation of RB, liberation of E2F, an E2F-induced increase in the amount of cyclin E, and cyclin E/CDK2-induced degradation of the CDK inhibitor p27$^{Kip1}$.

During the G1 phase, **origin of replication complexes** bind to **origins of replication** (see Fig. 3.3) of DNA.

## 1.2. The p53 Tumor Suppressor Pathway

The **checkpoint** for DNA integrity depends primarily on **p53**, a protein that senses DNA damage signals (Fig. 8.4).

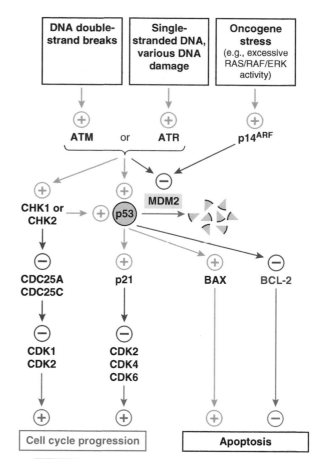

**Fig. 8.4**    **DNA damage and the p53 pathway.**

In the absence of DNA damage, the enzyme **MDM2** ubiquitylates p53 so that p53 is degraded inside proteasomes (ubiquitylation and proteasomes are described in Section 1.2 in Chapter 35).

In the presence of DNA damage, the protein kinases **ATM** and **ATR** phosphorylate p53 and MDM2; this leads to an increase in the concentration of p53 (see Fig. 8.4). p53 acts as a transcription factor and increases the concentration of the CKI **p21**. p21 then inhibits **CDK4/6** and **CDK2**, leading to cell cycle arrest (see also Fig. 8.1). The DNA damage–induced arrest of the cell cycle is redundant in that ATM also activates **checkpoint kinase 2** (**CHK2**) and ATR activates **checkpoint kinase 1** (**CHK1**; see also Section 5 in Chapter 2). These checkpoint kinases also detect DNA damage and then prevent the activation of the cyclin B/CDK1 complex that is needed for mitosis.

Besides DNA damage, **oncogenes** can also increase the activity of p53 (see Fig. 8.4). Oncogenic mutations of *RAS*, *RAF*, or *ERK* genes lead to increased synthesis of p14$^{ARF}$. p14$^{ARF}$ then sequesters MDM2 into the nucleolus, thereby increasing the survival of p53.

In neoplasms, sensing of DNA damage or oncogenic stress by p53, followed by cell cycle arrest, is often impaired. Most tumors contain p53 mutations, and most of these mutations impair the binding of p53 to DNA. That is, the mutations make it impossible for p53 to act as a transcription factor that produces mRNAs for proteins that arrest the cell cycle or promote apoptosis. Tumorigenic mutations that impair the p53 tumor suppressor pathway are frequently found in the genes *ATM*, *CDKN2A* (encoding p14$^{ARF}$ and p16$^{Ink4a}$), and *MDM2*.

**Li-Fraumeni syndrome** is an inherited cancer syndrome caused by heterozygosity for a mutant *TP53* gene, which encodes p53. In neoplasms, the second *TP53* allele is mutated or otherwise made nonfunctional. All affected patients develop tumors before age 70 years; the first tumor is generally diagnosed at age ~30 years in women and ~40 years in men. The tumors can occur in a number of tissues, such as bone, hematopoietic tissue, breast, brain, and adrenal glands.

Several **cell cycle checkpoints** exist: one for intact DNA in late G1, one for completeness of DNA replication in G2, and another for proper alignment of chromosomes in M phase. The G1 checkpoint depends on both the p53 and RB pathways: p53 enhances the transcription of inhibitors of cyclin D/CDK4 and cyclin D/CDK6; less RB is phosphorylated and more RB binds to E2F; and E2F is no longer free to stimulate gene transcription that would favor progress in the cell cycle. The restriction point is considered to be a separate process from the G1 checkpoint (independence from growth factors vs. integrity of DNA), but the two checkpoints depend on each other through the intertwining of RB and p53 pathways.

## 1.3. The WNT/β-Catenin Pathway

WNT signaling pathways play roles in development, establishment of cell polarity, and stem cell maintenance. WNT signaling is divided into **canonical** and noncanonical signaling, which work with and without **β-catenin**, respectively. Only the canonical pathway with β-catenin is presented here.

Humans make 19 different **WNT** proteins, which are palmitoylated (see Fig. 11.9 and Section 1.5 in Chapter 11) and glycosylated (see Figs. 7.7 and 7.8 and Section 4.2 in Chapter 7). After a cell secretes a WNT protein, WNT acts either on the same cell or a nearby cell.

Humans make 10 different **Frizzled** proteins, which are the receptors for WNT and are also G protein–coupled receptors.

In the absence of a WNT signal, free **β-catenin** is phosphorylated and ubiquitylated by a protein complex that includes the adenomatous polyposis coli (**APC**) protein; once ubiquitylated, APC is degraded inside proteasomes (see Fig. 35.1 and Section 1.2 in Chapter 35).

In the presence of a WNT signal, β-catenin is no longer phosphorylated, ubiquitylated, and degraded. Instead, β-catenin binds to a transcription factor of the T-cell factor/lymphoid enhancer factor (TCF/LEF) family (i.e., TCF7, TCF7L1, TCF7L2, or LEF1), which then moves into the nucleus and increases the transcription of certain genes that encode proteins that favor cell proliferation, such as the gene for cyclin D1.

β-Catenin also plays a role in connecting **actin filaments** of neighboring cells via adherens junctions (Fig. 8.5). Actin filaments are part of the cytoskeleton and help determine and

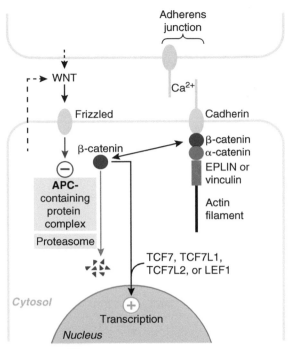

**Fig. 8.5**    The WNT/β-catenin pathway.

maintain cell shape. The adherens junctions consist of membrane-anchored **cadherins** (in two different cells) that bind to each other in the presence of Ca$^{2+}$, as well as β-catenin, α-catenin, and EPLIN or vinculin that connect cadherin to the actin filaments.

During the G0 phase, β-catenin is mostly at the cell membrane in adherens junctions, and its concentration in the cytosol is very low due to degradation in proteasomes (see Fig. 8.5). During the S and G2 phases, the concentration of soluble β-catenin increases; then, as cells enter the G0 or G1 phase, the concentration decreases again.

In many **tumors**, particularly pancreatic adenomas and colorectal carcinomas, WNT signaling is active regardless of the presence of WNT. This is commonly due to a genetic alteration that leads to loss of APC function (and hence survival of free β-catenin even in the absence of a WNT signal), but it can also be caused by the absence of cadherins.

## 1.4. Role of MYCs

The **MYC** transcription factors (MYC or c-MYC, N-MYC, and L-MYC) regulate the transcription of ~15% of all genes, many of which encode proteins that play a role in cell growth or cell cycle progression.

Normally, signals from the **RAS/RAF/ERK pathway** (see Fig. 8.3) or the **WNT pathway** (see Fig. 8.5) enhance the rate of transcription of *MYC* genes (Fig. 8.6). In turn, the MYC proteins partner with the transcription factor MAX to bind to E-box promoter elements, which contain the sequence CANNTG (N, any nucleotide).

MYC favors transcription of the genes that encode CDK4, cyclins, or enzymes of nucleotide biosynthesis, but it represses

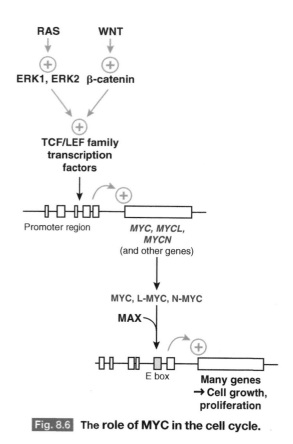

**Fig. 8.6**  The role of MYC in the cell cycle.

the transcription of the genes that encode the CDK inhibitors p21 and p27.

In tumors, excessive MYC activity can be due to translocation (joining a different promoter to a *MYC* gene), gene amplification, or mutation of one of the *MYC* genes. Furthermore, increased MYC activity may be due to increased upstream signals from the **WNT pathway** (see Fig. 8.5) or the **RAS/RAF/ERK pathway** (see Fig. 8.3). Among gene amplifications, amplification of the *MYCN* and *MYCL* genes (encoding N-MYC and L-MYC, respectively) is especially common. MYC-overexpressing tumors are generally very sensitive to nutrient deprivation.

## 1.5. Apoptosis

**Apoptosis** is a process of regulated cell suicide that can be initiated by extracellular or intracellular signals. Extracellular signals for apoptosis are particularly important in development and function of the immune system. Intracellular signals that induce apoptosis derive from **DNA damage response, hypoxia,** or **oxidative stress**. Apoptosis is the net result of an interplay of proapoptotic and antiapoptotic factors. Apoptosis is an important defense against the formation of a neoplasm.

During apoptosis, intracellular **caspases** become active, degrade proteins, and activate DNA degradation. Caspases contain a cysteine (C) residue in their catalytic site, and they cleave substrates that contain an aspartate (Asp) residue.

Humans express 11 different caspases, always as inactive precursors (i.e., zymogens, proenzymes, or procaspases) that are activated through proteolysis. Caspases are organized into cascades in which one caspase activates another caspase, thereby greatly amplifying the initial enzyme activity.

Among the caspases, **initiator caspases** (caspases 2, 8, 9, and 10) play a role early in the signaling pathway. **Effector caspases (executioner caspases;** caspases 3 and 7) catalyze terminal steps and degrade several hundred different proteins that contain an N-Asp-x-x-Asp sequence by hydrolyzing the protein after the second Asp.

Apoptosis can be divided into an **extrinsic pathway** that depends on plasma membrane receptors and an **intrinsic pathway** that depends on mitochondria. Intrinsic and extrinsic pathways use different initiator caspases, but they have common effector caspases.

The intrinsic pathway depends on the **permeabilization** of the outer mitochondrial membrane and the release of **cytochrome C** from the intermembrane space of mitochondria. The permeabilization of the outer mitochondrial membrane in turn depends on the balance of proapoptotic proteins, such as **BAX**, versus antiapoptotic proteins, such as **BCL2**. In a perfectly healthy cell, the antiapoptotic BCL2 prevails over the proapoptotic BAX, in part by forming an inactive BCL2-BAX dimer. When proapoptotic signals prevail (described later in this chapter), mitochondria release cytochrome C (in oxidative phosphorylation, cytochrome C normally carries electrons from complex III to complex IV; see Fig. 23.3 and Section 1.2 in Chapter 23).

In the presence of DNA double-strand breaks, **p53** becomes active and favors apoptosis via both the extrinsic and intrinsic pathways (see Figs. 8.4 and 8.7). In response to DNA damage, ATM, ATR, CHK1, and CHK2 increase p53 activity. p53 then activates the extrinsic pathway by favoring the transcription of the FAS ligand and the FAS receptor, which in turn leads to the activation of initiator caspases (caspases 8 or 10) and effector caspases (caspases 3 or 7). The effector caspases not only degrade proteins but also activate a **DNase** that cuts DNA in the linker regions between nucleosomes, generating fragments of ~180 base pairs. p53 activates the intrinsic pathway of apoptosis by stimulating the transcription of the **BAX** gene and the *BBC3* gene, which encodes the protein **PUMA**. PUMA neutralizes BCL2 and activates the proapoptotic BAX. BAX moves into the outer membrane of mitochondria, rendering the membranes permeable to cytochrome C. Cytochrome C in the cytosol then favors the formation of an **apoptosome**, activation of an initiator caspase, and activation of effector caspases (see Fig. 8.7).

Apoptosis results in the fragmentation of a cell into numerous membrane-enclosed vesicles that are phagocytosed by neutrophils and macrophages.

In neoplasms, genetic and epigenetic alterations frequently lead to a loss of proapoptotic factors and a gain in antiapoptotic factors to favor cell survival despite abnormal DNA. These alterations also render tumor cells resistant to chemotherapy-induced apoptosis.

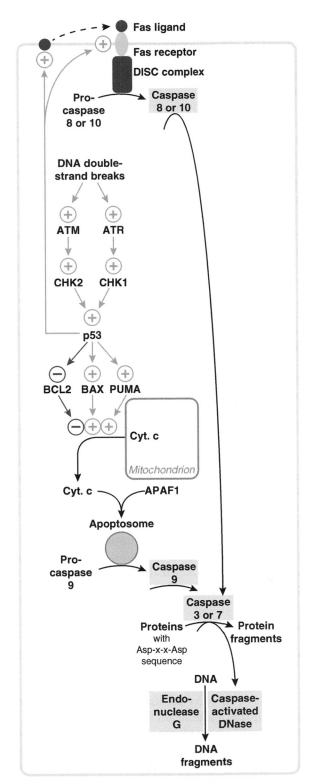

## 1.6. Control of S, G2, and M Phases of the Cell Cycle

During S phase, DNA is replicated, cyclin D is degraded, and **cyclin E/CDK2** and later **cyclin A**/CDK2 complexes provide the main CDK activity (see Fig. 8.1). Overexpression of cyclins

E1 and E2 is tumorigenic and is observed in tumors of the uterus or ovaries.

The **Cip/Kip** family proteins inhibit CDK2, as well as other CDKs. The Cip/Kip family includes **p21$^{Cip1}$**, **p27$^{Kip1}$**, and **p57$^{Kip2}$** (noted as p21, p27, and p57). The DNA damage sensed by p53 leads to increased synthesis of p21$^{Cip1}$ (see Fig. 8.4). The removal of a growth factor stimulus induces the synthesis of p27$^{Kip1}$, which is responsible for inducing and maintaining quiescence (G0; see Fig. 8.1).

The main CDK for transition from G2 to M phase is the **cyclin B/CDK1** complex. The cyclin B/CDK1 complex already forms during S phase, but it is inactive because of inhibitory phosphorylation by kinases named WEE1-like protein kinase 1 and 2, and by translocation to the cytosol. In late G2 phase, a **CDC25 phosphatase** activates CDK1 by dephosphorylating it, and the cyclin B/CDK1 complex moves to the nucleus.

In the presence of DNA damage, CHK1 phosphorylates and inhibits CDC25, which in turn keeps CDK1 inactive and makes entry into M phase impossible.

## 2. GENETIC ALTERATIONS IN CANCER CELLS

*Tumors and normal cells contain many mutations; a relatively small number of driver mutations among them is responsible for tumorigenesis. A single allele of an oncogene (representing a gain of function) is sufficient to favor tumorigenesis, but both alleles of a tumor suppressor must usually be altered to lose tumor suppressor function and favor tumorigenesis. Tumor cells typically contain approximately two to eight driver mutations, of which one is an oncogene and the rest are tumor suppressors. Age is a major risk factor for cancer. Smoking further increases cancer risk via the formation of mutagenic DNA adducts. Obesity is a risk factor for a limited number of cancers, notably cancer of the endometrium. Isolation and analysis of circulating tumor cells hold promise in making a prognosis and determining the optimal treatment.*

### 2.1. Genetic Alterations That Favor Neoplasia

Cancer is the consequence of multiple abnormalities of the genome of somatic cells. This damage is caused by inadequate or faulty repair of DNA damage and replication errors. Most of the mutations seen in tumors are single nucleotide substitutions, and most of these are missense mutations. In adults, solid tumors typically contain ~50 mutations that alter the amino acid sequence of proteins (when DNA repair is impaired, tumors show an even larger number of mutations). Some of the clinically significant mutations increase proliferation, and others inhibit apoptosis.

In a simple binary classification, **driver mutations** are key to neoplasia, whereas **passenger mutations** have few consequences. Currently, ~150 known driver mutations exist. A typical tumor contains two to eight driver mutations. For a type of cancer (e.g., colon cancer), tumors differ appreciably in their genetic abnormalities.

Compared with nonmalignant cells, tumors often show **aneuploidy** (i.e., a number of chromosomes that is not divisible by 23) and other **chromosome alterations**, such as partial deletions, translocations, and gene amplification. Most of the chromosome alterations are likely benign.

**Oncoproteins** from **oncogenes** favor the formation of neoplasms. Oncoproteins may be normal proteins that are expressed in unusual abundance because of **gene amplification** or a chromosome **translocation** that links the gene to a promoter that results in an increased rate of transcription. Alternatively, oncoproteins may be mutant proteins encoded by oncogenes that in turn derive from **proto-oncogenes**; for example, the gene for a growth factor receptor (a proto-oncogene) may be mutated to an oncogene so that the mutant receptor signals even in the absence of a growth factor. A single copy of an oncogene is sufficient to be tumorigenic.

**Tumor suppressors** act against tumorigenesis. In neoplasms, the tumor suppressor function can be lost by mutation or epigenetic effects. Mutations may cause a loss of function because of missense mutation, loss of heterozygosity (see Section 4.2 in Chapter 2), truncation, or aberrant splicing. For example, mutations in the *TP53* gene, which encodes p53, often impair DNA binding by p53. Epigenetic silencing of tumor suppressor expression may be due to DNA methylation, histone modification, or micro-RNAs (miRNAs; see Section 3 in Chapter 7). Common targets of promoter methylation are the genes *CDKN2A* (encoding the CKIs p14 and p16), *MLH1* (encoding a DNA mismatch repair protein), and *BRCA1* (encoding a homologous recombination repair protein).

Most often, the function of both alleles of a tumor suppressor needs to be lost for tumorigenesis to occur. The function of the two alleles may be lost by different mechanisms. Sometimes, only one allele of a tumor suppressor gene needs to be mutated for a tumor to develop, because the mutant allele shows a dominant negative effect or because there is haploinsufficiency when only a single functional allele is present.

**Oncogenic miRNAs** are miRNAs that degrade tumor suppressor mRNAs, and **tumor suppressor miRNAs** are miRNAs that degrade oncogene mRNAs. Because miRNAs enhance the degradation of multiple mRNAs, their effects may be tissue specific and difficult to predict.

Mutations in tumor suppressors, proto-oncogenes, or oncogenes can each be driver mutations.

Tumors typically have only about one oncogene mutation, whereas the remaining one to seven driver mutations concern the loss of tumor suppressor function.

Most of the major cancer-causing mutations affect the function of one out of about a dozen **pathways**. The most commonly affected pathways in cancer are the RB pathway (see Fig. 8.2 and Section 1.1) and the p53 pathway (see Fig. 8.4 and Section 1.2).

The function of **RB** is lost in almost all tumors. RB controls the G1/S phase transition (Figs. 8.1 and 8.2). RB function can be lost via mutations that abolish the interaction of RB with E2F (e.g., point mutations that generate a truncated protein, deletion of a DNA segment that includes the *RB1* gene), via

inhibition by a protein from a virus (e.g., papillomavirus protein E7), or via inappropriate phosphorylation of RB due to excessively high activity of CDK2, CDK4, or CDK6 (due to overexpression of cyclin D or cyclin E or loss of the inhibitory activity of p16 or p27).

The function of **p53** is also frequently lost in tumors. In the presence of DNA damage, p53 halts the cell cycle at the G1/S cell cycle checkpoint (see Figs. 8.1 and Fig. 8.4). The function of p53 may be lost due to a mutation in the DNA-binding domain, sequestration in the cytosol, degradation by increased MDM2 activity, degradation induced by the papilloma virus protein E6, or loss of the MDM2 inhibitor p14$^{ARF}$. With reduced p53 function, apoptosis is also reduced.

The PI3K/AKT pathway (see Fig. 8.3) is often activated, sometimes by the loss of PTEN activity.

Most of the targeted **antineoplastic agents** on the market today are inhibitors. Some of these inhibitors are used to impair the function of oncoproteins, such as protein kinases. For the most part, no drugs are available to remedy loss of tumor suppressor function directly. However, the loss of tumor suppressor activity generally results in increased activity of another protein downstream in the pathway that can sometimes be inhibited with a drug.

Many **heritable cancer syndromes** are inherited in an **autosomal dominant** fashion and are due to the inheritance of only one functional copy of a tumor suppressor allele. The mode of inheritance of any disease depends on the definition of the disorder. In heritable cancer syndromes, the disease is defined as an unusually early onset and an unusually high probability of developing a particular neoplasm. For a neoplasm to form, the function of both alleles of a tumor suppressor gene generally needs to be lost. The occurrence of an inactivating mutation depends on time. In a person who has only one allele to lose to inactivation, cancer occurs sooner than in a person who has two alleles to lose; hence the dominant pattern of inheritance.

## 2.2. Effect of Age on Tumorigenesis

The risk of being diagnosed with cancer greatly increases with age (Fig. 8.8), presumably because mutations accumulate with time. In fact, tumors in children generally contain fewer mutations than those in older adults. Furthermore, even normal, aged skin contains a significant fraction of tumorigenic driver mutations. By 85 years of age, ~50% of individuals develop cancer. One could surmise that if a person becomes old enough, he/she will die of cancer, but it turns out that according to mathematical predictions, even a 120-year-old person still has a ~20% chance of not dying of cancer.

A large portion of the age-dependent cancer risk is associated with the number of stem cell divisions, presumably because of associated replication errors. Cancer is thus a result of chance, and additional mutations due to smoking, exposure to ultraviolet (UV) radiation, excessive alcohol consumption, or obesity (see the following text) further increase this chance.

Tumors that are thought to be promoted by **mutagens**, such as smoking-induced lung cancer or UV light–induced

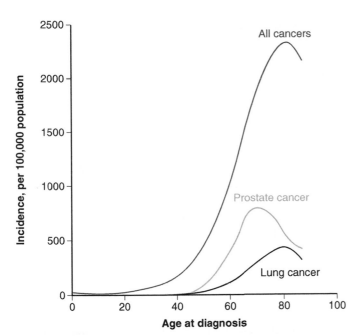

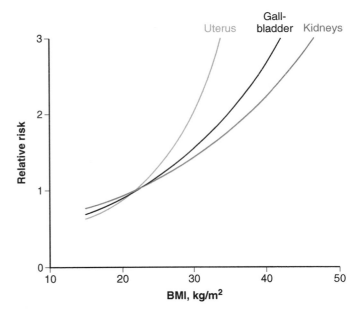

**Fig. 8.8** **Age as a key risk factor for cancer.** Age-specific Surveillance, Epidemiology, and End Results (SEER Program) incidence rates in the United States, 2009–2013. (Data from Howlader N, Noone AM, Krapcho M, et al, eds. SEER Cancer Statistics Review, 1975-2013, National Cancer Institute. Bethesda, MD. Available at http://seer.cancer.gov/csr/1975_2013.)

**Fig. 8.9** **Relative risk for cancer in select organs.** Records of ~5 million people in the United Kingdom (~9% of all inhabitants) from 1987–2012 were analyzed. (Data from Bhaskaran K, Douglas I, Forbes H, dos-Santos-Silva I, Leon DA, Smeeth L. Body-mass index and risk of 22 specific cancers: a population-based cohort study of 5·24 million UK adults. *Lancet.* 2014;384:755-765.)

melanoma, contain an especially high number of mutations. For instance, non-small-cell lung carcinomas from smokers have ~10 times the number of mutations found in the same tumors from nonsmokers.

Although clinical signs of a malignancy appear within a short time span, tumors are years or decades in the making.

## 2.3. Smoking and Cancer

Smoking increases a person's chance of developing cancer of the oral and nasal cavities, lungs, esophagus, pancreas, bladder, and other organs. Worldwide, ~20% of all cancer deaths are attributed to smoking tobacco.

**Tobacco smoke** contains some 20 known carcinogens, which can be grouped into **polycyclic aromatic hydrocarbons (PAH)** and the **nitrosamine** 4-(methylnitrosamino)-1-(3-pyridyl)-1-butanone. The most studied PAH is the highly carcinogenic **benzo[a]pyrene** (see Chapter 2). The carcinogens are modified in the body and then exert their toxic effect by forming adducts with DNA, predominantly at G or A. Repair of these adducts occurs via nucleotide excision repair (NER; see Fig. 2.7 and Section 3 in Chapter 2). If the adducts escape proper DNA repair, they may lead to a permanent mutation. Among the many permanent mutations, some lead to the formation of an oncogene and others lead to the loss of tumor suppressor function.

Smoke from a **water pipe** (**shisha**, **hookah**) is a major health hazard because significant amounts of carcinogens emanate from the charcoal that is used to heat the tobacco, and these carcinogens are inhaled with the smoke. For a comparable amount of nicotine consumed, smoke from a water pipe contains ~10 times more benzo[a]pyrene than smoke from a cigarette.

Despite the fact that smoking vastly increases a person's risk for **lung cancer**, no more than ~20% of smokers develop lung cancer.

**Chewing tobacco** contains N-nitrosamines that give rise to cancer of the oral cavity.

## 2.4. Obesity, Alcohol, and Cancer

Obesity is a gender-specific risk factor that affects a person's risk for certain neoplasms, especially in the uterus, gallbladder, kidneys, and liver (Fig. 8.9; calculation of body mass index [BMI] is explained in Section 5.1 in Chapter 39; a BMI >30 kg/m² indicates obesity). In contrast, the incidence of melanoma or bladder cancer does not markedly depend on adiposity.

The most thoroughly tested explanation of a link between obesity and cancer exists for cancer of the endometrium. The main difference between an obese and a lean person is the mass of adipose tissue. Adipose tissue converts circulating androstenedione into **estrone** (see Fig. 31.5 and Section 2.4 in Chapter 31), which constitutes the biggest source of estrogens after menopause. The obesity-induced, elevated concentration of estrone favors the growth of estrogen-dependent tumors.

Other proposed explanations for an obesity-induced increase in cancer risk state that the obesity-induced increased concentration of **insulin** or **hormones** released from the adipose tissue (e.g., more **leptin**, less **adiponectin**) favor growth-promoting signaling pathways, such as PI3K/AKT and RAS/RAF/ERK (see Fig. 8.3).

The effect of ethanol (alcohol) consumption alone (and in combination with smoking) on the risk of cancer in the mouth, pharynx, larynx, and esophagus is described in Section 4.5 in Chapter 30.

From the above, it is evident that counseling of patients regarding smoking, BMI, and alcohol consumption should be an integral part of health care.

## 2.5. Circulating Tumor Cells

**Circulating tumor cells** (CTCs) are cells that have been shed by a tumor or its metastases and entered the bloodstream. CTCs are of interest with regard to prognosis and monitoring therapy. After the removal of a primary tumor, CTCs are an indicator of the abundance of residual tumor cells.

In the laboratory, CTCs are enriched and identified on the basis of the presence and absence of certain cell surface proteins. CTCs are very rare. A blood sample that tests positive for CTCs typically contains more than four cells per 7.5 mL of blood in a blood collection tube. It is now possible to analyze the DNA in a single CTC.

Currently, CTCs can be used to make a prognosis and choose a treatment for cancer of the breast, prostate, or colon.

## 3. EXAMPLES OF COMMON NEOPLASMS

*Inherited BRCA mutations are one cause of hereditary breast and ovarian cancer (HBOC) syndrome. The most common targeted treatments of breast cancer involve the use of a selective estrogen receptor modulator, an aromatase inhibitor, or inhibition of the human epidermal growth factor receptor 2 (HER2). Many tumors of the lung test positive for the overexpression of kinases that can be inhibited pharmacologically. Prostate tumors are genetically very diverse and often contain a translocation that places a promoter with an androgen response element next to a transcription factor. Accordingly, patients with advanced prostate cancer are commonly given androgen deprivation therapy. Sporadic colorectal cancers frequently lack a functional APC protein and thus resemble tumors in patients with familial adenomatous polyposis (FAP; caused by a heritable monoallelic loss of APC function). Alternatively, sporadic colorectal cancers lack a functional DNA mismatch repair pathway and thus resemble tumors in patients with Lynch syndrome (caused by monoallelic inherited loss of a mismatch repair gene). Metastatic melanoma is commonly treated with immunotherapy. The growth of tumors that test positive for a RAF mutation can transiently be impeded with kinase-specific inhibitors. About half of the cases of familial melanoma are caused by mutations in a gene that encodes an inhibitor of cell cycle progression.*

Much of the detail we know about the genetic changes that occur in various tumors is based on massive parallel sequencing (next generation sequencing; see Section 5.2 in Chapter 4). Such sequencing is now gaining entry into clinical use, most often in the form of select cancer gene panels. The major current challenges are to learn to interpret the implications of observed mutations and to determine the most effective treatments. Health care providers will have to know the meaning and limitations of past and current tests, particularly when dealing with patients who have a hereditary cancer syndrome.

It is now apparent that there are about a dozen pathways that consistently function abnormally in cancer (see Section 2.1). Patients who have a hereditary mutation in one of these pathways commonly have an increased chance of developing tumors in multiple organs. Hence, a family history of cancer in one organ can be caused by several different heritable cancer syndromes; affected family members therefore need to be tested for mutations in multiple pathways. As an example, a patient who seems to have Lynch syndrome frequently also meets the criteria for testing for HBOC. Increasingly, *gene panels* and massive parallel sequencing are used to screen for multiple genetic alterations (see Section 6 in Chapter 4).

Currently, the most successful treatment of cancer is removal of the tumor by **surgery**. However, metastases are often in sites that cannot readily be accessed by surgery. At present, there are not sufficient means to detect small groups of precursor cells before they give rise to cancer. However, some premalignant conditions can successfully be detected, such as adenomatous colon polyps by colonoscopy and cervical dysplasia by colposcopy.

## 3.1. Breast Cancer

By histology, breast tumors are commonly divided into **ductal carcinomas** and **lobular carcinomas** (Figs. 8.10 and

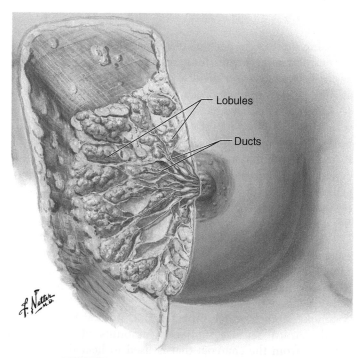

Lobules

Ducts

**Fig. 8.10** **Structure of the female breast.**

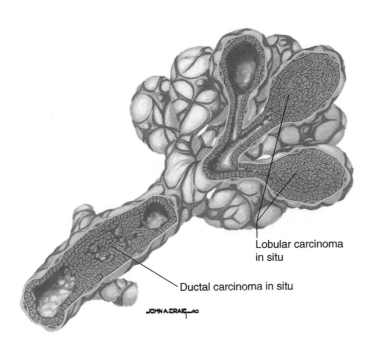

**Fig. 8.11** **Ductal and lobular carcinoma.**

Lobular carcinoma in situ

Ductal carcinoma in situ

JOHN A.CRAIG—AD

8.11), implying that the tumor cells arise from the epithelium of either ducts or lobules. Sometimes, tumors are designated as **mixed** ductal and lobular carcinoma. Furthermore, tumors are divided into **in situ carcinomas**, which are limited to growth within the epithelium of the ducts or lobules, and **invasive carcinomas** (**infiltrative carcinomas**), which have grown beyond the confines of the ducts and lobules into connective tissue of the breast. About 25% of all breast tumors are ductal carcinomas in situ, ~60% are invasive ductal carcinomas, and ~5% are invasive lobular carcinomas.

In the United States, ~12% of all women eventually develop invasive breast cancer. About 90% of these patients have **sporadic** breast cancer, whereas ~10% have an **inherited** mutation that is known to be associated with an increased cancer risk.

Mutations in the **BRCA1** and **BRCA2** genes are the main contributors to **HBOC** syndrome, accounting for ~50% of cases. The BRCA1 and BRCA2 proteins play a role in homologous recombination repair of double-strand breaks (see Section 4.2 of Chapter 2). Another ~8% of HBOC is due to mutations in other genes, such as PALB2, CHEK2, and the mutated genes that cause other known hereditary cancer syndromes, such as TP53 (Li-Fraumeni syndrome), PTEN (Cowden syndrome), STK11 (Peutz-Jeghers syndrome), or ATM. This leaves many more genetic causes of HBOC to be discovered. In the United States, at least 1 in 400 persons has inherited a pathogenic BRCA1 or BRCA2 mutation (among Ashkenazy Jews, the incidence is ~1:40). Among women with breast cancer, the prevalence of a heritable BRCA mutation is ~2%.

By 70 years of age, a woman who has inherited a BRCA1 or BRCA2 mutation has an ~55% chance of developing breast cancer and an ~25% chance of developing ovarian cancer

(rates are somewhat higher for BRCA1 and lower for BRCA2 mutations).

Clinically, the importance of diagnosing HBOC lies in increased surveillance, testing of relatives, and adjustments to therapy.

The most common mutations in sporadic breast tumors as determined by massive parallel sequencing (see Section 5.2 in Chapter 4) are in the **TP53** and **PIK3CA** genes. p53 becomes active in response to DNA damage and then arrests the cell cycle via an increased expression of p21 (see Fig. 8.4). The PIK3CA gene encodes the catalytic subunit of PI3K (see Fig. 8.3). Mutations in PIK3CA generally lead to increased activity in the PI3K/AKT/mTOR pathway, which inhibits apoptosis and promotes protein synthesis.

Breast tumors of patients with a germline nonfunctional BRCA allele generally show loss of BRCA function via a somatic alteration.

The primary treatment of breast cancer is **surgical** removal of the lesion; depending on the nature of the tumor, **adjuvant radiation therapy** and **adjuvant systemic therapy** are added to destroy any remaining tumor cells. Radiation therapy uses ionizing radiation, which induces single- and double-strand breaks (see Section 4 in Chapter 2). Systemic therapy often includes an anthracycline and cyclophosphamide regimen, followed by taxane treatment (abbreviated **AC-T regimen**). **Anthracyclines** are DNA intercalators, and the most commonly used drug is doxorubicin, which also inhibits topoisomerase II (see Section 5 in Chapter 1). **Cyclophosphamide** is a nitrogen mustard that induces intrastrand and interstrand DNA crosslinks (see Section 4.2 in Chapter 2). The **taxanes** inhibit the degradation of microtubules, which are part of the cytoskeleton; microtubules serve as lines for intracellular cargo transport, are degraded in preparation for prophase, are attached to kinetochores during prometaphase, and then serve as tracks for motor proteins that pull apart chromatids during anaphase. Tumor tissue is commonly tested for **estrogen receptors** (**ER**), **progesterone receptors** (**PR**), and **HER2**, because the results predict the effectiveness of targeted therapies. The physiological roles of estrogens and progesterone are described in Section 2.4 of Chapter 31. HER2 forms a heterodimer with an epidermal growth factor–stimulated **epidermal growth factor receptor** (**EGFR**) and then activates the RAS/RAF/ERK and PI3K/AKT/mTOR pathways (see Fig. 8.3). If the tumor is ER positive and PR positive, hormone therapy most often involves the use of a **selective estrogen receptor modulator**, such as **tamoxifen**; sometimes, an **aromatase inhibitor** is used (aromatase is needed for the synthesis of estrogens; see Fig. 31.5 and Section 2.4 in Chapter 31). If a tumor is HER2 positive, treatment with one or two different monoclonal **HER2 antibodies** (**trastuzumab, pertuzumab**) or with **lapatinib,** an inhibitor of the tyrosine kinase activity of both **HER2** and **EGFR,** is common. Tumors that test negative for ER, PR, and HER2 are called **triple negative**.

In clinical trials, perhaps half of all patients who have a germline BRCA mutation and then develop breast cancer benefit from using a poly (ADP-ribose) polymerase (**PARP**)

**inhibitor**. PARP inhibition impairs the base excision DNA repair pathway (BER; see Section 1 in Chapter 2). Because of redundancy in DNA repair pathways, cells with functional BRCA1 and BRCA2 survive in the presence of PARP inhibitors. However, cells without functional BRCA1 and BRCA2 undergo apoptosis when a PARP inhibitor inhibits BER (this finding is sometimes referred to as an example of **synthetic lethality**).

## 3.2. Lung Cancer

**Smoking** increases a person's risk for lung cancer 15- to 30-fold. In the United Kingdom, by the age of 75 years ~13% of all lifelong smokers die of lung cancer. Smokers account for ~90% of all lung cancers. Quitting smoking (compared with continued smoking) cuts the smoking-induced risk for lung cancer in half every 10 years.

In the absence of a clear driver mutation that can be targeted pharmacologically, lung cancer is treated with **platinum drugs** and a **topoisomerase inhibitor**. This is sometimes followed by radiation therapy.

Tumors that contain certain tyrosine kinase driver mutations can be treated with **tyrosine kinase inhibitors**. Thus, patients with an EGFR driver mutation can be given erlotinib or gefitinib (which reversibly inhibit the tyrosine kinase activity of the EGFR), or they can be treated with afatinib (which irreversibly inhibits the tyrosine kinase activities of EGFR and HER2). Patients with an anaplastic lymphoma kinase (ALK, a receptor tyrosine kinase) fusion oncogene can be treated with the protein kinase inhibitors crizotinib and ceritinib.

**Bronchogenic carcinoma** accounts for ~95% of all lung cancer and is subdivided as follows.

**Small-cell lung carcinoma** (**SCLC**, oat cell carcinoma) makes up ~20% of all lung cancer and is mostly related to smoking (see Fig. 1.11). Small-cell tumors show a high rate of mitosis and are also very sensitive to systemic chemotherapy, but they still have the lowest rate of 5-year survival among all patients with lung cancers. SCLC is commonly treated with platinum drugs, which generate intrastrand and interstrand adducts that are repaired by NER and by homologous recombination repair, respectively (see Figs. 2.8 and 2.10 and Sections 3 and 4.2 in Chapter 2).

**Non-small-cell lung carcinoma** (**NSCLC**) makes up ~70% of all lung cancers and is further subdivided into the following three types:

1. **Squamous cell carcinoma** (epidermoid carcinoma; Fig. 8.12) accounts for ~35% of all lung cancers and is related to smoking. About 80% of the tumors contain *TP53* mutations; ~70% contain deletions, promoter methylation, or mutations of the *CDKN2A* gene (encoding the CDK inhibitors p16^Ink4a and p14^Arf); ~50% contain alterations of the PI3K/AKT pathway; and ~35% contain alterations of the RTK/RAS/RAF/ERK pathway.
2. **Adenocarcinoma** (**AC**) occurs in ~25% of all lung cancers and is typically near the periphery of the lung (Fig. 8.13). About 80% of these tumors occur in smokers and ~20% in

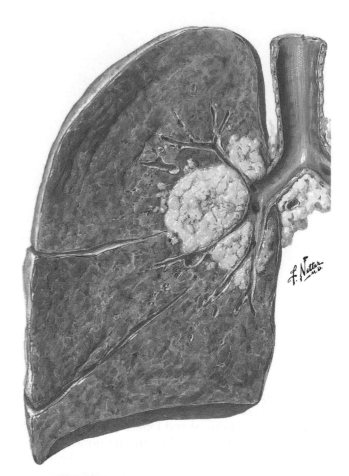

**Fig. 8.12** **Squamous cell lung carcinoma.**

nonsmokers. AC is the most common form of lung cancer in nonsmokers. Lung adenocarcinomas in smokers have about 10-fold the number of mutations in never-smokers. AC is genetically very diverse and difficult to treat successfully. Individualized treatment may be more successful than the standard chemotherapy. Genetic analysis for selected key pathogenic mutations and mutation-matched treatment is now the standard of care. About 75% of the ACs show alterations in the RTK/RAS/RAF pathway (whereby *EGFR* and *KRAS* are key contributors), ~65% have an abnormality in the p53 pathway (almost all attributable to *TP53* mutations), and ~65% have an altered regulation of the cell cycle (e.g., due to a *CDKN2A* alteration). A small fraction of tumors contains a translocation that generates an **ALK** fusion oncogene (for treatment, see earlier discussion).

3. **Large-cell anaplastic carcinoma** (Fig. 8.14) accounts for ~10% of all lung cancers and is usually related to smoking. It has a 5-year survival rate of ~10%, which is the lowest among all NSCLCs.

## 3.3. Prostate Cancer

In the United States, the lifetime risk for prostate cancer in men (Fig. 8.15) is ~14%, which is slightly higher than the lifetime risk for breast cancer in women.

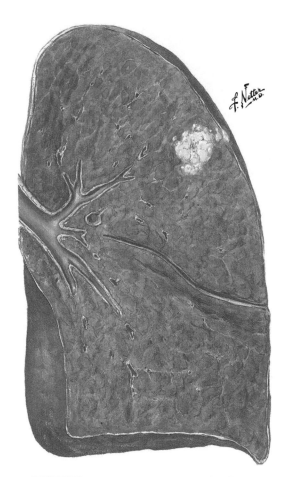

**Fig. 8.13** **Adenocarcinoma of the lung.**

Within the prostate gland, prostate cancer often exists in several distinct foci with the largest focus called the index tumor. The size of the tumor and a histology-derived Gleason grade determine the prognosis.

The main genetic alterations of prostate tumors are **translocations** that place an androgen-regulated promoter next to the gene for the transcription factor ERG or other members of this family. A typical prostate tumor has ~90 chromosome alterations. The genetic makeup of these tumors is very diverse, giving rise to numerous subtypes. Compared with other tumors, prostate tumors have relatively few point mutations.

Aside from surgery and radiation, the treatment of advanced prostate cancer often involves **androgen deprivation therapy**. The concentration of testosterone can be greatly lowered by either surgical or chemical castration (see Section 2.2 in Chapter 31). Taxanes (inhibitors of microtubule degradation; see Section 3.1) are often used as well.

### 3.4. Colorectal Cancer

In the United States, the lifetime risk for colorectal cancer is ~5%.

Colorectal carcinomas arise from adenomatous **polyps** that in turn give rise to **adenomas** that show some dysplasia and increased proliferation. Colonoscopies with the removal of polyps and adenomas can significantly reduce the incidence of colorectal cancer.

Most patients with colorectal cancer have the sporadic form, but ~5% of all patients with colorectal cancer have the heritable cancer syndromes Lynch syndrome, *MUTYH*-associated polyposis (MAP), or FAP.

Patients with **FAP** have a nonfunctional ***APC*** allele in their germline and have lost the function of the second allele in neoplasms. In the United States, FAP affects ~1 in 8000 people. Of all patients with colorectal cancer, ~0.5% have FAP. About 70% of persons have a parent with FAP, and ~30% have FAP due to a de novo mutation, often in the germline of a parent; either way, each offspring of an affected patient has a 50% risk of receiving the faulty *APC* allele. Almost all pathogenic *APC* alleles lead to truncation of the expressed APC protein.

APC is a tumor suppressor that plays a role in the degradation of **β-catenin** (see Fig. 8.5, Section 1.3). In the absence of a WNT signal, β-catenin is degraded. In the presence of a WNT signal, such as during development, APC no longer degrades β-catenin; β-catenin then binds to TCF/LEF family transcription factors, moves to the nucleus, and stimulates the transcription of certain genes that help advance the cell cycle, including *MYC* (see Fig. 8.6). When mutant APC is no longer able to guide the degradation of β-catenin, the cell behaves as if a WNT signal were present that favors cell proliferation.

Patients who have FAP are born with only one functional *APC* allele. Somatic alteration of the second allele (the only functional one) leads to numerous polyps, and if these are not removed, colorectal cancer develops earlier than in persons with two functional APC alleles. Systemic therapy of polyps with the nonsteroidal antiinflammatory drug **sulindac** reduces the average number and size of colorectal polyps.

For patients who have FAP, prophylactic removal of the colon, typically in the patient's 20s, is common. Without colectomy, patients develop hundreds to thousands of adenomas in their colon, and their risk of colorectal cancer is close to 100% by the age of 40 years (Fig. 8.16). Depending on the specific mutation in the *APC* gene, FAP is also associated with polyps in the upper gastrointestinal tract, tumors in the brain (especially medulloblastoma), epidermoid cysts, desmoid tumors, and osteomas (most often in the face).

About 85% of **sporadic** colorectal tumors (Fig. 8.17) have lost the function of APC (as in FAP). Most sporadic colorectal tumors have ~60 mutations that affect the amino acid sequence of a protein. Most of these colorectal tumors have also lost the function of p53 (see Fig. 8.4), and ~40% of the tumors show an increased activity of KRAS (see Fig. 8.3).

Approximately 1% of patients with colorectal cancer have the heritable disorder **MAP** caused by inherited homozygosity or compound heterozygosity for a loss-of-function mutation in the *MUTYH* gene. This hereditary cancer syndrome is unusual in that it shows an autosomal recessive pattern of inheritance. The *MUTYH* gene encodes the **DNA MYH glycosylase,** which is one of the many DNA glycosylases that contribute to BER of DNA (see Section 1 in Chapter 2). The phenotype of MAP is generally milder than that of FAP, although there is great variability.

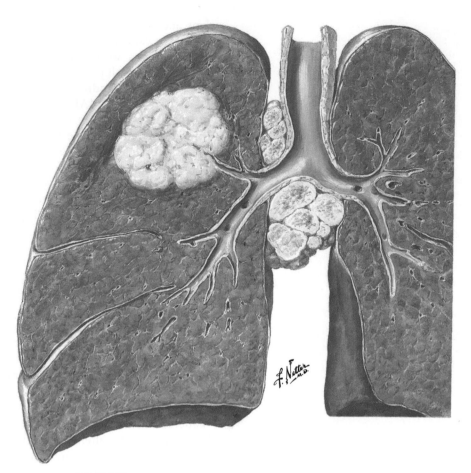

**Fig. 8.14** Large-cell anaplastic carcinoma of the lung.

**Lynch syndrome (hereditary nonpolyposis colon cancer)** is caused by a problem with DNA mismatch repair (see Section 2 in Chapter 2). This hereditary cancer syndrome accounts for ~3% of all colorectal tumors and is thus considerably more common than FAP. About 70% of patients who have Lynch syndrome inherit a mutant *MLH1* or *MSH2* allele, and the remainder have mutant alleles of the *PMS2* or *MSH6* genes (see Table 2.1 in Chapter 2). With time, some somatic cells, for instance in the colon, acquire a genetic alteration that leads to loss of the remaining functional allele, which impairs mismatch repair. This leads to replication errors throughout the genome, but especially in **short tandem repeats (microsatellites**; e.g., $A_{26}$ or $C_8$).

Besides colorectal cancer (see Fig. 2.5), patients with Lynch syndrome also have a much higher risk of developing other cancers, notably cancer of the endometrium, upper urinary tract, stomach, and small intestine.

About 15% of **sporadic** colon cancers show impaired mismatch repair (as in Lynch syndrome) and as a result contain ~700 mutations that change an amino acid sequence (this is ~10 times the number of mutations in mismatch repair competent cells; see earlier discussion). This type of sporadic colon cancer, as well as colorectal tumors in patients with Lynch syndrome, is sometimes called the **mutator phenotype**. Besides the loss of mismatch repair, WNT signaling (see Fig.

8.5) is almost always activated (mostly via loss of APC function), and the RAS/RAF/ERK pathway (see Fig. 8.3) is overly active (mostly due to activating mutations in the *BRAF, KRAS,* and *NRAS* proto-oncogenes).

Screening for defective mismatch repair is typically performed with **microsatellite analysis** or **immunohistochemical staining** for mismatch repair proteins, as described in Section 2 in Chapter 2.

Massive parallel sequencing (see Chapter 4) of a panel of genes known to cause hereditary colon cancer is now an option in genetic counseling.

Systemic treatment for metastatic colorectal cancer typically involves a cocktail of chemotherapeutic drugs, such as **fluorouracil** (see Fig. 37.7 and Section 5.1 in Chapter 37), **leucovorin** (to amplify the effect of fluorouracil; see Fig. 37.7 and Section 5.1 in Chapter 37), and either the platinum drug **oxaliplatin** (a regimen known as FOLFOX; see also Fig. 2.8 and Section 3 in Chapter 2) or the topoisomerase I inhibitor **irinotecan** (a regimen known as FOLFIRI; see Section 5 in Chapter 1). Patients whose tumors have a mismatch repair deficiency are not treated with fluorouracil because of a lack of benefit (the mechanism is unclear).

Therapy of metastatic colon cancer is often amplified with drugs that target the **EGF receptor** or vascular endothelial growth factor (**VEGF**) signaling. VEGF leads to growth of

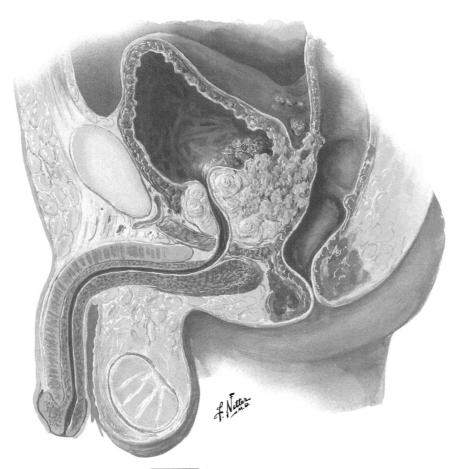

**Fig. 8.15**  **Prostate cancer.**

new blood vessels, such as into tumor tissue. Antibodies that target the EGFR are most effective in the setting of wild-type *RAS* genes (*RAS* is downstream of the EGFR; see Fig. 8.3).

### 3.5. Melanoma

In the United States, a person's lifetime risk for melanoma of the skin is ~2%.

Melanoma of the skin originates from **melanocytes** in the epidermis, which produce melanin pigments (see also Figs. 35.14 and 35.15). Melanomas (Fig. 8.18) are often recognized by their irregular borders, size (>6 mm in diameter), varied color, and change in appearance over time.

**UV radiation**, low-level skin **pigmentation, freckling**, and a large number of **nevi** are significant risk factors for cutaneous malignant melanoma. Clothing and sunscreen can significantly attenuate outdoor UV irradiation and reduce melanoma risk, as can self-examination of the skin for lesions.

Melanomas are classified on the basis of their shape, size, and invasion of other tissue layers. Locally confined melanomas are readily amenable to surgery, whereas highly metastasized melanomas have a poor prognosis.

Many patients with metastatic melanoma are treated with **immunotherapy**. Pharmacological immunotherapy favors the recognition of melanoma cells by T cells, followed by the destruction of tumor cells.

About 35% of patients with melanoma have a $\textbf{\textit{BRAF}}^{\textbf{V600}}$ **mutation** that activates *BRAF* constitutively. **Vemurafenib** and **dabrafenib** inhibit $\textit{BRAF}^{V600}$ and generally cause shrinkage of tumors, but this is unfortunately followed by relapse due to drug resistance. Similarly, the drug **trametinib**, which inhibits **MAP/ERK kinase** (downstream of *BRAF*; see Fig. 8.3), is initially effective but eventually becomes ineffective. A longer period of remission is obtained with the combination of a BRAF inhibitor and an ERK inhibitor.

About 25% of melanomas contain an activating mutation in the *NRAS* gene (NRAS is upstream of BRAF in the RTK/RAS/RAF/ERK pathway; see Fig. 8.3). Currently no approved drugs that inhibit mutant NRAS are available. Inhibition of the downstream kinase BRAF is (surprisingly) counterproductive.

**Familial melanoma** is a hereditary cancer syndrome that in ~50% of patients is due to an inherited mutant $\textbf{\textit{CDKN2A}}$ gene, which encodes **p16$^{\text{Ink4a}}$** and p14ARF. The prevalence of familial melanoma is ~4%. p16$^{\text{Ink4a}}$ normally inhibits cyclin D/CDK4 and cyclin D/CDK6 (see Figs. 8.1 and 8.2). p14$^{\text{ARF}}$ normally inactivates MDM2 and thus stabilizes p53 (see Fig. 8.4). Most pathogenic mutations of the *CDKN2A* gene lead to loss of only p16$^{\text{Ink4a}}$ function, but patients with these mutations also have an increased risk for **pancreatic cancer**.

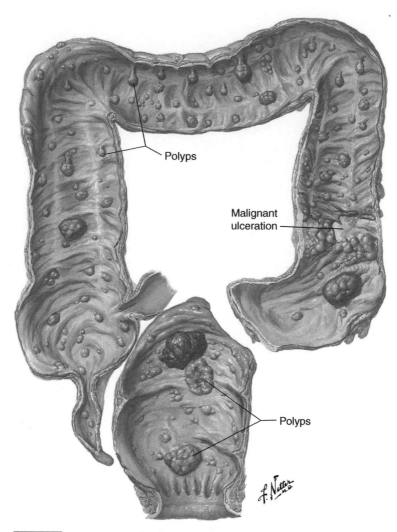

**Fig. 8.16** **Familial adenomatous polyposis of the large intestine.**

## 4. GLUCOSE USE BY TUMORS

*Tumors use considerably more glucose than normal cells. Positron emission tomography (PET) scanning of patients after the infusion of a radioactive glucose analog helps locate metastases.*

Even well-oxygenated tumor cells generate comparable amounts of adenosine triphosphate (ATP) via anaerobic and aerobic glycolysis, whereas normal cells produce almost all of their ATP via aerobic glycolysis. This observation is commonly referred to as the **Warburg effect**. No widely accepted explanation is yet found for the Warburg effect.

**PET** with radioactively labeled **2-fluoro-deoxyglucose** (2FDG) takes advantage of the increased glucose use of tumor cells (Fig. 8.19; 2FDG uptake is described in Section 6.3 in Chapter 19). PET studies are commonly used to reveal metastases.

### SUMMARY

- Quiescent cells are in the G0 phase. The activation of growth factor receptors induces a transition from the G0 to the G1 phase via synthesis of cyclin D, activation of CDK4 and CDK6, and phosphorylation of RB, which in turn releases E2Fs that alter transcription such that more cyclin D and E are expressed.

- p52 becomes active in response to phosphorylation by the kinases ATM, ATR, CHK1, or CHK2, which in turn become active in response to DNA damage. Activated p52 acts as a transcription factor that increases the transcription of genes that encode the CDK inhibitor protein (CKI) p21 and the proapoptotic BAX.

- WNT signaling via Frizzled receptors leads to an increase in the concentration of β-catenin, which in turn activates transcription factors of the TCF/LEF family. The TCF/LEF transcription factors enhance the transcription of the *MYC* gene and many other genes. MYC in turn is a transcription factor that affects the transcription of a large number of genes.

- About half of the patients with hereditary breast and ovarian cancer syndrome have inherited a defective *BRCA1* or *BRCA2* allele. Genetic alterations in cells of the breast and in other tissues that lead to the loss of function of the remaining BRCA allele are tumorigenic. Through

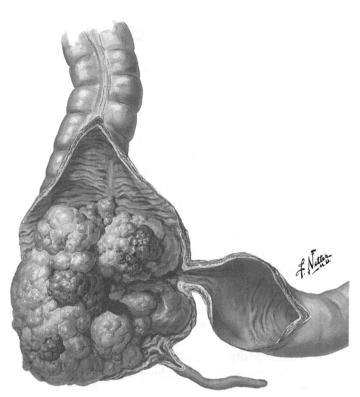

Fig. 8.17 **Carcinoma of the cecum.**

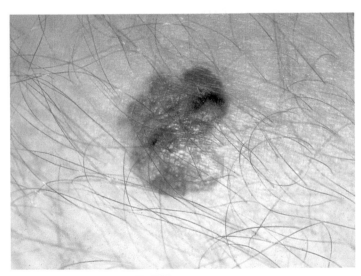

Fig. 8.18 **Melanoma.**

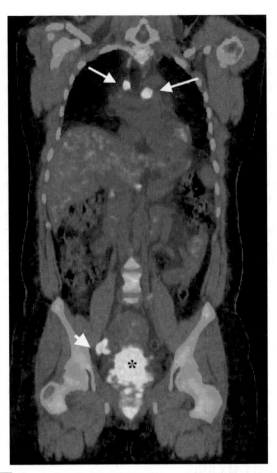

Fig. 8.19 **A coronal fused image of 2-$^{18}$F-deoxyglucose–based positron emission tomography and computed tomography (obtained with x-rays) of a patient with squamous cell carcinoma of the cervix.** The *asterisk* marks the primary tumor. The *short arrow* indicates a nearby adenoma, and the *long arrows* indicate lymph nodes in the mediastinum. (From Viswanathan C, Bhosale PR, Shah SN, Vikram R. Positron emission tomography-computed tomography imaging for malignancies in women. *Radiol Clin North Am.* 2013;51:1111-1125.)

synthetic lethality, PARP inhibitors are especially toxic to tumor cells that lack functional BRCA1 or BRCA2.

■ Lung cancers of smokers contain many more mutations than cancers of nonsmokers. Small-cell lung cancer develops mostly in smokers, is treated with platinum drugs, and is associated with a low rate of survival. Squamous cell carcinomas are also related to smoking and frequently show mutations in *TP53* and *CDKN2A*. Lung adenocarcinomas (ACs), which occur in both smokers and nonsmokers, are genetically very diverse but often contain mutations in *EGFR*, *KRAS*, *TP53*, and *CDKN2A*.

■ Tumors of the prostate usually contain a large number of translocations, and their growth is driven by androgens. The tumors are genetically highly diverse. Pharmacological treatment of advanced prostate cancer often includes androgen deprivation and taxanes (inhibitors of microtubule depolymerization).

■ Familial adenomatous polyposis (FAP) is caused by heterozygosity for a loss-of-function *APC* allele. APC plays a role in degrading β-catenin in the cytosol. Somatic loss of the second, functional *APC* allele is tumorigenic. Affected patients have hundreds to thousands of polyps in their colon and develop colon cancer unless they have a colectomy. Most patients with sporadic colorectal cancer also have lost the function of their APC protein.

■ *MUTYH*-associated polyposis (MAP) is due to an autosomal recessively inherited loss of DNA MYH glycosylase activity and resembles an attenuated form of FAP.

■ Lynch syndrome is caused by heterozygosity for a loss-of-function allele for one of the mismatch repair proteins (most often MLH1 or MSH2). Somatic loss of the second, functional allele is tumorigenic. This causes microsatellite instability. A minority of patients with sporadic colorectal cancer also have lost the function of the mismatch repair pathway. Fluorouracil is ineffective in these patients.

■ The risk for malignant melanoma of the skin rises with freckling, number of nevi, and exposure to sunlight. Furthermore, ~2% of the population has a mutation in the *CDKN2A* gene that causes familial melanoma because of the loss of p16[Ink4a] function; p16 normally inhibits cyclin D–activated CDK4 and CDK6. Patients who are heterozygous for loss of p16 are also at an increased risk of pancreatic cancer. About one-third of patients with sporadic melanoma have constitutively active V600E mutant BRAF, and metastases of such tumors are best treated with a combination of a BRAF inhibitor and a MEK inhibitor.

■ Tumor cells often use more glucose than normal cells, and 2-18F-deoxyglucose-based PET is used to locate metastases.

## FURTHER READING

■ Aoude LG, Wadt KA, Pritchard AL, Hayward NK. Genetics of familial melanoma: 20 years after CDKN2A. *Pigment Cell Melanoma Res.* 2015;28:148-160.

■ Cancer Genome Atlas Research Network. Comprehensive molecular profiling of lung adenocarcinoma. *Nature.* 2014;511:543-550.

■ Fearon ER. Colon and rectal cancer. In: Mendelsohn J, Gray JW, Howley PM, Israel MA, Thompson CB, eds. *The Molecular Basis of Cancer.* 4th ed. Philadelphia, PA: Elsevier-Saunders; 2015:499-513.

■ Hecht SS. Tobacco smoke carcinogens and lung cancer. *J Natl Cancer Inst.* 1999;91(14):1194-1210.

■ Mukherjee S. *The Emperor of all Maladies: A Biography of Cancer.* New York: Scribner; 2010.

■ Renehan AG, Zwahlen M, Egger M. Adiposity and cancer risk: new mechanistic insights from epidemiology. *Nat Rev Cancer.* 2015;15:484-498.

■ Roos WP, Thomas AD, Kaina B. DNA damage and the balance between survival and death in cancer biology. *Nat Rev Cancer.* 2016;16:20-33.

■ Roy-Chowdhuri S, de Melo Gagliato D, Routbort MJ, et al. Multigene clinical mutational profiling of breast carcinoma using next-generation sequencing. *Am J Clin Pathol.* 2015;144:713-721.

■ Tomasetti C, Vogelstein B. Variation in cancer risk among tissues can be explained by the number of stem cell divisions. *Science.* 2015;347:78-81.

■ Vogelstein B, Papadopoulos N, Velculescu VE, Zhou S, Diaz LA Jr, Kinzler KW. Cancer genome landscapes. *Science.* 2013;339:1546-1558.

# Review Questions

1. Which one of the following alterations of the genome most favors a neoplasm?

   **A.** A mutation that gives rise to E2F that has increased affinity for RB
   **B.** Amplification of the *CCND1* gene, which encodes cyclin D1
   **C.** Amplification of the *CDKN2A* gene
   **D.** Amplification of the *TP53* gene
   **E.** Loss of the *MDM2* gene

2. A 50-year-old patient with cancer of the colon and which one of the following characteristics is most likely to have Lynch syndrome?

   **A.** Colon tumor that does not stain for MLH1
   **B.** Colon tumor that shows microsatellite instability
   **C.** Has a grandfather who died of colon cancer at age 70 years
   **D.** Heterozygosity for a loss-of-function mutation in the *MSH2* gene in blood lymphocytes

3. Cowden syndrome is a heritable disorder that is caused by which of the following?

   **A.** Amplification of *MYC*
   **B.** Heterozygous deletion of *CDKN2A*
   **C.** Heterozygous loss-of-function mutation in *PTEN*
   **D.** Methylation of *RB1* promoter
   **E.** Methylation of *TP53* promoter

4. A 50-year-old patient underwent colonoscopy for the first time and was found to have colon cancer, as well as ~100 adenomas in the colon. Neither the parents nor the grandparents of the patient ever had colon cancer. The most likely diagnosis for this patient is which of the following?

   **A.** FAP
   **B.** Lynch syndrome
   **C.** *MUTYH*-associated polyposis
   **D.** Sporadic colorectal cancer

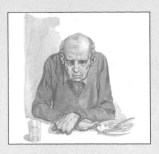

# Chapter 9

# Structure of Proteins and Protein Aggregates in Degenerative Diseases

## SYNOPSIS

■ Proteins are made of linear chains of amino acids. During translation, 21 different amino acids can be incorporated into the nascent peptide chain. Many of these amino acids can be modified after translation.

■ The sequence, posttranslational modification, and diversity of chemical properties of amino acids give rise to an amazing variety of proteins.

■ Proteins are held in their three-dimensional shape through numerous means, such as hydrogen bonds, hydrophobic effects, electrostatic interactions, van der Waals interactions, and chemical crosslinks (e.g., disulfide bridges).

■ The three-dimensional structures of proteins contain common elements; two such abundant elements are the α-helix and the β-sheet.

■ In the course of evolution, mixing and matching let many motifs (e.g., a sequence of amino acids that binds a nucleotide) become part of proteins that now serve diverse functions.

■ Proteins often contain domains that have a defined structure, regardless of flanking sequences. Each one of these domains has a function (e.g., binding DNA or holding and enclosing a substrate in an enzyme).

■ Proteins fold during and after synthesis, sometimes with the assistance of chaperone proteins.

■ The physiological, three-dimensional structure of proteins is only marginally stable. When this structure is lost, the protein no longer has the same function, and it is said to be denatured. By themselves, many denatured proteins cannot regain their original physiological shape.

■ Some proteins or portions of proteins normally have no discernible higher-order structure.

■ Denaturation of proteins in the stomach helps their digestion in the stomach and intestine, and it also kills pathogens. Similarly, in health care, denaturation and modification of proteins are used extensively to destroy pathogens.

■ Pathologic intracellular or extracellular aggregation of proteins is found in a number of diseases, for instance in Alzheimer disease, Parkinson disease, and amyloidosis due to chronic dialysis.

## LEARNING OBJECTIVES

*For mastery of this topic, you should be able to do the following:*

■ Explain the forces that hold most proteins in their native shape.

■ Draw a standard cartoon of an α-helix, a parallel β-sheet, and an antiparallel β-sheet. Indicate the location of the amino acid side chains relative to these images.

■ Describe the forces and secondary structures that favor aggregation of proteins.

■ Describe the changes in protein structure that occur when proteins are denatured.

■ Describe the effects of commonly used disinfectants (e.g., iodine, alcohols, hydrogen peroxide, and heat) on proteins.

■ Describe the nature and basic structure of amyloid, and indicate techniques to make amyloid visible.

## 1. AMINO ACIDS AS BUILDING BLOCKS OF PEPTIDES AND PROTEINS

*Amino acids consist of a constant $NH_3^+$–CH–COO⁻ group and a variable side chain. The diversity of chemical properties of side chains and the orientation of amino acids in space give rise to a great range of functions of peptides and proteins. Amino acids can be ordered into groups, the most important of which are nonpolar, polar uncharged, and polar charged.*

### 1.1. General Comments About Amino Acids

Peptides, polypeptides, and proteins are polymers of amino acids, in which the amino acids are linked via peptide bonds (see Section 2). A dipeptide consists of two amino acids, a tripeptide of three, a tetrapeptide of four, etc. The name **peptide** is commonly used for polymers that contain fewer than 50 amino acids, and the name **protein** is used for polymers that contain 50 or more amino acids. The term **polypeptide** is used for peptides or proteins that contain more than ~15 amino acids. However, there are no generally agreed-upon definitions.

Amino acids have the general structure $H_2N$–CH(R)–COOH; R represents the so-called **side chain** (Fig. 9.1). Different amino acids have different side chains. In solution, at a neutral pH, $H_2N$– becomes protonated to $H_3N^+$–, and –COOH is deprotonated to –COO⁻ (see the discussion of charged amino acids below). In peptides and proteins, the structure $H_2N$–CH–COOH becomes part of the peptide backbone.

There are L- and D-isomers of chiral amino acids (see Fig. 9.1). Glycine is not chiral, because R=H so that the central C-atom has two identical substituents. The "central" C-atom (called $C_\alpha$) of the other amino acids has four *different* substituents and is *chiral*. In the human body, practically all amino acids in peptides and proteins are of the **L-isomer**. In humans, the D-isomer has been found only in free amino acids to date (e.g., D-serine and D-aspartate, which play a role in signaling in the nervous system).

Messenger RNA encodes the synthesis of peptides and proteins from 21 different amino acids. The names of these amino acids, as well as their three- and one-letter abbreviations, are listed in Table 9.1. The DNA trinucleotide sequences that code for these amino acids are shown in Table 8.1. **Selenocysteine** is encoded by a combination of a UGA stop codon and a

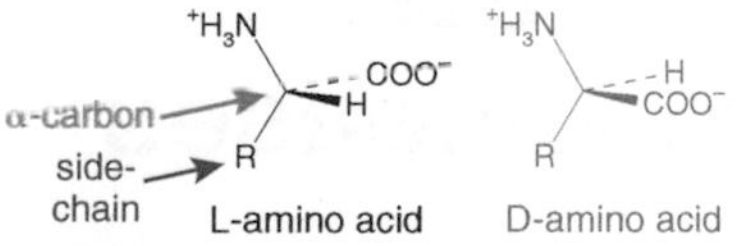

**Fig. 9.1** **L- and D-amino acids.**

**Table 9.1** **Names and Abbreviations of the Genetically Encoded Amino Acids**

| 1-Letter Abbreviation | Full Name | 3-Letter Abbreviation |
|---|---|---|
| A | Alanine | Ala |
| C | Cysteine | Cys |
| D | Aspartate | Asp |
| E | Glutamate | Glu |
| F | Phenylalanine | Phe |
| G | Glycine | Gly |
| H | Histidine | His |
| I | Isoleucine | Ile |
| K | Lysine | Lys |
| L | Leucine | Leu |
| M | Methionine | Met |
| N | Asparagine | Asn |
| P | Proline | Pro |
| Q | Glutamine | Gln |
| R | Arginine | Arg |
| S | Serine | Ser |
| T | Threonine | Thr |
| U | Selenocysteine | Sec |
| V | Valine | Val |
| W | Tryptophan | Trp |
| Y | Tyrosine | Tyr |

selenocysteine insertion sequence (SECIS) in the 3′-UTR of an mRNA. Examples of proteins that contain selenocysteine are glutathione peroxidase (see Chapter 21) and thioredoxin reductase (see Chapter 37).

## 1.2. Classification of Amino Acids

Fig. 9.2 shows the structures of the genetically encoded L-amino acids. Differences in the structure are confined to the side chain, except for proline, which also contains a bond between the main-chain amino group and the side chain (strictly speaking, it is therefore an imino acid).

The group of **nonpolar amino acids** contains a variety of subgroups. **Glycine** is the smallest of all amino acids, as its side chain is –H. Glycine provides the greatest flexibility for the three-dimensional course of a protein backbone. **Aliphatic** amino acids (**alanine, valine, leucine, isoleucine**) are progressively more hydrophobic as the nonpolar surface area of their side chain increases. Aliphatic amino acid side chains commonly participate in hydrophobic effects and van der Waals interactions (see Section 3). These occur for instance within the protein, between membrane proteins and membrane lipids, between proteins and organic compounds that are important to protein function, and between enzymes and substrates. Amino acids with **sulfur** in their side chain include **methionine** and **cysteine**. Methionine is commonly the first (i.e., N-terminal) amino acid of a newly synthesized protein, but this residue is often removed during posttranslational processing. Two cysteine side chains can become oxidized to form a **disulfide bond** (–S–S–, also called a **disulfide bridge**). Such disulfide bonds are often an important determinant of the final structure of a protein. **Phenylalanine** and **tryptophan** are nonpolar amino acids that have hydrophobic **aromatic** side chains. The aromatic side chains need a relatively large amount of space. The benzene rings of Phe and Trp can hold a small ion or a methyl group or benzene ring of another molecule in place. The side chain of **proline** is linked to the N-atom of the invariant $NH_2^+$–CH–COO$^-$ group, creating a ring, which reduces the flexibility of the $NH_2^+$–CH–COO$^-$ group and imposes additional steric constraints on the peptide backbone. For this reason, as detailed in Section 4.1, proline induces a kink into α-helices. On the other hand, proline, like glycine, can help form a sharp turn of the peptide chain, and it is therefore often found in such turns (see Section 4). **Selenocysteine** is found in a few enzymes that use this residue near their catalytic site. Examples are given above.

The group of **polar, uncharged amino acids** includes the amino acids that have either a hydroxyl group or an amido group in their side chain. **Tyrosine**, like phenylalanine and tryptophan mentioned above, has an aromatic side chain, but its side chain is also polar due to the hydroxyl group. The hydroxyl group can be phosphorylated or sulfated. Phosphorylation of tyrosine plays a prominent role in growth factor signaling (see Chapters 26 and 33). **Serine** and **threonine** also carry a hydroxyl group on their side chain, and this hydroxyl group can be conjugated with a phosphate, sulfate, or a polysaccharide. Phosphorylation of Ser or Thr is a widespread regulatory means of altering the properties of a protein. **Glutamine** and **asparagine** contain amido groups (–CO–NH$_2$). The NH$_2$ group can *donate* one or two hydrogen atoms while the C=O group can *accept* one or two hydrogen atoms to form one or more hydrogen bonds (see Section 3.2). These side chains are very hydrophilic because they can form hydrogen bonds with water.

The group of **polar, charged amino acids** includes aspartate, glutamate, lysine, arginine, and histidine. The side chains

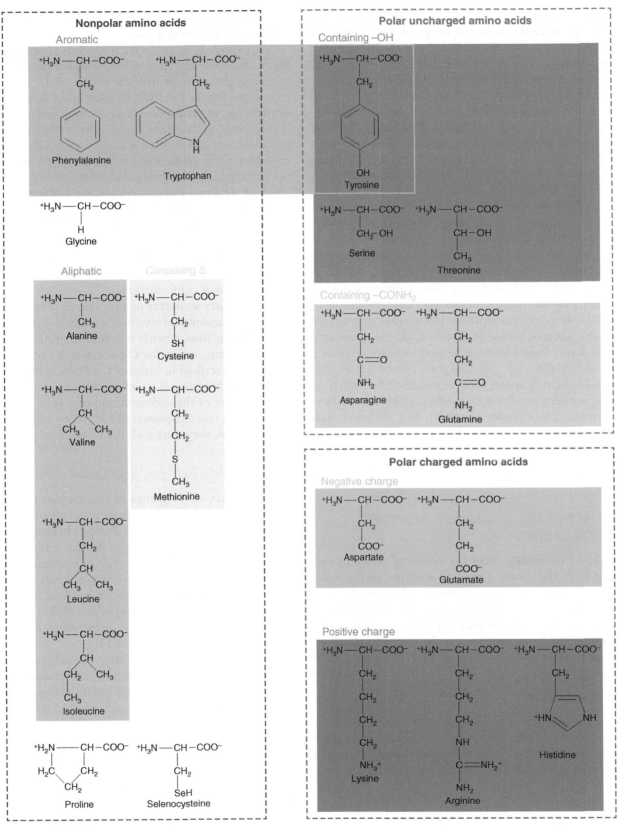

**Fig. 9.2** **Structures of the amino acids that ribosomes incorporate into nascent peptide chains.**

of **aspartate** and **glutamate** end in $-COO^-$. The pK for the carboxyl group ($-COOH$) is in the range of 4 to 5. At a pH *larger* than the pK, most of the carboxyl groups *lose* a proton and are **negatively** charged ($-COO^-$). The negatively charged carboxyl groups of glutamate and aspartate often interact electrostatically with other groups. In addition, the carboxyl group also forms hydrogen bonds. Glutamate and aspartate are frequently found near the catalytic centers of enzymes or at sites of protein-protein interaction. **Lysine** and **arginine** have **positively** charged side chains. The pK for the amino group ($-NH_2$) of lysine is ~10, and the pK for $=NH$ in the guanidino group $[-NH-C(NH)-NH_2]$ of arginine is ~12. At a pH *lower* than these pK values, most of the amino and guanidino groups gain a proton and are positively charged ($-NH_3^+$, $NH-C(NH_2^+)-NH_2$), as shown in Fig. 9.2. The side chains of lysine and arginine (like those of glutamate and aspartate mentioned above) form electrostatic interactions as well as hydrogen bonds. In DNA-binding proteins, lysine and arginine frequently coordinate the negatively charged phosphate moieties of the deoxyribonucleotides. In enzymes that require the prosthetic groups biotin or lipoic acid, the prosthetic group is covalently linked to the side chain amino group of a lysine near the catalytic site (see Chapters 10 and 22). In histones, the side chain of lysine is often modified by methyl or acetyl groups; these modifications affect DNA compaction and transcription (see Chapters 1 and 6). At a pH lower than ~6 to 7 (depending on the exact environment in a particular protein), most of the side chains of **histidine** are also positively charged. Histidine is often the donor and acceptor of $H^+$ in the active site of enzymes that catalyze $H^+$ transfer.

## 2. PEPTIDE BONDS, DISULFIDE BRIDGES, AND CROSSLINKS

*A peptide bond covalently links the carboxyl group of one amino acid with the amino group of another amino acid, thus giving rise to peptides and proteins. The peptide bond (C–N in –CO–NH–) has partial double-bond character, thereby limiting the conformational flexibility of peptides and proteins. Peptides or proteins can be linked by disulfide bridges or crosslinks.*

### 2.1. Peptide Bonds

In peptides, the carboxyl group of one amino acid (shown in black in Fig. 9.3) is linked to the amino group of another amino acid (shown in blue) via a **peptide bond** (an amide bond). The **peptide backbone** of peptides or proteins refers to the peptide-linked, repeated sequence $-N-CH-CO-$ that is common to all amino acids.

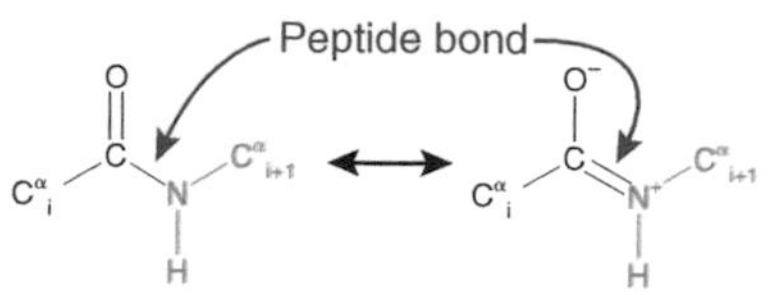

The peptide bond (C–N in –CO–NH–) has partial double-bond character and cannot rotate freely (see Fig. 9.3); the other bonds in the peptide backbone, $N-C_\alpha$ and $C_\alpha-C$, are true single bonds, but their rotation is limited by **steric hindrance** (i.e., atoms are not allowed to encroach on each other's space). Nonetheless, there is sufficient flexibility that the polypeptide chain can assume a huge variety of conformations, anywhere from an unlikely, fully extended conformation to the common, folded, functional, energetically favorable, and compact structure (for protein folding, see Section 4).

Amino acids with *small* side chains (e.g., glycine) afford the peptide backbone greater conformational flexibility than amino acids with *bulky* side chains (e.g., tryptophan). Proline, which has a *ring-locked* imino group instead of a rotatable amino group, locally constrains the backbone to an especially limited range of conformations.

The **primary structure** of a peptide or protein is the linear **sequence** of amino acid residues from the N- to the C-terminus. At the **N-terminus**, a newly synthesized protein has an amino [$^+H_3N-$] group, and at the **C-terminus**, a carboxyl [$-COO^-$] group. As described in Chapter 1, a DNA sequence is written $5' \rightarrow 3'$. The N-terminal amino acids of a protein are encoded on the 5'-side of the coding strand of a gene and the 5'-side of an mRNA (see Chapters 6 and 7). When ribosomes synthesize a protein, they start with the N-terminal amino acid.

## 2.2. Disulfide Bridges and Other Crosslinks

The side chain –S–H groups of two *cysteine* residues can be oxidized to form an –S–S– bond, which is called a **disulfide bridge** or a **disulfide bond**. A disulfide bridge can form both within a single polypeptide (e.g., human serum albumin; see Fig. 9.6), and also between subunits of a protein complex (e.g., between the subunits of the insulin receptor).

The side chains of *lysine* can be oxidized and then **crosslinked**; this happens with collagen and elastin in the extracellular matrix, for example, and gives rise to large and tough structures (see Chapters 12 and 13).

Besides an occasional covalent crosslinkage (sometimes between protein subunits), the three-dimensional structure of a folded, native protein is stabilized by scores of noncovalent interactions between atoms (see Sections 3 and 4).

## 3. FORCES THAT DETERMINE THE CONFORMATION OF PROTEINS AND PEPTIDES

*Numerous interactions between atoms stabilize the three-dimensional structure of peptides and proteins. These interactions consist of hydrogen bonds, hydrophobic effects, electrostatic interactions, and van der Waals interactions.*

### 3.1. Hydrophobic Effects

When hydrophobic molecules enter water, they disturb the normal, hydrogen-bonded structure of water. The tendency of

**Fig. 9.3** **Nature of the peptide bond.** The peptide bond is shown in the trans configuration, which is the most common. A cis-configuration (180-degree rotation around C-N) occurs mostly with proline.

the overall system to assume the lowest possible energy state makes the hydrophobic molecules stick together when they face water. This allows for maximal hydrogen bonding among water molecules. (Likewise, a few drops of cooking oil in water tend to coalesce into a single puddle.)

Hydrophobic effects amount to ~90% of the forces that keep a protein in the shape of a globule. The remaining drive toward the normal physiological shape of a protein derives from hydrogen bonding, ionic interactions, and van der Waals forces (see below).

Hydrophobic effects are an important driving force not only for the conformation of each single protein but also for the interaction of proteins with other molecules. For instance, proteins can interact with other proteins via **leucine zippers**, which are often found in transcription factors (Fig. 6.6). A protein can be anchored in a *lipid membrane* by hydrophobic effects between amino acid side chains and fatty acid tails or cholesterol in the membrane. In proteins that are enzymes, hydrophobic amino acid side chains often form a water-free environment for the chemical reaction that the enzyme catalyzes. In yet other proteins, hydrophobic effects often contribute substantially to the binding of *organic compounds*, thereby influencing their characteristics (e.g., heme in hemoglobin; see Chapter 14).

Approximately equal amounts of hydrophobic amino acids are generally found on the surface and in the interior of proteins. It is often erroneously suggested that hydrophobic amino acids are found almost exclusively in the interior of proteins. However, even the partial burying of hydrophobic side chains is energetically favorable, and therefore hydrophobic side chains on the protein surface help a protein assume a compact, globular shape. Furthermore, the chemical properties of many hydrophobic amino acid side chains are quite complex. Thus, the side chains of tryptophan and tyrosine have both a hydrophobic portion (the benzene ring) and a hydrophilic portion (the >N–H in the second ring of tryptophan, and the –OH on the benzene ring of tyrosine) that can participate in hydrogen bonding (>NH and –OH are hydrogen donors; –O– is a hydrogen acceptor). Hence, tryptophan and tyrosine are often found at the interface between the hydrophobic portion of the membrane lipid bilayer and the more hydrophilic phospholipid head groups (i.e., between the hydrophobic tails of the fatty acids in phospholipids and the carbonyl groups that are part of the –CO–O– ester link between fatty acids and the glycerol moiety of phospholipids; see Chapter 11).

## 3.2. Hydrogen Bonds

Hydrogen bonds form when two electronegative atoms each partially bind to a hydrogen atom. To this end, a **hydrogen donor**, such as –OH or –NH, must interact with a **hydrogen acceptor**, such as –O or –N. If a hydrogen bond forms between –N–H and O–, it is often schematically drawn as –N–H·····O–. Carbon atoms are not sufficiently electronegative to participate in hydrogen bonds.

The peptide backbone contains hydrogen donors in the –N–H and hydrogen acceptors in the =O of each amide group (–CO–NH–; Fig. 9.4); however, for steric reasons the donor and acceptor must come from different amino acid residues (see Sections 4.1 and 4.2).

The amino acid *side chains* contain the hydrogen donors –O–H (in Ser, Thr, Tyr), –N–H (in Trp, Asn, Gln, Lys, Arg, His), –S–H (in Cys), and –Se–H (in Sec), as well as the hydrogen acceptors =O (in Asn, Gln, Asp, Glu), –O– (in Ser, Thr, Tyr), and –N= (in His). *Water* can act as both a hydrogen donor and hydrogen acceptor.

Formation of a hydrogen bond generally liberates ~6% as much energy as the formation of a covalent C–C bond. The reaction of a hydrogen donor with an acceptor *within* a polypeptide is energetically more favorable than with *surrounding water* molecules. Hydrogen bonding between atoms of the peptide backbone stabilizes peptide α-helices and β-sheets (see Sections 4.1 and 4.2).

## 3.3. Electrostatic Interactions

Electrostatic interactions are the result of the attraction of unlike charges and the repulsion of like charges. Atoms of the peptide backbone are essentially uncharged, except for the amino and carboxyl termini. The amino acid side chains of Asp and Glu are *negatively* charged (see Fig. 9.2), while those of Lys and Arg (and sometimes His) are *positively* charged. The water molecule is a dipole: its O-atom carries approximately two-thirds of a negative charge, and its hydrogen atoms each carry approximately one-third of a positive charge. If a charged amino acid is brought into water, water molecules orient around the amino acid based on charge attraction and repulsion. For instance, if the –COO⁻ group of a glutamate side chain faces water, water molecules order such that their H atoms are closest to the negative charge of –COO⁻, while their O-atoms are farthest from the negative charge of –COO⁻.

Removing a *single* charge from the protein surface and burying it inside a protein carries a very high energy penalty (~50% as much energy as the formation of a covalent C–C bond). Therefore, almost all charged residues are on the surface of a protein, and if a charged residue is in the protein interior, it almost always interacts with a nearby opposite charge.

Arginine and lysine carry their positively charged groups on the tip of a somewhat hydrophobic side chain. In membrane proteins, much of this chain can be located next to the hydrophobic portion of membrane lipids (see Chapter 11), and the positively charged portion can interact with the negatively charged phosphate groups of phospholipids (fittingly, arginine and lysine are said to "snorkel").

## 3.4. Van der Waals Interactions

The term van der Waals forces is used inconsistently. Originally, the term referred to all attractive forces between molecules that influence the behavior of gasses. Van der Waals forces in the original sense includes interactions between molecules that have a permanent, induced, or temporary **dipole**. A molecule has a dipole when the center of its positive charge

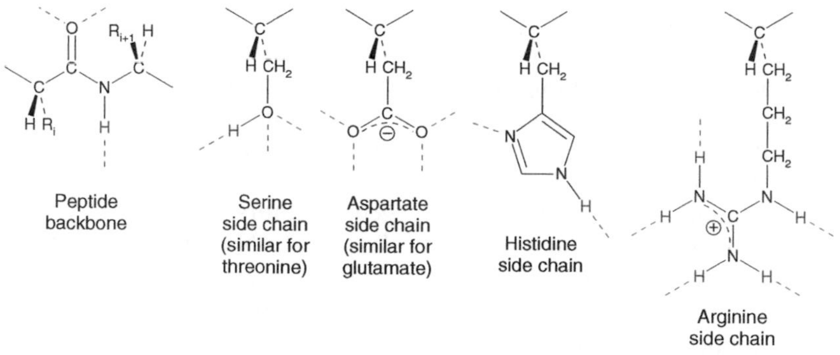

**Fig. 9.4** **Hydrogen bonding in proteins.** The maximum number of hydrogen bonds that can be expected to form are shown in red. In nature, atoms that are shown here to form two hydrogen bonds often form only one hydrogen bond.

differs from the center of its negative charge (i.e., typically, when a more electronegative atom attracts electrons more than a less electronegative atom). In this case, the dipole is *permanent* (e.g., a carbonyl group, which carries a slight excess negative charge on O and a slight excess positive charge on C). A dipole is *temporary* when it is simply due to the movement of electrons around nuclei (an example would be a molecule of $H_2$, which has two nuclei and two electrons). A dipole is said to be *induced* if it occurs in response to the nearby appearance of a charge (e.g., the charge of an amino acid side chain such as glutamate or lysine).

In this book, the term van der Waals interactions is used to describe weak, short-range interactions that result from a combination of the following forces: attraction between the positively charged *nucleus* of one atom and the negatively charged *electrons* of another atom, electrostatic interactions between atoms that carry a slight charge due to the presence of a dipole moment, and the repulsion of electrons between filled electron orbitals.

Favorable van der Waals interactions can occur between all types of atoms, are extremely sensitive to the distance between atoms, and require close packing of atoms.

## 3.5. Coordination of Metal Ions

Metal ions (e.g., $Ca^{2+}$, $Mn^{2+}$, $Fe^{2+}$, $Fe^{3+}$, $Zn^{2+}$, or $Cu^{2+}$) often coordinate with amino acid side chains. A well-known example of this are the **Zn-fingers** of steroid hormone receptors, which bind to DNA, and in which four residues ($\geq 2$ Cys, remainder: His) coordinate $Zn^{2+}$. One $\alpha$-helix (see Section 4.1) of a single Zn-finger commonly binds into the large groove of DNA and reads ~3 bases.

## 3.6. Entropy

Entropy is a force that works against the stability of the native conformation of proteins. All chemical systems tend to maximize their entropy. Proteins have the greatest amount of entropy when the constituent chemical groups move freely in space. However, in the native structure of proteins, atoms are packed closely together (driven by the forces described in Sections 3.1 to 3.5), and chemical groups thus have reduced

freedom of motion. When a protein is heated to an unphysiologically high temperature, the protein gains entropy. The increased motion annihilates noncovalent attractive forces (from hydrophobic effects to van der Waals interactions), and the protein loses its native structure. The protein then is in a **denatured state** (see Section 6).

Many pathogenic **mutations** appreciably diminish the stability of a protein by reducing the favorable interactions of functional groups and atoms. Stability can be tested by exposing the protein (typically an enzyme) in vitro to an unphysiologically high temperature.

## 4. ELEMENTS OF THE THREE-DIMENSIONAL PROTEIN STRUCTURE

*There are a few very common conformations of the peptide backbone. The most prominent of these are the α-helix and the β-sheet. About two-thirds of the amino acids in globular proteins are a part of an α-helix or a β-sheet. α-Helices are compact structures in which the peptide backbone forms a spiral along a central cylinder, and the side chains project from the cylinder toward its periphery. β-Sheets consist of peptide segments that line up next to each other in a parallel or antiparallel fashion. Both helices and sheets owe their stability to hydrogen bonds between peptide –N–H and –C=O groups. The peptide segments that connect helices and sheets are called loop structures. They usually have an ordered three-dimensional structure. With the exception of short loops, they differ from protein to protein.*

### 4.1. α-Helix

The peptide backbone makes up the core of an α-helix, while the amino acid side chains point toward the periphery of the helix (Fig. 9.5).

Very generally, approximately one-third of all amino acid residues in proteins are part of α-helices; however, this fraction varies widely between proteins. A typical α-helix in a globular protein contains ~12 amino acids and has ~3 turns (a globular protein has a length less than ~4 times its width).

The core of the α-helix is packed tightly enough so that van der Waals interactions can take place between atoms. In

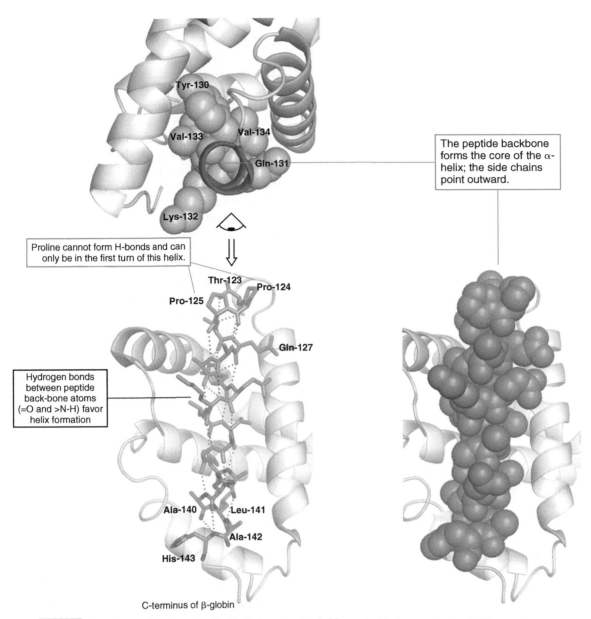

The peptide backbone forms the core of the α-helix; the side chains point outward.

Proline cannot form H-bonds and can only be in the first turn of this helix.

Hydrogen bonds between peptide back-bone atoms (=O and >N-H) favor helix formation

C-terminus of β-globin

**Fig. 9.5** **Conformation of an α-helix in human β-globin.** β-Globin is a constituent of human hemoglobin A (see Chapter 16). Amino acids in the C-terminal helix of β-globin are shown in orange. At lower left, the orange helix winds its way down from the top. For Ala-140 to His-143 (bottom of the orange helix), N-atoms are shown in blue and O in red. Each β-globin contains several additional α-helices (some are shown in gray). The image on the right shows the same C-terminal helix with space-filled atoms (using van der Waals radii). The image at the top shows a view down the long axis of the same helix. The atoms for amino acid residues 130-134 (midway down the helix) are space filled. Note that there is no empty space in the center of the helix. (Based on Protein Data Bank [www.rcsb.org] file 1HBB from Kavanaugh JS, Rogers PH, Case DA, Arnone A. High-resolution X-ray study of deoxyhemoglobin Rothschild 37 beta Trp—Arg: a mutation that creates an intersubunit chloride-binding site. *Biochemistry.* 1992;31:4111-4121.)

addition, each peptide backbone amide nitrogen [–(CO)–NH–] forms a hydrogen bond with a carbonyl oxygen [>C=O] four residues away from it on the peptide chain. The α-helix has 3.6 amino acid residues per turn, and it rises by 5.4 Å (54 nm) per turn. The long axes of the *hydrogen bonds* have approximately the same direction as the long axis of the helix. Fig. 9.5 illustrates these principles for β-globin.

Amino acids at the end of a *helix* must find special partners to form hydrogen bonds. Amino acids such as glycine and proline are particularly well suited for capping a helix.

**Proline**, owing to its structure (lack of an –NH when in a peptide bond), interrupts the hydrogen bonding within an α-helix, except in the first turn of a helix. The *mutation* of an amino acid residue inside a helix to proline is usually deleterious because it creates a kink or a break in the helix and thus likely changes the structure of other parts of the protein.

In cartoons of protein structures, helices are commonly shown as screws or cylinders. Fig. 9.6 shows the structure of human serum albumin as an example of such renderings.

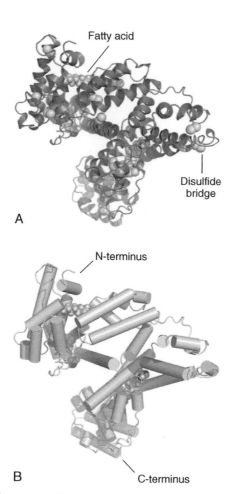

Fatty acid

Disulfide
bridge

A

N-terminus

B                    C-terminus

**Fig. 9.6** **Cartoons of human serum albumin complexed with fatty acids.** α-Helices are shown as spirals in **A** and as cylinders in **B**. **A** also shows disulfide bridges (S atoms are space filled). Four bound fatty acid molecules are shown with space-filled atoms. (Based on Protein Data Bank [www.rcsb.org] file 1BJ5 from Curry S, Mandelkow H, Brick P, Franks N. Crystal structure of human serum albumin complexed with fatty acid reveals an asymmetric distribution of binding sites. *Nat Struct Biol.* 1998;5:827-835.)

The sequence of amino acids is often such that one side of the helix is markedly hydrophobic, while the other side is markedly hydrophilic. An example is the **leucine zipper** motif (see Fig. 6.6) that can dimerize due to stabilizing hydrophobic effects.

**Membrane-spanning regions** of proteins are often α-helical (Fig. 11.8 shows an example). In *ion channels*, one side of such a helix sometimes contains mostly hydrophobic amino acid residues, while the other contains primarily hydrophilic residues. The hydrophobic side of the helix then faces the hydrophobic core of the membrane, and the hydrophilic side may form part of a hydrophilic transmembrane pore.

Two or more rather long α-helices can form a **coiled coil** (Fig. 9.7). Such structures are found, for example, in some transcription factors that dimerize on DNA promoters (see Chapter 6) and in SNARE complexes, which play a role in docking secretory vesicles to the plasma membrane. These SNARE complexes play a role, for example, in neurotransmission, in peptide hormone secretion (see Chapter 26), and in intracellular trafficking (e.g., inserting GLUT4 glucose transporters into the plasma membrane; see Chapter 18). Coiled coils owe their stability largely to hydrophobic effects.

Many collagens form a **triple helix** (see Fig. 13.1), a structure that is very different from an α-helix.

## 4.2. β-Sheets

**The prefixes** α- and β-, for helix and sheet, respectively, have historic roots. *Helices* were first found in an α-keratin, and *sheets* were first found in a β-keratin (a great many keratins are now known; they are found in hair, skin, and nails, and also as part of intermediate filaments in virtually every cell). The α-helix and β-sheet structures of proteins were first described in 1951, while the DNA double helix was discovered in 1953.

For a β-sheet to form, two or more strands (called **β-strands**) of one or more proteins must interact. In each strand, the carbonyl-O atoms of consecutive amino acids alternatingly point in opposite directions (like odd zippers with teeth that point into opposite directions; Fig. 9.8).

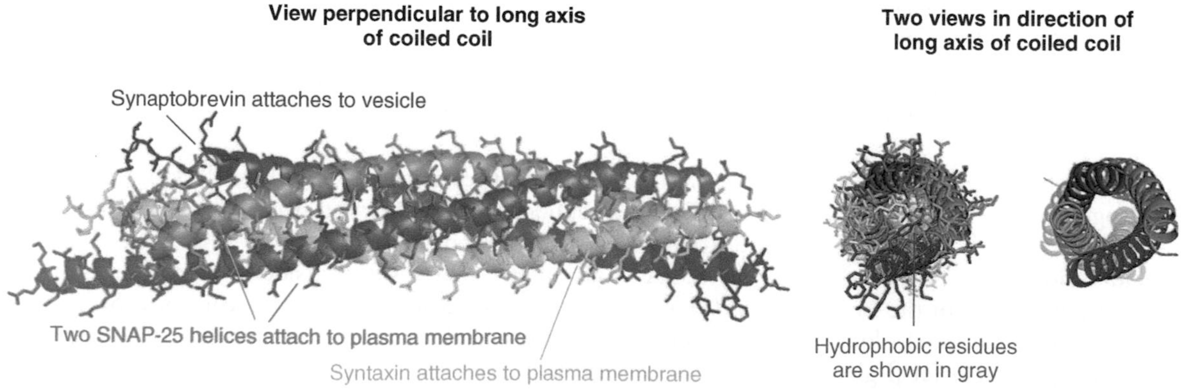

**View perpendicular to long axis of coiled coil**

**Two views in direction of long axis of coiled coil**

Synaptobrevin attaches to vesicle

Two SNAP-25 helices attach to plasma membrane

Syntaxin attaches to plasma membrane

Hydrophobic residues are shown in gray

**Fig. 9.7** **SNARE proteins can form a coiled coil.** (Based on Protein Data Bank [www.rcsb.org] file 1SFC from Sutton RB, Fasshauer D, Jahn R, Brunger AT. Crystal structure of a SNARE complex involved in synaptic exocytosis at 2.4 A resolution. *Nature.* 1998;395:347-353.)

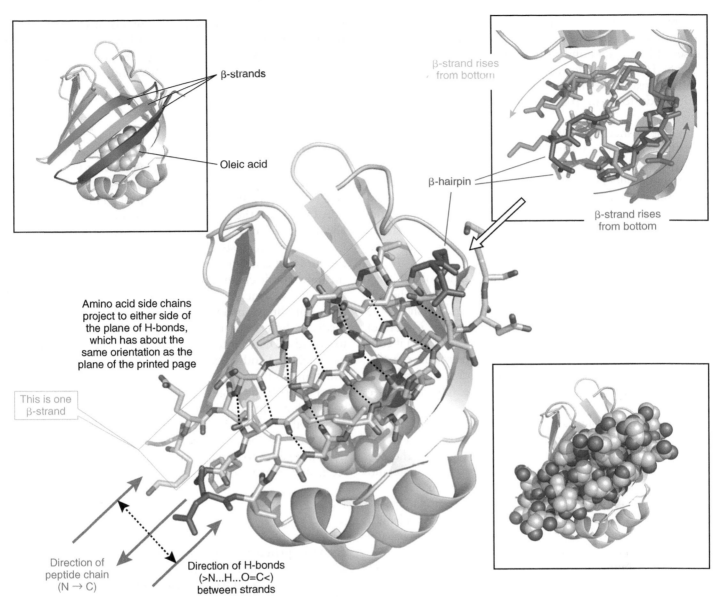

β-strands

Oleic acid

β-strand rises from bottom

β-hairpin

β-strand rises from bottom

Amino acid side chains project to either side of the plane of H-bonds, which has about the same orientation as the plane of the printed page

This is one β-strand

Direction of peptide chain (N → C)

Direction of H-bonds (>N...H...O=C<) between strands

**Fig. 9.8** **Model of the crystal structure of human brain fatty acid binding protein in complex with oleic acid.** This protein contains 10 β-strands (insert at top left; shown as ribbon arrows) that participate in β-sheet formation. The three strands at the top left are shown in the central panel as stick models with C-, N- and O-atoms in gray, blue, and red, respectively. H-atoms are not shown. The backbone O-atoms are carbonyl oxygens (>C=O), and the backbone N-atoms are linked to an H-atom (not shown); these H-atoms participate in hydrogen bonds (black dotted lines). The hydrogen bonds are approximately in a plane that is perpendicular to the line of sight. By contrast, the amino acid side chains project above and below the plane that is perpendicular to the line of sight. The solid gray arrows at the lower left indicate the direction of the strands (from N- to C-terminus); the three highlighted strands show an antiparallel organization. The highlighted strands are 10, 8, and 9 amino acid residues long. Two amino acid residues that connect adjacent antiparallel strands are hairpins and are shown in magenta. Oleic acid is shown with space-filled atoms (H-atoms are omitted). Oleic acid is in a folded conformation owing to its double bond and the influence of the protein environment. The inset on the top right shows a view down the long axis of the middle strand (light purplish blue). The strands on either side (cyan and dark blue) are not perfectly parallel to the center strand. Hence, their peptide backbones follow slightly different directions, creating a curvature in the β-sheet (this is common). The side chains point to opposite sides of the β-sheet. The inset on the lower right shows all atoms of the three selected β-strands in a space-filled cartoon (H-atoms are not shown, and the view of oleic acid is almost completely obstructed). Every other side chain of the three β-strands points in the direction of the viewer. (Based on Protein Data Bank [www.rcsb.org] file 1FE3 from Balendiran GK, Schnutgen F, Scapin G, et al. Crystal structure and thermodynamic analysis of human brain fatty acid-binding protein. *J Biol Chem.* 2000;275:27045-27054.)

Carbonyl-O atoms and amide-NH atoms on each strand then form interstrand hydrogen bonds. Two β-strands thus form one set of hydrogen bonds, three strands form two sets, and so forth. Hence, an increase in the number of interacting strands increases the number of hydrogen bonds per strand, which tends to favor β-sheets of unlimited size (see also below).

In some β-sheets the strands run **parallel**, in others they run **antiparallel** with regard to the N→C-terminal direction of the peptide backbone. If the strands of a single polypeptide run in antiparallel fashion, just two extra amino acids suffice to accomplish a turn (called a **β-hairpin**; see Fig. 9.8 and Section 4.3). However, if such strands run in parallel fashion, a much larger intervening sequence must cover the distance from the end of one β-strand to the beginning of the next β-strand.

In cartoons of protein structures, the strands of a β-sheet are commonly shown as flat ribbons, and an arrow at the end sometimes indicates the N→C direction. Fig. 9.8 shows the structure of the β-sheet in the **fatty acid binding protein** of brain. The β-sheet consists of *antiparallel* strands, and it coils into a cylindrical structure. This protein increases the effective solubility of fatty acids in the cytosol, and it also protects the cell from the detergent effects of the fatty acids (see Chapter 27).

When a drawing shows two ribbons (i.e., β-strands) next to each other, hydrogen bonds link the ribbons and lie in the approximate plane of the two ribbons (see Fig. 9.8). The side chains point at a right angle to the plane of the ribbon, and they alternate between the two sides of the ribbon.

*Globular* proteins often have parallel *and* antiparallel β-sheet structures. *Fibrous* proteins (proteins that have a length >10 times their width) sometimes have *antiparallel* but usually not *parallel* β-sheet structures.

β-Sheets are normally curved. Several β-strands can form a single, curved, almost cylindrical β-sheet that is called a **β-barrel**. Alternatively, two or more β-sheets plus connecting loops can form the sides of a polygonal body; this arrangement of β-sheets is called a **β-helix**. Yet another type of structure is called a **β-propeller**; each blade is made up of a β-sheet, whereby the β-strands closest to the center of the propeller are the shortest and those farthest away from the center the longest.

## 4.3. Loops

The term *loop* refers to the portion of a polypeptide chain that connects elements of secondary structure (i.e., α-helices and β-sheets). Loops or coils vary tremendously in size and may either move around fairly freely or else have a fixed structure that is neither helical nor sheetlike. In renderings of protein structure, loops are typically shown as thin lines. In globular proteins, approximately one-third of all amino acid residues are a part of loops.

A short **β-turn** typically consists of four amino acid residues and can accomplish a ~180-degree change of direction of the peptide backbone. In a β-sheet with antiparallel β-strands, the first and last residue of a β-turn are often part of the β-sheet; the second and third residues then form a β-hairpin (see Section 4.2 and Fig. 9.8). The second residue (i.e., the residue right after one β-strand) is often Gly, Asp, Asn, or Pro.

## 4.4. Motifs and Domains

A **motif** is a protein sequence pattern that is preserved through evolution and conveys a predictable property to a variety of proteins. For instance, Gly*Gly**Gly (* = any single amino acid residue) is a motif that helps a protein bind to a nucleotide. Obviously, these motifs are embedded in (and structurally dependent on) neighboring amino acid residues.

A **domain** consists of a contiguous stretch of amino acid residues that can function independently of other portions of the polypeptide chain and that is also physically distinct from them. For instance, among nuclear receptors (see Fig. 6-5) a ligand-binding domain binds a ligand, a dimerization domain mediates dimerization of the receptor when a ligand is bound to it, and a DNA-binding domain allows the protein to hold on to DNA. Another example is glucokinase, which contains two domains that move toward each other when glucose binds (see Fig. 10.2; the large domain is blue, the small domain is gold with a helix highlighted in red).

Sometimes, domains are connected by **hinges**, which are short and flexible segments that allow movement of one domain relative to another; such movements are often a prerequisite for enzyme catalysis.

## 4.5. Primary, Secondary, Tertiary, and Quaternary Protein Structure

The term **primary structure** refers to the sequence of amino acids in a protein (e.g., Met–Leu–Ser–Ala–).

The term **secondary structure** refers to elements repeatedly seen in the three-dimensional structure of proteins. This term includes helices and sheets. Some authors also consider common structures (e.g., β-turns) a part of the secondary structure, while others count them as a tertiary structure (see below).

The term **supersecondary structure** is sometimes used and refers to the structure of just a few (often three) α-helices and β-sheets.

The term **tertiary structure** refers to a description of the relative location of all atoms of a protein in space. Some of these atoms are part of α-helices, β-sheets, β-turns, other loops, motifs, or domains.

The term **quaternary structure** is used for the description of the composition and three-dimensional structure of a protein complex. Hemoglobin is an example of such a protein complex. As detailed in Chapter 16, hemoglobin consists of a heterotetramer of globin subunits, (e.g., two molecules of α-globin and two molecules of β-globin, each with a heme group bound to it; see Fig. 16.7). The conformation of any one globin subunit affects the conformation of all other globin subunits.

## 5. UNSTRUCTURED PROTEINS

*Some proteins or regions of proteins lack a recognizable secondary structure, which may provide advantages to protein modification and binding to other proteins.*

Compared with structured, globular proteins, intrinsically disordered proteins or disordered regions of proteins contain fewer hydrophobic amino acids and more polar amino acids. They also contain more charged amino acids. Therefore the hydrophobic effect, which contributes much to the stability of a structured protein, has significantly less effect on the structure of intrinsically disordered regions. Furthermore, intrinsically disordered proteins contain more glycine and more proline amino acids than well-structured proteins. Glycine adds flexibility (and entropy). Proline attenuates the formation of α-helices and β-sheets.

The lack of structure in intrinsically disordered regions of proteins may facilitate **posttranslational modification** by enzymes and may help **binding** to other molecules. Phosphorylation, sulfation, or acetylation may affect the charge distribution significantly and thus alter dramatically the behavior and conformation of intrinsically disordered proteins. Intrinsically disordered regions generally bind to other molecules with high specificity. They often also show a relatively low binding affinity, and they unbind relatively rapidly. Many intrinsically disordered regions have enough flexibility to bind to several different molecules.

An example of an intrinsically disordered region of a protein is the 51-residue sequence at the C-terminus of HIF-1α. Some of the amino acids in this region take on α-helical structure only when bound to transcription coactivators in the nucleus (the function of HIF-1α is described in Section 1.4 and in Fig. 16.5).

**Amylin**, produced by pancreatic β-cells, is another example of a peptide that has an intrinsically disordered region (see Section 8.4).

## 6. PROTEIN FOLDING

*Proteins fold soon after synthesis, sometimes with the help of chaperones. Disulfide bonds form with the help of an enzyme.*

The backbone of a protein can, in theory, assume a huge number of different conformations, even though peptide bonds can adopt only a limited number of torsion angles (see Section 2.1). During and after synthesis, a protein tends to assume a conformation of low energy. This is usually also a conformation with a low amount of internal motion (i.e., a situation of tight packing). However, some native proteins are not in their lowest state of energy; the lowest state may be an aggregated state, to which the proteins do not normally have kinetic access.

It seems likely that crude elements of a secondary structure form right after protein synthesis, and that a few key amino acid residues then form contacts with other residues so that the polypeptide chain quickly adopts a three-dimensional structure that is roughly similar to its native state. Then the protein may settle into its final, compact, native structure; sheets and helices, as well as interactions between amino acid residues that are distant in the primary sequence, become tighter. At this point, electrostatic and van der Waals interactions, which strongly depend on the three-dimensional conformation of a protein, convey specificity to a particular protein conformation. In large proteins, domains are thought to fold first and interact afterward.

The native structure of proteins is only marginally stable. In fact, it is commonly observed that **mutant** proteins have a shorter lifetime than normal proteins; part of this reduction in lifetime can be attributed to decreased stability.

Some proteins do not fold into the correct shape all by themselves but instead depend on **chaperone** proteins that use energy from ATP hydrolysis to guide proteins into the correct folding pattern. Some chaperones detect unfolded or incorrectly folded proteins by exposed patches of hydrophobic amino acid side chains. As described in Chapter 7, chaperone proteins either refold misfolded proteins or lead them to degradation in proteasomes.

When small proteins that do not normally need chaperones for folding are artificially unfolded in vitro, they often refold in less than 1 second.

Members of the protein disulfide isomerase family catalyze **disulfide bond** formation between cysteine side chains.

## 7. DENATURATION OF PROTEINS

*Proteins are intentionally denatured as part of disinfection.*

Denaturation of a protein is defined as a loss of its native (physiological) three-dimensional structure. However, a denatured protein may still have some secondary structure, such as α-helices or β-sheets. Once a protein has been denatured in vitro, it often cannot refold to its original native structure. Possible reasons for this are that the protein originally started folding already during biosynthesis so that N-terminal residues could fold before C-terminal residues could interfere, that the protein folded with the assistance of chaperones, and that the protein underwent posttranslational proteolytic or other processing after the normal folding process.

For most proteins, the difference in free energy between the normal physiological and the denatured state is on the order of only ~10 kcal/mol. This amount of energy is roughly equivalent to forming two hydrogen bonds de novo or burying two phenylalanine side chains in the protein interior instead of completely exposing them to water.

Chaperones can unfold proteins inside cells for **transport** from one compartment to another (e.g., from the cytosol to the nucleus, or from the cytosol to mitochondria via specialized pores in the membranes of these organelles).

Denaturation of proteins is often used as a means of **disinfection**. An unphysiologically high **temperature**, as is used in pasteurization, cooking, and sterilization, leads to the loss of the normal protein conformation. This is in large part due to a temperature-induced increase in entropy that destabilizes hydrogen bonds, hydrophobic interactions, electrostatic interactions, and van der Waals forces.

A change in **pH** may also cause denaturation. This happens physiologically in lysosomes and endosomes in all cells, as well as in the lumen of the stomach. Pathologically, for example, it happens when the eyes are exposed to lye (concentrated NaOH).

**Iodine**-containing disinfectants (e.g., betadine and isodine; so-called iodophors) iodinate proteins.

**Alcohols** (e.g., 70% to 90% ethanol or isopropanol), by replacing water as a solvent, lead to diminished hydrogen bonding between the protein and solvent, reduced hydrophobic effects, and decreased shielding of electrical charges by the solvent.

**Bleach** and similar disinfectants release hypochlorous acid and hypochlorite (HOCl and ClO⁻, respectively), which chlorinate the α-carbon of amino acids. "**Bleach alternatives**" are made to release hypochlorous acid and hypochlorite at a somewhat acidic pH instead of the strongly alkaline pH of regular bleach (i.e., sodium hypochlorite).

**Detergents** can solubilize hydrophobic side chains and thereby alter the conformation of a protein.

## 8. DISEASES THAT ARE ACCOMPANIED BY EXCESSIVE PROTEIN AGGREGATION

*Pathologic aggregation of proteins into fibrillar structures is a hallmark of degenerative diseases such as Alzheimer and Parkinson diseases. Increased formation of hydrogen bonds and sequestration of hydrophobic residues from water both drive aggregation of proteins into fibrils.*

### 8.1. Formation of Extracellular Amyloid Fibrils

**Amyloid fibrils** are fibrillar aggregates of proteins that stain with **Congo Red**. The term *amyloid* is partially a misnomer. In the nineteenth century, Virchow found that he could stain these fibers with iodine, like starch, and he named them amyloid fibers (in Greek, *amylin* means *starch*). Shortly after that, it became clear that amyloid fibers not only contain carbohydrates, but also proteins. Amyloid fibrils are roughly 100 Å (10 nm) in diameter and have a length up to greater than 100 times their diameter (i.e., a length up to ≥1 μm; for comparison, a red blood cell has a diameter of 7–8 μm). Fibrils may contain thousands of protein molecules.

Amyloid fibrils form as a result of a pathologically increased concentration of one or more normal proteins, the presence of a mutant protein, the presence of a seed structure, or the absence of an inhibitor of aggregation.

All amyloid fibrils contain **β-strands** and **β-sheets** in a **cross-β motif**. The β-sheets and the cross-β motif extend over the length of the fibril. The direction of the β-strands of individual molecules is perpendicular to the length of the fibril. Fig. 9.9 shows an example of an amyloid fibril. Amyloid fibrils can serve as seeds to which additional molecules are added such that the entire fibril has the same longitudinal architecture. A single type of peptide can often give rise to several different amyloid fibril structures.

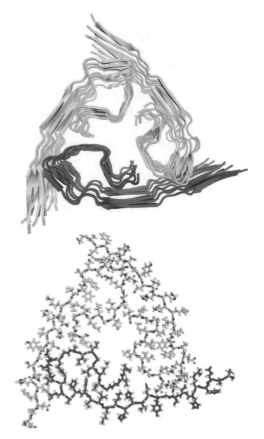

**Fig. 9.9** **Model of Aβ40 fibrils grown in vitro using seeds from the brain of an Alzheimer patient.** The long axis of the fibril is parallel to the line of sight. The fibril resembles a stack of pancakes for which each pancake consists of three Aβ40 molecules (cyan, green, or magenta) stabilized mostly by hydrophobic effects due to nonpolar amino acid side chains. The stack, in turn, is stabilized mostly by hydrogen bonds between backbone atoms of successive molecules. (From Tycko R. Amyloid polymorphism: structural basis and neurobiological relevance. *Neuron.* 2015;6(8):632-645.)

The formation of amyloid fibrils is energetically favorable for many proteins, but other low-energy states, as well as kinetic barriers, can prevent proteins from becoming part of amyloid.

About 25 different proteins are known to give rise to amyloid fibrils in vivo, and the peptide cores of all of these fibrils are decorated by a number of other molecules (e.g., heparan sulfate proteoglycan, apolipoprotein E, and serum amyloid P). **Heparan sulfate proteoglycan** is a normal part of the extracellular matrix (see Chapter 13); the negatively charged sulfate and carboxyl groups of its carbohydrate chains bind to positively charged amino acid side chains (e.g., Arg, Lys, or His) of several protein molecules in the fibril. **Apolipoprotein E** is a constituent of many lipoprotein particles (see Chapters 28 and 29). **Serum amyloid P protein** is a glycoprotein that is synthesized in the liver, secreted into the blood, and eventually eliminated by the liver. Its half-life in serum is ~1 day. During inflammation, the concentration of amyloid P in the serum increases up to 1,000-fold. The normal physiological function of serum amyloid P is incompletely understood. Serum amyloid P belongs to the pentraxin family. This family of proteins plays a role in opsonizing and neutralizing pathogens as part of the innate immune system that then informs the adaptive immune system. Serum amyloid P protein can stabilize fibrils by binding simultaneously to the monosaccharides of several molecules of the glycosylated, amyloidogenic protein.

Amyloid fibrils are insoluble in water, and extracellular proteases and phagocytic cells do not appreciably degrade amyloid fibrils.

The formation of amyloid fibrils is associated with impaired function and the death of nearby cells, but the exact pathogenesis is only poorly understood. Amyloid fibrils themselves or much smaller oligomers of their constituents impair cellular function, perhaps by changing the permeability of the cell membrane. In addition, an ever-increasing amount of extracellular amyloid can displace the cells and eventually reduce the supply of nutrients. Common sites of amyloid deposition and cell death are the brain, heart, kidney, and joints.

When patients are suspected of having an amyloid disease (see below), the ultimate **diagnosis** often rests on demonstrating plaques of long, unbranched amyloid fibrils using stains and a light microscope, as well as an electron microscope. To this end, biopsy material may come from gum tissue, abdominal subcutaneous fat, or a kidney. If an amyloid disease involves the brain exclusively, such an analysis is commonly performed postmortem. Currently, amyloid fibrils are identified on the basis of appearance (**plaques** under the light microscope, fibrils of ~10 nm diameter in the **electron microscope** and a length on the order of μm regardless of core protein), staining with **Congo red** ("Congophilia"; if so stained, appearing either red or green in the polarized light microscope when the plane of polarized light is parallel or perpendicular to the long axis of the fibril, respectively, which is due to the orientation of the repeating β-sheets in the fibril). Antisera can be used to determine the protein that gives rise to the amyloid fibrils. Laser microdissection of plaques in a biopsy, followed by mass spectrometry, is another useful option.

## 8.2. Formation of Intracellular Aggregates

Intracellular aggregates are known to be formed through several mechanisms that range from hydrophobic effects to cross–β-sheet formation. In patients who have sickle cell disease, fibers inside the red blood cells form through an aggregation of hemoglobin S (for an extensive discussion, see Section 3.2 in Chapter 17 and Figs. 17.5 and 17.6). Through the formation of a cross-β structure, normal proteins can give rise to **neurofibrillary tangles**, amyloid fibrils, or **intranuclear inclusions**. The aggregation is driven by the same basic forces as in extracellular aggregation (see Section 8.1).

The neurofibrillary tangles of patients with Alzheimer disease, familial frontotemporal dementia with parkinsonism, Down syndrome, or amyotrophic lateral sclerosis contain aggregated, abnormally phosphorylated, and acetylated **tau protein**. Tau is a microtubule-associated protein that stabilizes microtubules. Microtubules are cablelike structures inside

cells on which motor proteins "run." The motor proteins move intracellular organelles as well as chromosomes or chromatids during meiosis and mitosis. The aggregation of tau is thought to cause a deficiency of free tau, which renders the microtubules less stable, and thus impairs transport along axons so that the neurons no longer work properly. **Tauopathy** is a term used for a disease that is accompanied by the formation of fibrils containing tau.

## 8.3. Alzheimer Disease

The extracellular amyloid fibrils seen in Alzheimer disease and in Down syndrome consist of amino acid residues 1-40 and 1-42 of the **Aβ-protein**. These polypeptides are derived from the **amyloid precursor protein (APP)** through the action of β- and γ-secretase (these secretases are proteases). Aβ protein is found throughout the body, but fibrils of Aβ are restricted to the synapses and the basement membranes of the blood vessels in the brain.

The major **hereditary** forms of Alzheimer disease are caused by mutations in the genes for **APP, presenilin 1**, and **presenilin 2**. The mutations in the *APP* gene typically affect amino acids outside the Aβ(1-42)-protein but adjacent to the secretase cleavage sites. Mutations in the presenilins give rise to altered γ-secretase activity.

The gene for APP is on chromosome 21, and patients with **Down syndrome** have three copies of chromosome 21. Patients with Down syndrome show amyloid deposits by 40 years of age.

For research studies, the amount of Aβ-amyloid in brain can be assessed by **proton emission tomography (PET)** using a radioactive ($^{18}$F-labeled) dye.

Patients with the **apolipoprotein E4** isoform are more likely to have **sporadic Alzheimer disease**. Compared with those who are homozygous for the E3 allele (~60% of the population), each E4 allele approximately doubles the risk and causes onset roughly 5 years earlier. The apolipoprotein E4 allele is the most important factor in a person's risk for sporadic Alzheimer disease. In the United States, ~2% of the population is homozygous for the E4 allele, and ~20% is heterozygous.

Besides extracellular fibrils made of Aβ (Fig. 9.10), most patients with Alzheimer disease also have intracellular fibrils made of **tau**, and yet other intracellular fibrils made of α-synuclein (**Lewy bodies**; see Parkinson disease in Section 8.5). The tau protein in the intracellular fibrils is aberrantly phosphorylated and acetylated, and it cannot fulfill its normal role in stabilizing microtubules.

## 8.4. Type 2 Diabetes

In many patients who have **type 2 diabetes** or an insulinoma, pathologic fibrils of **amylin** form in the *extracellular* space predominantly of the islets of Langerhans in the pancreas. Amylin is a 37-amino acid peptide hormone that is an intrinsically partially disordered peptide (see Section 5). It is also called **islet amyloid polypeptide (IAPP)**. Amylin plays a role

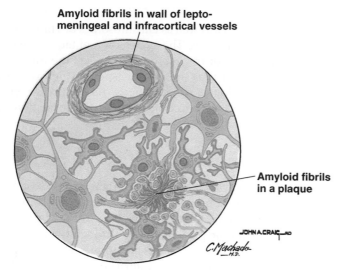

**Amyloid fibrils in wall of lepto-meningeal and infracortical vessels**

**Amyloid fibrils in a plaque**

**Fig. 9.10** Extracellular plaques containing β-amyloid in the brain of a patient with Alzheimer disease.

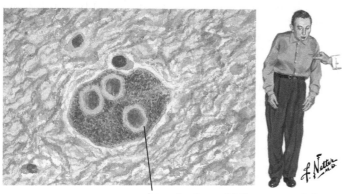

**Lewy body containing α-synuclein**

**Fig. 9.11** Pathologic aggregation of α-synuclein in Parkinson disease.

in regulating glucose metabolism (see Chapters 26 and 39). Together with insulin, amylin is stored inside β-cell secretory vesicles; it is therefore also secreted together with insulin. Inside β-cell secretory vesicles, insulin (but not proinsulin) binds to amylin and thereby keeps amylin from aggregating into fibrils. Inside secretory vesicles, there are ~100 molecules of insulin per molecule of amylin. In the bloodstream, the concentration of amylin is too low to permit appreciable aggregation into fibrils. Hence, aggregation is confined to the extracellular space near β-cells. It appears likely that *oligomers* of amylin are pathogenic, interact with the plasma membrane, and perhaps alter membrane permeability, resulting in β-cell death. Whether such a mechanism is responsible for some of the deterioration of β-cell function that is characteristic of type 2 diabetes remains to be seen. Like other amyloid fibrils, fibrils of amylin contain a cross-β structure.

**Pramlintide** is a synthetic, especially soluble *analog* of amylin that is used to treat patients with **type 1** or **type 2 diabetes** (see Chapter 39). Pramlintide greatly reduces the excursion of the blood glucose concentration after a meal; in

fact, when patients take pramlintide they require less insulin to control blood glucose.

## 8.5. Parkinson Disease

Parkinson disease can arise as a result of various genetic mutations. Through pathways that remain largely unknown, many patients accumulate fibrils (also called **Lewy bodies**; Fig. 9.11) *inside* cells of the substantia nigra. The fibrils contain mostly **α-synuclein**, a protein that is made in the synapse. The disease is accompanied by a loss of neurons in the substantia nigra. The substantia nigra normally sends messages to the basal ganglia via dopaminergic synapses.

Patients with Parkinson disease show a tremor at rest but not during voluntary movements. They also have rigid muscles, move slowly, and have little expression on their face. Parkinson disease usually becomes clinically apparent in the sixth to eighth decades of life.

In the United States, more than 2% of the population has Parkinson disease. Most of this disease is sporadic. Some of the **hereditary** forms of Parkinson disease are due to missense mutations in α-synuclein.

### SUMMARY

- Proteins are synthesized from 21 different amino acids, which are linked by peptide bonds (–CO–NH–). The arrangement in space of these amino acids determines the properties of a protein.
- On average, in the native, folded state, approximately two-thirds of the amino acid residues of a protein are part of α-helices or β-sheets. The amino acids that are not part of helices and sheets are generally part of turns and loops. Tight turns have a common structure, but the longer loop regions usually differ appreciably in structure from protein to protein.
- The native, three-dimensional structure of proteins is a result of H-bonding, hydrophobic effects, electrostatic interactions, and van der Waals interactions between the atoms of amino acids.
- Thermodynamics favor the aggregation of β-strands into infinitely large β-sheets. In nature, such aggregation is usually prevented, often by steric means. However, there are many diseases, collectively called amyloid diseases, that are associated with the aggregation of proteins into ~10 nm diameter, very long fibrils, called amyloid fibrils. Patients with Alzheimer disease form extracellular amyloid fibrils that contain the Aβ-protein; these fibrils, in turn, give rise to plaques. Neurons of patients with Alzheimer disease also contain intracellular fibrils of tau protein, which in turn form neurofibrillary tangles. Extracellular fibrils containing amylin (also called IAPP) are found in patients with type 2 diabetes. In patients with Parkinson disease, α-synuclein gives rise to intracellular fibrils in cells of the substantia nigra; the fibrils aggregate into Lewy bodies.

## FURTHER READING

- Finkelstein AV, Ptitsyn OB. Protein Physics: A Course of Lectures, ed 2. London: Academic Press; 2016:528. These authors take a rigorous chemical approach that is suitable for those who want to learn more about protein structure.
- Protein Data Bank: <www.rcsb.org>. This databank provides free access to data for thousands of protein structures.
- Tycko R. Amyloid polymorphism: structural basis and neurobiological relevance. *Neuron*. 2015;86:632-645.

# Review Questions

1. The termini of proteins are usually found near the surface of the protein. The most likely reason for this is which of the following?

    A. Neither the first nor the last residue of a polypeptide chain can be part of a hydrogen-bonded α-helix or β-sheet.
    B. Proteins fold *after* synthesis by ribosomes has started but *before* it has ended.
    C. The higher mobility of side chains near the termini prevents their participation in van der Waals interactions.
    D. The termini are charged, and there would be a large energy penalty for burying these charges in the protein interior.

2. The codons GGA, GGC, GGG, and GGU all encode the amino acid glycine. In turn, the codons GUA, GUC, GUG, and GUU all encode the amino acid valine. Mutation of the first nucleotide (G) of a codon for Gly is usually much more damaging to the function of a protein than mutation of the first nucleotide (G) of a codon for Val. Which of the following is the best explanation for this finding?

    A. Compared with glycine, valine poses greater constraints on the conformation of the peptide backbone.
    B. Glycine is more likely to be exposed on the surface of a protein than valine.
    C. Glycine residues give rise to greater hydrophobic effects than valine residues.
    D. The side chain of valine is much smaller than that of glycine.

3. Aminolevulinic acid (ALA), which derives from glycine, has the following structure:

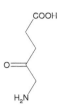

In dermatology, ALA is sometimes applied to a skin area as an acidic solution or cream. Application of an electric current then moves ALA through the stratum corneum into the underlying epidermis. What is the charge of ALA that moves under these conditions?

A. −2
B. −1
C. 0
D. +1
E. +2

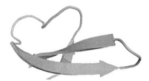

4. The figure above shows the structure of a defensin. The antiparallel β-sheet (indicated by two long flat ribbons) is most likely primarily stabilized by which of the following?

    A. Electrostatic interactions among oppositely charged atoms of the two β-strands
    B. Hydrogen bonds between amino acid side chains of the two β-strands
    C. Hydrogen bonds between O and N in the peptide backbone of the two β-strands
    D. Hydrophobic effects due to the presence of aliphatic and aromatic amino acid side chains among the two β-strands
    E. Van der Waals interactions between neighboring atoms of amino acid side chains

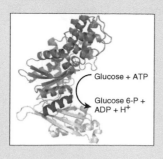

Glucose + ATP

Glucose 6-P + ADP + H⁺

## Chapter 10

# Enzymes and Consequences of Enzyme Deficiencies

## SYNOPSIS

- Enzymes catalyze chemical reactions by lowering the activation energies of these reactions.
- Most enzymes are proteins, but some consist of RNA or a mixture of RNA and protein. Some enzymes need coenzymes (organic nonprotein molecules) for catalysis.
- Thermodynamics determine whether a reaction from reactants to products is energetically possible.
- Physiological or pathological changes in the concentrations of reactants and products allow many reactions in the human body to change direction; such reactions are said to be *reversible*. Other reactions are favorable in only one direction under conditions that are compatible with life; these reactions are termed *physiologically irreversible*.
- Regulatory circuits control the activities of many of the enzymes that catalyze physiologically irreversible reactions.
- The three-dimensional arrangement of amino acids in enzymes provides specificity for the binding of substrates.
- The Michaelis-Menten equation describes how enzymatic activity depends on the substrate concentration. This equation is valid for some enzymes.
- Some enzymes show cooperativity and thus are described by a *modified* Michaelis-Menten equation. Such enzymes become significantly active only above a threshold concentration of the substrate.
- The activity of certain enzymes is regulated by activators, by inhibitors, and/or by covalent modification, such as phosphorylation.
- In all pathways, the enzyme with the lowest rate of reaction limits flux through the pathway. An enzyme deficiency tends to lead to an *increased* concentration of all upstream reactants and a *decreased* concentration of all downstream products.

## LEARNING OBJECTIVES

*For mastery of this topic, you should be able to do the following:*

- Examine available resources to determine whether two enzymes catalyze the same reaction or different reactions.
- Define the terms zymogen, proenzyme, ribozyme, coenzyme, cofactor, prosthetic group, apoenzyme, holoenzyme, isozyme, catalytic cycle, and enzyme unit.
- Describe the relationship between thermodynamics and the feasibility of enzyme catalysis of a chemical reaction.
- Explain how an enzyme can increase the rate of a reaction.
- Compare and contrast physiologically reversible and physiologically irreversible reactions in the human body.
- Explain the effect of temperature and pH on an enzyme-catalyzed reaction.
- Compare and contrast the key-lock theory and the induced fit theory of enzymatic action.
- Use the Michaelis-Menten equation to relate $K_m$, enzyme activity, and substrate concentration to each other.

- Compare and contrast the properties of enzymes that show simple Michaelis-Menten type kinetics and enzymes that show cooperativity.
- Define allostery and provide an example.
- Compare and contrast how competitive and noncompetitive inhibitors affect the rate of enzyme catalysis, taking into account the concentration of substrate.
- List an example each of feedback and feed-forward regulation.
- Predict the effects of a partial or a complete enzyme deficiency on the concentrations of the intermediates of a metabolic pathway.
- Explain why the activity of certain enzymes in the blood is of interest in the diagnosis of disease.

## 1. NOMENCLATURE OF ENZYMES

*The names of enzymes end in -ase. Different naming systems exist, of which the "recommended names" are used here. Enzymes are most often proteins and sometimes require inorganic or organic, nonpeptidic cofactors for catalysis. A few enzymes consist of RNA or a mixture of RNA and protein.*

Enzymes are characterized by the suffix **–ase**. Each enzyme can be identified in three different ways: (1) the **recommended name**, which is generally the historically grown name (e.g., hexokinase; Table 10.1); (2) the "**systematic name**," which describes the chemical function of an enzyme (e.g., ATP:D-hexose 6-phosphotransferase; Table 10.2); and (3) the **enzyme classification number** (e.g., EC 2.7.1.1), which is based on the systematic naming system. This text generally uses only the recommended names, although such a name is occasionally at odds with the physiological function of an enzyme. With the recommended names, some enzymes are named after the *compound they degrade* (e.g., glucose 6-phosphatase, which degrades glucose 6-phosphate to glucose and phosphate; see Chapters 24 and 25). Others are named more descriptively after the *reaction they catalyze* (e.g., alcohol dehydrogenase, which removes hydrogen from alcohol [see Chapter 30], or aminotransferase, which transfers an amino group from an amino acid to a keto acid [see Chapter 35]). Some enzymes are named after the *reactions they catalyze in test tubes*, but not in the human body.

Virtually all enzymes are **proteins**. However, a small number of RNAs can also catalyze chemical reactions. These RNAs are collectively called **ribozymes**, RNA enzymes, or catalytic RNAs. Physiologically important ribozymes typically catalyze reactions that involve RNA as a substrate (e.g., RNA processing by spliceosomes [see Chapter 6] or protein

**Table 10.1**  **Classification of Enzymes by Recommended Name**

| Recommended Name | Systematic Name | Reaction Catalyzed* | Examples |
|---|---|---|---|
| Kinase | ATP (substrate): phosphotransferase | $A–OH + ATP \leftrightarrow A–P_i + ADP$ | Hexokinase, cAMP-dependent protein kinase = protein kinase A |
| Phosphatase | Phosphohydrolase | $A–P_i + H_2O \leftrightarrow A–OH + H–P_i$ | Glucose 6-phosphatase, phosphoprotein phosphatase |
| Synthase | Oxidoreductase, transferase, ligase (depending on the reaction) | $A + B \leftrightarrow C + D$ | Methionine synthase, thymidylate synthase |
| Dehydrogenase | Oxidoreductase | $AH_2 + B \leftrightarrow A + BH_2$ | Glucose 6-phosphate dehydrogenase, malate dehydrogenase, alcohol dehydrogenase |
| Reductase | Oxidoreductase | $AH_2 + B \leftrightarrow A + BH_2$ | Hydroxymethylglutaryl coenzyme A reductase (HMG-CoA reductase), dihydrofolate reductase |
| Peptidase | Most often: hydrolase | $A + H_2O \leftrightarrow B + C$ | Trypsin, elastase, carboxypeptidase |

*The reactions are written in the direction that corresponds to the recommended name. The reactions are shown as being reversible ($\leftrightarrow$) because enzymes work in both directions. The concentrations of reactants and products affect the direction of the reaction.
ATP, adenosine triphosphate; cAMP, cyclic adenosine monophosphate; HMG-CoA, 3-hydroxy-3-methylglutaryl coenzyme A.

**Table 10.2**  **Classification of Enzymes by Systematic Name**

| Systematic Name | EC Number | Reactions Catalyzed (Sample) | Examples (Recommended Names) |
|---|---|---|---|
| Oxidoreductase | EC 1.x.x.x. | $AH_2 + B \leftrightarrow A + BH_2$ | Glycerol-3-phosphate dehydrogenase, lactate dehydrogenase, malate dehydrogenase |
| Transferase | EC 2.x.x.x. | $AB + C \leftrightarrow A + BC$ | Hexokinase, various amino acid transaminases |
| Hydrolase | EC 3.x.x.x. | $A + H_2O \leftrightarrow B$ | 3′,5′-Cyclic-nucleotide phosphodiesterase, methenyltetrahydrofolate cyclohydrolase |
| Lyase | EC 4.x.x.x. | $X \leftrightarrow A + B$ (a bond must be broken by hydrolysis or oxidation; or: a new double bond or a new ring must be formed) | Fructose-bisphosphate aldolase, fumarate hydratase, argininosuccinate lyase |
| Isomerase | EC 5.x.x.x. | $X–A–B–Y \leftrightarrow Y–A–B–X$ | Triose-phosphate isomerase, UDP-glucose 4-epimerase, prostaglandin D synthase, phosphoglycerate mutase |
| Ligase | EC 6.x.x.x. | $A + B + C \leftrightarrow A–B + D + E$ | Various amino acid tRNA ligases, DNA ligase, ubiquitin-protein ligase, argininosuccinate synthase, pyruvate carboxylase |

EC, enzyme classification number; UDP, uridine diphosphate.

synthesis by ribosomes [see Section 3 in Chapter 7]). Unless specifically stated otherwise, in this chapter the term "enzyme" refers to a protein.

A **zymogen** or **proenzyme** is a precursor protein to an active enzyme that has little or no enzymatic activity; however, once it is processed posttranslationally, often by limited proteolysis, it becomes competent for catalysis. For instance, the pancreas secretes enzymatically inactive trypsinogen, chymotrypsinogen, and proelastase, which become active trypsin, chymotrypsin, and elastase, respectively, in the lumen of the intestine (see Chapter 34).

A **coenzyme** is an organic molecule that binds to an enzyme (transiently or permanently) and participates in catalysis. Coenzymes are typically needed for oxidation-reduction reactions and as temporary acceptors in the transfer of chemical groups. An example is lipoic acid, which participates in the oxidative decarboxylation of pyruvate by pyruvate dehydrogenase (see Chapter 22). Lipoic acid is covalently bound to the side chain amino group of a lysine residue of pyruvate dehydrogenase. Lipoic acid transiently accepts a $CH_3-CH(OH)-$ group, presents it for oxidation to $CH_3-CO-$, and transfers $CH_3-CO-$ to yet another coenzyme, coenzyme A. Many enzymes contain tightly bound **metal ions** in their active sites; these metal ions are *not* usually called coenzymes.

Some terms in enzymology are poorly defined and consequently used in different ways. Thus, coenzymes are often also called **cofactors**. Sometimes, the distinction between **substrate** and coenzyme becomes blurry. For instance, $NAD^+$ and NADH are substrates of many different dehydrogenases, but some scientists also refer to them as coenzymes or cofactors. Some coenzymes are called **prosthetic groups**. In general, the term prosthetic group implies that the coenzyme is tightly or covalently bound to the enzyme and does not dissociate from the enzyme during catalysis. An example of such a prosthetic group is biotin, which is linked covalently to a lysine residue in all human carboxylases (see Section 3 in Chapter 22 and Section 2 in Chapter 27). Other examples are lipoic acid (mentioned in the preceding paragraph) and heme in cytochromes (see Chapters 14 and 23).

The term **apoenzyme** refers to a coenzyme-dependent enzyme that does not have a coenzyme bound to it, while the term **holoenzyme** refers to such an enzyme that has its coenzyme bound to it, usually tightly. Alternatively, a holoenzyme may be an enzymatically functional assembly of two or more molecules.

**Isozymes (isoenzymes)** are enzymes that catalyze the same reaction yet differ in their amino acid sequences. Often, isozymes differ in their maximal velocity of catalysis (i.e., $V_{max}$, see Section 3) and in the concentration of substrate that is needed for half-maximal activity (i.e., $K_m$ or $S_{0.5}$; see Section 3). An example of this are the hexokinases, which phosphorylate glucose; hexokinases I, II, III, and IV are half-maximally active at glucose concentrations of about 0.03, 0.3, 0.03, and 5 mM, respectively. Some isoenzymes are derived from different genes; others originate from a single gene through alternative use of transcription start sites, alternative RNA splicing, or different posttranslational processing (see Chapters 6 and 7).

## 2. ENZYME CATALYSIS OF CHEMICAL REACTIONS

*The observed high specificity of the binding of substrates to enzymes is due to steric effects and numerous functional group interactions between enzymes and substrates. An enzyme-catalyzed reaction is faster than an uncatalyzed reaction because it has a lower activation energy. Temperature and pH profoundly influence the activity of enzymes.*

**Chemical thermodynamics** allow one to determine whether a chemical reaction can take place, based on an analysis of the temperature, concentration, and standard Gibbs free energy ($G^0$) of the reactants and products. Only reactions that lead to an overall lowering of Gibbs free energy (those with a **negative $\Delta G$**) occur spontaneously. The **change in Gibbs free energy** during a reaction ($\Delta G$) depends on the energy state of the atoms and the bonds between them, the movement of atoms and molecules in space (e.g., rotation, tumbling, and oscillation), and the concentrations of reactants and products. Only those reactions can occur spontaneously that result in a decrease in Gibbs free energy; enzymes do not change this fact.

When a chemical reaction is at **equilibrium**, there is no net force to drive it toward either reactants or products. At equilibrium, the thermodynamic driving force $\Delta G$ is therefore zero. In cells, there is usually some flux in all metabolic pathways; hence, virtually no reaction is exactly at equilibrium. However, a large number of reactions are *close* to equilibrium. Examples of such reactions are the isomerization of glucose 6-phosphate and fructose 6-phosphate in glycolysis (see Chapter 19) and gluconeogenesis (see Chapter 25), as well as the redox reaction between malate and oxaloacetate in the citric acid cycle (see Chapter 22).

An enzyme accelerates the rate of a thermodynamically feasible reaction by lowering the **activation energy** of the reaction. Many thermodynamically feasible reactions do not happen because their activation energy is too high. For instance, glucose and ATP in water at pH 7 do not appreciably react with each other. However, the enzyme hexokinase changes the reaction path so that the activation energy is low enough for the reaction to occur with high frequency at normal body temperature.

The activation energy of a reaction is set largely by the energy level of the transition state that has the highest Gibbs free energy. Hence, the activation energy is also called the **transition state barrier** (Fig. 10.1). Since enzymes only affect the reaction path but not the nature of the reactants or products, enzymes do not affect the position of the equilibrium between the reactants and products.

**Temperature** affects enzymes in two opposing manners. An increase in temperature facilitates a reaction by increasing the number of molecules that have sufficient energy to cross the transition state barrier. On the other hand, most human enzymes lose their *structure* as the temperature rises. The net result is that most enzymes have their highest activity near the physiological core body temperature.

**pH** affects enzymatic activity via the degree of protonation of amino acid side chains and peptide termini; these, in turn, affect the formation of hydrogen bonds and electrostatic interactions. Often, it is the protonation of residues near the catalytic site that is most important in determining the pH optimum of an enzyme. These residues can serve as proton donors or acceptors. The pH may also affect the protonation of a substrate. Enzymes tend to have the highest activity at the pH at which they normally should be active. For many enzymes that normally reside in the lumen of the intestine, the blood, extracellular space, cytosol, endoplasmic reticulum, secretory vesicles, mitochondria, or nucleus, the optimal pH is in the range of 7 to 8. For many enzymes that must be active in the lumen of the stomach or inside lysosomes, the optimal pH is in the range of 4 to 5. Some of these enzymes become inactive when they are exposed to a near-neutral pH. However, many

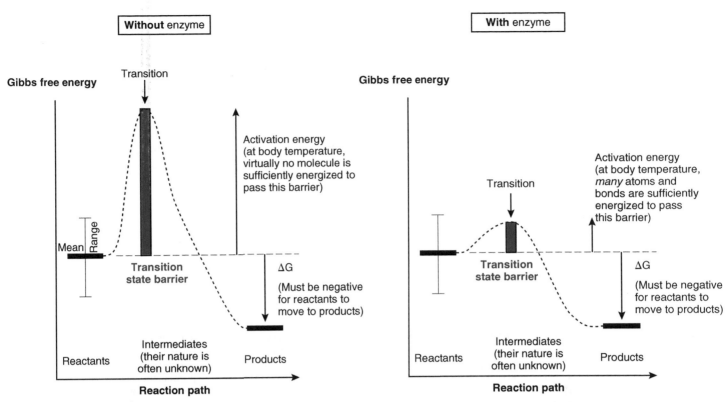

**Fig. 10.1** **The effect of an enzyme on the energy diagram of a chemical reaction.** The means of the Gibbs free energy of intermediates on the reaction path are plotted (the thermal energy of individual molecules varies a bit around the mean).

other enzymes are highly active even far from their normal physiological pH.

Most enzymes accept only a narrow range of substrates. Specificity stems from the substrate-binding site, as well as the catalytic mechanism. Substrates are bound with high specificity through a three-dimensional network of electrostatic effects, hydrophobic effects, hydrogen bonds, and van der Waals interactions, as already described for the protein-protein interactions in Section 3 in Chapter 9. Since enzymes consist of L-amino acids, which are chiral, enzymes themselves are chiral (i.e., they have a handedness). Indeed, most enzymes can distinguish the **enantiomers** of substrates if the chiral center of the substrate is near the substrate binding site.

Based on the observed specificity of enzymes for substrates, the **key-lock theory** of the late nineteenth century postulates that the catalytic sites of enzymes fit substrates precisely like a negative fits its corresponding positive. This theory can indeed explain many interactions among enzymes, substrates, and inhibitors, although it presents enzymes and substrates as static, inflexible structures. Based on a more thorough understanding of chemical structures and the interactions of substrates and enzymes, the **induced fit theory** of the mid-twentieth century improved on the key-lock theory. This theory expressly takes into account that the three-dimensional structure of enzymes and substrates is not rigid but pliable. The induced fit theory postulates that the binding of a substrate may induce an appreciable *change* in the orientation of the reactive groups of the active site of an enzyme and that catalysis often occurs only when these reactive groups have a specific orientation.

Fig. 10.2 shows the structure of an enzyme that uses an induced fit mechanism.

Enzymes **catalyze** chemical reactions by providing a reaction path that has a lower transition state barrier than the uncatalyzed reaction and therefore occurs more readily. This can be accomplished by the following means. Some enzymes induce a conformational strain in a substrate as they bind it. A change in enzyme conformation, often induced by the binding of a substrate, sometimes brings the substrate and cofactor into a particularly favorable alignment. Other enzymes preferentially bind substrate molecules that have assumed an optimal orientation and configuration that favors a reaction and thus lowers the transition state barrier. Enzymes facilitate catalysis in a three-dimensional structure that provides well-positioned chemical groups (including those on cofactors), reaction-dependent movement of these chemical groups, or a space that may be free of water or have only one or two strategically placed water molecules. Regarding the latter, binding of a substrate sometimes induces a movement of an enzyme domain that encloses the substrate in a chamber made up of amino acids that no longer have a connection to bulk water. In many enzymes, substrates, cofactors, and intermediates are bound in such a way as to stabilize the transition state.

Enzymes are sometimes organized into **complexes** with closely spaced active sites (e.g., carbamoyl-phosphate synthase II/aspartate carbamoyltransferase/dihydroorotase in pyrimidine nucleotide de novo synthesis; see Chapter 37), or with prosthetic groups that pass intermediates from active site to

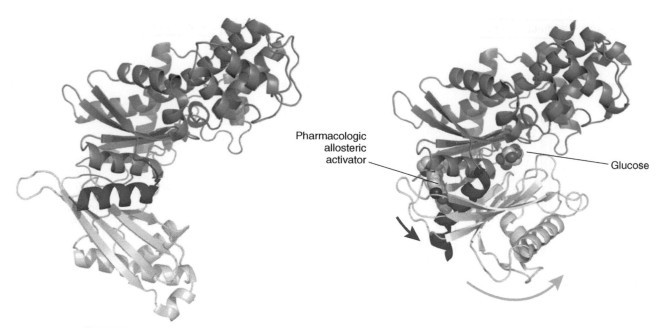

**Fig. 10.2** **Induced fit in glucokinase.** In the insulin-secreting pancreatic β-cells, glucokinase serves as a glucose sensor (see Chapter 26). In the liver, glucokinase produces glucose 6-phosphate mostly in the fed state (see Chapter 19). *Left,* Pure glucokinase. *Right,* Glucokinase with glucose and a pharmacological allosteric activator. The larger domain (blue) is shown in the same position. Upon binding glucose, the smaller domain (gold) rotates by ~100 degrees relative to the larger domain, and the end of the C-terminal helix (red) moves away from the larger domain, with glucokinase thereby enclosing glucose in a chamber. (Based on Protein Data Bank [www.rcsb.org] files 1V4T and 1V4S from Kamata K, Mitsuya M, Nishimura T, Eiki J, Nagata Y. Structural basis for allosteric regulation of the monomeric allosteric enzyme human glucokinase. *Structure.* 2004;12:429-438.)

active site (e.g., fatty acid synthase; see Chapter 27). Such arrangements are favorable due to reduced diffusion, degradation, or competition of substrates, as well as reduced interaction of substrates with the surrounding fluid.

**Amino acid side chains** of enzymes can participate in catalysis. For instance, Cys can form covalent bonds via the sulfur atom of its sulfhydryl group and Ser via the oxygen atom of its hydroxyl group. Similarly, reversible protonation and deprotonation can occur on a nitrogen atom of the 5-membered ring of His, on an oxygen atom of the carboxyl group of Asp or Glu, or on the oxygen atom of the hydroxyl group of Ser (for structures of amino acids, see Chapter 9).

Enzymes differ vastly in the time it takes to complete a **catalytic cycle**. A catalytic cycle starts, for example, with the binding of substrate and ends with the release of the product and formation of the enzyme in its initial state. G-proteins by themselves may take up to about 7000 seconds (~2 hours) to complete a catalytic cycle (hydrolysis of GTP to GDP; see Chapter 33). Glucokinase needs about 0.02 seconds to phosphorylate glucose to glucose 6-phosphate (see Chapter 19), while fumarase needs only about 0.001 seconds to convert fumarate + $H_2O$ to malate (see Chapter 22), and carbonic anhydrase needs just about 0.000002 seconds to convert $CO_2$ + $H_2O$ to $HCO_3^-$ + $H^+$ (see Chapter 16).

The **turnover number** of an enzyme (often called $k_{cat}$) is the maximal number of catalytic cycles an enzyme performs in 1 second. For instance, if a catalytic cycle takes 0.001 seconds, the turnover number is $1/0.001$ s $= 1000$ s$^{-1}$.

## 3. ENZYME ACTIVITY AS A FUNCTION OF THE CONCENTRATION OF SUBSTRATES

*The Michaelis-Menten equation describes the activity of simple enzymes as a function of substrate concentration. A modified form of this equation describes the behavior of enzymes that show cooperativity toward a substrate.*

The **Michaelis-Menten** equation describes enzyme activity as a function of the concentration of a single substrate. This equation is valid only when the concentration of the product is negligible, and the concentration of the enzyme-substrate complex stays constant.

$$\frac{v}{V_{max}} = \frac{s}{s + K_m}$$

In the above equation, **v** is the rate at which the enzyme gives rise to the product (moles/time). $V_{max}$ is the maximal rate at which the enzyme can make a product (this is assumed to happen at an infinitely high substrate concentration, but in practice there are limits to the substrate concentration, such as substrate solubility and effects of the solution on enzyme structure). The concentration of substrate is denoted by s. $K_m$ is the concentration of substrate at which the enzyme gives rise to the product at **half** its **maximal** rate (i.e., $v/V_{max} = 0.5$). A graph of values that fit this equation is shown in Fig. 10.3. $V_{max}$ and $K_m$ are the characteristic properties of individual enzymes.

If an enzyme has **two substrates**, the Michaelis-Menten equation still applies if the concentration of one substrate is

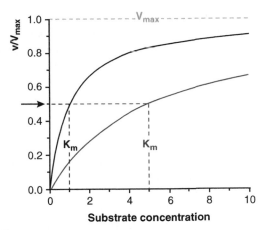

**Fig. 10.3** Activity of two different enzymes as a function of the substrate concentration and as predicted by the Michaelis-Menten equation.

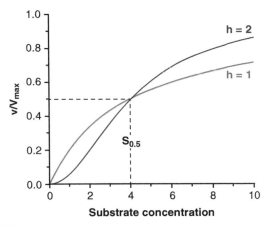

**Fig. 10.4** Enzyme activity as predicted by a modified Michaelis-Menten equation for enzymes that show cooperativity toward their substrate. No cooperativity: blue. With cooperativity: red.

**Table 10.3** Substrate Concentration and Enzyme Activity as Predicted by the Michaelis-Menten Equation

| Substrate Concentration | Relative Enzyme Activity ($v/V_{max}$) |
|---|---|
| $0.1 \times K_m$ | 0.09 |
| $1 \times K_m$ | 0.50 |
| $10 \times K_m$ | 0.91 |
| $100 \times K_m$ | 0.99 |

held constant and that of the other varied. Furthermore, the product of $v/V_{max}$ for substrate 1 and $v/V_{max}$ for substrate 2 is often a useful approximation of the rate of a reaction that has two substrates.

An equation of the same mathematical form as the Michaelis-Menten equation also applies to the binding of molecules to proteins, such as the binding of insulin to the insulin receptor, or of cobalamin to intrinsic factor. Thereby, actual binding replaces v, and the maximum amount of binding replaces $V_{max}$. $K_s$, the concentration at which binding to the protein is half-maximal, replaces $K_m$, the substrate concentration at which an enzyme is half-maximally active.

According to the Michaelis-Menten equation, enzymatic activity is **not directly proportional** to the substrate concentration. A few key numbers are listed in Table 10.3. (Note that if the substrate concentration is far below the $K_m$, and less than $0.01 \times K_m$, the reaction rate v is nearly proportional to the substrate concentration s.)

Under physiological circumstances, the substrate concentration is often below the $K_m$ of an enzyme. Hence, most enzymes normally work at only a fraction of their maximal catalytic capacity, and they therefore have a lot of reserve capacity.

The higher the $K_m$ of an enzyme for a substrate, the higher the concentration of the substrate must be to achieve a certain $v/V_{max}$.

The Michaelis-Menten equation is valid whether the rate-limiting step in the enzyme catalysis is the association between the enzyme and the substrate or the reaction from enzyme-substrate complex to the product. In the latter case, the $K_m$ is a measure of the **substrate affinity** of an enzyme.

Enzyme activity is usually stated in **enzyme units** (**U**). One U is the amount of an enzyme that produces 1 μmol of product per minute. The conditions for this enzyme activity are not standardized across the board, but must be stated in each report. In general, a unit refers to a measured $V_{max}$.

Some enzymes consist of **several interacting subunits** with mutually dependent conformations: binding of substrate to one subunit induces a conformational change in another subunit, thereby changing its catalytic properties. This phenomenon is called **cooperativity**. The activity of enzymes that show cooperativity toward a substrate can be described by a **modified Michaelis-Menten equation** as follows:

$$\frac{v}{V_{max}} = \frac{(s)^h}{(s)^h + (S_{0.5})^h}$$

In this equation, $S_{0.5}$ is the concentration of substrate at which the enzyme shows half-maximal activity; the term $S_{0.5}$ is used in place of $K_m$ because it denotes not *one* substrate molecule binding to the enzyme and reacting, but a mean of *several* substrate molecules binding and reacting. h is also called the **Hill coefficient** or **cooperativity coefficient**. It does not have to be an integer. If h is larger than 1, the enzyme is said to display **positive cooperativity**. A linear plot of the activity of such an enzyme versus substrate concentration shows an S-shaped relationship (Fig. 10.4). (Negative cooperativity is not discussed here.)

Examples of enzymes that have cooperativity are **glucokinase**, which has a Hill coefficient of about 1.5 (see Chapters 19 and 26), and phosphofructokinase 1 (see Chapter 19) and amidophosphoribosyltransferase (see Chapter 38), which have Hill coefficients of about 2.

A formula similar to that for enzyme cooperativity is found for the cooperative binding of ligands to proteins under equilibrium conditions, such as oxygen to hemoglobin (hemoglobin saturation with $O_2$ = hemoglobin-bound $O_2$/maximal amount of hemoglobin-bound $O_2$ = $O_2^h/[O_2^h + P_{50}^h]$; see Chapter 16).

A physiologically important difference between an enzyme that follows Michaelis-Menten kinetics and one that shows cooperativity is that the latter may be turned off more fully at substrate concentrations below $S_{0.5}$ (see Fig. 10.4).

## 4. ACTIVATORS AND INHIBITORS OF ENZYMES

*Inhibitors and activators of enzymes play major roles in the physiological and pharmacological regulation of enzymes. Such modifiers bind in the active site of an enzyme, a regulatory site that is remote from the active site, or any other place on the enzyme. Among the inhibitors, competitive inhibitors compete with the substrate for binding to the active site, while noncompetitive inhibitors do not show such competition.*

Many enzymes are controlled by reversibly binding inhibitors and activators. A substrate binds to a site that is variably referred to as the **substrate binding site**, **active site**, or **catalytic site**. Activators typically bind to a site at some distance from the substrate binding site; in this case, they are *allosteric activators* (see Fig. 10.2 and Table 10.4). Inhibitors that compete with the substrate for a binding site are called *competitive* **inhibitors**. Inhibitors that bind to a site at some distance from the substrate binding site(s) are allosteric inhibitors. Some of these inhibitors are called *noncompetitive* **inhibitors** (there are also mixed and uncompetitive inhibitors, which are not discussed here). Physiological noncompetitive inhibitors often bind to specific regulatory sites on enzymes.

If an enzyme is exposed to a competitive inhibitor, the substrate competes with the inhibitor. A high concentration of the substrate can, therefore, make the presence of inhibitor irrelevant to enzyme activity. A competitive inhibitor increases the apparent $K_m$, but it has no effect on the $V_{max}$ of an enzyme. In contrast, a noncompetitive inhibitor decreases the $V_{max}$, but it has no effect on the $K_m$.

In enzymology, the adjective "allosteric" is often misused as a substitute for "cooperative." In a strict sense, an allosteric activator or inhibitor (also called allosteric effector) by definition binds to an enzyme at some distance from the catalytic site. Most allosterically regulated enzymes are also multimeric complexes of several identical subunits, and they do show cooperativity (see Section 3). However, this does not mean that all allosterically regulated enzymes must show cooperativity (cooperativity usually means that the conformation of one subunit affects the conformation of other subunits in a multimeric enzyme complex).

If an enzyme accepts **different substrates into the same site**, each substrate acts as a *competitive inhibitor* of the other

substrate. For instance, alcohol dehydrogenase accepts ethanol, ethylene glycol ("antifreeze"), and methanol as substrates. In methanol- or ethylene glycol-poisoned patients, ethanol can therefore be used to diminish the formation of a toxic product from either methanol or ethylene glycol (see Chapter 36).

While practically all physiological and most pharmacologically used inhibitors act reversibly, others act irreversibly. Among these **irreversible inhibitors**, some simply dissociate from the enzyme extremely slowly, and they are thus irreversible only for practical purposes. Truly irreversible inhibitors react with an enzyme by forming a covalent bond that cannot be split readily. These inhibitors can modify any portion of the enzyme. In terms of enzyme kinetic analysis, they never exhibit purely competitive inhibition. Some of these irreversible inhibitors resemble substrates but then trap the enzyme irreversibly in one phase of its catalytic cycle. These latter inhibitors are also called **suicide inhibitors**; Table 10.4 provides three examples. An enzyme that has reacted with a suicide inhibitor cannot regain its catalytic activity and must be degraded and replaced.

The commonly used terms feedback inhibition, product inhibition, and feed-forward activation are based on knowledge of metabolic pathways. **Feedback inhibition** refers to the inhibition of the activity of an enzyme by a downstream product. **Product inhibition** refers to the inhibition of an enzyme by its product. Some scientists view product inhibition as a form of feedback inhibition. Others reserve the term feedback inhibition for inhibitors that are not the immediate product of the reaction in question, and they therefore do not consider product inhibition to be a form of feedback inhibition. **Feed-forward activation** refers to the activation of an enzyme by an upstream metabolite. The following are examples of feedback inhibition, product inhibition, and feed-forward activation in glycolysis (see Chapter 19): glucose 6-phosphate product inhibits hexokinase, ATP feedback inhibits phosphofructokinase 1, and fructose 1,6-bisphosphate feed-forward activates pyruvate kinase.

Some enzymes change activity in response to **covalent modification**. The best-known examples are enzymes that are influenced by **phosphorylation** (the addition of a phosphate group) at one or more key residues. Kinases add phosphate groups, and phosphatases remove them. Examples are glycogen synthase and glycogen phosphorylase (see Chapter 24).

## 5. ENZYME ACTIVITY AND FLUX IN METABOLIC PATHWAYS

*For convenience, enzyme-catalyzed reactions are categorized into physiologically reversible and irreversible reactions. The irreversible reactions occur physiologically in only one direction, regardless of the concentrations of the reactants and products. These reactions commit molecules to pathways, and the activity of enzymes that catalyze them is often regulated by the concentration of a product of the pathway. A partial deficiency of an enzyme of a metabolic pathway may limit flux through every step of the pathway.*

**Table 10.4** **Examples of Commonly Encountered Activators and Inhibitors of Enzymes**

| Type and Subtype | Pathway | Example |
|---|---|---|
| **Allosteric activator** | Glycolysis | Fructose-2,6-bisphosphate activates phosphofructokinase 1 by increasing its affinity for the substrate fructose-6-phosphate (see Chapter 19). |
| | Glycogen synthesis | Glucose 6-phosphate activates glycogen synthase in part by increasing its affinity for the substrate UDP-glucose (see Chapter 24). |
| | Signaling | cAMP activates cAMP-dependent protein kinase by causing the dissociation of regulatory subunits that inhibit catalytic subunits (see Chapter 33). |
| | Synthesis of urea | N-acetylglutamate induces an active conformation of carbamoylphosphate synthase I, which catalyzes an early step in the elimination of nitrogen as urea (see Chapter 35). |
| **REVERSIBLE INHIBITORS** | | |
| **Competitive inhibitor** | Cholesterol synthesis | The widely used **statin** drugs inhibit HMG-CoA reductase by binding to the active site in place of HMG-CoA (see Chapter 29). |
| | Synthesis of dTMP | The antineoplastic drug **methotrexate** inhibits dihydrofolate reductase by binding to the same site as the substrate dihydrofolate (see Chapter 37). |
| **Noncompetitive inhibitor** | Glycolysis | ATP allosterically inhibits phosphofructokinase 1 by decreasing its affinity for the substrate fructose-6-phosphate (see Chapter 19). |
| **IRREVERSIBLE INHIBITORS** | | |
| **Suicide inhibitor** | Synthesis of dTMP | The body converts the antineoplastic/cancer chemotherapeutic drug **5-fluorouracil** to 5F-dUMP, which reacts in place of dUMP (i.e., 5H-dUMP) with thymidylate synthase and $N^5$, $N^{10}$-methylene tetrahydrofolate, leading to an intermediate that cannot go forward or backward in the reaction sequence (see Chapter 37). |
| | Formation of urate | Xanthine oxidase normally converts hypoxanthine to xanthine and then to urate. **Allopurinol** gets converted to oxypurinol, which inhibits xanthine oxidase irreversibly (see Chapter 38). |
| | Acidification of stomach | An $H^+$, $K^+$-ATPase normally pumps $H^+$ out of parietal cells and into the lumen of the stomach (see Chapter 34). **Omeprazole** and related proton pump inhibitors form a covalent bond with a cysteine residue of the $H^+$, $K^+$-ATPase that is very long lived. |

ATPase, adenosine triphosphatase; cAMP, cyclic adenosine monophosphate; dTMP, deoxythymidine monophosphate; dUMP, deoxyuridine monophosphate; HMG-CoA, 3-hydroxy-3-methylglutaryl coenzyme A; UDP, uridine diphosphate.

In clinical biochemistry, it is useful to divide enzyme-catalyzed reactions into groups of physiologically reversible and irreversible reactions.

All chemical and enzyme-catalyzed reactions can only proceed in the direction of liberating Gibbs free energy (see Section 2). In theory, reactants and products of any chemical reaction can be chosen such that the reaction proceeds forward or backward (i.e., every chemical reaction is reversible). Enzymes also catalyze reactions in both directions. However, inside an organism, only a relatively narrow range of concentrations of the reactants and products is compatible with life.

This text uses the terms reversible and irreversible as follows. Physiologically **reversible reactions** are often close to equilibrium and they can proceed forward or backward, depending on the prevailing concentrations of the reactants and products (these reactions generally have a change in Gibbs free energy, $\Delta G$, between 0 and about $-20$ kJ/mol). **Physiologically irreversible** reactions are far from equilibrium and proceed only in one direction because the concentration of the products relative to that of the reactants is never high enough to reverse the reaction (these reactions generally have a change in Gibbs free energy, $\Delta G$, between about $-20$ and $-130$ kJ/mol). In the liver, for example, the reversible reactions in glycolysis proceed in one direction in the fed state (see Chapter 19), and in the opposite direction in the fasting state (see Chapter 25); in the fasting state, enzymes that catalyze the irreversible reactions of glycolysis are made quite inactive and enzymes that catalyze *different* irreversible reactions for gluconeogenesis are made active.

Irreversible reactions commit chemicals to pathways, and the rate of these reactions does not depend on the concentration of the products. In the pathway shown in Fig. 10.5, reaction 1 irreversibly feeds A into the pathway. Such a reaction is typically regulated, often via inhibition from a downstream product (i.e., feedback inhibition; see Section 4). Furthermore, such a reaction often also limits flux through the pathway (flux is the number of molecules that pass through per unit of time). In glycolysis, for example (see Chapter 19), A is fructose 6-phosphate, and B is fructose 1,6-bisphosphate; reaction 1 is

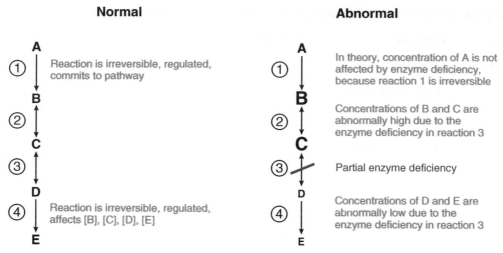

**Fig. 10.5** **Normal and abnormal regulation of flux through a metabolic pathway.** Single-headed arrows indicate irreversible reactions; double-headed arrows indicate reversible reactions.

catalyzed by phosphofructokinase 1, and this enzyme is regulated by the concentrations of AMP and ATP. These nucleotides can be viewed as feedback regulators since glycolysis lowers the concentration of AMP and maintains or increases the concentration of ATP.

In the pathway discussed above (see Fig. 10.5), B is converted to C and then to D by the reversible reactions 2 and 3. Under normal circumstances, there is usually an excess of enzyme activity to catalyze such reactions. Additionally, the activity of enzymes that catalyze these reactions is not regulated. The relative concentrations of B, C, and D depend largely on chemical thermodynamics, and to a lesser degree on the rate of flux through the pathway (at a low rate of flux, the concentrations of B, C, and D are closer to equilibrium than at a high rate of flux). Examples of reversible reactions in glycolysis are those shown with bidirectional arrows in Fig. 19.2 in Chapter 19.

In the pathway shown in Fig. 10.5, reaction 4, which is irreversible, determines the concentrations of intermediates B, C, and D. The rate of the irreversible reaction 4 depends only on the concentration of D. If the rate of reaction 4 is less than that of reaction 1, the concentration of intermediates B, C, and D increases, which also enhances the rate of reaction 4. Thus, the concentrations of B, C, and D depend on the amount of enzyme that catalyzes reaction 4, as well as on the kinetic properties of this enzyme. An example of reaction 4 in glycolysis is the conversion of phosphoenolpyruvate to pyruvate, which is catalyzed by pyruvate kinase (see Chapter 19). Some intermediates of glycolysis are needed for other pathways so that a control of the concentrations of these intermediates becomes important. Indeed, the activity of pyruvate kinase is controlled not just by the amount of enzyme that is present and active, but also by an intermediate of the pathway, fructose 1,6-bisphosphate (e.g., B in the pathway of Fig. 10.5).

**Steady state** is defined as a state in which the concentrations of reactants and products do not change. Many

metabolic reactions can be considered to be very close to steady state. If a linear pathway of metabolism is in steady state, every reaction also shows the same flux. If the pathway shown in Fig. 10.5 is in a steady state, flux through the reaction A → B is therefore the same as through reaction B → C, and so forth. In cells, steady state is typically achieved within seconds. Samples taken from patients (e.g., blood) are expected to reflect steady-state conditions.

If there is a partial or complete **deficiency** of the enzyme that catalyzes reaction 3 in the pathway shown in Fig. 10.5, there is an increase in the concentrations of B and C, and a decrease in the concentrations of D and E. The concentration of A is not affected because it is followed by an irreversible reaction, the rate of which is not influenced by the concentration of product B. Again, steady state is generally reached within seconds. If a patient has a deficiency in enzyme 3, the build-up of B and C, or the depletion of D and E, can have clinical significance.

## 6. ENZYMES IN THE BLOOD THAT HAVE DIAGNOSTIC SIGNIFICANCE

*Data on the activity of certain enzymes in the blood provide the clinician with information about tissue damage.*

Tissues normally lose a small fraction of their enzymes into the bloodstream. Tissue damage enhances this loss. Measurements of the activities in the blood of some of these enzymes provide the clinician with useful data (Table 10.5). In blood, these enzymes play no physiological role.

## 7. ENZYME-LINKED IMMUNOSORBENT ASSAY

*Enzyme-linked immunosorbent assays (ELISAs) allow the measurement of a very small amount of an antigen or antibody due to the high sensitivity with which enzyme activity of an enzyme-antibody or the enzyme-antigen conjugate can be measured.*

## Table 10.5 Enzymes in the Blood That Are Useful for Diagnosis

| Enzyme | Interpretation of Abnormal Activity |
|---|---|
| γ-Glutamyl transpeptidase | Elevation may indicate liver damage. |
| Alanine aminotransferase | Elevation may indicate liver damage. |
| Aspartate aminotransferase | Elevation may indicate damage to liver or heart. |
| Alkaline phosphatase | Elevation may indicate obstructive liver disease or a bone disorder.* |
| Creatine kinase | Elevation may indicate damage to skeletal or cardiac muscle. Isozymes exist, and isozyme composition can be determined. |
| Lactate dehydrogenase | Elevated total activity may indicate damage to one of many tissues. Isozymes exist. |
| Amylase | Elevation may indicate an obstruction of the pancreatic duct or damage to the pancreas. |
| Lipase | Elevation may indicate damage to the pancreas. |

*Normally elevated in pregnant women due to loss from the placenta.

ELISAs are carried out with an enzyme that is covalently linked to an antigen or an antibody. In the simplest form of the assay (Fig. 10.6), an antigen is immobilized on the surface of a small container, an enzyme-antibody conjugate is added, and the activity of the bound enzyme is then measured (often by measuring a light-absorbing or a fluorescent product). One such application is the measurement of ferritin in serum (see Section 7 in Chapter 15). Alternatively, antibodies in a patient's serum are adsorbed, an antigen-enzyme conjugate is added, and the activity of the bound enzyme is measured. This method is currently used to measure antibodies against the hepatitis C virus or the human immunodeficiency virus.

## SUMMARY

- Enzymes can be identified by systematic name as oxidoreductases, transferases, hydrolases, lyases, isomerases, or ligases; they can also be identified by an enzyme classification (EC) number that is based on these categories. However, clinically relevant enzymes are for the most part still identified by their recommended names, which often have historical roots.

- Enzymes often contain nonpeptidic molecules as coenzymes. When such coenzymes are tightly or covalently bound, they are often called prosthetic groups; examples are biotin, heme, and lipoic acid.

- Isoenzymes (isozymes) are enzymes that catalyze the same reaction but differ in their amino acid sequence. Often, isoenzymes also differ in their kinetic properties; the hexokinases are an example.

- Enzymes act as catalysts. An enzyme speeds up a thermodynamically feasible reaction (one with a negative ΔG) by decreasing its activation energy. Enzymes do not change the position of the chemical equilibrium.

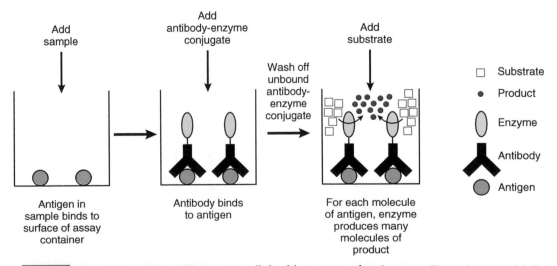

**Fig. 10.6  Basic principle of the enzyme-linked immunosorbent assay.** The antigen may bind directly to the surface of the assay container, or to antibodies with which the surface has been precoated. The product is usually measured by the absorbance of light, fluorescence upon excitation with light, or emission of light (luminescence).

- Enzymes have a pH and temperature optimum.
- The lock-and-key theory is an older and the induced-fit theory a more recent attempt to model enzyme-substrate interactions.
- The Michaelis-Menten equation is $v/V_{max} = s/(s + K_m)$. The $K_m$ is the concentration of substrate s, at which the enzyme works at half its maximal velocity (i.e., s, at which $v/V_{max} = 0.5$). A doubling of substrate concentration does not usually lead to a doubling of enzyme activity because the v (or $v/V_{max}$) versus s plots are not linear.
- For enzymes that show cooperativity for a substrate, the Michaelis-Menten equation can be modified and written as $v/V_{max} = s^h/(s^h + S_{0.5}^h)$. $S_{0.5}$ is the substrate concentration at which the enzyme works at half its maximal velocity. h is the Hill coefficient.
- An enzyme unit (U) is usually the amount of enzyme that produces product at the rate of 1 μmol/min (based on the calculated $V_{max}$).
- Allosteric regulatory sites are by definition located at a site of the enzyme that is removed from the catalytic (or active) site. Competitive inhibitors compete with the substrate for binding to the catalytic site, while noncompetitive inhibitors bind to another site. Some drugs are suicide inhibitors (i.e., they typically bind to the catalytic site and then irreversibly inhibit the enzyme).
- The flux in metabolic pathways is often regulated by feed-forward activation, feedback inhibition, or product inhibition.
- In a linear metabolic pathway, a partial enzyme deficiency leads to an *increase* in the concentrations of metabolites that precede the impaired reaction (except metabolites that are upstream of an irreversible reaction) and a *decrease* in the concentrations of metabolites that follow the impaired reaction.
- The activities of some enzymes in the bloodstream are indicative of damage to a specific tissue. These activities are reported as U or IU per volume of the blood, plasma, or serum.
- Enzyme-linked immunosorbent assays (ELISAs) are used to measure low concentrations of proteins of clinical interest. These assays derive their specificity from antigen-antibody interactions, and their sensitivity from an antigen- or antibody-linked enzyme that produces many molecules of product for each protein molecule of interest.

### FURTHER READING

- Biomolecular Movies and Images for Teaching. Induced fit and hexokinase. <http://www.chem.ucsb.edu/~molvisual/ABLE/induced_fit/index.html>.
- BRENDA: The Comprehensive Enzyme Information System. <http://www.brenda-enzymes.org>. This site provides a list of enzymes along with names, reactions, kinetic parameters, and a set of links to literature data.
- Cook PF, Cleland WW. *Enzyme Kinetics and Mechanism.* London: Garland Science; 2007.
- Copeland RA. *Enzymes: A Practical Introduction to Structure, Mechanism, and Data Analysis.* 2nd ed. New York: Wiley-VCH; 2000.
- Fersht A. *Structure and Mechanism in Protein Science: A Guide to Enzyme Catalysis and Protein Folding.* New York: WH Freeman; 1999.
- Jencks WP. *Catalysis in Chemistry and Enzymology.* New York: McGraw-Hill; 1969.
- Koshland DE. Application of a theory of enzyme specificity to protein synthesis. *Proc Natl Acad Sci USA.* 1958;44:98-104.
- Skloot R. Some called her Miss Menten. *Pittmed Mag.* 2000;2(4):18-21. Available at: <http://pittmed.health.pitt.edu/oct_2000/miss_menten.pdf>.

# Review Questions

1. An enzyme that is normally active in the cytoplasm is tested both at pH 7 and at pH 5. Then the enzyme activities at these two conditions are compared. None of the catalytically active amino acid side chains has ionizable groups. At pH 5, protons most likely behave like which one of the following?

   A. Allosteric activator
   B. Competitive inhibitor
   C. Irreversible inhibitor
   D. Noncompetitive inhibitor
   E. Suicide inhibitor

2. Dihydrofolate reductase catalyzes the reaction DHF + NADPH + $H^+$ → THF + $NADP^+$. The inhibitor methotrexate binds to the catalytic site of dihydrofolate reductase in place of DHF. The graph below shows the activity of dihydrofolate reductase with and without methotrexate. Which of the following is the major effect of methotrexate?

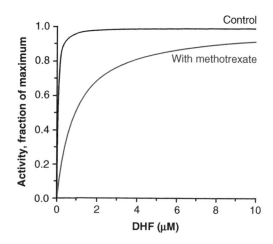

   A. Decrease of the $K_m$ of dihydrofolate reductase for DHF
   B. Decrease of the $V_{max}$ of dihydrofolate reductase
   C. Increase of the $K_m$ of dihydrofolate reductase for DHF
   D. Increase of the $V_{max}$ of dihydrofolate reductase

3. An enzyme was purified from fibroblasts of a healthy patient. In addition, this enzyme was also purified from the fibroblasts of a patient who has a disorder of metabolism. As judged by electrophoresis and staining of the protein, the purity of both enzymes was 97%. Results of the kinetic analyses of equal concentrations of purified protein are shown in the graph below. Based on these data, the mutant enzyme causes disease chiefly by having which of the following?

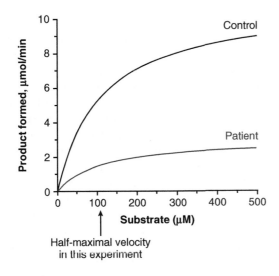

**A.** A decreased $K_m$

**B.** A decreased $V_{max}$

**C.** An increased $K_m$

**D.** An increased $V_{max}$

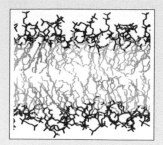

# Chapter 11

# Biological Membranes

## SYNOPSIS

■ The membranes that enclose cells and their subcellular compartments consist of phospholipids, glycosphingolipids, cholesterol, and proteins that are lipid embedded or bound to the membrane surface. The extracellular side of plasma membranes contains many sugar residues, which are covalently linked to phospholipids and membrane proteins.

■ Plasma membranes and the membranes that delimit most organelles contain two layers. Lipids and proteins in each layer diffuse laterally.

■ Substances that are sufficiently hydrophobic (including oxygen and many currently used orally effective drugs) can cross biological membranes. However, charged or highly hydrophilic compounds do not diffuse through membranes; rather, such compounds cross membranes only with the aid of transport proteins.

■ Some transport proteins facilitate passive transport of substances across membranes; others use the energy from nucleotide hydrolysis or from an electrochemical gradient to transport compounds actively across a membrane.

## LEARNING OBJECTIVES

*For mastery of this topic, you should be able to do the following:*

■ Describe the structure and content of a biological bilayer membrane, list at least five types of lipids in such membranes, describe the membrane distribution of these lipids, and characterize the processes that maintain or destroy membrane lipid asymmetry, paying special attention to phosphatidylserine.

■ List the means by which proteins can be anchored in a membrane.

■ Explain how ethanol, $O_2$, $CO_2$, $NH_3$, $K^+$, $Na^+$, and glucose are transported across membrane bilayers.

■ Compare and contrast the transport mechanism and transport rate of channels or pores, transmembrane carrier proteins, and pumps; then, provide an example of each.

## 1. STRUCTURE AND COMPOSITION OF MEMBRANES

*Membranes form barriers to hydrophilic substances and thus, compartmentalize metabolic reactions, signaling, electrical charges, and so forth. Membranes consist of a bilayer of lipids, into which proteins are embedded. The major membrane lipids are diacylglycerophospholipids, cardiolipin, plasmalogens, sphingomyelin, gangliosides, and cholesterol. Proteins often use α-helices to span membranes. Other proteins are anchored to the membrane via a phospholipid, a fatty acid, or a prenyl group.*

### 1.1. Physiological Roles of Membranes

The term **membrane** is usually reserved for lipid **bilayers**, such as the plasma membrane, the inner and outer nuclear and mitochondrial membranes, and the membranes that delimit lysosomes, the smooth and rough endoplasmic reticulum, peroxisomes, secretory vesicles, and synaptic vesicles. In contrast, lipid storage droplets inside cells and lipoprotein particles in the blood are delimited by a **monolayer** of phospholipids (as well as proteins) (see Chapters 28 and 29).

Membranes delimit cells and subcellular compartments. Membranes can separate synthesis and degradation (e.g., in the liver, fatty acid synthesis in the cytosol from fatty acid degradation in the mitochondria; see Chapter 27). They can delimit zones for regulation or signaling (e.g., $Ca^{2+}$ signaling in the cytosol, whereby the extracellular space, mitochondria, and the endoplasmic reticulum play accessory roles; see Chapter 33). They can serve as a scaffold for forming enzyme complexes (e.g., adenylate cyclase and protein kinase A; see Chapter 24) and serve as a reservoir for phospholipids that are needed in signaling (e.g., by phospholipases; see Chapter 33) or for biosyntheses (e.g., of prostaglandins; see Chapter 32). They can also act as electrical insulators between ions and thus participate in energy production (see Chapter 23) or electrical signaling (e.g., in pancreatic endocrine cells; see Chapter 26).

### 1.2. Structure of Lipids

Lipid bilayer membranes contain phospholipids, sphingolipids, cholesterol, and proteins. A classification of phospholipids and sphingolipids is shown in Fig. 11.1. Phospholipids and sphingolipids can contain various fatty acids. Section 1 in Chapter 27 provides an introduction to saturated, cis-unsaturated, and trans-unsaturated fatty acids.

The **phospholipids** always contain a phosphomonoester or a phosphodiester (see Fig. 11.1). Among them, the **diacylglycerophospholipids** are **esters** of glycerol and two fatty acids. The most abundant diacylglycerophospholipids in membranes are **phosphatidylcholine** (popularly called **lecithin**), **phosphatidylserine**, **phosphatidylethanolamine**, and **phosphatidylinositol**. Phosphatidylinositol can be phosphorylated and then hydrolyzed as part of signal transmission (see Chapter 33).

The **plasmalogens** are also phospholipids, but they contain a **vinyl ether** and an ester (see Fig. 11.1). The plasmalogens carry the prefix plasmenyl (e.g., in plasmenylethanolamine). Plasmalogens probably serve as **antioxidants**. Their vinyl

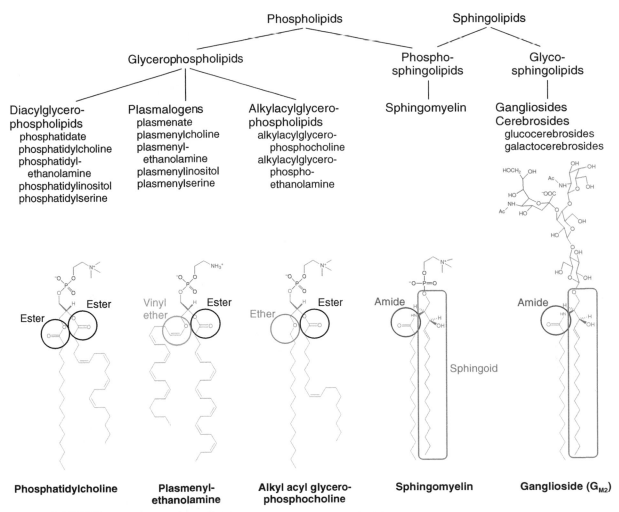

**Fig. 11.1** **Classification of phospholipids and sphingolipids.** For each molecule shown, the fatty acid content may vary significantly.

ether more readily reacts with reactive oxygen radicals than does an ester in a diacylglycerophospholipid. As a result, plasmalogens protect polyunsaturated fatty acids (e.g., arachidonic acid and docosahexaenoic acid) from a radical attack. Of all the phospholipids in the brain and cardiac and skeletal muscle, 20% or more are plasmalogens. In **myelin**, most of the phospholipids are plasmalogens, and without plasmalogens, nerve conduction is profoundly impaired. Many **peroxisome disorders** impair plasmalogen biosynthesis and thus the function of the nervous system.

The diacylglycerophospholipids and plasmalogens have similar **head groups** (i.e., choline, serine, ethanolamine, or inositol) (Fig. 11.2).

**Cardiolipin** in the inner membrane of mitochondria is a unique glycerophospholipid in that it contains *four* fatty acids (see Fig. 11.3). When the function of mitochondria is compromised, cardiolipin moves to the outer mitochondrial membrane and becomes a signal for **apoptosis** of the cell. Antibodies to cardiolipin are found in the autoimmune disorder **antiphospholipid syndrome**, which has a prevalence of about 0.5% and leads to vascular thrombosis (blood clot forming inside a blood vessel).

In **alkylacylglycerophospholipids**, one substituent of glycerol is an alkyl group, and the other substituent is an acyl group. Hence, alkylacylglycerophospholipids contain a plain ether (not a vinyl ether) and an ester.

The **sphingolipids** (see Fig. 11.1) contain a **sphingoid**, which is synthesized from serine and a fatty acid. The sphingolipids are divided into two categories, the **phosphosphingolipids** and the **glycosphingolipids**. The phosphosphingolipids are also phospholipids because they contain a phosphate group. The most common phosphosphingolipid is **sphingomyelin**. Glycosphingolipids are found primarily in the outer leaflet of the plasma membranes. The most commonly encountered glycosphingolipids are the **gangliosides**, which contain one or more sialic acid residues (usually N-acetylneuraminic acid). Gangliosides are particularly abundant in the plasma membranes of neurons, and their degradation is impaired in **Tay-Sachs disease**.

**Ceramides** consist of a sphingoid that is acylated on its amino-nitrogen. Ceramides, in contrast to sphingomyelin, contain no phosphate or head group. Ceramides play a role in signaling. Ceramides can be synthesized from serine and palmitate; they can be produced directly from sphingomyelin, or

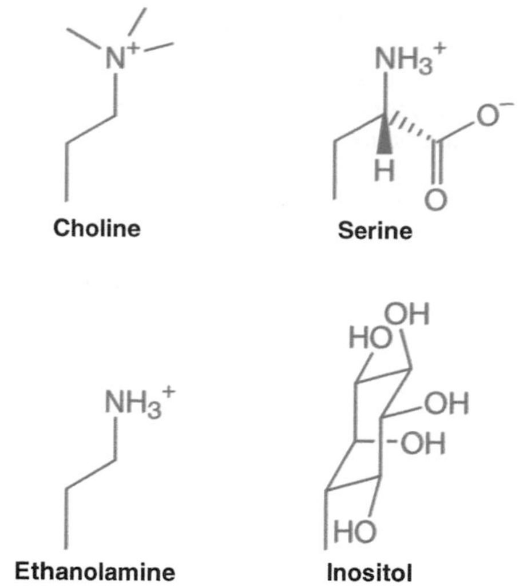

Choline

Serine

Ethanolamine

Inositol

**Fig. 11.2** **Structure of head groups in diacylglycerophospholipids and plasmalogens.**

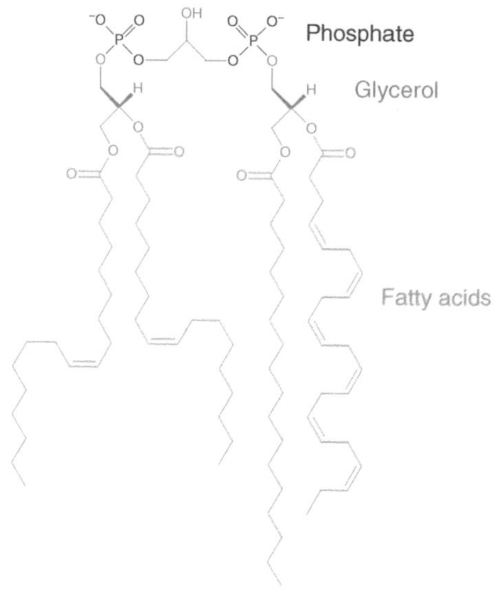

Phosphate

Glycerol

Fatty acids

**Fig. 11.3** **Structure of a cardiolipin.** Various fatty acids can be part of cardiolipin.

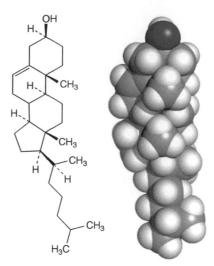

**Fig. 11.4** **Structure of cholesterol.** The hydroxyl group is hydrophilic and is primarily located at the water interface of membranes, while the remaining portion of cholesterol is hydrophobic and preferentially associates with sphingomyelin. In this space-filled model, C is gray, H white, and O red. (Based on svn.cgl.ucsf.edu/chimera/trunk/devel/RasMol/RasMol_Scripts/BILAYR1P/CHOLESTE.pdb.)

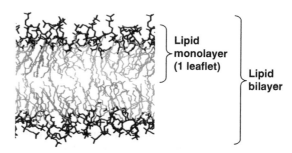

Lipid monolayer (1 leaflet)

Lipid bilayer

**Fig. 11.5** **Basic structure of a lipid bilayer membrane.** A computer simulation of a bilayer that consists of phosphatidylcholine that contains two 14-carbon saturated fatty acids. The head groups are shown in black, and the rest of each molecule is shown in gray. (Modified from Robinson AJ, Richards WG, Thomas PJ, Hann MM. Head group and chain behavior in biological membranes: a molecular dynamics computer simulation. *Biophys J.* 1994;67:2345–2354.)

they can be generated from a sphingoid that is released from lysosomes, which degrade sphingolipids (this is called the salvage pathway).

**Lysophospholipids** are phospholipids (glycerophospholipids or sphingolipids) that have lost one of their constituent fatty acids. This is commonly due to the action of various phospholipases, such as in the digestive tract (see Chapter 28) or in signaling (see Chapter 33). When present in the plasma membrane at a sufficiently high concentration, lysophospholipids lead to cell lysis (hence their name).

Membranes also contain **cholesterol** (Fig. 11.4). Membranes of different organelles differ in their lipid composition. Cholesterol is commonly found in plasma membranes, as well as in the membranes of lysosomes and the trans-Golgi, but it is scarce in the endoplasmic reticulum membrane.

## 1.3. Composition and Structure of Bilayer Membranes

The lipid **bilayer** of membranes (Fig. 11.5) contains phospholipids, sphingolipids, and cholesterol. The lipid bilayer consists of an inner and an outer **leaflet**, each of which is a monolayer of lipids. The lipids in each monolayer are **amphipathic**; their hydrophobic portions aggregate to form the hydrophobic core of the membrane; their hydrophilic portions (phosphate- and head groups; see Fig. 11.1) face the water phase on either side of the membrane. Such bilayer membranes also form spontaneously in vitro from lipid mixtures in water. (Triglycerides are not sufficiently amphipathic to form bilayer membranes.)

Lipid bilayer membranes form a **barrier** against hydrophilic substances, while they permit the passage of many uncharged, lipophilic substances (see Section 2).

Membrane **proteins** are embedded into one or both lipid layers (see Section 1.5). Some of these proteins help transport hydrophilic substances across membranes (see Section 2.2).

**Detergents** can destroy membranes by solubilizing proteins and lipids into mixed micelles. This is the basis of the antimicrobial effect of soap.

**Liposomes** (lipid vesicles) are used as vehicles for drug delivery. Liposomes consist of a spherical lipid bilayer membrane that encloses a small amount of liquid. Liposomes are made in the laboratory. They are much smaller than cells. Drug-loaded liposomes have a tendency to accumulate in the extracellular space of tumor tissues, owing to leaky capillaries; there, liposomes act as slow-release vesicles, either in the extracellular space or after uptake into cells. Macrophages tend to take up most of the liposomes. Coating liposomes with polyethylene glycol (PEG) dramatically prolongs the time they are circulating.

In biological membranes, at physiological temperature, phospholipids and sphingolipids are free to diffuse within their leaflet, but they cannot readily flip from one leaflet to the other. Proteins that are embedded in the membrane (see Section 1.5) likewise can diffuse within the plane of the bilayer membrane, but they cannot flip from one side of the membrane to the other. This state in which the long axis of the phospholipids always points in the same direction, yet molecules can move laterally, is also called a liquid crystalline state. In contrast, at a considerably lower temperature, the lipids enter a gel state in which lipids and membrane proteins have greatly reduced lateral mobility.

**Unsaturated fatty acids** increase membrane **fluidity** (i.e., they favor a liquid crystalline state). In contrast, **saturated fatty acids** lower membrane fluidity.

Under physiological conditions, **cholesterol** increases the mechanical strength of the membranes and reduces their permeability to water and small molecules. Cholesterol binds most strongly to phospholipids with saturated acyl chains, which are predominantly found in sphingomyelin and to a lesser extent in phosphatidylcholine). Under physiological circumstances, cholesterol has the effect of ordering lipids and condensing the bilayer, hence the increased strength and decreased permeability.

Commonly found **fatty acids** in phospholipids include palmitic (16:0; for nomenclature, see Section 1 in Chapter 27), stearic (18:0), oleic (18:1), linoleic (18:2), arachidonic (20:4), and docosahexaenoic acid (22:4). Within the same membrane, phosphatidylcholine, phosphatidylserine, phosphatidylethanolamine, and sphingomyelin often differ appreciably in their fatty acid composition.

The two leaflets of plasma membranes have a different **lipid composition**. Among phospholipids, sphingomyelin and phosphatidylcholine predominate in the **outer leaflet**, while phosphatidylserine and phosphatidylethanolamine are found mostly in the **inner leaflet** (Table 11.1 provides an example).

The distribution of **cholesterol** between the membrane leaflets is approximately equal or skewed in favor of the sphingomyelin-rich outer leaflet. However, cholesterol also spontaneously flips between the membrane leaflets. Plasma

**Table 11.1   Asymmetrical Distribution of Phospholipids in Human Red Blood Cell Membranes**

| Phospholipid | % of Total | |
| --- | --- | --- |
|  | Inner Leaflet | Outer Leaflet |
| Sphingomyelin | 2 | 20 |
| Phosphatidylcholine | 7 | 20 |
| Phosphatidylserine | 13 | 2 |
| Phosphatidylethanolamine | 23 | 7 |
| Others | 3 | 3 |

Data from Zachowski A. Phospholipids in animal eukaryotic membranes: transverse asymmetry and movement. *Biochem J.* 1993;294:1-14.

membranes contain approximately equal numbers of cholesterol and phospholipid molecules.

When **phosphatidylserine** moves from the inner to the outer leaflet of the plasma membrane, it acts as a signal. Macrophages in the reticuloendothelial system of the spleen, for example, recognize phosphatidylserine on the surface of **senescent red blood cells** and then remove these cells. Elsewhere in the body, macrophages similarly recognize an increased concentration of phosphatidylserine in the outer leaflet of the membrane of cells that undergo **apoptosis** (programmed cell death; see Chapter 8). In **platelets**, an increased concentration of phosphatidylserine in the outer leaflet of the membrane plays a role in activating other platelets, a prerequisite for blood clotting.

Biological membranes contain **membrane rafts**. There are two types of rafts: (1) short-lived planar rafts and (2) long-lived caveolae. The **planar rafts** are thought to consist mainly of saturated phospholipids and sphingolipids, cholesterol, and membrane proteins that either have a glycophosphatidylinositol anchor (and face the extracellular space) or a fatty acid anchor (and face the cytosol; see Section 1.5). The planar rafts are most likely very small (a diameter of <1% of the diameter of a red blood cell) and short lived (a half-life in the millisecond range). **Caveolae** are flask-like invaginations of the plasma membrane that are particularly abundant in adipocytes, vascular endothelial cells, and smooth muscle cells. Caveolae play a role in signaling, membrane maintenance, and endocytosis. The invaginations are created and stabilized by integral and peripheral membrane proteins (e.g., the caveolins and cavins; see Section 1.5).

### 1.4. Transport of Lipids Inside Membranes

Several enzymes move phospholipids between membrane leaflets (Fig. 11.6). The transport of phospholipids from the outer leaflet to the inner leaflet is also called flipping, and the transporters responsible for this are called **flippases**.

Cytosol    **Membrane**    Extracellular space

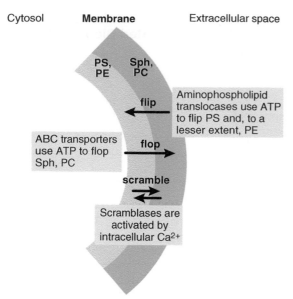

PS, PE    Sph, PC

**flip**

Aminophospholipid translocases use ATP to flip PS and, to a lesser extent, PE

ABC transporters use ATP to flop Sph, PC

**flop**

**scramble**

Scramblases are activated by intracellular $Ca^{2+}$

**Fig. 11.6**  **Enzymes that maintain or abolish the asymmetric distribution of phospholipids in bilayer membranes.** *ABC,* ATP binding cassette; *ATP,* adenosine triphosphate; *PC,* phosphatidylcholine; *PE,* phosphatidylethanolamine; *PS,* phosphatidylserine; *Sph,* sphingomyelin.

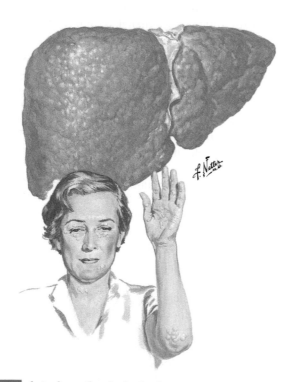

**Fig. 11.7**  **Intrahepatic cholestasis.** The disorder leads to jaundice and xanthomas of the face, neck, palms, and elbows.

Conversely, outward transport is called flopping and is accomplished by **floppases**. **Scramblases** move phospholipids between leaflets in either direction.

Mutant **multidrug resistance protein 3 (MDR3)** is a floppase encoded by the *ABCA4* gene and gives rise to a form of **intrahepatic cholestasis** (Fig. 11.7). MDR3 transports phosphatidylcholine from the inner to the outer leaflet of the

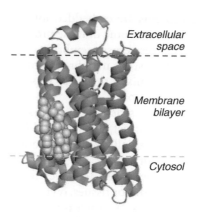

**Fig. 11.8**  **Part of the human $\beta_2$-adrenergic receptor.** Two molecules of cholesterol are shown as spheres, with the O of the hydroxyl group shown in red. To obtain a crystal for analyses, one amino acid residue was mutated, and a 26-residue cytosolic loop was replaced by another protein (not shown). (Based on Protein Data Bank file 3D4S. From Hanson MA, Cherezov V, Griffith MT, et al. A specific cholesterol binding site is established by the 2.8 A structure of the human beta2-adrenergic receptor. *Structure.* 2008;16:897-905.)

plasma membrane. Secretion of phospholipids from the liver into bile is important to attenuate the toxic effects of bile salts and to prevent the formation of cholesterol stones. Severely affected patients develop cirrhosis and liver failure, and they are at risk for a cholangiocarcinoma.

## 1.5. Membrane Proteins

Proteins can be part of, or tied to, a membrane in many different ways. Some proteins contain one or more **helices** with hydrophobic amino acids that **span** the membrane (e.g., the human $\beta$-adrenergic receptor) (Fig. 11.8). Less commonly, proteins span a membrane with $\beta$-**sheets** that form a $\beta$-**barrel** (aquaporin is an example). Other proteins anchor themselves with a loop or helix of hydrophobic amino acids in only one membrane leaflet. Proteins with amino acid membrane anchors are called **integral** (or **intrinsic**) **membrane proteins**. In the lab, detergents can free such integral membrane proteins; physiologically, proteases can cut off a domain that protrudes from the membrane. For example, in the brain, the extracellular domain of the amyloid precursor protein is freed by a secretase (see Chapter 9). Yet, other proteins bind to lipids or proteins in the plasma membrane largely via electrostatic interactions, so that in the lab they can be removed from the membrane with a concentrated salt solution. These latter proteins are called **peripheral membrane proteins**. An example of such a protein is cubilin (see Fig. 36.9), which binds to the integral membrane protein amnionless and plays a role in cobalamin absorption. Other such peripheral membrane proteins play a role in signaling (see Chapter 33) by binding to specific lipids, such as phosphatidylinositol 4,5-bisphosphate (PIP2), phosphatidylinositol (3,4,5)-trisphosphate (PIP3), phosphatidylinositol 4-phosphate (PI4P), or diacylglycerol (DAG). Finally, there are proteins that are anchored in the membrane by a posttranslationally added

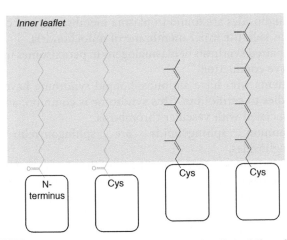

**Fig. 11.9** **Proteins tethered to the inner leaflet of the plasma membrane.**

lipid, (e.g., a fatty acid, an isoprene, or a glycosylphosphatidylinositol). Some of these proteins can be cut loose from their anchor, and some can even be reanchored.

Posttranslationally acquired inner-leaflet lipid anchors for proteins (Fig. 11.9) may consist of a **myristoyl** group (a 14-carbon fatty acid), a **palmitoyl** group (a 16-carbon fatty acid), a **farnesyl** group (a 15-carbon isoprene), or one to two **geranylgeranyl** groups (a 20-carbon isoprene). Proteins that contain a farnesyl or geranylgeranyl group are called **prenylated**. Some prenylated proteins also carry a palmitoyl anchor. The synthesis of isoprenes has several steps in common with the synthesis of cholesterol, and isoprene synthesis, like cholesterol synthesis, is inhibited by the **statin** drugs (see Fig. 29.4 and Section 2.1 in Chapter 29). The products of several proto-oncogenes and oncogenes (e.g., Ras proteins) have isoprene anchors. Statin use is associated with a lower risk of certain cancers. Whether statins also have a place in cancer treatment remains unknown. Prenylation is irreversible, but certain proteins can extract prenylated proteins from a membrane or deliver them to a membrane. Palmitoylated proteins can be released from their membrane anchor.

On the cytosolic side of the plasma membrane, the **cytoskeleton**, a network of cytosolic and transmembrane proteins, shapes and stabilizes the membrane.

**Glycosylphosphatidylinositol (GPI)** can anchor proteins in the outer leaflet of the plasma membrane (Fig. 11.10). Proteins with GPI anchors are on the extracellular face of the plasma membrane, and GPIases can cut the anchor so as to release the protein into the extracellular space.

**Paroxysmal nocturnal hemoglobinuria** is caused by an attack of the innate immune system on circulating red blood cells that lack GPI-anchored proteins that normally suppress this immune reaction. In most patients, this is an acquired mutation of hematopoietic stem cells. The product of the mutated gene normally catalyzes the first step in the synthesis of the GPI anchor. Formation of blood clots is the main problem in this disease.

The luminal side of intestinal enterocytes and blood vessel endothelial cells contains proteins in the plasma membrane that are glycosylated so extensively that the glycosyl residues

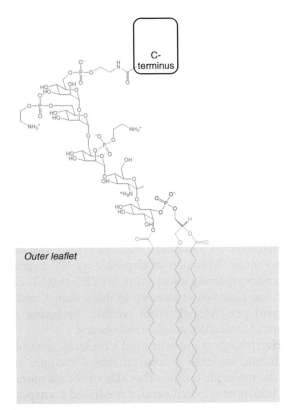

**Fig. 11.10** **Glycosylphosphatidylinositol-anchored proteins are tethered to the outer leaflet of the plasma membrane.**

form part of a **glycocalyx**, the thickness of which may be many times that of the membrane itself.

## 2. MOVEMENT OF MOLECULES ACROSS MEMBRANES

*Membranes are permeable to moderately hydrophobic substances, but they are a barrier to hydrophilic substances, particularly charged species. Some transport proteins form pores through which molecules can move, while many other transport proteins bind a molecule, undergo a conformational change, and then release the molecule on the other side of the membrane. Some of these latter proteins transport a second, different molecule in the same or opposite direction, and some are powered by ATP hydrolysis.*

### 2.1. Simple Diffusion of Molecules Through the Hydrophobic Core of the Lipid Bilayer

Some substances can cross a lipid bilayer by **simple diffusion**. Such substances must be soluble in the water phase on either side of the membrane, and they must also be sufficiently lipophilic to shed water and dissolve in the hydrophobic core of the lipid bilayer membrane. Substances that have a net electrical charge are usually too hydrophilic to dissolve in the hydrophobic membrane core. Indeed, as a rule in metabolism, charged molecules do not cross membranes by simple diffusion. Examples of molecules that pass through membranes by simple diffusion are $O_2$, $CO_2$, $NH_3$, ethanol, and many orally taken drugs.

## 2.2. Transport of Molecules Through Transport Proteins in Membranes

Charged, appreciably hydrophilic, or large molecules may cross a lipid bilayer only with the help of a transport protein. The transport protein may simply provide a means for the molecule to move down an electrochemical gradient (a combination of an electrical charge gradient and a chemical concentration gradient). If this is the case, such movement is called **facilitated diffusion**.

Some transport proteins provide (at least temporarily) a **pore** (also called a **channel**), through which specific molecules can move. Examples of channels are $Na^+$ channels and the water-transporting aquaporins. $Na^+$, $K^+$, and $Cl^-$ can move through ion channels at rates up to more than 1 million ions per second per channel. Pores provide the fastest mode of transport of molecules across a membrane.

**Carrier** transport proteins bind a molecule on one side of a membrane, undergo a conformational change, and then release the molecule on the other side of the membrane. This type of transport is called **carrier-mediated transport** and is a form of facilitated diffusion. In general, carriers operate at a much lower transport rate than pores. GLUT-type glucose transporters are an example of a carrier (see Chapter 18).

Some carrier transport proteins move molecules against their electrochemical gradient by using energy either from nucleotide hydrolysis or the electrochemical gradient of another molecule; this is called **active transport** and is a subcategory of carrier-mediated transport. Some of the proteins that catalyze active transport are also called **pumps**. Examples of active transport are the $Na^+$-coupled amino acid transporters (see Chapter 34) and the $Na^+$: $K^+$-ATPase, a pump that uses ATP to move $Na^+$ and $K^+$ ions in opposite directions (against their respective electrochemical gradients).

Carrier transport proteins that facilitate the simultaneous transport of two different molecules in the same direction are also called **cotransporters** or **symporters** (or symport); those that transport in opposite directions are called **antiporters** (or antiport) or **exchangers**. An example of a cotransporter is the $Na^+$-coupled glucose transporter (SGLT1) in the epithelium of the small intestine (see Chapter 18). An example of an exchange transporter is the antiporter for aspartate and glutamate in the inner mitochondrial membrane that is part of the malate-aspartate shuttle (see Chapters 19, 23, and 25).

## SUMMARY

- Bilayer membranes enclose cells, subcellular organelles, and intracellular vesicles. These membranes may contain cholesterol, glycerophospholipids, and sphingolipids.
- Phosphatidylcholine, phosphatidylethanolamine, phosphatidylserine, phosphatidylinositol, plasmenylethanolamine, plasmenylcholine, and sphingomyelin are all phospholipids that are commonly found in biological bilayer membranes.

Gangliosides are found in plasma membranes, and cardiolipin is in the inner membrane of mitochondria.

- Impaired synthesis of plasmalogens in peroxisomes impairs nerve conduction.
- Patients who have antiphospholipid syndrome have antibodies to cardiolipin. This syndrome is common, and it is associated with vascular thrombosis.
- Common sphingolipids are sphingomyelin and gangliosides.
- Cholesterol is a major constituent of the plasma membrane. It increases the mechanical strength of the membrane and decreases its permeability to water and small molecules.
- The leaflets of bilayer membranes often differ in phospholipid composition (e.g., phosphatidylserine is predominantly in the inner leaflet, while gangliosides and sphingomyelin are in the outer leaflet of plasma membranes). In part, such asymmetry is a result of leaflet-specific synthesis in the endoplasmic reticulum or mitochondria. However, lipid transporters also actively maintain phospholipid asymmetry. Aminophospholipid transporters are flippases that move phosphatidylserine and phosphatidylethanolamine from the outer leaflet of the plasma membrane to the inner leaflet. Conversely, certain ABC transporters are floppases that move sphingomyelin and phosphatidylcholine from the cytosolic leaflet to the outer leaflet of the plasma membrane.
- Impaired flopping of phosphatidylcholine from the inner to the outer plasma membrane leaflet leads to a form of intrahepatic cholestasis.
- Scramblases can move phosphatidylserine to the outer membrane leaflet, where it is a signal for platelet activation or apoptosis.
- Membranes contain short-lived planar rafts and comparatively long-lived invaginated rafts in the form of caveolae that play a role in signaling and membrane traffic.
- Membrane proteins can contain sequences that span the membrane several times, or they can contain a peptide anchor that penetrates only one membrane leaflet. Proteins can also acquire posttranslationally a membrane anchor of myristic acid, palmitic acid, farnesol, or geranylgeranol for anchoring in the inner leaflet of the plasma membrane. Yet other proteins acquire a glycosylphosphatidylinositol (GPI) anchor for anchoring in the outer leaflet of the plasma membrane.
- $O_2$, $CO_2$, and ethanol cross membranes without the aid of a transporter. Channels or pores rapidly transport small molecules, such as $Na^+$, $K^+$, $Cl^-$, and water. Carriers more slowly transport a variety of molecules, sometimes with the help of an electrochemical gradient or the input of energy from ATP hydrolysis. Certain carrier transport proteins are called antiports, exchangers, symports, or cotransporters.

## FURTHER READING

- Kovtun O, Tillu VA, Ariotti N, Parton RG, Collins BM. Cavin family proteins and the assembly of caveolae. *J Cell Sci.* 2015;128:1269-1278.

# Review Questions

1. Which of the following best describes the reason that phosphatidylserine by itself fails to cross the plasma membrane?

   A. Phosphatidylserine contains an ether-linked alkenyl chain.
   B. Phosphatidylserine contains two hydrophobic isoprenes.
   C. Phosphatidylserine is a glycolipid.
   D. Phosphatidylserine is electrically charged.

2. An antiporter that transports amino acids with a positively charged side chain between the extracellular space and the cytosol in exchange for the efflux of amino acids with an uncharged side chain is most likely also which of the following?

   A. A flippase
   B. A glycolipid
   C. A membrane-spanning protein
   D. An aminophospholipid translocase

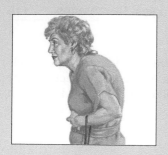

# Chapter 12

# Collagen, Collagenopathies, and Diseases of Mineralization

## SYNOPSIS

- Various types of collagens provide tensile strength in bone, tendons, and ligaments or filter fluids in the kidney glomeruli.
- Collagen α-chains are synthesized inside cells as precursors of mature collagen molecules. The precursors aggregate into trimers that form a collagen triple helix. The trimers are exported into the extracellular space. In some types of collagen, after proteolysis of flanking prosequences, the triple helices assemble to form fibrils or networks. Covalent cross linking further improves the stability of these complexes.
- The deposition of calcium phosphate within collagen fibrils, a process called mineralization, stiffens bone.
- Achondroplasia is caused by mutations that activate a fibroblast growth factor receptor, which in turn leads to decreased production of collagen in bone, causing short stature.
- The more severe forms of osteogenesis imperfecta are most often due to mutations in type I collagen that impair the formation of a triple helix, which greatly weakens bones and leads to numerous fractures.
- Most patients who have the classical Ehlers-Danlos syndrome have a mutant type V collagen that leads to hyperextensible and fragile skin.
- Insufficient mineralization of bone causes rickets in children and osteomalacia in adults.
- Paget disease of bone is associated with certain foci of excessive growth and other foci of excessive destruction in one or multiple bones.
- In persons with osteoporosis, loss of bone mineral density increases fracture risk.
- Mutations in some of the network-forming type IV collagen chains cause thin basement membrane nephropathy (which causes hematuria) or Alport syndrome (a disorder that leads to early kidney failure).
- Mutations in an anchoring fibril-forming type VII collagen α-chain cause dystrophic epidermolysis bullosa, a severe blistering disease.

## LEARNING OBJECTIVES

*For mastery of this topic, you should be able to do the following:*

- Explain how fibrillar collagens are synthesized inside the cell and how they form fibrils in the extracellular space. Describe the role of ascorbate in this process.
- Compare and contrast the structure of a collagen triple helix with the structure of an α-helix (e.g., an α-helix in hemoglobin).
- Name the cause and signs of achondroplasia.
- List signs of vitamin C deficiency and explain why this deficiency is associated with poor wound healing.
- Describe the mineralization of collagen fibers and explain how mineralization is abnormal in rickets, osteomalacia, and osteoporosis.

- Explain why mutation of a Gly residue to another amino acid in a collagen triple helix is usually inherited in an autosomal dominant fashion.
- Describe the signs of classical Ehlers-Danlos syndrome, define the cause of this disorder, and explain the pattern of inheritance.
- Compare and contrast signs and symptoms of rickets and osteomalacia, and describe the main causes of these disorders.
- Describe the signs, symptoms, and broad cause of Paget disease of bone and list the most common treatment option.
- Describe the signs of osteogenesis imperfecta, define the most common cause of this disorder, list treatment options, and explain the most common pattern of inheritance.
- Compare and contrast the signs, causes, and treatment options of thin basement membrane nephropathy, Alport syndrome, and Goodpasture syndrome. Explain the pattern of inheritance of thin basement membrane nephropathy and Alport syndrome.
- Compare and contrast the causes of dystrophic epidermolysis bullosa and of epidermolysis bullosa acquisita.

## 1. BIOSYNTHESIS AND DEGRADATION OF FIBRILLAR COLLAGENS

*Protein synthesis produces fibrillar procollagens inside the endoplasmic reticulum. In the endoplasmic reticulum, many proline and some lysine residues are hydroxylated in vitamin C–dependent reactions. Three procollagen chains associate near their C-termini, and a triple helix forms. After secretion into the extracellular space, peptidases cleave the N- and C-terminal propeptides. A dioxygenase oxidizes some lysyl and hydroxylysyl residues to aldehydes. Triple helices aggregate and become cross-linked, forming microfibrils. The microfibrils in turn aggregate into fibrils and fibers. Collagens are resistant to most proteases. Matrix metalloproteinase-1 cleaves fibrillar collagens, which causes the helix to unwind and thereby become susceptible to degradation by other proteases.*

### 1.1. Overview of Types of Collagen

Collagens are the major component of the extracellular matrix and amount to about 30% of the protein mass in a human.

Many different collagens are known; they are numbered in the order of discovery. The collagens are commonly grouped into fibrillar and nonfibrillar collagens.

**Fibrillar collagens** provide mechanical strength, for instance, in bone, tendons, ligaments, and cartilage. This group encompasses collagens I, II, III, V, and XI. Mutations in some of these collagens cause diseases such as osteogenesis imperfecta (brittle bones; see Section 2.4) or Ehlers-Danlos syndrome (hyperelastic skin, hyperextensible joints; see Section 2.5).

**Nonfibrillar collagens** serve a variety of purposes. In this chapter, they are grouped into network-forming collagens and collagens of anchoring fibrils. **Network-forming collagens** are present in the sheet-like basement membranes, including the kidney glomeruli, where they help filter fluids. The main representative of this group is collagen type IV. Mutations in some of the type IV collagen chains cause thin basement membrane nephropathy or Alport syndrome (a disorder that leads to early kidney failure). The collagens of **anchoring fibrils,** such as type VII collagen, anchor the basement membrane to collagen fibrils that are present in the underlying connective tissue. Mutations in this collagen give rise to dystrophic epidermolysis bullosa (a severe skin-blistering disorder).

All collagens contain a **triple-helix domain,** which is formed from three collagen **α-chains** (β is only used in reference to a *pair* of cross-linked α-chains). Some collagen triple helices contain three *identical* α-chains (e.g., type II collagen). Other collagens contain two to three *different* α-chains (e.g., type IV collagen); in this case, the different α-chains are distinguished as α1, α2, and so on. Humans have close to 50 different genes that encode collagen α-chains.

According to the common **terminology** for **collagen protein,** α-chains are described in the form "αn(#)," such as α2(IV), where "n" is a number for the type of α-chain and "#" is a Roman number for the type of collagen that results from the assembly of several α-chains. Human **collagen-coding genes** are named in the form "COL#An," where "#" is an Arabic number for the type of collagen (e.g., 4 for collagen type IV), "A" stands for α-chain, and "n" is still the number that follows the character α in the naming of collagen protein α-chains. For example, the collagen α-chain α2(IV) is the product of the gene *COL4A2*.

## 1.2. Biosynthesis and Posttranslational Modification of Fibrillar Collagens

Collagen is synthesized from **preprocollagen.** Fig. 12.1 provides an overview of the posttranslational processing of preprocollagen. Further details are provided below.

The pre- or **signal** sequence ensures transfer of the growing peptide chain into the endoplasmic reticulum. Inside the endoplasmic reticulum, a signal peptidase cleaves the signal sequence (see Fig. 7.6 and Section 3 in Chapter 7).

The fibrillar procollagens contain a central domain that eventually participates in the formation of a triple helix; this domain contains many repeats of Gly-X-Y, where X is most often proline and Y is most often hydroxyproline. Another common amino acid in the Y-position is lysine. Inside the endoplasmic reticulum, **procollagen-proline 4-dioxygenases** (**proline 4-hydroxylases**) and **procollagen-lysine 5-dioxygenases** (**lysine 5-hydroxylases**) hydroxylate

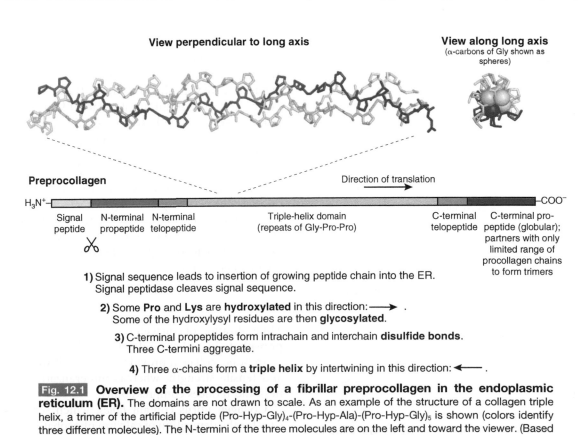

**View perpendicular to long axis**

**View along long axis**
(α-carbons of Gly shown as spheres)

**Preprocollagen**

H₃N⁺—    —COO⁻

Signal peptide | N-terminal propeptide | N-terminal telopeptide | Triple-helix domain (repeats of Gly-Pro-Pro) | C-terminal telopeptide | C-terminal propeptide (globular); partners with only limited range of procollagen chains to form trimers

Direction of translation →

**1)** Signal sequence leads to insertion of growing peptide chain into the ER. Signal peptidase cleaves signal sequence.

**2)** Some **Pro** and **Lys** are **hydroxylated** in this direction: —→ . Some of the hydroxylysyl residues are then **glycosylated**.

**3)** C-terminal propeptides form intrachain and interchain **disulfide bonds.** Three C-termini aggregate.

**4)** Three α-chains form a **triple helix** by intertwining in this direction: ←— .

**Fig. 12.1** **Overview of the processing of a fibrillar preprocollagen in the endoplasmic reticulum (ER).** The domains are not drawn to scale. As an example of the structure of a collagen triple helix, a trimer of the artificial peptide (Pro-Hyp-Gly)₄-(Pro-Hyp-Ala)-(Pro-Hyp-Gly)₅ is shown (colors identify three different molecules). The N-termini of the three molecules are on the left and toward the viewer. (Based on Protein Data Bank file 1CGD of Bella J, Brodsky B, Berman HM. Hydration structure of a collagen peptide. *Structure.* 1995;3:893-906.)

many Y-position prolines and also some lysine side chains (Fig. 12.2). Hydroxylation proceeds from the N-terminus (which is synthesized first) toward the C-terminus. The extent to which lysine residues are hydroxylated varies greatly among collagens and tissues. The proline- and lysine-hydroxylating enzymes require **vitamin C** (**ascorbate, ascorbic acid**; see Section C below).

Some of the **hydroxylysyl** residues are **O-glycosylated** in the endoplasmic reticulum and in the Golgi.

Once the proline and lysine dioxygenases have reached the C-terminus of the procollagen α-chains, a **protein disulfide isomerase** forms disulfide bridges in the C-terminal propeptide.

Once the folded C-termini of three collagen α-chains aggregate, the **triple helix** forms from the C-terminal side (Fig. 12.2 and Section 2.3), assisted by peptidyl-prolyl cis-trans isomerase. The isomerase can produce the required trans configuration of the peptide bond. The triple helix is stabilized by hydrogen bonds, water bridges, hydrophobic interactions, and van der Waals interactions.

Replacement of glycine residues in a collagen triple helix is strongly pathogenic, whereas replacement of some amino acids in positions X and Y is less damaging. In the triple helix, the glycine residues of one chain are always opposite the X or Y positions of the other chains. Nonglycine residues impair triple-helix formation because there is no room for a side chain larger than –H (as in Gly). Charged or hydrophobic amino acids in positions X and Y influence the lateral aggregation of collagen triple helices in the extracellular space (see below and Fig. 12.3). Compared to helix formation, lateral aggregation is less dependent on the amino acid side chain structure.

The procollagen trimers are sorted through the Golgi apparatus and emerge from the Golgi inside secretory vesicles. Collagen molecules that are not part of a triple helix (i.e., surplus chains, mutant chains) are degraded. The procollagen trimers are then secreted into the extracellular space.

In the extracellular space, **procollagen N-endopeptidases** and **procollagen C-endopeptidases** cleave the N- and C-terminal propeptides of procollagens (see Figs. 12.1 and 12.3). The remaining triple-helix domains, framed by N- and C-terminal **telopeptides**, spontaneously aggregate into **microfibrils**, helped by telopeptides and by patches of charged or hydrophobic amino acid side chains in X and Y positions within the triple-helix domains. It is a quirk of the collagen research field that a *trimeric* complex of collagen molecules that is formed in the extracellular space is called a collagen *monomer* in a context of multimonomer fibrils.

**Collagen microfibrils** (diameter ~0.003 μm) aggregate into **collagen fibrils** of various diameters, which in turn aggregate into **collagen fibers** that may reach a diameter of ~10 μm (by comparison, the diameter of a red blood cell is ~7 to 8 μm). The dermatan sulfate-containing proteoglycan (see Fig. 13.4 and Section 2.1 in Chapter 13) **decorin** binds to collagen microfibrils in regular intervals and thereby determines spacing between microfibrils, as well as fibril shape. Furthermore, **glycosylation** of hydroxylysyl residues may alter the lateral aggregation of collagen triple helices. The fibers can be as long as a tendon.

**Lysyl oxidases** in the extracellular space can oxidize a lysyl or hydroxylysyl side chain in each one of the telopeptides of collagens I, II, or III. (These lysyl *oxidases* are not to be confused with the lysine *hydroxylases* in the endoplasmic reticulum as mentioned above.) Oxidation of lysine residues yields **allysine** residues, and oxidation of hydroxylysine residues yields **hydroxyallysine** residues. These residues spontaneously participate in intramolecular and intermolecular cross-linking reactions with lysine residues in telopeptides and triple-helix regions of neighboring molecules (Fig. 12.3). When there is a pulling force on collagen fibers, the collagen monomers normally slide past each other. Cross-links decrease such sliding and therefore increase the tensile strength but decrease the elasticity of collagen fibers. Furthermore, if there are too many cross-links, the capacity of the fibrils to absorb energy decreases. (The lysyl oxidases described here are also involved in oxidizing lysyl side chains in elastin; see Section 1.1 in Chapter 13.)

## 1.3. Mineralization of Fibrillar Collagens in Bone

Mineralization of collagen refers to the deposition of **calcium phosphate** in and around collagen fibers.

In bone, collagen provides the overall structure, flexibility, and tensile strength, whereas mineralization increases stiffness and reduces compressibility.

Collagen fibrils contain *holes*, which serve as nucleation sites for the deposition of calcium phosphate. As shown in Fig. 12.3, there is a gap between consecutive collagen triple helices in a fibril. These gaps are connected into channels so that

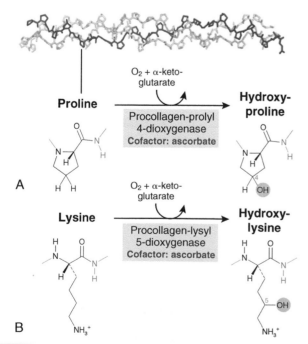

**Fig. 12.2** **Posttranslational formation of hydroxyproline and hydroxylysine in procollagen.** Numbers in enzyme names refer to amino acid carbons (1 is at the –CO– end).

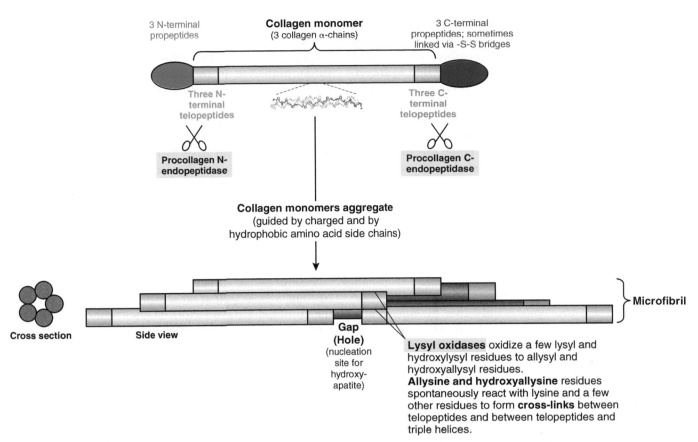

**Fig. 12.3** **In the extracellular space, processing of procollagen trimers and the aggregation of collagen triple helices yields collagen microfibrils.** Relative to their length, the collagen trimers are shown at 10 times their actual width. Furthermore, for simplicity, the trimers are shown as cylinders, when in reality the trimers are twisted around each other.

the collagen fiber can be mineralized after assembly. Electrically charged amino acid side chains pointing into the holes facilitate the binding of the first calcium cations and phosphate anions; that is, they facilitate nucleation of a **hydroxyapatite** crystal. The hydroxyapatite crystals are only approximately two-thirds the thickness and in their longest dimension one-third the length of a collagen triple helix.

Bone-forming osteoblasts contain **bone alkaline phosphatase** on their surface and release some of it into the blood. The enzyme contributes to alkaline phosphatase activity commonly measured in serum for diagnostic purposes. Children have higher serum alkaline phosphatase activity than adults. Adults who have excessive osteoblast activity (e.g., in Paget disease of bone or in osteomalacia; see Sections 2.5 and 2.6) also have elevated serum alkaline phosphatase activity.

Bone is the main **reservoir** of calcium phosphate and serves as a reservoir for these ions; however, it can cover only a portion of daily needs for phosphate (the remainder has to be absorbed from food).

### 1.4. Degradation of Fibrillar Collagens

Degradation of fibrillar collagens occurs during growth, bone remodeling, wound healing, and arthritis. Fibrillar collagens normally have half-lives of many weeks or months.

Most proteases cannot degrade an intact collagen triple helix. Proteolysis of collagen triple helices is catalyzed by the **matrix metalloproteinases** MMP-1, MMP-2, MMP-8, MMP-13, and MMP-14 (the prefix *metallo-* indicates that these enzymes contain a metal, such as $Zn^{2+}$). These enzymes are secreted into the extracellular space as procollagenases; there, other proteases cleave the N-terminus, yielding active collagenases. The collagenases cleave the $\alpha1$ or $\alpha2$ chain of a type I collagen monomer at a bond approximately three-fourths of the length of a collagen molecule. The resulting fragments then unfold, and the chains are degraded further by other proteases (e.g., gelatinases).

The extracellular matrix contains a reservoir of **tissue inhibitors of metalloproteinases**, as well as other protease inhibitors. Tissue inhibitors of metalloproteinases inhibit matrix metalloproteinases (such as collagenases) by binding into their active site.

## 2. DISEASES OF BONE THAT ARE ASSOCIATED WITH FIBRILLAR COLLAGENS

*Various mutations in the type I collagen genes cause osteogenesis imperfecta, which is characterized by inadequate production of the extracellular matrix in bone. Severe forms of the disease cause death in utero or shortly after birth; less severe forms can result in lifelong disability. Mutations in type V collagen cause the classic Ehlers-Danlos syndrome manifesting as hyperelastic, poorly healing skin. Patients who have a vitamin C deficiency have decreased hydroxylation of extracellular matrix proteins. These patients bruise easily and show impaired wound healing. Paget disease of bone is caused by increased turnover of bone and the deposition of abnormal new bone, causing fissures and bone pain. Osteomalacia is a syndrome of "weak" bones due to deficient mineralization, which in turn commonly has its origins in a deficiency of circulating vitamin D or phosphate. Patients who have osteoporosis have an abnormally low bone mineral content.*

## 2.1. Overview and General Comments

The majority of mutations in **collagen** genes cause disease when present in a *heterozygous* state, either by *haploinsufficiency* of the remaining normal allele, or by a *dominant-negative* effect of the mutant allele (see Table 5.1 and Section 2 in Chapter 5). Dominant-negative effects can be explained with the following example. If a heterozygous patient synthesizes a mutant $\alpha 1(I)$-procollagen chain at a normal rate, the chance that three normal type I collagen $\alpha$-chains [i.e., two $\alpha 1(I)$-chains and one $\alpha 2(I)$-chain] come together to form a normal triple helix is only 25%. [On the other hand, if the mutation were in the $\alpha 2(I)$-chain, the chance would be 50%.] If triple helices that contain one or more mutant $\alpha$-chains are exported into the extracellular space, most collagen microfibrils and practically all collagen fibers contain one or more mutant $\alpha$-chains.

Most mutations in collagen **processing enzymes** cause disease only when present in a homozygous or compound heterozygous state.

Fig. 12.4 provides an overview of the location of the molecular defect in collagen synthesis, mineralization, and degradation that is observed in the diseases of bone that are discussed in this section.

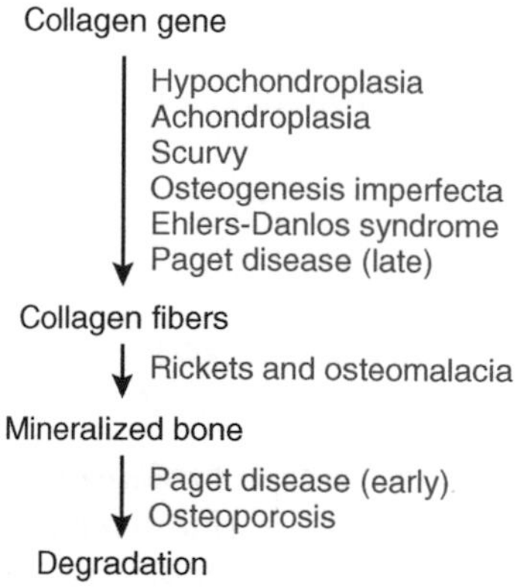

## 2.2. Hypochondroplasia and Achondroplasia

Hypochondroplasia and achondroplasia are caused by activating mutations in the fibroblast growth factor receptor-3 (FGFR3). When active, this receptor stops growth of bones. About 80% of affected patients have a de novo mutation, and the others inherited the mutation in autosomal dominant fashion. Each of these dysplasias occurs in ~1:15,000 births. Persons who have hypochondroplasia or achondroplasia make up most of the people who have markedly short stature.

Persons who have achondroplasia have short arms and legs, a large head, and altered facial features (Fig. 12.5). Those with hypochondroplasia have milder symptoms than those who have achondroplasia. In an affected fetus, short limbs are noticeable by ultrasound late in pregnancy.

FGFR3 signals through the RAS-RAF-MEK-ERK pathway (see Fig. 8.3), as well as other pathways. After binding one of the fibroblast growth factors, FGFR3 forms a dimer that has tyrosine kinase activity. While ligand-activated FGFR3 receptors can stimulate the growth of many types of cells (e.g., fibroblasts), it inhibits the growth of matrix-producing chondrocytes in the growth plates via cell cycle inhibition (the mechanism is not well understood).

The most common mutations that give rise to hypochondroplasia and achondroplasia are a glutamine to lysine mutation (N540K) and a glycine to arginine mutation (G380R) in FGFR3, respectively. The mutant amino acid side chains lead to a modest increase in the fraction of dimerized (and thus active) receptors, even in the absence of a fibroblast growth factor.

Collagen gene

    Hypochondroplasia
    Achondroplasia
    Scurvy
    Osteogenesis imperfecta
    Ehlers-Danlos syndrome
    Paget disease (late)

Collagen fibers

    Rickets and osteomalacia

Mineralized bone

    Paget disease (early)
    Osteoporosis

Degradation

**Fig. 12.4**   **Diseases that involve collagen.**

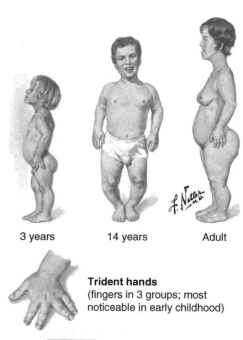

3 years    14 years    Adult

**Trident hands**
(fingers in 3 groups; most noticeable in early childhood)

**Fig. 12.5**   **Achondroplasia.**

## 2.3. Vitamin C (Ascorbate) Deficiency

We obtain ascorbate mostly from **plants** (see Table 12.1). Plants in turn synthesize relatively large amounts of ascorbate via a pathway that starts with glucose 6-phosphate. The structure of ascorbate (vitamin C) is shown in Fig. 21.7. The concentration of ascorbate inside cells is in the submillimolar to millimolar range. Ascorbate is needed for the hydroxylation of proline and lysine residues (see Fig. 12.2).

In the United States, the **recommended daily dietary allowance** for vitamin C for people who are at least 19 years old is 90 mg for men, 75 mg for nonpregnant women, 85 mg for pregnant women, and 120 mg for lactating women. Smokers should take in an extra 35 mg per day.

Ascorbate crosses human cell membranes via one of the **sodium-dependent vitamin C transporters** (SVCT-1 or SVCT-2; genes are named *SLC23A1* and *SLC23A2*, respectively), whereas dehydroascorbic acid crosses it via one of the **glucose transporters** (GLUT-1, GLUT-3, or GLUT-4). Inside cells, dehydroascorbic acid is reduced to ascorbate. Normally, SVCTs provide cells with most of their ascorbate; however, during oxidative stress or inflammation, uptake of dehydroascorbate via GLUTs becomes more important. The intracellular concentration of ascorbate in the brain is ~3 mM and that of muscle is about ~0.5 mM.

**Vitamin C deficiency**, characterized by a concentration of ascorbate in serum of less than 11 μM, is common worldwide. Vitamin C deficiency is most common among refugee populations, among people who consume few vitamin C–rich fruits and vegetables, and among smokers (oxidants in smoke react with ascorbate). Patients who had gastric bypass surgery often become deficient in vitamin C unless they take a vitamin C supplement. A marked deficiency also often occurs in patients who receive renal dialysis. These patients are asked to exclude potassium-rich foods from their diet; however, some of these foods also happen to be important sources of vitamin C. To make matters worse, these patients lose a large amount of ascorbic acid through dialysis.

In patients with vitamin C deficiency, the rate of hydroxylation of prolyl and lysyl side chains is diminished; **collagen** therefore forms at a decreased rate. With a decrease in the rate of hydroxylation, triple-helix formation is delayed and slowed. Furthermore, collagens produced by ascorbate-deficient cells have decreased thermal stability and tensile strength. Indeed, patients severely deficient in vitamin C bruise easily, their gums may bleed, and their wounds heal poorly (Fig. 12.6).

**Table 12.1**    **Sources of Vitamin C (Ascorbate)**

| Food | Vitamin C Content (mg/100 g Edible) |
|---|---|
| Pepper, sweet, red, raw | 128 |
| Kiwi, green | 75 |
| Cauliflower, boiled | 73 |
| Cabbage, raw | 72 |
| Cabbage, boiled | 38 |
| Strawberries | 57 |
| Pineapple | 36 |
| Orange juice | 33 |
| Tomato | 20 |
| Potato, boiled in skin | 13 |
| Apple | 6 |
| Walnuts | 1 |
| Pasta (dry) | 0 |
| Milk (whole, from cow) | 0 |

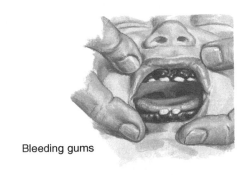

Bleeding gums

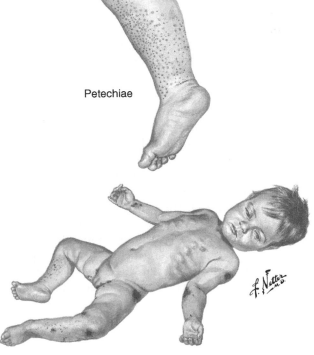

Petechiae

Multiple spots of subcutaneous bleeding

**Fig. 12.6**    **Deficiency of vitamin C (ascorbate).**

Petechiae occur, especially around hair follicles. Patients report joint pain and often have swollen joints. Vitamin C–deficient patients are also at an increased risk for cardiovascular disease.

## 2.4. Osteogenesis Imperfecta

In ~90% of patients, osteogenesis imperfecta (**brittle bone disease**) is caused by an **autosomal dominantly** inherited mutation in one allele of the **COL1A1** or **COL1A2** gene; these genes encode the type I collagen α-chains. More than 1,500 pathogenic mutations are known. The remaining patients have mutations in genes, the products of which interact with type I collagen, and these latter mutations are generally inherited in autosomal recessive fashion. Osteogenesis imperfecta occurs in ~1 in 15,000 newborns.

**Haploinsufficiency** due to a mutation in the **COL1A1** gene usually leads to the mildest form of osteogenesis imperfecta (see Fig. 12.7). A single functional COL1A1 allele is not sufficient to give rise to normally structured bone, although all of the collagen is normal. The frequency of fractures varies widely. In affected children, fractures in the arms and legs may occur when they start to walk.

In general, **dominant-negative mutations** in the **COL1A1** or **COL1A2** gene lead to a more severe phenotype than a mutation that causes haploinsufficiency (Fig. 12.7). In dominant-negative mutations, an amino acid substitution impairs the formation of a collagen triple helix and therefore also the formation of all higher-order structures, such as bone. The substitution is often in a glycine codon. As shown in Fig. 12.1, at glycine positions, there is no room for an amino acid side chain in the collagen triple helix. Some of these mutations also lead to an accumulation of misfolded proteins in the endoplasmic reticulum, a decrease in the rate of translation (except mRNAs that encode chaperones), and eventually apoptosis. Dominant-negative mutations result in disease that ranges from thin bones and fractures in utero (which can be seen by ultrasound), followed either by death on the first day of life or lifelong deformities, to normal stature at birth but fragile teeth and osteoporosis in adulthood. About half of these patients also develop hearing loss at an unusually early age.

Clinically, a finding of **bluish sclerae**, which is especially noticeable at birth and during the early years of life, should raise suspicion that the patient has osteogenesis imperfecta.

**Bisphosphonates** are widely used in the treatment of osteogenesis imperfecta. These drugs (e.g., pamidronate, zoledronate) bind to hydroxyapatite crystals and then cause apoptosis of osteoclasts, which degrade bone. Bisphosphonate therapy increases bone mineral density; in some patients, it also reduces the rate of fractures. Bisphosphonates are not used in patients who have a type of osteogenesis imperfecta that is caused by defective mineralization.

## 2.5. Ehlers-Danlos Syndrome

Ehlers-Danlos syndrome (EDS) is a collection of diseases with various causes. EDS is classified based mostly on clinical find-

**Mild form**

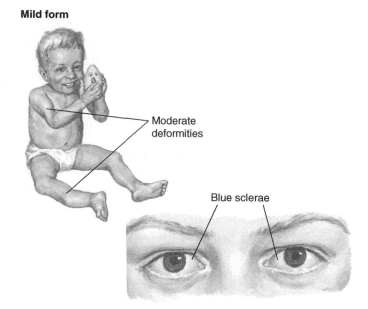

**Severe form**

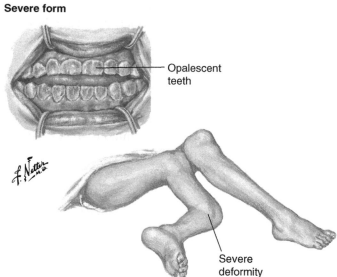

**Fig. 12.7** **Osteogenesis imperfecta.** *Top,* Haploinsufficiency of the α1(I)-chains leads to a mild form of the disease. The sclerae are typically blue at birth. Most fractures occur as the child starts to walk; however, these fractures heal rapidly. *Bottom,* Dominant-negative mutations lead to broken bones in utero and after birth. Bone deformities and fragility typically require multiple surgeries and may prevent patients from walking.

ings. Common signs include altered skin, joint hypermobility, and ready bruising (Fig. 12.8). The prevalence of EDS in all its varieties is ~1 in 7,000. The most common forms of EDS are classic EDS and hypermobility EDS, which show autosomal dominant inheritance.

About 90% of patients who have **classic EDS** have a mutation in one allele of the **COL5A1** or **COL5A2** gene. Type V collagen consists of two different α-chains. Most pathogenic alleles result in haploinsufficiency. In women who are pregnant with an affected fetus, the membranes, which are of fetal origin, commonly rupture prematurely. Walking is delayed in children. The skin of affected patients is fragile. Scars from

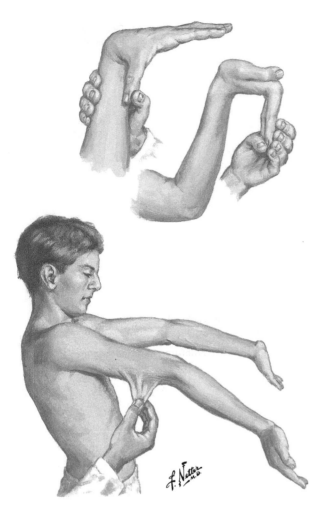

**Fig. 12.8** Joint hypermobility and skin hyperelasticity in Ehlers-Danlos syndrome.

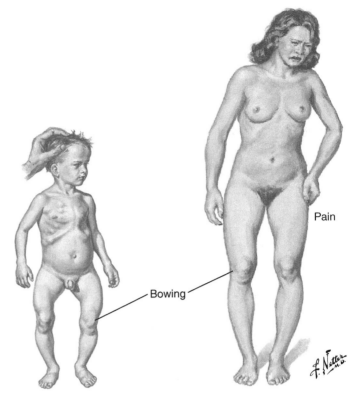

**Fig. 12.9** Rickets and osteomalacia.

minor falls start in early childhood and have the appearance of cigarette paper. After surgery, sutures must be left in place about twice the normal length of time.

The cause of most forms of **hypermobility EDS** is still unknown. Patients typically have musculoskeletal pain, recurrent joint dislocation, and mitral valve prolapse.

## 2.6. Rickets and Osteomalacia

**Rickets** and **osteomalacia** are mainly due to decreased **mineralization** of matrix proteins; in turn, this is generally due to a vitamin D deficiency, a calcium deficiency, or phosphate deficiency (Fig. 12.9). The term *rickets* is usually reserved for the syndrome seen in children; the term *osteomalacia* is reserved for adults. In affected patients, bones develop painful fissures even after minor trauma, and the skeleton may deform (more so in children).

Worldwide, **vitamin D deficiency** is often due to malnutrition. However, in developed countries there are many other prevalent causes, such as low exposure to sunlight, disease-induced decreased absorption in the intestine, or chronic kidney disease (see also Section 5 in Chapter 31). In the absence of adequate calcitriol (the active form of vitamin D

that acts as a signal), there is decreased absorption of calcium in the intestine and kidneys as well as decreased release from bones.

A **dietary calcium deficiency** that causes rickets occurs mostly among children in developing countries. In adults, a calcium deficiency is predominantly associated with osteoporosis (see Section 2.8) rather than osteomalacia.

A **phosphate deficiency** can develop in patients who absorb too little phosphate due to gastrointestinal disease or who have excessively high concentrations of the phosphaturic hormone **fibroblast growth factor 23 (FGF23)**. The concentration of circulating FGF23 is elevated in patients who have a (usually benign) **tumor** that secretes FGF23 and in patients who have **X-linked hypophosphatemia** (~1 in 20,000 births) due to a mutation in the *PHEX* gene. Patients can be treated with phosphate and calcitriol (the activated form of vitamin D), unless they have hypercalcemia.

Basic laboratory evaluation of rickets includes measurements of serum calcium, phosphate, alkaline phosphatase, and calcidiol (the form of vitamin D that is stored in blood; see Section 5 in Chapter 31).

## 2.7. Paget Disease of Bone (Osteitis Deformans)

Paget disease of bone (Fig. 12.10) is accompanied by increased bone remodeling and an abnormal structure of bone. There are foci of excessive degradation and other foci of excessive formation of new bone that has an abnormal structure. Degradation predominates early in the disease, whereas bone formation prevails later on.

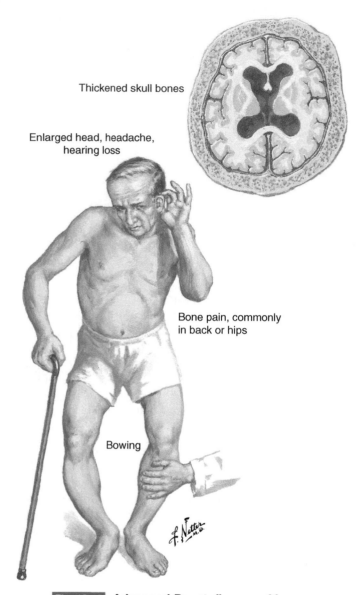

Thickened skull bones

Enlarged head, headache, hearing loss

Bone pain, commonly in back or hips

Bowing

**Fig. 12.10**  **Advanced Paget disease of bone.**

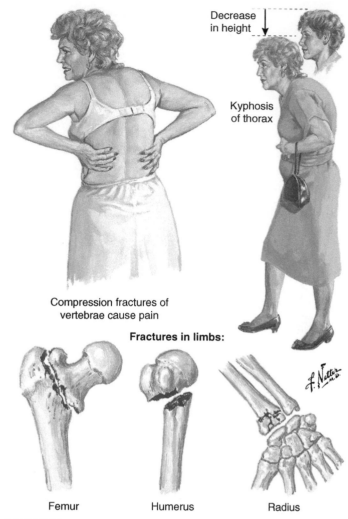

Decrease in height

Kyphosis of thorax

Compression fractures of vertebrae cause pain

**Fractures in limbs:**

Femur          Humerus          Radius

**Fig. 12.11**  **Common fracture sites in osteoporosis.** Osteoporosis is also accompanied by a decrease in body height.

Paget disease of bone is found in ~2% of persons aged 60 years and older. Most commonly, a diagnosis is incidentally made based on an x-ray image. The disease is almost twice as prevalent among men as among women. At diagnosis, almost all patients are older than 55 years.

About half of the patients who have familial Paget disease have a mutation in the **sequestosome**-1 (*SQSTM1*) gene. The mechanism of pathogenesis is unclear.

Patients who have Paget disease of bone may have pain, deformities, deafness, decreased bone strength, and neurologic deficits. The disease may affect only one bone, or it may be systemic and affect multiple bones. In the long term, patients are at an increased risk of developing a **sarcoma** in bone.

Most patients who have Paget disease are treated with **bisphosphonates**, which inhibit osteoclast activity (for details on these drugs, see Section 2.8). Disease activity can be monitored with measurements of serum **alkaline phosphatase** activity, which reflects osteoblast activity.

## 2.8. Osteoporosis

**Osteoporosis** is associated with changes in the structure of bone that reduce bone strength and increase fracture risk (Figs. 12.11 and 12.12). This is the most common disorder of bone.

Bone mass peaks in a person's early twenties and gradually decreases afterward, thus increasing the risk of fracture. Women experience an additional loss of bone mass when the concentration of estrogens drops because of menopause. In persons with osteoporosis, common fracture sites are the wrist, hip, and vertebrae.

**Bone mineral density** is commonly assessed at the neck of the femur and at the lumbar vertebrae levels using **dual x-ray absorptiometry** (**DXA scan**). Low bone mineral density is associated with increased fracture risk.

Bone undergoes ongoing resorption by **osteoclasts** and formation by **osteoblasts** to remove microdamage and maintain

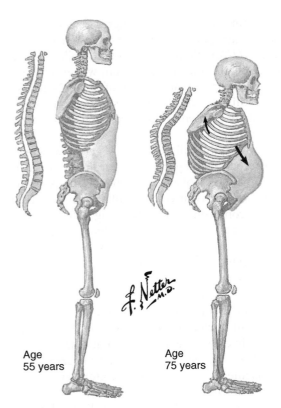

**Fig. 12.12** **Skeletal changes in osteoporosis.**

Age 55 years

Age 75 years

strength. An imbalance between resorption and formation leads to bone with abnormal mechanical properties. Furthermore, an increased rate of remodeling leads to decreased secondary mineralization, which decreases bone strength.

The formation of osteoclasts from precursor cells depends in large part on the protein **RANKL** on the surface of osteoblasts; RANKL activates the receptor **RANK** on the surface of osteoclasts. **Osteoprotegerin** is a glycoprotein that binds to RANKL and thereby prevents RANKL from activating RANK.

In women before menopause, the high concentration of estrogens inhibits the formation of RANKL while promoting the formation of osteoprotegerin. Thus the net effect of estrogens is to reduce the formation and activation of osteoclasts.

Apart from aging, bone mass also decreases in response to **vitamin D deficiency** (see Section 2.6), **hyperparathyroidism**, and prolonged use of systemic **glucocorticoids** (e.g., **prednisone**) at a high concentration. Parathyroid hormone stimulates the release of calcium from bone as part of the regulation of the concentration of calcium in the blood. Glucocorticoids inhibit osteoblast activity and increase osteoclast activity via increased synthesis of RANKL and RANK.

The nonpharmacological treatment of osteoporosis involves weight-bearing **exercise**, adequate intake of **calcium** and **vitamin D**, **smoking** cessation, abstention from excessive **alcohol** use, and limitation of the risk of **falls**.

The options for pharmacological treatment of osteoporosis include inhibition of osteoclast activity with a bisphosphonate, an antibody to RANKL, or the estrogen agonist/antagonist raloxifene, as well as activation of osteoblast activity through intermittent exposure to a parathyroid hormone analog.

The nitrogen-containing **bisphosphonates** (**zoledronate**, **risedronate**, **alendronate**) induce **apoptosis** of osteoclasts. Alendronate and risedronate are taken orally on a weekly basis, whereas zoledronate is injected intravenously (IV) once a year, often for 3 years. These bisphosphonates tightly and selectively bind to hydroxyapatite in bone, where the longest acting among them stay for many years. Once these bisphosphonates are taken up into an osteoclast, they inhibit **farnesyl pyrophosphate synthase** in the cholesterol synthesis pathway (see Fig. 29.4). The reduction in farnesyl pyrophosphate production reduces the conjugation of signaling proteins with farnesylpyrophosphate and geranylgeranyl pyrophosphate (see also Section 1.5 in Chapter 11), leading to apoptosis.

Bisphosphonates are also used to prevent the increased destruction of bone that accompanies Paget disease of bone (see Section 2.7) or osteomalacia (see Section 2.6); they are effective in the treatment of osteogenesis imperfecta (see Section 2.4), and they can be coupled to a radioactive element (e.g., a γ-emitting isotope of technetium) for detection of bone metastases.

The estrogen agonist/antagonist (formerly selective estrogen receptor modulator [SERM]) **raloxifene** is an option for the prevention and treatment of osteoporosis in women. Raloxifene also reduces the incidence of invasive **breast cancer**; however, it can cause hot flashes and thromboembolisms.

**Denosumab** is an antibody that binds to **RANKL** and thus prevents the formation and activation of osteoclasts. Denosumab is injected subcutaneously every 6 months.

**Teriparatide** is a recombinant fragment of **parathyroid hormone**. Teriparatide is injected subcutaneously every day. This generates a pattern of exposing bone to waves of teriparatide, which activates osteoblasts more than osteoclasts (this is contrary to chronic exposure to a high concentration of parathyroid hormone, which activates osteoclasts more than osteoblasts).

## 3. TYPE IV COLLAGEN: A NETWORK-FORMING COLLAGEN

*Like the fibrillar collagens described previously, the network-forming type IV collagens also contain a long triple helix; however, instead of fibrils, they form a meshwork. Mutations in some of the type IV collagen genes cause thin basement membrane disease or Alport syndrome. An autoimmune reaction to the α3(IV) chain causes Goodpasture syndrome.*

Like the fibrillar collagens, type IV collagen contains a long triple-helix region, as well as N- and C-terminal propeptides. However, the triple-helix trimers (i.e., collagen monomers; see Fig. 12.3) form mesh-like networks. Type IV collagen is the primary collagen of all **basement membranes (basal lamina)**. A basement membrane is a sheet of extracellular matrix that affects tissue permeability, serves as a base for the attachment of epithelial cells, and allows passage of leukocytes. For instance, in the skin, the basement membrane separates the epidermis from the underlying dermis (Fig. 12.15). In the small intestine, the basolateral portion of the epithelial cells that absorbs nutrients is attached to the basement membrane. Besides collagen, basement membranes also contain laminins; these are proteins and are not discussed here.

There are six different α-chains for type IV collagen, which are matched up to form three different networks.

The **α1/α2 network** contains collagen that consists of two α1- and one α2-chain. It is found in most basement membranes.

The **α3/α4/α5 network** contains collagen that consists of one α3-, one α4-, and one α5-chain. It is found especially in filtration barriers, such as in glomeruli (see Fig. 12.13). It is also found in membranes in the cochlea (i.e., in the inner ear).

The C-termini of triple helices aggregate end to end, and the N-termini aggregate into tetramers, thus forming a mesh.

The **α1/α2/α5/α6 network** contains collagen that consists of two α1-chains and one α2-chain, which in turn is linked to another collagen that consists of two α5-chains and one α6-chain. This collagen network is found in basement membranes that are frequently stretched, such as in vessels, viscera, and the epidermis.

Mutations in the collagen type IV genes cause **Alport syndrome (hereditary nephritis)**, which has a prevalence of ~1 in 8,000. About 85% of affected patients have **X-linked** Alport syndrome, which is caused by a mutation in the **COL4A5** gene on the X chromosome. The remaining ~15% of patients have **autosomal recessively** inherited Alport syndrome and are homozygous or compound heterozygous for mutations in either the **COL4A3** or the **COL4A4** gene. In total, hundreds of pathogenic mutations in collagen type IV genes are known. The rate of de novo mutations is ~15%.

Starting in childhood, patients with Alport syndrome have **hematuria** and **progressive proteinuria**. Without treatment, they typically develop **end-stage renal disease** in their early twenties. These patients often also have **hearing loss**.

The **basement membrane of the glomeruli** not only contains a type IV collagen α3/α4/α5 network but also a type IV collagen α1/α2 network. As glomeruli develop, the α1/α2 network of type IV collagen is laid down first. Later, podocytes replace this network with a α3/α4/α5 network, which provides greater long-term stability.

In patients with Alport syndrome, the α3/α4/α5 network of type IV collagen is typically absent from the glomerular basement membrane. With time, the original α1/α2 network undergoes proteolysis and increasingly fails to retain large molecules. Accompanying fibrosis eventually impairs kidney function.

Women with autosomal recessively inherited Alport syndrome and men with X-linked or autosomal recessively inherited Alport syndrome have a fairly similar, severe set of symptoms. Because of random and patchwise inactivation of one X chromosome, women who are heterozygous for X-linked Alport syndrome have a clinical course that is anywhere from mild to severe.

The **treatment** of Alport syndrome involves a reduction in **blood pressure** via the renin-angiotensin-aldosterone system (see Fig. 31.17 and Section 4.1 in Chapter 31) to reduce fibrosis and delay the onset of kidney failure. First-line treatment with an **angiotensin-converting enzyme inhibitor**, such as ramipril, and second-line addition of an **angiotensin receptor blocker**, such as losartan, is common.

**Thin basement membrane nephropathy (TBMN, familial hematuria)** is due to heterozygosity for a pathogenic mutation in the **COL4A3** or **COL4A4** gene; that is, affected patients are carriers for autosomal recessive Alport syndrome. TBMN is a much milder disease than Alport syndrome. Affected patients have intermittent or persistent hematuria (based on examination with a microscope) and minimal proteinuria; otherwise, kidney function is nearly normal. About 1% of the population has TBMN due to a mutant type IV collagen.

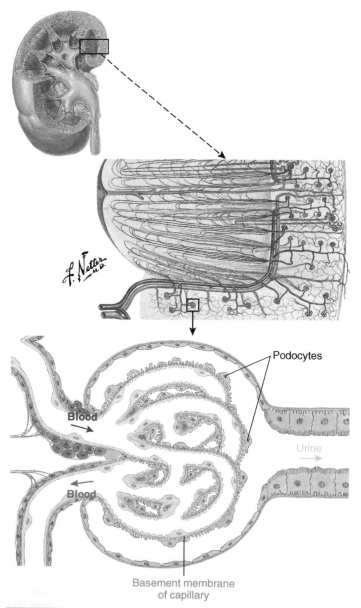

Podocytes

Blood

Urine

Blood

Basement membrane
of capillary

**Fig. 12.13** **The basement membrane of the capillaries in the glomeruli of the kidneys contains type IV collagen.** *Top,* Numerous glomeruli in the parenchyma of a kidney. *Bottom,* A single glomerulus.

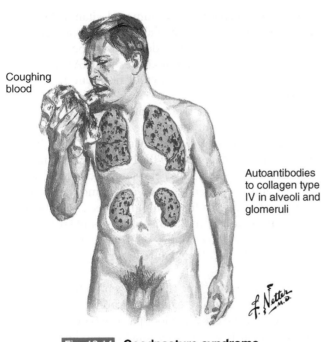

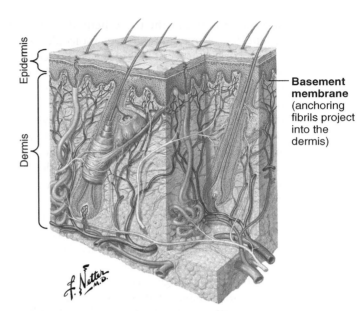

**Fig. 12.14**  **Goodpasture syndrome.**

**Fig.12.15**  **Cross section of skin.** Collagen type VII forms anchoring fibrils that anchor the basement membrane in the underlying dermis.

**Goodpasture syndrome** (also called **antiglomerular basement membrane disease**) is most often the consequence of an autoimmune reaction against the C-terminal domain of the α3-chain of type IV collagen. About 1 in 15,000 people eventually develop Goodpasture syndrome. Smokers and persons exposed to breathing hydrocarbons (e.g., gasoline fumes) are most likely to be affected. In the alveoli and glomeruli, autoantibodies to type IV collagen bind to basement membranes, and proteases from macrophages and neutrophils destroy the α3/α4/α5 collagen network. Affected patients often have cough, shortness of breath, proteinuria, and hematuria; smokers may even cough up blood (Fig. 12.14). Affected patients are treated with **plasmapheresis** (to remove autoantibodies) and **immune suppression** (to inhibit formation of autoantibodies). These patients commonly have a shortened life expectancy.

## 4. TYPE VII COLLAGEN: THE COLLAGEN OF ANCHORING FIBRILS

*Anchoring fibrils connect the epidermis to the underlying dermis. These anchoring fibrils consist of type VII collagen. An altered structure of anchoring fibrils is the cause of various types of epidermolysis bullosa, which is characterized by blistering of the skin and mucous membranes following mild mechanical trauma.*

**Type VII collagen** consists of a trimer of α1(VII)-chains. Collagen type VII forms the **anchoring fibrils** that connect the basement membrane of the epidermis to the underlying papillary dermis (Fig. 12.15).

**Dystrophic epidermolysis bullosa** (**DEB**) is caused by a mutation in the *COL7A1* gene, which encodes the α-chain

that forms a homotrimer that is **type VII collagen**. More than 300 pathogenic mutations are known.

In patients who are affected with DEB, the skin and mucous membranes are fragile and blister after minor trauma. Upon healing, the blisters form scars. Electron microscopy reveals that the tissue separates below the lamina densa (the lamina densa is a part of the basement membrane). The anchoring fibrils may be altered, reduced in number, or completely absent.

*Dominantly* inherited forms of DEB are due to mutations in glycine codons of type VII collagen.

*Autosomal recessively* inherited forms of DEB have varied causes. The **Hallopeau-Siemens** type, the most severe of all forms of DEB, is due to mutations that truncate the collagen type VII α-chain. The resulting mRNA is degraded by nonsense-mediated RNA decay (see Section 3 in Chapter 7). On analysis, there is no immunoreactive type VII collagen.

Besides DEB, there are several other forms of epidermolysis bullosa (e.g., simplex, junctional). Those diseases are due to mutations in other proteins of the epidermal-dermal junction, which are not discussed in this book.

**Epidermolysis bullosa acquisita** is an autoimmune disease that is caused by **antibodies** against **type VII collagen** (usually the N-terminal propeptide). Disease onset is typically during adulthood.

## SUMMARY

- Fibrillar collagens are synthesized as procollagens. In the endoplasmic reticulum, using ascorbate (vitamin C) as a cofactor, proline and lysine dioxygenases hydroxylate some proline and lysine residues in the triple-helix domain and in the telopeptides. Three procollagen molecules then aggregate. These trimers are secreted into the extracellular space. There, procollagen endopeptidases remove the propeptides, and the remaining trimeric complexes, now called collagen monomers, aggregate into collagen microfibrils. Lysyl oxidases oxidize some lysyl and hydroxylysyl residues, producing allysine and hydroxyallysine residues, which spontaneously form cross-links with lysyl and other residues in neighboring telopeptides and triple-helix regions. The cross-links increase the tensile strength of collagen microfibrils but decrease their elasticity.

- In holes (gaps) between collagen monomers, collagen fibers in bone are mineralized with hydroxyapatite, which increases stiffness and reduces compressibility. Bone serves as a reservoir of calcium and phosphate.

- The triple-helix region of collagens is resistant to most proteases. However, collagenases, a subclass of matrix metalloproteinases, do cleave a collagen α-chain in a triple helix about three-fourths of its length from the N-terminal end. Subsequently, the triple helix unravels, and the α-chains are digested by other enzymes. Tissue inhibitors of metalloproteinases inhibit collagenases and other matrix metalloproteinases.

- Achondroplasia and hypochondroplasia are caused by an activating mutation in the fibroblast growth factor receptor-3 (FGFR3) that leads to cessation of osteoblast activity, diminished collagen production, and short stature. About 80% of mutations occur de novo. Inheritance is autosomal dominant.

- Vitamin C (ascorbate) deficiency causes a decreased rate of collagen Pro and Lys hydroxylation, which in turn leads to decreased secretion of collagen and decreased cross-linking of collagen monomers.

- Osteogenesis imperfecta is due to a mutation in collagen α1(I)- or α2(I)-chains. Owing to the formation of structurally impaired trimers, microfibrils, and so forth, most of these mutations show dominant-negative effects. Affected patients have an increased rate of bone fractures, in severe cases already in utero.

- Most forms of classic Ehlers-Danlos syndrome (EDS) are caused by mutations in collagen type V that cause abnormally elastic skin, easy bruising, and delayed healing of sutured skin.

- Rickets and osteomalacia are due to demineralization of collagen in bone, often due to a vitamin D deficiency or an excessive need for calcium and phosphate from the bone reservoir.

- Early in the disease, Paget disease of bone shows mostly foci of increased bone degradation; later in the disease, foci of bone formation predominate. The disease is associated with bone pain, an enlarged head, and impaired hearing. It is more common among men and inherited in autosomal dominant manner.

- Osteoporosis is associated with reduced bone mineral density (measurable with a DXA scan) and an increased risk for bone fractures. Patients should be advised about exercise, supplementary calcium and vitamin D, smoking cessation, and moderation of alcohol use. Options for pharmacological treatment include bisphosphonates, the estrogen agonist/antagonist raloxifene, the RANKL antibody denosumab, and the parathyroid hormone fragment and analog teriparatide.

- Type IV collagen is a typical network-forming collagen. It is found in basement membranes.

- Mutations in type IV collagen can cause thin basement membrane nephropathy (TBMN, familial hematuria), a disorder accompanied by persistent microscopic hematuria. Patients of either sex who are homozygous or compound heterozygous for such mutations, and patients who are hemizygous for mutations in an X-linked type V collagen gene can have Alport syndrome. Alport syndrome typically leads to kidney failure in adults as well as hearing loss.

- Autoantibodies to type IV collagen, often induced by smoking and exposure to hydrocarbon vapors (e.g., from gasoline), are the cause of Goodpasture syndrome. The syndrome primarily affects lung function and, in severe cases, kidney function as well.

- Type VII collagen is part of the anchoring fibrils that link the epidermis of the skin to the underlying dermis. Mutations in type VII collagen can cause dystrophic epidermolysis bullosa (DEB, a severe blistering disease).

## FURTHER READING

- Al-Rashid M, Ramkumar DB, Raskin K, Schwab J, Hornicek FJ, Lozano-Calderón SA. Paget disease of bone. *Orthop Clin North Am.* 2015;46:577-585.

- Drake MT, Clarke BL, Lewiecki EM. The pathophysiology and treatment of osteoporosis. *Clin Ther.* 2015;37:1837-1850.

- Goldsweig BK, Carpenter TO. Hypophosphatemic rickets: lessons from disrupted FGF23 control of phosphorus homeostasis. *Curr Osteoporos Rep.* 2015;13:88-97.

- Harrington J, Sochett E, Howard A. Update on the evaluation and treatment of osteogenesis imperfecta. *Pediatr Clin North Am.* 2014;61:1243-1257.

- Krejci P. The paradox of FGFR3 signaling in skeletal dysplasia: why chondrocytes growth arrest while other cells over proliferate. *Mutat Res Rev Mutat Res.* 2014;759:40-48.

- Landis WJ, Jacquet R. Association of calcium and phosphate ions with collagen in the mineralization of vertebrate tissues. *Calcif Tissue Int.* 2013;93:329-337.

- Lupsa BC, Insogna K. Bone health and osteoporosis. *Endocrinol Metab Clin North Am.* 2015;44:517-530.

- National Osteoporosis Foundation. <www.nof.org>. This site contains updated treatment recommendations for physicians.

- Savige J. Alport syndrome: its effects on the glomerular filtration barrier and implications for future treatment. *J Physiol.* 2014;592:4013-4023.

# Review Questions

1. A woman and her male partner both have hematuria (determined by microscopy). Biopsies of their kidneys showed thinning of the basement membrane. Compared with the general population, these patients are at a much increased risk of having offspring with which of the following?

   A. Alport syndrome
   B. Ehlers-Danlos syndrome
   C. Marfan syndrome
   D. Osteoarthritis
   E. Osteoporosis

2. A 20-year-old male patient has persistent hematuria. His mother also has hematuria, but his father does not. This patient most likely has which one of the following disorders?

   A. Autosomal recessive Alport syndrome
   B. Ehlers-Danlos syndrome
   C. Goodpasture syndrome
   D. X-linked Alport syndrome

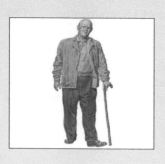

## SYNOPSIS

■ Elastic fibers, consisting mainly of elastin and fibrillin, can be stretched and will recoil. Abnormal elastic fibers are found in patients with emphysema, α-1-antitrypsin deficiency, Marfan syndrome, or Williams syndrome.

■ Proteoglycans are proteins that are heavily glycosylated with glycosaminoglycans (polysaccharides containing aminated sugars), such as heparan sulfate, keratan sulfate, chondroitin, and dermatan sulfate. Proteoglycans are synthesized inside the cell and then secreted. In the extracellular space, various proteins bind to specific portions of the glycan chains. Proteoglycans take up compressive forces (e.g., in knee joints and intervertebral disks).

■ Hyaluronic acid, another glycosaminoglycan, is a long polysaccharide that is synthesized inside the cell and extruded into the extracellular space. Hyaluronic acid serves as a lubricant and as a scaffold for binding proteoglycans.

■ Osteoarthritis is associated with degradation of joint cartilage, which contains proteoglycans.

■ The main degradation of glycans of proteoglycans occurs inside lysosomes. Such degradation is impaired in patients who have a heritable mucopolysaccharidosis. In these patients, glycosaminoglycans accumulate in lysosomes, thereby damaging the central nervous system, liver, heart, lungs, or various other tissues.

■ Remodeling of the extracellular matrix takes place in wound healing, in fibrosis, and during pregnancy-induced changes of the cervix.

## LEARNING OBJECTIVES

*For mastery of this topic, you should be able to do the following:*
■ Describe the signs, major pathology, and treatment of Marfan syndrome.
■ Describe the consequence of haploinsufficiency for elastin.
■ Describe the pathogenesis of emphysema as it relates to elastic fibers.
■ Describe the signs, diagnosis, and treatment of hereditary α-1-antitrypsin deficiency.
■ Outline the synthesis and structure of proteoglycans.
■ Outline the synthesis, structure, and roles of hyaluronate.
■ Describe the fate of cartilage in patients who have osteoarthritis.
■ Describe the general cause of the mucopolysaccharidoses, and list successful approaches to treatment of type I mucopolysaccharidosis (Hurler syndrome).
■ Define fibrosis and explain how it can impair organ function.

## 1. ELASTIN AND FIBRILLINS

*Elastic fibers allow the extracellular matrix to stretch and recoil. Elastic fibers consist mostly of elastin and to a lesser extent fibrillin that forms microfibrils. The microfibrils may serve as guides for the deposition of elastin. Like the collagens, a precursor of elastin is intracellularly synthesized. After export, extracellular processing, and attachment to integrin, elastin becomes cross-linked. In patients who have emphysema, excessive degradation of elastin impairs lung function. In patients with Marfan syndrome, a mutant fibrillin alters production and maintenance of elastic fibers. This can lead to life-threatening rupture of a major artery.*

### 1.1. Synthesis of Elastic Fibers

Elastin is predominantly found in large arteries, lung, ligaments, tendons, skin, and elastic cartilage (e.g., in the front of the rib cage; Fig. 13.1). In large arteries, elastic fibers form several cylindrical layers (called elastic lamellae) along the long axis of the vessel. These lamellae buffer pressure changes during the pumping cycle of the heart (large arteries also contain collagen fibers, which limit the stretching). In lung and in the cartilage of the auricles, elastic fibers form a lattice. In ligaments and tendons, the elastic fibers lie next to each other with the major axis parallel to the major physiological force.

**Elastic fibers** consist of **elastin** and **microfibrils**. Elastin makes up the core of an elastic fiber and constitutes about 90% of the weight of such a fiber. The microfibrils appear to serve as guides for the deposition of elastin. Some of these microfibrils are interspersed in the core of the elastic fiber, whereas others surround the mature elastic fiber like a sheath. The microfibrils have a diameter of about 0.01 μm (about three times the diameter of collagen microfibrils). Microfibrils contain many different proteins, including fibrillin-1 (see below).

Elastin is the product of cross-linked monomers of **tropoelastin**. Elastin is mainly synthesized by fibroblasts, smooth muscle cells, and some chondrocytes during development of the fetus and shortly after birth. Normally, elastin turns over slowly enough so that most of it lasts for a person's lifetime. There is only one gene for tropoelastin; however, tropoelastin RNA can be spliced in different ways, giving rise to several isoforms. During and after translation, **elastin-binding protein** binds tropoelastin, keeps it from aggregating, and thus chaperones it through the Golgi and into secretory vesicles. Tropoelastin has a globular shape. In the extracellular space, **lysyl oxidase** and **lysyl oxidase-like proteins** oxidize about 40 lysine side chains of tropoelastin to **allysine** side chains These side chains then form di-, tri- or tetravalent crosslinks to yield elastin. Lysyl oxidase also converts lysyl residues in *collagen* to allysyl residues (see Section 1.2 in

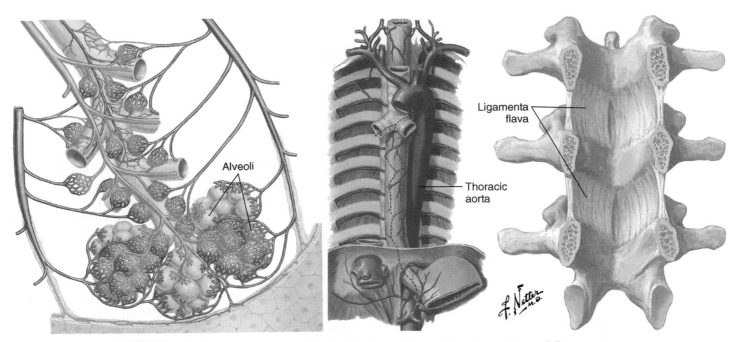

**Fig. 13.1** **Elastic fibers are prevalent in the lungs, large blood vessels, and ligaments.**

Chapter 12), which form crosslinks with collagen as well as elastin.

The **elasticity** of elastin is thought to be due to a stretching-induced decrease in entropy and an **entropy**-driven spontaneous return to the unstretched state. Current models assume that when elastin is stretched, hydrophobic amino acid side chains become exposed to water, or unordered sequences or β-turns become ordered (i.e., they lose some of their freedom to assume different conformations). In all of these cases, entropy decreases. When the stretching force vanishes, the natural tendency of molecules toward disorder (i.e., an increase in entropy) is thought to drive recoil.

Fibrillin-1 on the outside of elastic fibers binds **latent transforming growth factor β binding proteins**, which in turn bind the inactive precursor of the protein **transforming growth factor β (TGF-β)**. Matrix-bound inactive TGF-β serves as a reservoir for the production of active TGF-β. TGF-β affects various processes, including production and maintenance of the extracellular matrix.

## 1.2. Marfan Syndrome

Mutations in **fibrillin-1,** the most abundant protein of microfibrils in elastic fibers, cause the classic **Marfan syndrome**. Marfan syndrome is characterized by abnormalities of the skeleton, cardiovascular system, and the eyes (Fig. 13.2). There are more than 1,000 known pathogenic mutations of the fibrillin-1 gene (**FBN1**). In addition, within a family, the phenotype of the same mutation varies greatly. About 1 in 5,000 persons has Marfan syndrome.

The pathogenesis of Marfan syndrome is only partially understood and seems to be due to excessive **TGF-β** signaling (cause unclear), as well as structural deficiencies of microfibrils that contain mutant fibrillin-1 and may induce counterproductive repair mechanisms. The related Loeys-Dietz syndrome, which shows some of the same pathology, is most often caused by mutations in TGF-β receptors and unexpectedly also leads to excessive TGF-β signaling.

Patients with Marfan syndrome typically show increased **joint flexibility, skeletal abnormalities**, and, with increasing age, **lens dislocation** as well as **dilation of the aorta**. The ascending aorta and the root of the aorta dilate, leading to **dissection of the aorta** (a life-threatening emergency), **prolapse of the mitral valve,** and **regurgitation**. Dissection of the aorta is also a key feature of Loeys-Dietz syndrome.

The rate of dilation of the aorta is slowed by reducing the pulse pressure with the **β₁-adrenergic receptor antagonist atenolol** or the **angiotensin II receptor blocker losartan**; losartan also reduces excessive TGF-β signaling (and is an effective treatment for Loeys-Dietz syndrome).

Marfan syndrome is usually inherited in **autosomal dominant** fashion. About two-thirds of all patients inherit the mutation from an affected parent. About one-third of all patients have a de novo mutation, which occurred in the germline of an unaffected parent. Either way, offspring of an affected patient have a 50% chance of inheriting the faulty fibrillin-1 (FBN1) allele.

## 1.3. Supravalvular Aortic Stenosis

Patients with supravalvular aortic stenosis have an abnormally narrow ascending aorta as well as abnormally narrow coronary arteries, carotid arteries, renal arteries, and pulmonary arteries due to hemizygous loss of function of an allele of the **elastin** gene. Haploinsufficiency for elastin leads to narrowing of arteries via decreased production of tropoelastin,

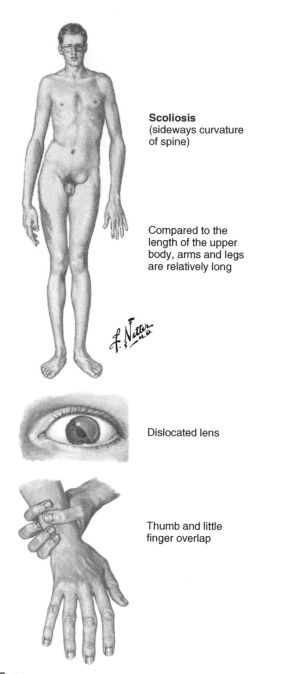

Scoliosis
(sideways curvature
of spine)

Compared to the
length of the upper
body, arms and legs
are relatively long

Dislocated lens

Thumb and little
finger overlap

**Fig. 13.2** **Signs of classic Marfan syndrome.** Affected patients frequently have scoliosis (pathologic sideways curvature of the spine). Compared with the length of the upper body, the arms and legs are relatively long. Many patients have a dislocated lens. When wrapping their hand around their wrist, the thumb and little finger overlap.

hyperproliferation of smooth muscle cells, and increased deposition of collagen.

Most often, haploinsufficiency for elastin is a consequence of **Williams syndrome**, a microdeletion on chromosome 7, which includes the elastin gene and occurs in ~1 in 10,000 births. Williams syndrome can be detected by prenatal screening using fluorescence in situ hybridization (see Section 1 in Chapter 4). The syndrome is associated with a low IQ and particularly outgoing behavior.

## 1.4. Degradation of Elastic Fibers, Emphysema, and α-1-Antitrypsin Deficiency

While turnover of elastic fibers is normally minimal, degradation of elastic fibers is enhanced in wounds. In wounds, neutrophils release the protease **elastase**. In healthy tissue, **α-1-antitrypsin** inhibits elastase as well as other proteases, including trypsin. α-1-Antitrypsin in the serum stems mostly from the liver.

**Emphysema** is a part of **chronic obstructive pulmonary disease (COPD)**, which is most often associated with **smoking**. COPD is characterized by persistent, pathologically reduced airflow. In the lungs of a patient with emphysema, the walls between alveoli are progressively and irreversibly destroyed, creating large spaces with a much-reduced surface for gas exchange (Fig. 13.3). Oxygen supplementation helps by increasing the net transfer of oxygen to blood.

Emphysema is accompanied by a marked loss of elastin in the lungs. Smoking attracts an increased number of **neutrophils** and **macrophages** into the lungs, where these cells release **elastases** that degrade elastin and other proteins of the extracellular matrix. In addition, smoking leads to the inhibition of the synthesis of several components of the extracellular matrix.

A **deficiency of α-1-antitrypsin** can lead to emphysema and sometimes liver disease. Worldwide, ~1 in 2,000 individuals is homozygous or compound heterozygous for a pathogenic allele of α-1-antitrypsin. In the United States, ~1 in 3,000 persons is *homozygous* for the Z allele (Glu342Lys, E342K) of α-1-antitrypsin. The α-1-antitrypsin of these patients has less than 10% of the normal inhibitory effect of α-1-antitrypsin; this is considered a severe deficiency. In the absence of an insult from the environment, antitrypsin deficiency may not damage the lungs. However, smokers develop symptoms of emphysema at ~40 years of age.

The **diagnosis** of α-1-antitrypsin deficiency is based on measurements of α-1-antitrypsin in serum, analysis of α-1-antitrypsin by isoelectric focusing, and genotyping by polymerase chain reaction–based methods. It is recommended that patients who have COPD (see above) be tested for α-1-antitrypsin deficiency, although only ~1% of all these patients have α-1-antitrypsin deficiency and even though antitrypsin deficiency is most common among the youngest patients. If a patient tests positive for antitrypsin deficiency, the patient's relatives should be informed about testing options.

Patients who can blow out only a reduced volume of air in 1 second and who have serum antitrypsin activity below a certain threshold are given **augmentation therapy** with weekly **intravenous antitrypsin**. The antitrypsin is made from pools of human plasma. Augmentation therapy delays the progression of emphysema.

A minority of patients with severe α-1-antitrypsin deficiency develop clinically apparent liver disease at 1 to 2 months of age; affected infants typically have persistent jaundice and an elevated concentration of liver enzymes in serum. Such liver disease is seen only with certain mutations, including the Z allele (i.e., E342K). The pathogenic mutant α-1-antitrypsin accumulates inside hepatocytes. Some of the patients with the

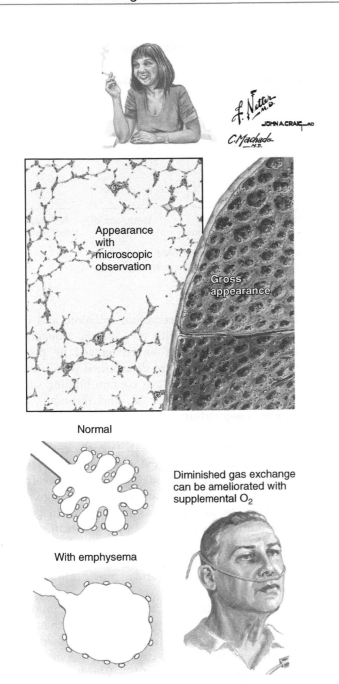

Normal

With emphysema

Diminished gas exchange can be ameliorated with supplemental O$_2$

**Fig. 13.3** **Destruction of alveoli in the lungs of patients with emphysema.**

Z allele eventually develop liver cirrhosis or hepatocellular carcinoma.

# 2. PROTEOGLYCANS AND GLYCOSAMINOGLYCANS

*Proteoglycans consist of a core protein that is linked to numerous long polysaccharide chains. These polysaccharides are glycosaminoglycans, which are subdivided into heparan sulfates, keratan sulfates, chondroitin sulfates, and dermatan sulfates. Modification of sugar residues in these polysaccharides creates specific binding sites for proteins, such as growth*

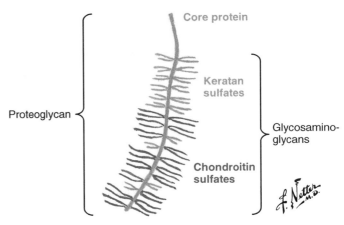

**Fig. 13.4** **Structure of a proteoglycan.**

*factors and coagulation factors. Chondrocytes can synthesize the polysaccharide hyaluronate and extrude it into the extracellular space. In the extracellular space, hyaluronate binds proteoglycans and other proteins. Degradation of glycosaminoglycans requires several sulfatases and hydrolases in lysosomes. A deficiency of any one of these enzymes leads to a mucopolysaccharidosis, whereby glycosaminoglycans accumulate in lysosomes and cause progressive damage, generally to the nervous system.*

## 2.1. Synthesis and Degradation of Proteoglycans Containing Heparan, Keratan, Chondroitin, or Dermatan Sulfate

Proteoglycans consist of a core **protein** to which **glycosaminoglycans** (**mucopolysaccharides**) are covalently linked (Fig. 13.4). Examples of core proteins are aggrecan, syndecan, perlecan, decorin, glypican, agrin, and collagen XVIII. Glycosaminoglycans are **polysaccharides** that contain aminated sugars (see below).

The glycosaminoglycans are subdivided into **heparan sulfates, keratan sulfates, chondroitin sulfates**, and **dermatan sulfates**, all of which contain dozens to hundreds of disaccharide repeats (Fig. 13.5). Each of these disaccharide repeats contains an aminated sugar: glucosamine or galactosamine. Sulfation of these glycosaminoglycans is highly variable and can change within a molecule from one disaccharide repeat to the next. A few sulfated sugar residues suffice to provide a specific binding site for a protein.

Heparan sulfates are ubiquitous, and keratan sulfates are found in the cornea and in cartilage. Chondroitin sulfates are the predominant glycosaminoglycan in cartilage, and dermatan sulfates predominate in skin (Fig. 13.6).

The **core protein** of a proteoglycan is synthesized by ribosomes that are bound to the endoplasmic reticulum. During synthesis, the nascent protein chain is translocated into the lumen of the endoplasmic reticulum. From the endoplasmic reticulum, the protein is transported into the Golgi apparatus. Starting in the endoplasmic reticulum and ending in the Golgi apparatus, a **tetrasaccharide** (first xylose, then galactose, galactose, and finally glucosamine) is added to hydroxyl

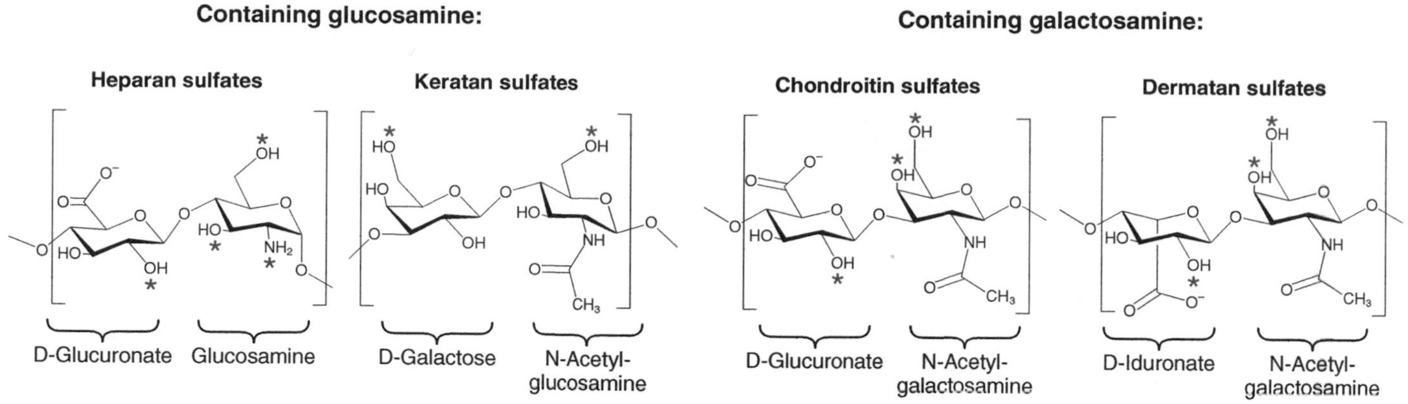

**Containing glucosamine:**

**Heparan sulfates**

**Keratan sulfates**

D-Glucuronate    Glucosamine

D-Galactose    N-Acetyl-glucosamine

**Containing galactosamine:**

**Chondroitin sulfates**

**Dermatan sulfates**

D-Glucuronate    N-Acetyl-galactosamine

D-Iduronate    N-Acetyl-galactosamine

**Fig. 13.5** **Basic structure of glycosaminoglycans.** Asterisks indicate possible sites of sulfation. Brackets enclose the most common disaccharide-repeating unit of different types of glycosaminoglycans.

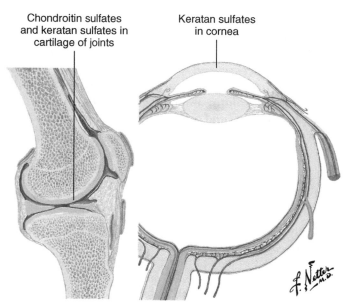

Chondroitin sulfates and keratan sulfates in cartilage of joints

Keratan sulfates in cornea

**Fig. 13.6** **Sites of proteoglycan deposition: the knee joint and the eye.**

groups of certain serine or threonine side chains of the core protein. In the Golgi apparatus, the tetrasaccharide is extended by the addition of monosaccharides to generate the repeating disaccharide units shown in Fig. 13.5. Uridine diphosphate sugars serve as substrates for all of these glycosylation reactions. The iduronate residues in heparan sulfate and dermatan sulfate are the result of C5 epimerization of glucuronate residues by an epimerase.

Several **sulfotransferases** sulfate some of the sugar residues; the sulfate derives from **3′-phosphoadenosine 5′-phosphosulfate** (PAPS; see Fig. 36.16 and Section 9 in Chapter 36). Sulfated sugar residues typically occur in clusters.

Proteoglycans emerge from the Golgi in secretory vesicles, which are released into the extracellular space. Proteoglycans can have an anchor in the plasma membrane, or they can at first be free in the extracellular space and then attach to the extracellular matrix. In the extracellular space, **6-O-endosulfatases** can remove 6-O-sulfate groups.

The aforementioned epimerization, sulfation, and desulfation yield polysaccharides with very specific sequence and sulfation patterns, which can be recognized by proteins. However, how these patterns are determined is still unclear. Heparan sulfates, for example, can contain binding sites for antithrombin, coagulation factor $X_a$, and thrombin, all of which influence **coagulation** (blood clotting). Throughout the extracellular matrix, glycosaminoglycans bind (and serve as reservoirs for) cytokines and growth factors depending on sulfation patterns. Many of these cytokines and growth factors are released during **matrix remodeling** or **wound healing**.

Proteoglycans are particularly abundant in **cartilage**, where they are produced by **chondrocytes** inside the cartilage. Cartilage in the human body includes *morphological* cartilage (e.g., in the nose), *elastic* cartilage (e.g., in front of the rib cage), *fibrocartilage* (e.g., in intervertebral disks), and *hyaline* cartilage (e.g., at the growth plate and in movable joints on top of bones, see Fig. 13.6).

Proteoglycans help cartilage, such as in knee joints and intervertebral disks (see Figs. 13.6 and 13.10), absorb mechanical energy and deform without fracturing. The proteoglycans are enclosed by a semipermeable capsule of other matrix proteins (mostly collagens; see Fig. 13.10). Within this capsule, the glycosaminoglycans maintain a sizable swelling pressure due to Donnan osmotic pressure. This pressure has its origins in osmotically active cations that neutralize sulfate and carboxylate groups on the glycosaminoglycans.

**Heparin** is an analog of heparan sulfate and is used as an anticoagulant. Heparin is isolated from the intestines of pigs. It contains more iduronate and sulfate groups than most heparan sulfates. Heparin and some heparan sulfates both have anticoagulant activity. The anticoagulant activity of the negatively charged heparin can be inhibited by **protamine**, a protein from salmon sperm that contains many positively charged arginine residues (protamine is also used to complex insulin; see Section 4.3 in Chapter 39).

In the extracellular space, glycosaminoglycans are hydrolyzed by both exoglycosidases and endoglycosidases. **Exoglycosidases** degrade glycosaminoglycans from one end, one residue at a time; **endoglycosidases** hydrolyze internal glycosidic bonds, thereby producing fragments that are ~40 sugar residues long. **Sulfatases** remove sulfate groups.

## 2.2. Hyaluronate, a Glycosaminoglycan That Binds to Link Proteins

Hyaluronate (**hyaluronic acid, hyaluronan**) is a long, unbranched polysaccharide that consists of hundreds to thousands of repeating units of glucuronyl N-acetylgalactosamine (Fig. 13.7) and serves as both a lubricant and a platform for the binding of certain proteins. Hyaluronic acid is a glycosaminoglycan like heparan sulfate, keratan sulfate, chondroitin sulfate, and dermatan sulfate. However, hyaluronate is not sulfated, and it is synthesized very differently from these other glycosaminoglycans; **hyaluronan synthases** are embedded in the plasma membrane and directly extrude hyaluronate into the extracellular space.

Free hyaluronate binds a large amount of water, is an excellent **lubricant**, and is found in synovial fluid, covering cartilage.

In the extracellular space, **link proteins** connect hyaluronate to extracellular matrix proteins (mostly proteoglycans; Fig. 13.8). These interactions generate huge complexes. Hyaluronic acid–protein complexes are found in skin and cartilage.

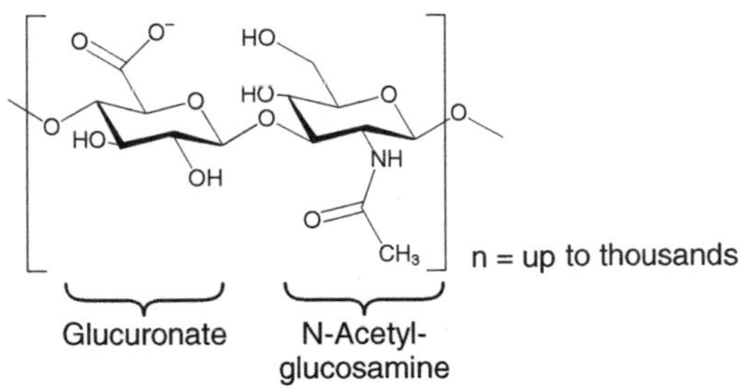

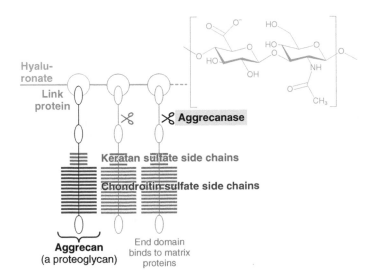

Glucuronate    N-Acetyl-glucosamine

**Fig. 13.7** **Basic building block of the polysaccharide and glycosaminoglycan hyaluronate.**

Hyaluronate  
Link protein  
**Aggrecanase**  
Keratan sulfate side chains  
Chondroitin sulfate side chains  
**Aggrecan** (a proteoglycan)    End domain binds to matrix proteins

**Fig. 13.8** **Structure of a hyaluronate-proteoglycan complex.** Each molecule of hyaluronate can bind up to ~100 molecules of link protein. Ovals in aggrecan indicate globular domains in the protein.

**Aggrecan** is one of the proteoglycans that is bound to hyaluronate via a link protein. Aggrecan contains glycosaminoglycans that consist of keratan sulfate or chondroitin sulfate.

In **hyaline cartilage** (e.g., in the knee joint; see Fig. 13.6), hyaluronate-proteoglycan complexes are trapped inside a matrix of collagen. Normal function of hyaline cartilage depends on hyaluronate and aggrecans of adequate length, adequate glycosylation of aggrecan, and adequate sulfation of keratan and chondroitin. An abnormality of any one of these parameters impairs the function of hyaline cartilage and can cause **arthritis**.

**Hyaluronidases** degrade hyaluronate (the glycosaminoglycan to which link proteins attach; see Fig. 13.8). Hyaluronic acid in the skin has a half-life of about 1 day; in cartilage, it has a half-life of 1 to 3 weeks. One type of hyaluronidase is anchored to the outside of plasma membranes; it cuts hyaluronate to fragments of about 100 sugar residues.

In the extracellular matrix, the **aggrecanases** ADAMTS4 and ADAMTS5 continuously degrade aggrecan, but remnants of aggrecan can remain on hyaluronate until the hyaluronate is degraded (see Fig. 13.8).

Chondrocytes, macrophages, keratinocytes, and other cells express plasma membrane receptors for fragments of hyaluronate through which the fragments are endocytosed. Receptors for hyaluronate fragments that reach the *circulation* are removed chiefly by receptors in the lymph nodes. Once the hyaluronate fragments reach the lysosomes, a hyaluronidase degrades them to tetrasaccharides. The tetrasaccharides are then hydrolyzed to monosaccharides, which are released into the cytosol.

## 2.3. Osteoarthritis

Osteoarthritis is characterized by a loss of joint **cartilage** that causes pain with movement (Fig. 13.9). This is the most common form of arthritis. Osteoarthritis affects mostly the hands, feet, knees, hips, and spine, and it is the leading indication for implantation of an artificial joint.

Early in the disease process, the osteoarthritic cartilage contains inordinately few proteoglycans, in part because the **aggrecanases** ADAMTS4 and ADAMTS5 degrade aggrecan.

There are many different causes of osteoarthritis; among them are inflammation of the joint, improper alignment of bones, joint laxity, injury, excess body weight, and, less commonly, mutations in the *COL2A1* gene (type II collagen is the most abundant protein in cartilage).

In osteoarthritis, inflammation causes granulocytes and chondrocytes to produce cytokines that induce chondrocytes to synthesize and release more matrix metalloproteinases and aggrecanases. These enzymes, in turn, gradually destroy joint cartilage. With the chronic nature of osteoarthritis, there is insufficient compensatory synthesis of the extracellular matrix.

Treatment aims to strengthen the joint, lessen the load on it, and decrease both pain and inflammation. These improvements may happen with orthoses, weight loss, exercise, intermittent heat treatment, acetaminophen, oral or topical nonsteroidal antiinflammatory agents, topical capsaicin, or

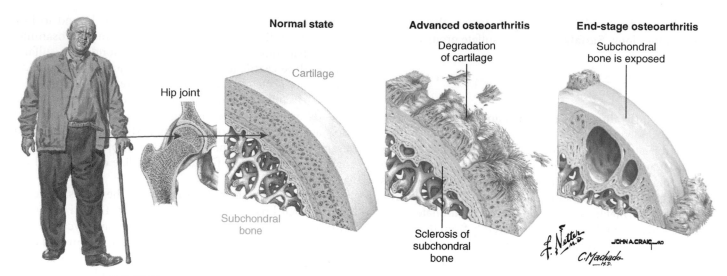

**Normal state**

Cartilage

Hip joint

Subchondral bone

**Advanced osteoarthritis**

Degradation of cartilage

Sclerosis of subchondral bone

**End-stage osteoarthritis**

Subchondral bone is exposed

**Fig. 13.9** Destruction of joint cartilage, calcification, and abnormal growth of bone in osteoarthritis.

glucocorticoids injected into the joint. Total joint replacement (arthroplasty) is used as a last resort.

**Degeneration of intervertebral disks** typically leads to low-back pain and is often considered a form of osteoarthritis (Fig. 13.10). Intervertebral disks allow motion of the spine in different directions while bearing a load. A disk consists of an annulus fibrosus and a nucleus pulposus. The annulus fibrosus contains mostly collagens (types I and II), which provide form to the disk. The nucleus pulposus is rich in proteoglycans, which bind water and provide resistance to compression; the nucleus also contains some collagen. Among the proteoglycans, the glycosaminoglycan side chains contain mostly chondroitin sulfate. With degeneration of the disk, the matrix of the nucleus pulposus loses proteoglycans and gains collagen.

**Glucosamine** and **chondroitin**, taken by mouth, are often used in the treatment of osteoarthritis. However, these saccharides are of uncertain benefit.

## 2.4. Mucopolysaccharidoses

The lysosomes of patients with a mucopolysaccharidosis are missing one of the many enzyme activities that are needed to degrade glycosaminoglycans (previously called **mucopolysaccharides**). The prevalence of mucopolysaccharidosis is ~1 in 30,000. Disease becomes apparent only if enzyme activity is less than ~2% of the normal. Because of inadequate degradation, glycosaminoglycans accumulate in lysosomes of most cells and eventually cause progressive organ damage. Affected patients may develop a dysmorphic face, hepatomegaly, splenomegaly, hernias, deafness, cardiomyopathy, lesions of the heart valves, airway obstruction, caries, or dysfunction of the central nervous system. Diagnosis relies heavily on measurements of enzyme activities in various cells or body fluids.

The most common forms of mucopolysaccharidosis are **Hurler syndrome** (a severe form and subtype of mucopolysaccharidosis type I) and **Sanfilippo syndrome** (mucopolysaccharidosis type III, which has four subtypes denoted A, B,

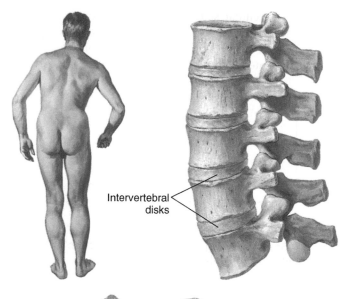

Intervertebral disks

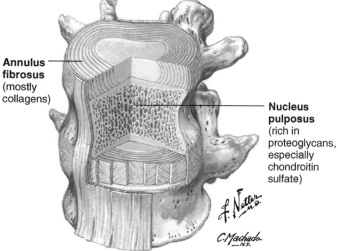

Annulus fibrosus (mostly collagens)

Nucleus pulposus (rich in proteoglycans, especially chondroitin sulfate)

Degeneration of disk is associated with loss of proteoglycan and gain of collagen

**Fig. 13.10** Structure of intervertebral disks.

C, and D). Both disorders are inherited in an autosomal recessive manner. Hurler syndrome is due to a deficiency of L-iduronidase, which hydrolyzes the terminal iduronate residue from dermatan sulfate and heparan sulfate. As a result, dermatan sulfate and heparan sulfate accumulate in lysosomes. Most severely affected patients have facial dysmorphism from birth and develop symptoms during the second year of life. Sanfilippo syndrome is caused by a deficiency in one of the four enzymes that play a role in degrading heparan sulfate; as a result, heparan sulfate accumulates in lysosomes. Besides the signs and symptoms common to all mucopolysaccharidoses (see above), most patients develop severe hyperactivity and aggression, seizures, sleep disturbance, and retinopathy.

**Intravenous enzyme replacement therapy** is available for mucopolysaccharidosis type I. The exogenous enzyme contains covalently linked mannose 6-phosphate (the localization signal for lysosomes), binds to mannose 6-phosphate receptors on the plasma membrane, is endocytosed, and ends up in lysosomes. However, infused enzyme does not readily cross the blood-brain barrier.

**Transplantation of hematopoietic stem cells** from bone marrow or cord blood is feasible for the treatment of patients with Hurler syndrome. Descendants of transplanted stem cells are thought to leak enzymes into their environment (including the enzyme missing from the host cells, L-iduronidase). Enzymes that contain mannose 6-phosphate then end up in lysosomes. Although transplantation reduces hepatomegaly, splenomegaly, and deterioration of the central nervous system, it does not prevent skeletal problems or retinopathy.

## 3. REMODELING OF THE EXTRACELLULAR MATRIX

*Alterations of the extracellular matrix that involve collagens, elastic fibers, and proteoglycans are involved in a number of physiologic and pathologic processes. During and after pregnancy, the cervix normally undergoes substantial remodeling of its extracellular matrix. Wound healing is accompanied by removal of extracellular matrix followed by resynthesis of matrix. Osteoporosis manifests itself in progressive weakening of bone. Fibrosis is characterized by excessive deposition of extracellular matrix to the detriment of organ function.*

### 3.1. Wound Healing

A few days after injury, a transient extracellular matrix forms that is gradually replaced by a stronger matrix (Fig. 13.11). Immediately after skin is wounded, **clotting** prevents further blood loss. Peaking about 1 day after injury, **neutrophils** move into the wound. Neutrophils remove bacteria and cellular debris, including proteins of the extracellular matrix. Unwounded tissue has a sufficient amount of extracellular protease inhibitors so that its extracellular matrix is not degraded. Within about a day, the neutrophils die by

**Immediately after incision and suturing**

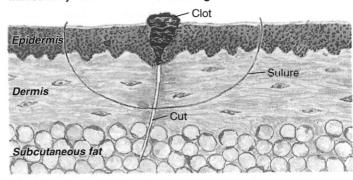

**24-48 hours**

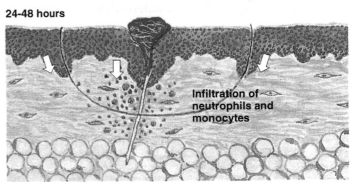

**5-8 days**

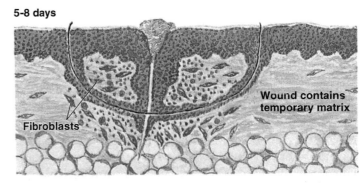

**10-15 days**

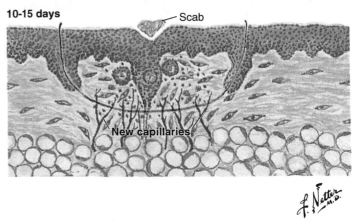

**Fig. 13.11** **Healing of sutured skin.**

apoptosis. One to three days after the initial injury, **monocytes** from the blood and from healthy tissue near the wound move into the wound and transform into macrophages. These macrophages phagocytose the remains of the neutrophils and also further degrade extracellular matrix in the wound.

About 3 to 7 days after injury, epithelial cells at the edge of the wound start to proliferate, and **fibroblasts** from surrounding healthy tissue migrate into the wound. The fibroblasts start to synthesize collagen. Initially, they produce a matrix of type I and type III collagen that has only very low tensile strength. Starting about 1 week after injury and then lasting months, the early collagen matrix is degraded and replaced by a stronger matrix, which contains about 80% type I collagen and about 20% type III collagen. However, collagen in the scar never attains the same organization as exists in uninjured skin. A few days after injury, responding to signals from fibroblasts, **keratinocytes** move from surrounding tissue into the wound, where they proliferate, differentiate, and reform the epidermis.

Within 3 months of injury, wounded skin regains about 80% of its original tensile strength. Thereafter, tensile strength does not increase significantly. Vitamin C deficiency, infection, hyperglycemia, hypoxia, ischemia, malnutrition, an elevated concentration of glucocorticoids, or a hereditary extracellular matrix disorder reduces the rate of healing and decreases the strength of scarred skin. If collagen synthesis is excessive, a hypertrophic scar (i.e., a keloid) forms.

## 3.2. Remodeling of the Cervix

During pregnancy, parturition, and the postpartum period, the cervix softens, ripens, dilates, and then repairs. Softening starts about 1 month after conception and lasts well into the third trimester. It results in reduced collagen cross-linking and reorganization of type I and type II collagen fibrils, which provide tensile strength. Ripening starts several weeks before labor and involves the addition of proteoglycans and hyaluronate; these compounds are thought to help disperse collagen. During labor, hyaluronidase activity in the cervix increases. Dilation of the cervix is also facilitated by invading leukocytes that release proteases, which degrade the extracellular matrix.

During the postpartum repair phase, proteoglycans are degraded, and dense connective tissue is formed once again. Premature ripening and dilation of the cervix are frequent causes of preterm deliveries.

## 3.3. Fibrosis

Fibrotic diseases are caused by overactive mesenchymal cells that generate an excessive, disorganized extracellular matrix. Fibrosis means replacement of normal tissue with scar tissue that has an abnormal extracellular matrix. For fibrosis to occur, there must be an interaction between the immune system and connective tissue that leads to an excessive wound healing response to injury. Wound healing normally involves activation of mesenchymal cells (i.e., hepatic stellate cells, mesangial cells, fibroblasts in the skin or in the lungs). Fibrosis can affect a variety of organs, such as the liver, kidneys, intestine, heart, lungs, skin, and eyes.

**Liver cirrhosis** (Fig. 13.12) can be caused by hepatitis virus B or C infection, excessive alcohol ingestion (see Section 4.4 in Chapter 30), hemochromatosis (see Fig. 15.10 and Section 9.2 in Chapter 15), cholestasis, or α-1-antitrypsin disease (see Section 1.4). Liver cirrhosis is seen in up to 10% of human autopsies; however, the condition often remains clinically silent. Cirrhosis is associated with proliferation of a fibrotic (i.e., poorly organized) extracellular matrix, of which collagen types I and III are the most abundant proteins. The outcome of liver cirrhosis can be portal hypertension and impaired hepatocellular function. Furthermore, most cases of liver cancer arise from liver cirrhosis. Fibrosis typically starts with injury to hepatocytes, such as by excessive alcohol consumption (with accumulation of acetaldehyde), a hepatotoxic drug (e.g., methotrexate), or excessive iron stores. The injury activates inflammatory cells that in turn activate matrix-producing hepatic stellate cells (lipocytes, Ito cells).

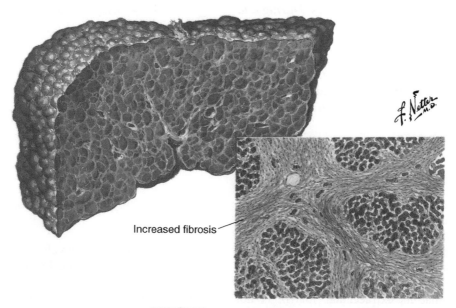

Increased fibrosis

**Fig. 13.12**   **Liver cirrhosis.**

## SUMMARY

- Elastic fibers consist mostly of elastin. The core and periphery of elastic fibers contain microfibrils, a major component of which is fibrillin. Mutations in fibrillin-1 can cause Marfan syndrome, which can be accompanied by dilation and dissection of blood vessels, skeletal abnormalities, and poor eyesight.
- Elastase degrades elastin. In chronic smokers, neutrophils and macrophages destroy elastin in the lungs, causing emphysema. $\alpha$-1-Antitrypsin is a natural inhibitor of elastase. A heritable deficiency of $\alpha$-1-antitrypsin affects about 1 in 2,000 individuals. Most patients predominantly have emphysema; some also have liver disease and are at a high risk of liver cirrhosis and hepatocellular carcinoma.
- Proteoglycans consist of a core protein and linked long glycosaminoglycans (carbohydrate chains) that consist of repeats of heparan sulfate, keratan sulfate, chondroitin sulfate, or dermatan sulfate. The sulfation of the saccharides is highly variable. Certain sequences of a few sulfated saccharides serve as binding sites for specific proteins. Proteoglycans are particularly abundant in cartilage, where they play a role in absorbing compressive forces. Heparin is used as an anticoagulant. It is typically isolated from pig intestine.
- Hyaluronic acid is also a glycosaminoglycan; however, it is not covalently linked to a core protein. Hyaluronic acid serves as a scaffold for link proteins to bind to, which in turn bind proteoglycans, such as aggrecan.
- Osteoarthritis is characterized by a gradual loss of cartilage from joints. It is unclear whether oral glucosamine and chondroitin have a beneficial effect.
- Deficiencies of enzymes that degrade glycosaminoglycans in lysosomes can cause one of the mucopolysaccharidoses (e.g., Hurler syndrome, Sanfilippo syndrome). Affected patients typically develop a dysmorphic face, hepatomegaly, splenomegaly, hernias, deafness, cardiomyopathy, lesions of the heart valves, airway obstruction, caries, or dysfunction of the central nervous system.

## FURTHER READING

- Baldwin AK, Simpson A, Steer R, Cain SA, Kielty CM. Elastic fibres in health and disease. *Expert Rev Mol Med.* 2013;15:e8.
- Campos MA, Lascano J. α1 Antitrypsin deficiency: current best practice in testing and augmentation therapy. *Ther Adv Respir Dis.* 2014;8:150-161.
- Cheng S, Mohammed TL. Diffuse smoking-related lung disease: emphysema and interstitial lung disease. *Semin Roentgenol.* 2015;50:16-22.
- The Marfan Foundation. <http://www.marfan.org/dx/home>. This site contains helpful information for the diagnosis of Marfan syndrome.

# Review Questions

1. A 30-year-old man with Marfan syndrome undergoes genetic testing in anticipation of preimplantation testing of embryos. Testing of the man's DNA is expected to reveal a pathogenic mutation in the gene for which one of the following proteins?

   A. $\alpha$-1-Antitrypsin
   B. Elastin
   C. Elastase
   D. Fibrillin-1
   E. TGF-$\beta$ receptor 1

2. A 39-year-old man with a 20-year history of smoking two packs of cigarettes per day is diagnosed with emphysema. His 40-year old brother has a similar history. Further testing for this patient should involve a search for a pathogenic mutation in the gene for which one of the following proteins?

   A. $\alpha$-1-Antitrypsin
   B. Elastin
   C. Elastase
   D. Fibrillin-1
   E. TGF-$\beta$ receptor 1

3. Which one of the following drugs is most likely useful in the treatment of Hurler syndrome?

   A. $\alpha$-1 proteinase inhibitor (antitrypsin)
   B. Chondroitin
   C. Glucosamine
   D. Laronidase (iduronidase)
   E. Losartan

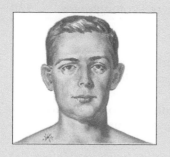

# 14

# Heme Metabolism, Porphyrias, and Hyperbilirubinemia

## SYNOPSIS

- Heme is an organic molecule that consists of a porphyrin ring that binds to and coordinates an iron ion (Fig. 14.1).
- Heme is a part of hemoglobin, myoglobin, and the cytochromes. Heme iron can bind oxygen or facilitate redox reactions.
- Most of the daily heme synthesis occurs in immature red blood cells and the liver. Other cells synthesize heme only at a low rate.
- Porphyrias are caused by deficiencies in enzymes of heme synthesis that lead to the accumulation of toxic intermediates. Some porphyrias primarily affect the nervous system, while others affect the skin.
- Lead poisoning is associated with decreased heme synthesis and damage to the nervous system.
- When heme-containing proteins are degraded, the amino acids and the heme iron are recycled, while the porphyrin moiety is converted to bilirubin glucuronates, which are secreted into bile.
- A high concentration of bilirubin in the blood indicates the premature death of red blood cells, reduced glucuronidation of bilirubin, or impaired excretion of bilirubin glucuronides.

## LEARNING OBJECTIVES

*For mastery of this topic, you should be able to do the following:*
- Describe the main inciting events, symptoms, pathology, and treatment of acute intermittent porphyria and porphyria cutanea tarda.
- Describe the effect of lead poisoning on the synthesis of heme and hemoglobin.
- Describe the main source and production of bilirubin and conjugated bilirubin, paying attention to the tissues in which this occurs as well as the transport of intermediates between these tissues.
- Interpret lab reports on bilirubin measurements.
- Define the signs and symptoms of hyperbilirubinemia.
- Define cholestasis and explain how it affects lab values for bilirubin.
- Compare and contrast the causes of neonatal jaundice and Gilbert syndrome.
- List the drugs that require special consideration when given to patients who have Gilbert syndrome or severe hyperbilirubinemia.
- List the proteins that remove heme and hemoglobin from blood plasma, and relate laboratory data for these proteins to hemolysis.

## 1. HEME SYNTHESIS

*Most of the body's heme synthesis occurs in two compartments: the bone marrow synthesizes heme while synthesizing hemoglobin, and the liver synthesizes heme as part of the synthesis of cytochrome P450 enzymes. At elevated concen-*

*trations, intermediates of heme synthesis are toxic. Cells synthesize heme only on demand.*

### 1.1. Use of Heme in Proteins

**Heme** is a prosthetic group that reversibly binds oxygen or accepts and donates electrons. Heme consists of a **porphyrin** (an organic molecule) and an **iron** ion (see Fig. 14.1). A **prosthetic group** is an organic, nonpeptidic molecule (e.g., heme) that binds to a protein (see Section 1 in Chapter 10).

Heme is found principally as the prosthetic group of **hemoglobin**, **myoglobin**, and the **cytochromes**, and also of **catalase**. In hemoglobin and myoglobin, heme reversibly binds oxygen (see Chapter 16). The cytochromes encompass cytochrome P450 enzymes, cytochrome $b_5$, and the cytochromes that are involved in mitochondrial respiration. **Cytochrome P450** enzymes are located in the membrane of the endoplasmic reticulum. These enzymes hydroxylate endogenous and exogenous compounds (e.g., steroids and most drugs). Hydroxylation makes these compounds more water soluble. Drug intake often leads to a marked increase in the synthesis of cytochrome P450 enzymes. **Cytochrome $b_5$** is involved in electron transfer, often from NADH. The cytochromes that are involved in **mitochondrial respiration** transport electrons from ubiquinol to oxygen. In all of these cytochromes, heme is the prosthetic group that reversibly accepts and donates electrons (see Chapter 23). **Catalase** is an enzyme that degrades hydrogen peroxide (it catalyzes the reaction $2\ H_2O_2 \rightarrow 2\ H_2O + O_2$; see Chapter 21).

### 1.2. Pathway and Regulation of Heme Synthesis

Most of the heme synthesis occurs in the bone marrow and the liver. A healthy person synthesizes approximately 0.3 g of heme per day. About 80% of the daily heme synthesis occurs in erythropoietically active bone marrow for the production of hemoglobin. About 15% of the daily heme synthesis occurs in the liver as part of the synthesis of cytochrome P450 enzymes and catalase.

Fig. 14.2 shows the **pathway** of heme synthesis. In essence, glycine and the citric acid cycle intermediate succinyl–coenzyme A (succinyl-CoA) give rise to aminolevulinic acid, eight molecules of which eventually give rise to a ring-shaped porphyrinogen. Removal of carboxyl groups and oxidation generates a more hydrophilic porphyrin, into which an iron ion is inserted (iron enters mitochondria via mitoferrin, see Section 5 in Chapter 15). The porphyrins, possessing an extensive system of conjugated double bonds, absorb visible light.

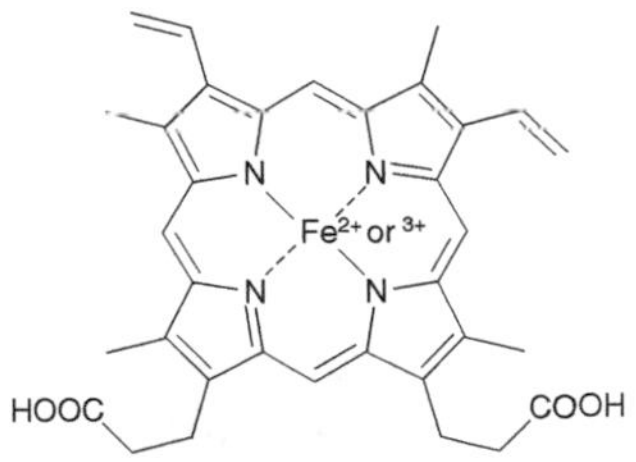

**Fig. 14.1** Heme.

Hemoglobin, for instance, looks reddish. Parts of heme synthesis take place in the mitochondria; others occur in the cytosol.

The physiological **regulation** of heme synthesis occurs chiefly at the level of **aminolevulinic acid synthase** (ALA synthase; see Fig. 14.2). In the first step in heme synthesis, ALA synthase inside mitochondria catalyzes the condensation of succinyl-CoA and glycine to **ALA** (5-aminolevulinic acid, $\delta$-aminolevulinic acid). As this is the first committed step (i.e., the first irreversible reaction) in heme synthesis, it is regulated. There are two types of ALA synthase that differ in regulation and are derived from different genes: the erythroid type and the housekeeping type.

The **erythroid-type ALA synthase** (ALA synthase 2) is synthesized only when **iron** is present. This ALA synthase is expressed chiefly in hemoglobin-synthesizing precursor cells of red blood cells (i.e., polychromatophilic erythroblasts and all reticulocytes; see Fig. 16.3). The mRNA for ALA synthase contains an **iron response element** (IRE; see Section 3 in Chapter 15). Only in the presence of iron can this mRNA be translated. In erythropoietic cells, the supply of iron is commonly borderline low. Iron-dependent synthesis of ALA synthase ensures that there is enough iron to insert into the penultimate product of the heme synthesis pathway (see Fig. 14.2). Otherwise, protoporphyrin IX would accumulate and damage cells (see below).

The activity of the **housekeeping-type ALA synthase** (ALA synthase 1) is regulated principally by feedback inhibition from free **heme** (see Fig. 14.2). This enzyme is expressed in most cell types, but it is most abundant in the liver. The liver needs heme mainly as a cofactor for the enzymes of the cytochrome P450 pathway (see above). Free heme is noxious to cells. As the concentration of free heme increases, the housekeeping ALA synthase is progressively more inhibited. Conversely, when a relatively large amount of heme is needed for cytochrome P450 synthesis, the concentration of free heme decreases, and the activity of ALA synthase increases.

Both ALA synthases use **pyridoxal phosphate** as a cofactor, which is derived from **vitamin B$_6$** (also called **pyridoxine**). Pyridoxal phosphate is also a cofactor for many aminotransferases (see Fig. 35.4). Indeed, the ALA synthases are also a type of aminotransferase. A vitamin B$_6$ deficiency can impair synthesis of red blood cells (see Section 2.6).

## 2. DISEASES ASSOCIATED WITH HEME SYNTHESIS

*Several diseases (mostly porphyrias) are associated with impaired heme synthesis. All of these diseases are uncommon, except for lead poisoning. The porphyrias can be categorized into those that damage primarily the nervous system (e.g., acute intermittent porphyria), those that damage the skin (e.g., porphyria cutanea tarda), and those that damage both the nervous system and the skin.*

### 2.1. General Considerations

A patient who produces an excessive concentration of any porphyrinogen or porphyrin is susceptible to **photo damage** of the skin. Hydroxymethylbilane can spontaneously cyclize to uroporphyrinogen. All **porphyrinogens** in heme synthesis (i.e., uro-, copro-, and protoporphyrinogen) readily and spontaneously oxidize to the respective **porphyrins** (Fig. 14.3; also see Fig. 14.2). When these porphyrins reach the skin via the bloodstream, they absorb sunlight and give rise to oxygen **radicals** that damage the skin. A system of several conjugated double bonds is needed for a molecule to absorb light from the sun (see Fig. 14.3). For this reason, only porphyrins (e.g., protoporphyrin, heme) appreciably absorb **sunlight**, while their precursors do not.

For diagnostic purposes, plasma, urine, and stool can be tested for intermediates of heme synthesis. If a patient has neurovisceral symptoms (see Section 2.3), urine tests for ALA and PBG are ordered. If the patient is photosensitive (see Section 2.4), plasma is first tested for total porphyrins. If this test is positive, urine and stools are tested for specific porphyrins. The most water-soluble **porphyrins** are excreted in the **urine**, while the less soluble ones are excreted in the **stool** (via the bile). Carboxyl groups (–COOH) increase the water solubility of porphyrinogens and porphyrins. Hence, at the extremes, uroporphyrin (the oxidation product of uroporphyrinogen, eight –COOH) are mostly found in urine, while protoporphyrin (the oxidation product of protoporphyrinogen, two –COOH) is found mostly in stool. Porphyrins with intermediate numbers of carboxyl groups distribute accordingly. Data on individual porphyrins usually help make a diagnosis.

**Lead poisoning** is common and inhibits heme synthesis; porphyrias (deficiencies of enzymes of the heme synthesis pathway) are uncommon. Acute intermittent porphyria is the most prevalent porphyria with damage predominantly to the nervous system, while porphyria cutanea tarda is the most prevalent porphyria with damage predominantly to the skin.

### 2.2. Use of Porphyrins for Photodiagnostic Purposes and Photodynamic Therapy

Exogenous aminolevulinic acid (ALA), or an analog, is used for photodiagnosis and photodynamic therapy. Normally, the rate of synthesis of ALA determines flux in the heme synthesis pathway. Exogenous ALA bypasses the control of ALA synthase, and cells convert this ALA to protoporphyrin IX. Protoporphyrin IX tends to accumulate more in tumor cells than in normal cells. ALA can be given orally. ALA or ALA esters can also be applied to the skin. ALA crosses plasma membranes with the help of transporters for dipeptides and amino acids.

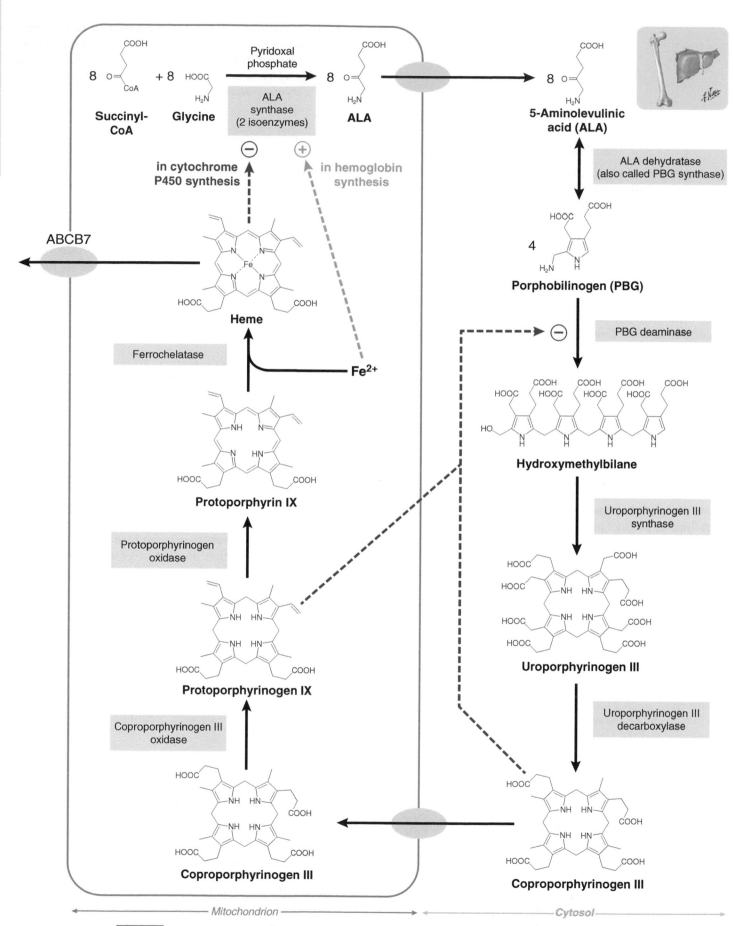

**Fig. 14.2**   **Biosynthesis of heme.** Most of the heme is synthesized in red blood cell precursors and in the liver.

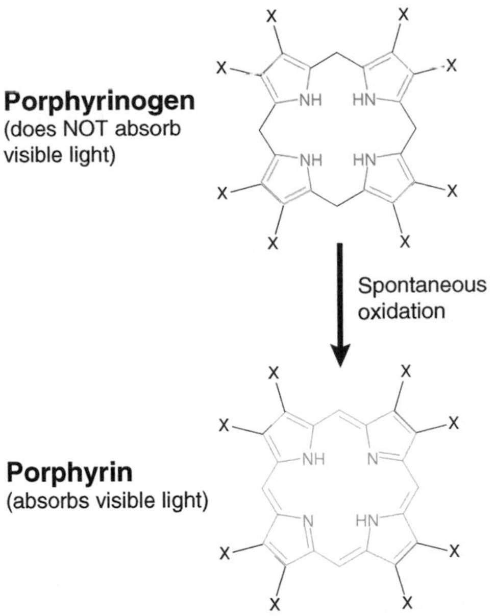

Porphyrinogen
(does NOT absorb
visible light)

Spontaneous
oxidation

Porphyrin
(absorbs visible light)

**Fig. 14.3** **Spontaneous oxidation of porphyrinogens to porphyrins.** Porphyrinogens possess only the isolated, relatively small, aromatic pyrrole rings (*blue*), while the porphyrins contain a more extensive system of delocalized electrons (*orange*). As a consequence, porphyrinogens do not absorb sunlight, whereas porphyrins do. X is $CH_3$, $CH{=}CH_2$, $CH_2{-}COOH$, or $CH_2{-}CH_2{-}COOH$.

**Fluorescence detection** after excitation with blue light is the most sensitive means of locating **protoporphyrin IX** for **diagnostic** purposes. This technique is chiefly used to locate **neoplasms**.

For **photodynamic therapy**, protoporphyrin IX formed inside cells is activated with blue or red light, depending on the desired tissue depth of activation (red light penetrates further into tissues). When protoporphyrin IX absorbs light, it rapidly reacts with oxygen ($O_2$) to produce the highly reactive **singlet oxygen** (an energy-rich form of $O_2$ that is a toxic "reactive oxygen species" [ROS]; see Chapter 21). Photodynamic treatment is used for the destruction of superficial or internal tumors (e.g., lung cancer and intraductal cholangiocarcinoma).

## 2.3. Diseases of Heme Synthesis That Primarily Affect the Nervous System

### 2.3.1. Acute Intermittent Porphyria

Acute intermittent porphyria is caused by reduced activity (<50% of normal) of **porphobilinogen deaminase**. This disorder is inherited in autosomal dominant fashion. In North America, at least one person in 10,000 has insufficient enzyme activity (approximately half of the normal amount), and most of these people have an attack sometime during their life. The disease starts in the liver and manifests itself as a disease of the nervous system. Episodic attacks are brought on by an increased demand for heme in the liver, such as by substances that induce the **cytochrome P450** system (e.g., barbiturates, contraceptives, sulfonamides, or alcohol). Under normal circumstances, the patient's liver has enough porphobilinogen deaminase activity to synthesize an adequate amount of heme.

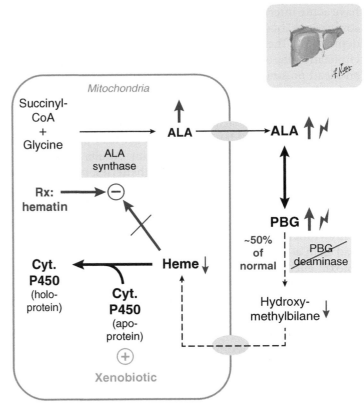

**Fig. 14.4** **Pathogenesis of an attack in a patient with acute intermittent porphyria.**

However, when demand for heme is increased, the liver of these patients does not have enough porphobilinogen deaminase activity. The resulting low concentration of heme deinhibits ALA-synthase and thus creates a detrimental accumulation of **ALA** (5-aminolevulinic acid) and **PBG** (porphobilinogen); see Figs. 14.2 and 14.4.

During an attack, patients with acute intermittent porphyria present with intense central **abdominal pain**. The abdominal pain may be due to the accumulation of PBG in the liver, as well as the neurotoxic effects of ALA excess and heme deficiency. Patients also present with vomiting, hypertension, and tachycardia. Furthermore, some patients have motor neuropathy (that may lead to respiratory paralysis), anxiety, depression, psychosis, or life-threatening seizures. Patients with acute intermittent porphyria are not photosensitive. During an attack, the urine contains abnormally high amounts of ALA (20–100 mg/day; normal, <7 mg/day) and PBG (50–200 mg/day; normal, <4 mg/day).

**Treatment** of acute intermittent porphyria includes inhibition of ALA synthase with a high dietary **carbohydrate** intake (oral or intravenous; mechanism of action not understood), intravenous **hematin** (**hydroxyheme**, sometimes called **hemin**) to replenish the heme pool and inhibit ALA synthase, and pain management.

### 2.3.2. Lead Poisoning and ALA Dehydratase-Deficient Porphyria

An **acquired** decrease in the activity of **ALA dehydratase** is seen in patients with **lead poisoning**. As with patients who have acute intermittent porphyria, patients who have lead poisoning can have abdominal pain, motor neuropathy, and depression. The concentration of lead in the blood helps the clinician differentiate between acute intermittent porphyria and lead poisoning.

Lead poisoning most often occurs through ingestion or inhalation of lead-containing particles or fumes. Some paints used to be made with lead (white lead carbonate and/or yellow lead chromate). Children sometimes get lead poisoning due to eating chips of old, lead-based paint. Adults get lead poisoning through workplace exposure (batteries, paints). While the blood of nonsymptomatic patients typically contains about 2-μg lead/dL (~0.1 μM), a concentration more than 10 μg/dL is a cause for follow-up and intervention. Children are especially vulnerable because they absorb and retain much more lead than adults, and they are also more sensitive to the neurotoxic effects of lead than adults. Long-term lead exposure increases an adult's risk for cognitive decline. Long-term exposure is best assessed by measuring lead in the tibia with a special radiographic procedure.

In patients who have blood lead levels more than about 45 μg/dL, **chelation therapy** may be indicated to remove lead from the body. This commonly involves the use of oral **succimer** (dimercaptosuccinic acid), intravenous or intramuscular **Ca$^{2+}$-EDTA** (ethylenediamine tetraacetic acid complexed with calcium), or, less commonly, intramuscular **dimercaprol** (dimercaptopropanol).

The **neurotoxic** effects of lead are complex and incompletely understood. Clearly, lead (Pb$^{2+}$) binds to ALA dehydratase in place of zinc (Zn$^{2+}$) and thereby inhibits ALA dehydratase activity; this inhibition causes a rise in the concentration of ALA. ALA then spills into the blood and from there into the nervous system. Lead may also bind to DNA-binding proteins that contain a certain subtype of Zn-finger, which would alter transcription. Besides these effects on Zn$^{2+}$-containing proteins, lead also binds into the Ca$^{2+}$-binding site of Ca$^{2+}$-activated protein kinase C and of synaptotagmin. Ca$^{2+}$-activated protein kinase C is involved in intracellular signal transmission, and synaptotagmin is involved in neurotransmitter release. Many other proteins that contain Zn$^{2+}$ or Ca$^{2+}$ are not affected by lead poisoning because their affinity for Pb$^{2+}$ is too low. Lead can also be toxic to the kidneys and cause **gout** (see Chapter 38).

An abnormally high concentration of ALA is also seen in patients with the extremely rare **hereditary** disease **ALA-dehydratase-deficient porphyria**. These patients, too, present with neuropathy.

## 2.4. Diseases of Heme Synthesis That Affect Only the Skin

### 2.4.1. Porphyria Cutanea Tarda

In porphyria cutanea tarda, **uroporphyrinogen III decarboxylase** activity is deficient (<20% of normal activity); Fig. 14.5. Porphyria cutanea tarda is the most prevalent porphyria that involves photosensitivity. Porphyria cutanea tarda is usually

an acquired disease of the liver but not of the blood-forming tissues. An elevated **iron** content of the liver appears to be a prerequisite. Additionally, iron overload (often due to hereditary hemochromatosis; see Chapter 15), hepatitis C, AIDS, certain drugs (e.g., estrogens), excessive alcohol intake, or smoking can lead to insufficient uroporphyrinogen III decarboxylase activity. It is currently thought that these coexisting conditions lead to the formation of an inhibitor of uroporphyrinogen III decarboxylase. Less frequently, the uroporphyrinogen III decarboxylase deficiency is inherited rather than acquired. In this case, even environmental influences of low potency can render a patient symptomatic.

Porphyria cutanea tarda involves **photosensitivity** but not neurologic symptoms. Patients with porphyria cutanea tarda are photosensitive because uroporphyrinogen III and partially decarboxylated intermediates between uroporphyrinogen III and coproporphyrinogen III are present at an abnormally high concentration. These porphyrinogens leak from the liver into the bloodstream and spontaneously oxidize to porphyrins, which have an extensive system of conjugated double bonds (see Fig. 14.3). In the skin, upon exposure to light, the porphyrins give rise to reactive oxygen radicals, which in turn damage the cells and cause blisters that take up to 1 month to heal, often with scarring (Fig. 14.6). From the blood, porphyrins reach the **urine** and give it a **red** to **purple** color.

Laboratory tests on 24-hour urine usually reveal elevated amounts of **uroporphyrin**, which has eight carboxyl groups, as well as porphyrins with seven, six, and five carboxyl groups (named **hepta-**, **hexa-**, and **penta-carboxyporphyrin,** respectively). These porphyrins are oxidized intermediates of the impaired decarboxylation reactions between uroporphyrinogen (eight carboxyl groups) and coproporphyrinogen (four carboxyl groups). Patients with porphyria cutanea tarda can synthesize heme at a near normal rate because the loss of uroporphyrinogen III is made up by increased synthesis, owing to reduced feedback inhibition from heme as well as protoporphyrinogen and coproporphyrinogen. The excretion of ALA and PBG in the urine is normal.

The treatment of porphyria cutanea tarda has three main objectives: (1) to improve liver function by treatment of underlying disorders, such as hepatitis C or iron overload (excess iron stores can be depleted with **phlebotomy**; see Chapter 15); (2) to reduce formation of porphyrin radicals in the skin by **avoidance of sun exposure** and the use of sunscreen lotion; and (3) to prevent damage to the skin by porphyrin radicals with oral supplements of β-**carotene**, an antioxidant (see Chapter 21).

### 2.4.2. Other Porphyrias That Affect the Skin but Not the Nervous System

Insufficient activity of **uroporphyrinogen III synthase** causes **congenital erythropoietic porphyria**, and insufficient activity of **ferrochelatase** causes **erythropoietic protoporphyria**. Neither of these porphyrias gives rise to neurovisceral symptoms.

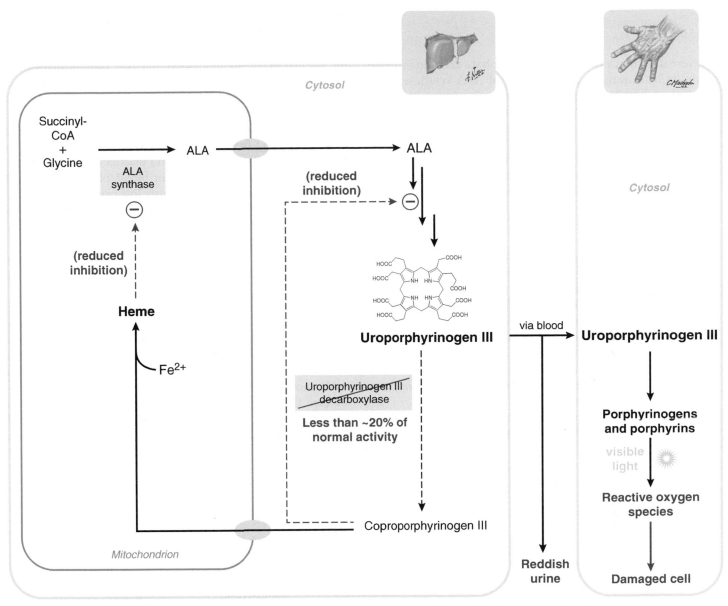

**Fig. 14.5** Pathogenesis of photosensitivity in a patient with porphyria cutanea tarda.

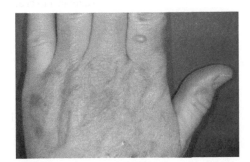

**Fig. 14.6** **Porphyria cutanea tarda.** (From Frank J, Poblete-Gutiér-rez P. Porphyria cutanea tarda: when skin meets liver. *Best Pract Res Clin Gastroenterol.* 2010;24:735–745.)

## 2.5. Porphyrias That Affects Both the Nervous System and the Skin

Insufficient activity of **coproporphyrinogen I oxidase** causes **hereditary coproporphyria**, and **protoporphyrinogen oxidase** causes **variegate porphyria**. These porphyrias lead to the accumulation of coproporphyrinogen and protoporphyrinogen, respectively, which feedback inhibit PBG deaminase, the enzyme that is deficient in acute intermittent porphyria (see Figs. 14.2 and 14.4). Hence, these porphyrias share symptoms of neurotoxicity. The accumulating porphyrinogens spontaneously oxidize to porphyrins (see Fig. 14.3), which render patients photosensitive, akin to those who have porphyria cutanea tarda (see above).

## 2.6. Diseases of Heme Synthesis That Cause Anemia but Not Neurotoxicity or Skin Damage

A severe **deficiency of pyridoxal phosphate** can impair heme synthesis by diminishing the activity of ALA synthase. Pyridoxal phosphate is derived from pyridoxine (vitamin $B_6$; see Fig. 35.4). Vitamin $B_6$ deficiency is rare. Women who use oral contraceptives and patients who regularly abuse alcohol are most at risk.

An extremely rare, heritable deficiency of the erythroid form of **ALA synthase** (see Fig. 14.2) causes **X-linked sideroblastic anemia**, which is characterized by life-threatening iron accumulation.

## 3. DEGRADATION OF HEME TO BILIRUBIN

*When red blood cells are degraded, the iron in heme is recycled, while the porphyrin moiety is degraded to bilirubin and eventually excreted. An excessive amount of bilirubin in the blood indicates reduced survival of red blood cells and/ or insufficient excretion of bilirubin. Excretion may be inadequate due to impaired conjugation with glucuronic acid in the liver or impaired secretion of conjugated bilirubin from the liver into the intestine.*

In a healthy patient, about 80% of heme degradation reflects degradation of **aged red blood cells** (i.e., greater than 120-day-old cells), and about 15% reflects the degradation of heme by enzymes in the liver and the kidneys. Less than 3% of heme degradation results from the degradation of excess heme in the normal erythropoietic bone marrow. Though myoglobin (a heme-containing and oxygen-binding protein in muscle) is abundant, it turns over too slowly to contribute significantly to heme degradation.

In blood plasma, **haptoglobin** and **hemopexin** bind free hemoglobin and free heme, respectively, and deliver these to the liver. Free hemoglobin in blood plasma stems from intravascular hemolysis. Free heme in blood plasma has leaked from cells or has been spontaneously lost from free methemoglobin, which in turn is formed from free hemoglobin in blood plasma. Removal of haptoglobin-hemoglobin complexes can occur at a much greater rate than de novo haptoglobin synthesis. Hence, a low concentration of haptoglobin in the serum indicates the presence of intravascular hemolysis.

The spleen removes aged red blood cells and turns the heme into bilirubin (Fig. 14.7). In an asplenic patient, the liver removes the aged red blood cells. **Macrophages** in the spleen (**Kupffer cells** in the liver) break down hemoglobin into globin and heme. Globin is then degraded into its component amino acids, most of which are eventually reused for protein synthesis (see Chapter 34). Heme oxygenase degrades heme into **iron** and **biliverdin**. The iron is recycled. Biliverdin is reduced to **bilirubin** and released into the bloodstream. Carbon

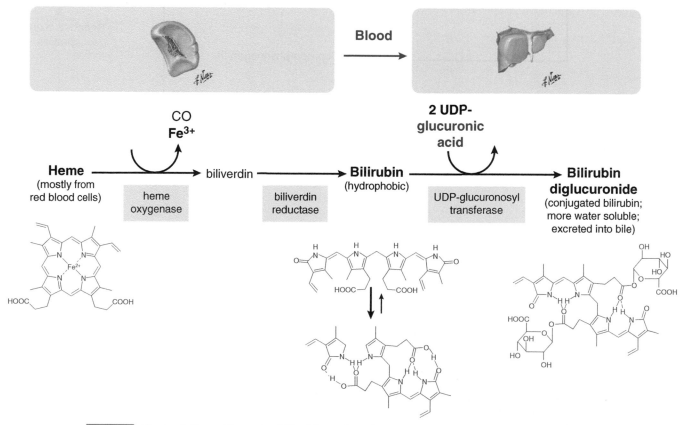

**Fig. 14.7** Degradation of heme to bilirubin and conjugation with glucuronic acid to bilirubin diglucuronide.

monoxide (CO) from the oxidation of heme is carried away in blood, bound to hemoglobin, and eventually exchanged for oxygen; CO production from heme degradation is normally too small to cause appreciable toxicity.

In water, bilirubin forms internal **hydrogen bonds** that conceal the hydrophilic groups from water (see Fig. 14.7), and thus render it poorly water soluble. Hence, in the bloodstream, bilirubin binds to **albumin** (a protein that is secreted by the liver and has a half-life in the blood of about 3 weeks). This complex does not pass through the glomerular membrane in the kidneys nor is it excreted into the bile.

Bilirubin is an abundant fat-soluble **antioxidant** (see Chapter 21). It protects **polyunsaturated fatty acids** from **peroxyl radicals** and proteins from **hydroxyl radicals** (see Chapter 21). However, besides this beneficial role, bilirubin at a high concentration is also neurotoxic (see the following discussion on kernicterus and Crigler-Najjar syndrome).

The liver takes up bilirubin from the blood, conjugates it, and excretes **bilirubin glucuronides** into the bile duct (see Fig. 14.7). **Bilirubin UDP-glucuronosyl transferase** in the membrane of the endoplasmic reticulum conjugates bilirubin with **glucuronic acid** to form conjugated bilirubin (i.e., bilirubin monoglucuronide and bilirubin diglucuronide). **Conjugated bilirubin** is more hydrophilic than bilirubin. (The UDP-glucuronic acid for the conjugation reaction is produced by the oxidation of UDP-glucose by UDP-glucose dehydrogenase.) Conjugated bilirubin (together with other glucuronides, such as those from drugs conjugated with glucuronic acid) is actively secreted into the **bile**.

Conjugation with glucuronic acid, catalyzed by a number of different UDP-glucuronosyl transferases, is a general and important pathway of **detoxification**. Another important pathway of detoxification is hydroxylation by the cytochrome P450 system (see Section 1.1).

## 4. LAB ASSAYS: DIRECT, TOTAL, AND INDIRECT BILIRUBIN

*The total and direct-reacting bilirubin in blood are commonly measured. If the total bilirubin is raised and if the direct/total bilirubin ratio is high, bile likely cannot flow out of the liver into the duodenum.*

Normally, 95% or more of the bilirubin in the blood is unconjugated and 5% or less is conjugated (Fig. 14.8). Most of the conjugated bilirubin is bilirubin diglucuronide.

In the laboratory, bilirubin is measured as the colored (green) product of a reaction with a **diazo reagent**. In alcohol, the diazo dye reacts with all of the bilirubin (conjugated and unconjugated). The result is reported as the **total bilirubin** (see Fig. 14.8). In water, the diazo dye also reacts with both conjugated and unconjugated bilirubin, but it reacts more quickly with conjugated (water-soluble) than unconjugated (fat-soluble) bilirubin. This reaction is not allowed to proceed to completion and is stopped after a few minutes. The result is called **direct bilirubin**. This fraction contains all of the conjugated and some of the unconjugated bilirubin.

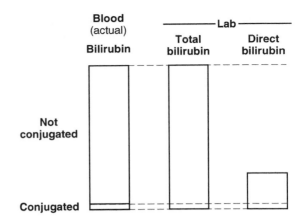

**Fig. 14.8** Relationship of bilirubin lab values to the actual concentrations of bilirubin species in the blood of a healthy patient.

A normal value for the total bilirubin is 0.1 to 1.0 mg/dL; for the direct bilirubin, it is 0.3 mg/dL or less. The direct bilirubin is always smaller than the total bilirubin.

The mathematical difference between the total bilirubin and the direct bilirubin is called the **indirect bilirubin**. Virtually all of the indirect bilirubin represents unconjugated bilirubin.

The lack of specificity of the direct bilirubin assay for conjugated bilirubin complicates the interpretation of abnormalities. Only a major elevation in conjugated bilirubin generates a lopsided direct bilirubin/total bilirubin ratio.

There is a convenient **15% rule of thumb** to interpret bilirubin measurements: If a patient has marked hyperbilirubinemia (e.g., >3 mg/dL), and **if the direct bilirubin is 15% or more of the total bilirubin,** the patient is said to have a **direct hyperbilirubinemia,** which is most likely due to **cholestasis** (i.e., the conjugated bilirubin cannot properly get out of the liver and into the duodenum).

A patient who has marked hyperbilirubinemia (e.g., >3 mg/dL) and a direct bilirubin of 15% or less of the total bilirubin is said to have an **indirect hyperbilirubinemia**. Such a patient either produces too much bilirubin or has a problem conjugating bilirubin.

Note that the 15% rule of thumb does not apply to patients who have a normal or only mildly elevated total bilirubin.

## 5. PROBLEMS WITH THE DEGRADATION OF HEME

*Jaundice is an indication of hyperbilirubinemia. Bilirubin, at a high concentration, is neurotoxic. Hyperbilirubinemia is commonly seen in newborns and in patients who have a hemolytic anemia, Gilbert syndrome, liver disease, or blockage of the bile system.*

### 5.1. General Considerations

**Jaundice** is due to a deposition of bilirubin in the sclerae and skin, which is visible when the total bilirubin in the blood is greater than ~3 mg/dL (see, for example, Figs. 14.10 and 14.12).

In patients with severe hyperbilirubinemia, **alternative pathways of bilirubin excretion** become appreciable. Unconjugated bilirubin can spontaneously oxidize to less hydrophobic products that can be excreted into the bile. Unconjugated bilirubin can also photoisomerize to a more water-soluble diastereomer, which is excreted in the urine (see neonatal jaundice and "bili-lights" below). Conjugated bilirubin can be filtered in the glomeruli and lost into the urine, thereby markedly darkening the urine.

## 5.2. Hyperbilirubinemia Due to Impaired Excretion of Conjugated Bilirubin

If conjugated bilirubin is not adequately secreted from the liver into the bile system and from there into the intestine, it may spill into the bloodstream, thereby giving rise to jaundice and a direct bilirubin that is **more than 15%** of the total bilirubin (Fig. 14.9).

### 5.2.1. Acquired Cholestasis

Cholestasis, a lack of adequate bile flow, causes an accumulation of conjugated bilirubin in the liver. Cholestasis may be due to a problem within the liver or outside of it (see Fig. 14.10).

**Intrahepatic cholestasis** may be due to **primary biliary cirrhosis**, an autoimmune disease seen in about 0.1% of women over 40 years of age and much less frequently among men. Primary biliary cirrhosis is associated with the destruc-

tion of interlobular (or microscopic) bile ducts. Intrahepatic cholestasis may also be due to **primary sclerosing cholangitis** (suspected to be of autoimmune origin) that causes persistent inflammation and stricturing of bile ducts.

**Extrahepatic cholestasis** is due to the physical obstruction of the common bile duct. The obstruction may be created by

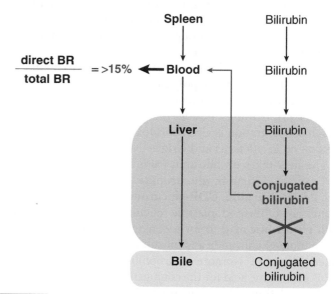

**Fig. 14.9** Deficient secretion of conjugated bilirubin (BR) from the liver into the bile and then the duodenum markedly increases the concentration of conjugated bilirubin in the blood, causing a direct hyperbilirubinemia.

**Intrahepatic cholestasis**

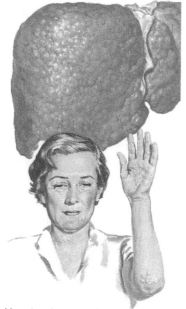

Hepatocytes cannot secrete conjugated bilirubin into bile ducts, or bile ducts are nonfunctional

**Extrahepatic cholestasis**

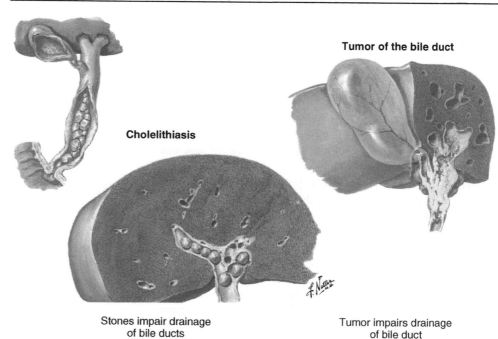

Cholelithiasis

Tumor of the bile duct

Stones impair drainage of bile ducts

Tumor impairs drainage of bile duct

**Fig. 14.10** Impaired bilirubin excretion may be due to intrahepatic or extrahepatic cholestasis. Either way, patients can develop jaundice.

gallstones or tumors (e.g., **pancreatic head cancer, carcinoma of the ampulla of Vater**) that obstruct the bile ducts.

### 5.2.2. Congenital Impairment of Hepatic Bilirubin Diglucuronide Secretion: Dubin-Johnson Syndrome

**Dubin-Johnson syndrome** is due to a hereditary deficiency in the transporter that excretes conjugated bilirubin and other glucuronides into the bile canaliculi. This transporter is variably called the **multidrug resistance-associated protein 2 (MRP2)** or the **ATP-binding cassette subfamily C member 2** and is encoded by the *ABCC2* gene. Dubin-Johnson syndrome is inherited in an autosomal recessive fashion. Prevalence is unclear but is thought to be much less than 1 in 1,000. It is reasonable to suspect Dubin-Johnson syndrome (or another heritable problem of bilirubin excretion) when laboratory data show direct hyperbilirubinemia but no abnormalities in other parameters that reflect liver function (e.g., enzymes, coagulation factors, or albumin). Patients with Dubin-Johnson syndrome are more sensitive to the antifolate drug methotrexate because their cells eject methotrexate at an abnormally low rate (see Section 5.3 in Chapter 37).

### 5.3. Hyperbilirubinemia Due to Increased Degradation of Heme

If a hyperbilirubinemia is caused only by increased degradation of heme, a patient has an indirect hyperbilirubinemia (i.e., the total bilirubin is elevated, and the direct bilirubin usually amounts to **less than 15%** of the total bilirubin, provided that the total bilirubin is greater than about 3 mg/dL; Fig. 14.11). Increased degradation of heme and subsequent increased production of bilirubin can be due to ineffective erythropoiesis or hemolytic disease.

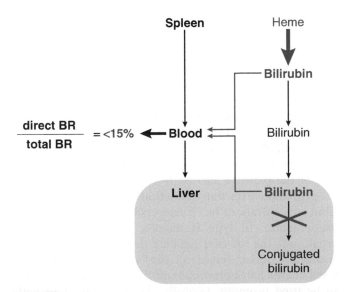

**Fig.14.11** **Excess production of bilirubin (BR) and inadequate conjugation of bilirubin can each lead to indirect hyperbilirubinemia in which the direct bilirubin is less than 15% of the total bilirubin.**

**Ineffective erythropoiesis** is associated with the destruction of heme-containing red blood cell precursors (i.e., polychromatophilic erythroblasts and reticulocytes; see Fig. 16.3). Ineffective erythropoiesis is seen in **lead poisoning** (see Section 2.3.2 above), **congenital erythropoietic porphyria** (see Section 2.4.2), **thalassemia major** (due to a problem with globin synthesis; see Chapter 17), and **megaloblastic anemia** (due to a problem with DNA replication; see Chapter 36).

**Hemolytic disease** is due to the premature destruction of red blood cells. Examples include **sickle cell anemia** (see Chapter 17), **glucose 6-phosphate dehydrogenase deficiency** (see Chapter 21), and **pyruvate kinase deficiency** (see Chapter 19).

### 5.4. Hyperbilirubinemia Due to Inadequate Conjugation of Bilirubin

The diseases discussed in this section (i.e., neonatal jaundice, Crigler-Najjar syndrome, Gilbert syndrome, and acquired deficiencies of bilirubin conjugation) are all associated with an indirect hyperbilirubinemia (i.e., with a direct bilirubin of <15% of the total bilirubin).

### 5.4.1. Neonatal Jaundice

Newborns (especially premature babies) often have insufficient amounts of **bilirubin UDP-glucuronosyl transferase**, since the liver starts synthesizing this enzyme only around the time of birth. As a result, these newborns have an abnormally high concentration of bilirubin in the blood, and they have neonatal jaundice (see Fig. 14.12). In utero, the fetus' enzyme deficiency is not a problem because bilirubin diffuses across the placenta and is conjugated in the mother's liver.

**Albumin** acts as a buffer for (unconjugated) bilirubin so that the concentration of free bilirubin rises significantly only when albumin is nearly saturated with bilirubin. For this reason, a total bilirubin concentration in blood plasma that does not rise beyond 20 mg/dL is usually safe. For comparison, a healthy 3-day-old baby has a bilirubin concentration of ~6 mg/dL.

**Kernicterus** (acute bilirubin encephalopathy; see Fig. 14.12) is a severe form of jaundice in which aggregates of (unconjugated) bilirubin and phospholipids form on the membrane surfaces of neurons, predominantly in the basal ganglia, which initiates an encephalopathy that may cause permanent brain damage (especially to the auditory system) or death. Since the aggregates form and dissolve slowly, there may be a lag time between changes in the concentration of bilirubin in the blood and changes in the degree of encephalopathy. With vigilance, kernicterus should be avoidable. Newborns with an unrecognized hemolytic disorder (e.g., glucose 6-phosphate dehydrogenase deficiency; see Chapter 21) are at an especially high risk of developing kernicterus.

In babies with hyperbilirubinemia, the physician must be careful not to introduce drugs (e.g., **sulfonamides**) or **fatty acids** that bind to albumin and thereby displace

**Jaundice**

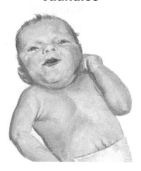

**Consequences of kernicterus**

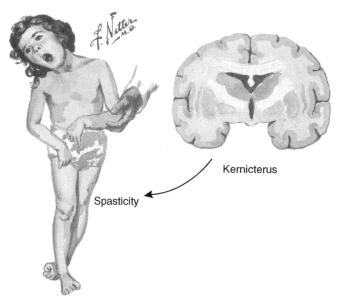

Spasticity

Kernicterus

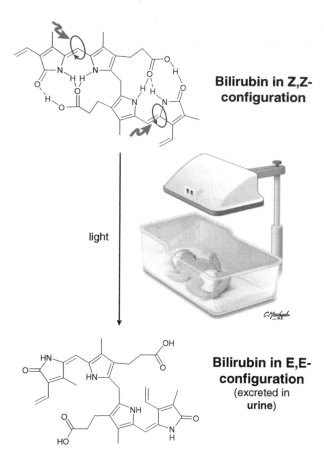

**Bilirubin in Z,Z-configuration**

light

**Bilirubin in E,E-configuration**
(excreted in urine)

Fig. 14.13 **Light can induce the isomerization of bilirubin to a more water-soluble diastereomer.**

Fig. 14.12 **Neonatal jaundice and kernicterus.**

(unconjugated) bilirubin. The physician also must be careful not to introduce drugs (e.g., **steroids**) that are detoxified by UDP-glucuronosyl transferase, the enzyme that conjugates bilirubin.

Patients with very high concentrations of (unconjugated) bilirubin can be treated in three main ways: (1) **exchange transfusion** can be used to remove bilirubin and red blood cells that are prone to hemolysis due to hemolytic disease; (2) an infusion of **albumin** can help bind some bilirubin, but it may also increase blood pressure; and (3) most importantly, **phototherapy** ("bili-lights") can be used to isomerize bilirubin in the skin in a water-soluble form (Fig. 14.13). Blue-green light appears to be suited best to this purpose. The physiological isomer of (unconjugated) bilirubin has the Z,Z-configuration. Light can excite bilirubin and allow the rotation of one or two double bonds to produce diastereomers of the E,Z-, Z,E-, or E,E-configuration. These latter diastereomers form fewer intramolecular hydrogen bonds than bilirubin in the Z,Z-configuration, and they expose more hydrophilic groups (–OH, =NH, =O) to water. As a consequence, these diastereomers do not bind to albumin as tightly as does

bilirubin in the Z,Z-configuration, and appreciable amounts of them can be filtered through the glomeruli and excreted via the urine.

## 5.4.2. Crigler-Najjar Syndrome

Crigler-Najjar syndrome is due to a very rare, inherited deficiency of bilirubin **UDP-glucuronosyl transferase**. In **type I** disease, the enzyme deficiency is nearly complete, and in the absence of treatment, patients die from kernicterus within a few years of life. This syndrome is occasionally seen among the **Amish** or **Mennonites**. The lifelong, extreme hyperbilirubinemia requires daily treatment with bili-lights. Bili-lights are less effective in adults than in babies because of less translucent skin and a smaller surface/volume ratio. Replacement of the patient's liver with a transplanted normal liver (i.e., orthotopic liver transplantation) can restore normal bilirubin concentrations but is irreversible and requires immunosuppression. In **type II** disease, the deficiency is only partial, and the affected patients develop kernicterus only episodically during trauma or sepsis. Early identification of these patients helps prevent brain damage because bili-lights can be used promptly. Globally, dozens of different pathogenic mutations have been identified in UDP-glucuronosyl transferase. Most of these mutations affect the amino acid sequence.

### 5.4.3. Gilbert Syndrome

Gilbert syndrome, seen in about 9% of the population, is due to a hereditary, marked deficiency of **bilirubin UDP-glucuronosyl-transferase**. The deficiency is much less severe than what is seen in Crigler-Najjar syndrome. The disease is usually due to an autosomal recessively inherited mutation in the **promoter** of the gene, which reduces gene expression to approximately one-third of the normal levels. Neonates with Gilbert syndrome have more pronounced and longer-lasting hyperbilirubinemia than neonates normally do. Children and adults with Gilbert syndrome show hyperbilirubinemia in the absence of liver disease (i.e., liver enzymes and coagulation are normal). Hyperbilirubinemia develops predominantly during periods of high rates of heme degradation (e.g., during illness or stress, or after **alcohol** consumption; mostly in males, possibly due to higher turnover of hemoglobin). Ongoing therapy is not necessary. Of clinical importance, however, is the fact that patients with Gilbert syndrome conjugate the topoisomerase inhibitor and anticancer drug **irinotecan** (see Chapter 1) abnormally slowly, which makes the drug more toxic to them.

### 5.4.4. Acquired Deficiency of Bilirubin Conjugation

Damage to liver cells can impair the conjugation of bilirubin. Causes of such damage may be acquired liver disease, liver ischemia, intrahepatic cholestasis, and extrahepatic cholestasis. In addition to conjugation, these diseases can also affect the excretion of conjugated bilirubin into the bile system, so that the direct bilirubin is 15% or more of the total bilirubin.

Acquired liver disease causing jaundice can be due to **fatty liver** disease (see Fig. 28.11), **viral hepatitis**, **autoimmune hepatitis**, **hemochromatosis** (see Figs. 15.4 and 15.10), **Wilson disease** (leading to copper overload of the liver), liver toxins (including some drugs), excessive **alcohol** ingestion, **carcinoma**, or **α1-antitrypsin deficiency** (possibly due to harmful accumulation of aggregates of mutant α1-antitrypsin in hepatocytes; jaundice then occurs mostly in affected newborns).

### SUMMARY

- Heme is synthesized mainly in the bone marrow for the benefit of erythropoiesis. Heme synthesis for red blood cells depends on the availability of iron.
- The second major site of heme synthesis is in the liver, where heme is needed chiefly for the cytochrome P450 system, which plays a role in the detoxification of metabolites and drugs. In the liver, heme synthesis is regulated primarily by the concentration of free heme.
- The two possible major manifestations of various porphyrias are skin damage and neurologic dysfunction with intense abdominal pain. Neurologic effects and abdominal pain are seen in a setting of ALA accumulation. Photodamage to the skin occurs when porphyrinogens or porphyrins accumulate.
- Acute intermittent porphyria is the most common porphyria that affects the nervous system but not the skin. The disease is due to a heritable ~50% decrease in the activity of PBG deaminase. The disease is inherited in autosomal dominant fashion. Acute attacks may be induced by an increased demand for the cytochrome P450 system and may be accompanied by life-threatening neurologic dysfunction.
- Porphyria cutanea tarda is the most common porphyria that affects only the skin. The disease is due to a deficiency of uroporphyrinogen decarboxylase in the liver, most often as a consequence of liver disease in a setting of elevated liver iron stores.
- The initial steps in the diagnosis of a porphyria involve measurements of ALA and porphobilinogen (PBG) in urine and the measurement of porphyrins in blood plasma.
- In the treatment of porphyrias, the synthesis of ALA can be inhibited with intravenous hematin and a high glucose intake, while photodamage by porphyrins can be prevented with light avoidance, sunscreen, and β-carotene. Iron overload can be reduced by phlebotomy.
- Most of the heme that is to be degraded stems from the removal of aged red blood cells in the spleen. The spleen degrades heme into iron and bilirubin. The iron is recycled, and the bilirubin is released into the bloodstream where it binds to albumin. The liver takes up bilirubin and conjugates it with glucuronic acid to form conjugated bilirubin, which it secretes into bile.
- Jaundice is caused by an excessive concentration of bilirubin in the bloodstream (the total bilirubin is more than ~3 mg/dL).
- In a hyperbilirubinemic patient, a direct bilirubin that is greater than 15% of the total indicates a problem with the excretion of conjugated bilirubin. This may be caused by the defective excretion of conjugated bilirubin into the bile ducts or by cholestasis, which in turn may be intrahepatic or extrahepatic. Intrahepatic cholestasis may be due to stricturing or destruction of the bile ducts, which happens with primary biliary cirrhosis and primary sclerosing cholangitis. Extrahepatic cholestasis may be due to obstruction of bile flow by gallstones or tumors.
- In a hyperbilirubinemic patient, a direct bilirubin that is less than 15% of the total indicates excessive production of bilirubin or inadequate conjugation of bilirubin. Excessive production of bilirubin occurs in ineffective erythropoiesis and hemolytic anemia. Inadequate conjugation of bilirubin is common in neonates, due to yet inadequate synthesis of bilirubin UDP-glucuronosyl-transferase. Inadequate conjugation is also observed in patients who have Gilbert syndrome and in patients who have the rare Crigler-Najjar syndrome.
- Liver disease, such as viral hepatitis or liver cancer, and bile duct blockage (by stones or tumor tissue) may affect both the conjugation of bilirubin and the excretion of bilirubin glucuronides.

- Kernicterus, a bilirubin encephalopathy with high mortality and morbidity, can occur at a high concentration of unconjugated bilirubin (generally >20 mg/dL).

## FURTHER READING

- Chiabrando D, Mercurio S, Tolosano E. Heme and erythropoieis: more than a structural role. *Haematologica*. 2014;99:973-983.
- Marion R: The girl who mewed. Discover; 1995. Available at <http://discovermagazine.com/1995/aug/thegirlwhomewed550>. This is an interesting and typical tale of what it takes to diagnose a rare disease such as acute intermittent porphyria; it is also a nice description of the disease.
- Roveri G, Nascimbeni F, Rocchi E, Ventura P. Drugs and acute porphyrias: reasons for a hazardous relationship. *Postgrad Med*. 2014;126:108-120.
- Schulenburg-Brand D, Katugampola R, Anstey AV, Badminton MN. The cutaneous porphyrias. *Dermatol Clin*. 2014;32:369-384.
- Subcommittee on Hyperbilirubinemia, American Academy of Pediatrics. Management of hyperbilirubinemia in the newborn infant 35 or more weeks of gestation. *Pediatrics*. 2004;114:297-316.
- Wallenstein MB, Bhutani VK. Jaundice and kernicterus in the moderately preterm infant. *Clin Perinatol*. 2013;40: 679-688.
- Warniment C, Tsang K, Galazka SS. Lead poisoning in children. *Am Fam Physician*. 2010;81:751-757.

# Review Questions

1. Which one of the following diseases is a son most likely to inherit from his father when his mother is neither a carrier nor affected by the disease?

   A. Acute intermittent porphyria
   B. Glucose 6-phosphate dehydrogenase deficiency
   C. Hemoglobin H disease
   D. Porphyria cutanea tarda
   E. Sickle cell anemia

2. A blood sample from an ill 50-year-old woman shows the following values: hematocrit, 39%; MCV, 90 fL; transferrin saturation, 35%; total bilirubin, 9.0 mg/dL; direct bilirubin, 6.3 mg/dL. These lab results are most consistent with which one of the following diseases?

   A. Acute intermittent porphyria
   B. Autoimmune destruction of bile ducts
   C. Gilbert syndrome
   D. Lead poisoning
   E. Mild glucose 6-phosphate dehydrogenase deficiency

3. Parenteral nutrition is instituted for a 4-day-old infant who has a total bilirubin of 18 mg/dL and a direct bilirubin of 3.0 mg/dL. Which one of the following macronutrients in the parenteral nutrition should be restricted in this patient?

   A. Carbohydrate
   B. Fat
   C. Protein

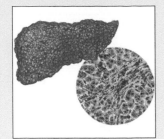

# Chapter 15

# Iron Metabolism: Iron-Deficiency Anemia and Iron Overload

## SYNOPSIS

- Iron is needed mostly for the synthesis of heme (see Chapter 14) in hemoglobin. Lesser amounts of iron are used to synthesize heme in myoglobin, the cytochromes P450, as well as the cytochromes and iron-sulfur clusters that participate in oxidative phosphorylation.
- When iron-containing proteins are degraded, the iron is recycled.
- There is no regulated process of iron excretion. Iron is lost mainly through bleeding, pregnancy, and lactation.
- To replace lost iron, healthy children and adults need to take in iron. Epithelial cells in the small intestine absorb a portion of dietary iron. A Western diet usually contains enough iron to meet normal needs.
- The liver secretes the hormone hepcidin, which regulates how much iron the intestinal epithelial cells release into the bloodstream. The amount of iron transferred into the blood is inversely related to the concentration of hepcidin. In addition, hepcidin also regulates the release of iron from other stores in the body.
- Iron homeostasis and body iron content can be assessed by measuring the serum concentration of iron, the total iron-binding capacity as a proxy for transferrin (an iron transport protein), and ferritin (an iron storage protein).
- Chronic blood loss or long-term dietary iron deficiency depletes tissue iron and eventually causes anemia.
- A long-term excess of iron uptake leads to iron overload, which can be associated with dysfunction of the liver, endocrine organs, joints, and the heart.
- Acute poisoning due to oral iron supplements first damages the gastrointestinal tract and then organs throughout the body.

## LEARNING OBJECTIVES

*For mastery of this topic, you should be able to do the following:*
- Describe the uptake of iron from the diet into the intestine, the release of iron from the intestine into the blood, the movement of iron around the body, storage of iron in tissues, the major use of iron, and loss of iron from the body. Describe the role of hepcidin in regulating iron flux.
- Calculate the transferrin saturation from the serum iron and total iron-binding capacity, and use this value together with other lab tests to assess a patient's iron status, paying special attention to iron deficiency, overload, and poisoning.
- Compare and contrast the daily amount of iron that is absorbed from dietary sources and the daily dose of supplemental iron that is used to prevent or treat iron deficiency, considering the patient's age, gender, and reproductive status.
- Describe the dangers of iron supplements to young children. Explain the biochemical processes that underlie the pathology of acute iron poisoning. Identify potential treatment methods for acute iron poisoning.
- Explain how ineffective erythropoiesis and transfusions can lead to an iron overload.

- Describe the genetic basis and inheritance pattern of the most common form of hereditary hemochromatosis. Describe current genetic testing for this disorder and list the prevalence of pathogenic genotypes.
- Compare and contrast phlebotomy and chelation therapy in the treatment of iron overload or acute iron toxicity. Identify disease conditions for which phlebotomy is usually appropriate. Identify disease conditions for which chelation therapy is usually appropriate.

## 1. THE BODY'S PRINCIPAL IRON STORES

*Most of the body's iron is contained in blood as part of heme. Free iron is toxic. In cells, nonheme iron is stored inside the storage protein ferritin and in its derivative hemosiderin. Most iron leaves the body as a result of bleeding, the delivery of a fetus, or lactation.*

**Iron** is principally found in **heme**, and heme, in turn, is principally found in red blood cells (Fig. 15.1). Heme is a small organic molecule that contains iron (see Fig. 14.1). Heme is found mostly in hemoglobin, myoglobin, in cytochrome P450, and in the cytochromes that participate in oxidative phosphorylation (see Chapter 23). Red blood cells and their **hemoglobin**-synthesizing precursors contain most of the body's heme; therefore, they normally also contain most of the body's iron, about 2.4 g in a healthy adult. As a rule, 1 mL of packed red blood cells contains ~1 mg of iron. Skeletal and cardiac muscle contain **myoglobin**, which uses heme to bind $O_2$ reversibly (see Chapter 16). Hepatocytes are rich in **cytochromes**, which also contain heme as a prosthetic group.

Inside cells, iron is stored inside **ferritin** in the cytoplasm (Figs. 15.1 and 15.2). Free iron can promote the production of free radicals (see Sections 9.1 and 9.6) that damage cellular constituents. Such undesirable reactions are minimized when iron is stored inside ferritin. The largest amounts of ferritin iron are found in the liver, the spleen, and the bone marrow (see Fig. 15.1).

**Macrophages** in the spleen, bone marrow, and, to a lesser degree, the liver (**Kupffer cells**) (Fig. 15.3) degrade heme from engulfed red blood cells and temporarily store the iron inside ferritin. Most of this iron is eventually transferred to red blood cell progenitor cells in the bone marrow, where it is again stored inside ferritin.

**Hemosiderin** is a membrane-enclosed, insoluble degradation product of ferritin that is normally found in the liver, the bone marrow, and to a lesser extent the spleen. Hemosiderin can be stained with Prussian blue for observation by light microscopy (Fig. 15.4).

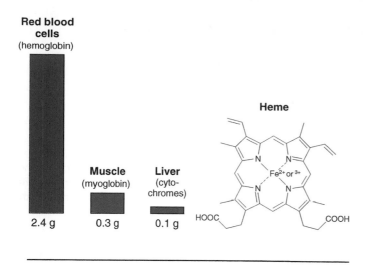

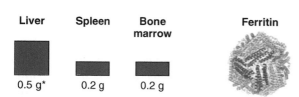

**Fig. 15.1** **In a healthy human body, most of the iron is inside circulating red blood cells as part of heme in hemoglobin.** *Includes iron in hemosiderin.

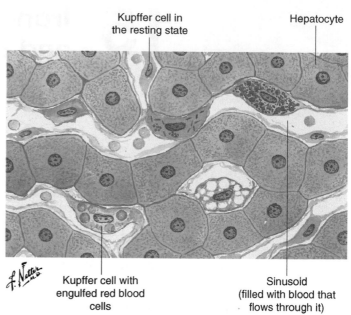

**Fig. 15.3** **Kupffer cells in liver sinusoids take up old red blood cells and store their iron inside ferritin.** Light microscopic image of a hematoxylin-eosin–stained thin section of human liver. The Kupffer cells degrade red blood cells, temporarily store the iron from their heme, and then release it. Normally, ~98% of liver iron is in the hepatocytes. (The dark brown cell is also a Kupffer cell.)

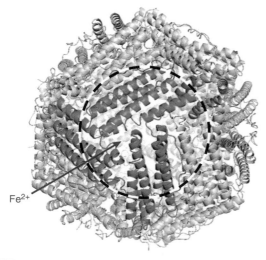

**Fig. 15.2** **Crystal structure–based model of human H-ferritin.** Ferritin consists of H- and L-chains in tissue-specific proportions. $Fe^{2+}$ enters through one of eight channels, is oxidized to $Fe^{3+}$ by $O_2$, and precipitates inside ferritin. The central cavity (outlined by a black dashed circle) can accommodate a maximum of ~4,000 atoms of $Fe^{3+}$. The release of iron may require degradation of ferritin by proteasomes or lysosomes. (Based on Protein Data Bank file 3AJO from Masuda T, Goto F, Yoshihara T, et al. The universal mechanism of iron translocation to the ferroxidase site in ferritin, which is mediated by the well conserved transit site. *Biochem Biophys Res Commun.* 2010;400:94-99.)

**Iron-sulfur proteins** play important roles in the citric acid cycle and oxidative phosphorylation but make up less than 3% of total body iron. Examples of iron-sulfur proteins are aconitase/IRP1 (see Section 3 and Chapter 22) and complexes I, II, and III in oxidative phosphorylation (see Chapter 23).

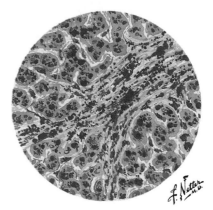

**Fig. 15.4** **Hemosiderin in an iron-overloaded liver.** During histological processing, iron was reacted with acid ferrocyanide to produce dark blue, insoluble Prussian blue. Stainable iron in the liver occurs in proportion to body iron stores. Processing of a sample from a *normal* liver gives rise to no or little Prussian blue (much less than shown here).

Iron-sulfur proteins are also called **nonheme iron proteins** since their iron ($Fe^{2+}$ or $Fe^{3+}$) is coordinated with inorganic sulfides ($S^{2-}$) or sulfides of cysteine side chains ($-S^-$).

## 2. ABSORPTION OF DIETARY IRON

*Intestinal epithelial cells take up iron from the diet either as heme (e.g., from red meat) or as the ferrous cation ($Fe^{2+}$; e.g., from plant sources or a supplement). The liver secretes the hormone hepcidin, which regulates the release of iron from intestinal epithelial cells into the bloodstream.*

Iron is absorbed mostly in the duodenum and jejunum, either as **heme**, or as a **ferrous iron ion** ($Fe^{2+}$; Fig. 15.5). Most

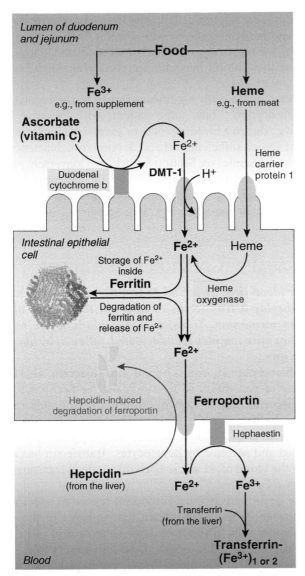

**Fig. 15.5** **Uptake of iron into enterocytes, temporary intracellular storage, and release of iron into the bloodstream.** Hepcidin regulates the release of iron into the bloodstream via ferroportin.

diets contain ~8 mg iron per 1,000 kcal, mostly as nonheme iron. Heme is found in meats. Iron supplements contain iron salts (mostly salts of $Fe^{2+}$, such as ferrous sulfate, $FeSO_4$). When chelated with **ascorbate** (vitamin C), such iron ions are taken up especially well.

The luminal surface of intestinal epithelial cells contains one transport system for heme and another for $Fe^{2+}$ (see Fig. 15.5). After heme has been taken up into intestinal epithelial cells, it is degraded by heme oxygenase (see Chapter 14), freeing $Fe^{2+}$. Much of the naturally occurring dietary nonheme iron is in the $Fe^{3+}$ form. The microvilli of the intestinal epithelial cells contain an enzyme (**duodenal cytochrome b**) that reduces ferric iron ($Fe^{3+}$) to ferrous iron ($Fe^{2+}$). Dietary ferrous iron ($Fe^{2+}$) is absorbed to a greater extent than dietary ferric iron ($Fe^{3+}$) because it does not require such reduction. The intestinal epithelial cells take up $Fe^{2+}$ through a **divalent metal transporter** (DMT1), which also transports manganese ions

(a required trace metal), and many other metals, including those that are toxic (e.g., cadmium or lead ions).

Intestinal epithelial cells either store $Fe^{2+}$ inside ferritin in the cytosol (after oxidation to $Fe^{3+}$; see Section 1 and Fig. 15.2) or export it into the blood. Intestinal cells take up much more iron from the gut lumen than they release into the bloodstream. $Fe^{2+}$ leaves intestinal cells via the iron transporter **ferroportin** (also referred to as solute carrier family 40 subfamily A member 1, abbreviated as SLC40A1), the availability of which is regulated by hepcidin (see Section 3). On the basolateral surface of the enterocytes, **hephaestin** or **ceruloplasmin** then oxidize extracellular $Fe^{2+}$ to $Fe^{3+}$, which binds to **transferrin** (see Section 4). Intestinal epithelial cells are shed when they are ~**2 to 3 days** old, and any iron in them is lost. Intestinal ferritin thus serves as a short-term iron reservoir that evens out changes in the iron content of the diet.

Iron transport in other cells has many similarities to intestinal epithelial cells. Peripheral cells usually acquire their iron from endocytosing transferrin that has iron bound to it, and once it is inside the endosomes, the iron dissociates from the transferrin receptor-transferrin-iron complex. While **DMT1** is in the plasma membrane of intestinal epithelial cells, in other cells it is also in the membrane of the endocytic vacuoles and transports released iron from the vacuoles into the cytoplasm. DMT1 also transports iron across the mitochondrial outer membrane. Finally, **ferroportin** also releases iron from splenic macrophages and Kupffer cells in the liver into the bloodstream. Hephaestin does not seem to be used by splenic macrophages, hepatocytes, and Kupffer cells in the liver to reduce $Fe^{2+}$ to $Fe^{3+}$; these cells use only ceruloplasmin.

## 3. REGULATION OF IRON RELEASE INTO THE BLOODSTREAM

*Iron-response proteins that bind to iron-responsive elements in mRNAs often regulate the expression of proteins that are involved in iron homeostasis. In addition, the liver secretes the peptide hormone hepcidin, which controls iron transport in the body. Hepcidin inhibits the release of iron into the bloodstream from intestinal epithelial cells, macrophages in the spleen, Kupffer cells in the liver, and macrophages in the bone marrow. Inflammation and high iron stores in the liver stimulate hepcidin secretion and thus diminish the concentration of iron in the blood. In contrast, ineffective erythropoiesis, anemia, and hypoxia minimize hepcidin secretion from the liver and thus enhance the release of iron from the intestine, spleen, or liver into the blood.*

The **iron-response proteins IRP1** and **IRP2** regulate the expression of some proteins that are involved in iron transport and storage. In the absence of iron, these proteins bind to **iron-responsive elements** (IREs) in mRNA and thereby either block translation or favor the survival of the mRNA. Conversely, in the presence of iron, the iron response proteins no longer have access to mRNA: IRP1 becomes a cytosolic aconitase that cannot bind an IRE, and IRP2 is degraded in proteasomes. Iron-dependent regulation of translation or degradation is observed for the mRNAs that encode DMT1, ferritin, ferroportin, transferrin receptor 1, or erythroid ALA synthase. Besides iron, the signaling by IRP1 and IRP2 also depends on the local **oxygen** concentration.

**Hepcidin** is a 25-amino acid peptide that binds to **ferroportin** and thereby causes ferroportin to be internalized and degraded. Hepatocytes synthesize hepcidin and then secrete it into the sinusoids, from where it reaches the central vein of the lobule and finally the systemic circulation. Hepcidin in effect prevents iron from leaving intestinal epithelial cells, macrophages in the spleen, Kupffer cells in the liver, or macrophages in the bone marrow; in this way, hepcidin lowers the concentration of transferrin-bound iron in the blood. The purpose of increased hepcidin secretion appears to be twofold: to prevent an overload of the body with dietary iron and to starve microorganisms of iron, which limits their growth.

The proteins **HFE**, **transferrin receptor 2**, and **hemojuvelin** are involved in regulating hepcidin synthesis. Mutations in these proteins (including hepcidin) are known causes of increased iron absorption (see Sections 9.1 and 9.2).

In healthy individuals, inflammation and high iron stores in the liver stimulate hepcidin secretion and thereby inhibit iron transport via ferroportin (Fig. 15.6). **Chronic inflammation**, via an increased concentration of interleukins (e.g., IL-1 and IL-6) in the blood, increases hepcidin secretion. Inflammation in this context can be caused by AIDS, tuberculosis, rheumatoid arthritis, inflammatory bowel disease, or malignancy, for example. An adverse effect of this regulation is that patients with chronic inflammation become anemic due to insufficient release of iron from stores (see Section 8.2 below). **High iron stores** in hepatocytes also lead to an increased secretion of hepcidin (but the secretion of hepcidin is abnormally low in patients who have hemochromatosis; see Section 9.2 below).

**Ineffective erythropoiesis**, **anemia**, and **hypoxia** *oppose* hepcidin secretion (see Fig. 15.6) and thus promote the uptake of dietary iron, as well as the release of iron from macrophages

in the spleen, Kupffer cells in the liver, and macrophages in the bone marrow. Patients with chronic ineffective erythropoiesis, anemia, or hypoxia tend to accumulate too much iron because they inhibit hepcidin secretion *even when liver iron stores are excessive.*

There are clinically significant **limits** to the regulation of iron absorption. Thus, some patients with excessive **blood loss** (e.g., due to a bleeding ulcer or excessive menstrual flow) cannot absorb sufficient iron and develop iron deficiency with or without anemia (see Section 8.1 below). Conversely, patients who ingest iron in very marked excess (acutely or over a long period) do not inhibit iron absorption sufficiently and eventually accumulate too much iron (see Section 9.1 below).

## 4. TRANSPORT OF IRON IN THE BLOOD

*In the blood, iron is bound to transferrin. Cells in need of iron display a transferrin receptor on the surface of their plasma membrane. Transferrin-iron binds to the receptor and the entire complex is endocytosed, followed by liberation of the iron.*

In blood plasma, iron is bound to **transferrin**. This lowers the rate of generation of free radicals (see Sections 9.1 and 9.6), prevents loss of iron by filtration in the kidneys, and makes the blood much less hospitable to microorganisms. Transferrin is a ~78,000 molecular weight protein that is synthesized and secreted by hepatocytes. Transferrin has a half-life in the blood of ~1 week. Each molecule of transferrin can bind two $Fe^{3+}$ ions.

The quantitatively most important release of iron into the bloodstream is the release from macrophages in the spleen and Kupffer cells in the liver. Under the control of hepcidin (see Section 3 and Fig. 15.5), these cells export iron as $Fe^{2+}$ (ferrous iron). In the bloodstream, **ceruloplasmin** (synthesized and secreted by hepatocytes) oxidizes $Fe^{2+}$ to $Fe^{3+}$ (ferric iron), and $Fe^{3+}$ then binds to transferrin. The release of iron from intestinal epithelial cells into the bloodstream is comparatively small; it only has to compensate for losses, which are normally small compared with the overall rate of iron recycling.

Almost all cells have **receptors for transferrin**. **Type 1** transferrin receptors (**TfR1**) are ubiquitous; the number of these receptors on the plasma membrane surface is proportional to a cell's iron needs. In contrast, **type 2** transferrin receptors (**TfR2**) are only minimally dependent on a cell's iron stores. TfR2 receptors are found in hepatocytes and, to a lesser degree, in immature erythroid cells, and in the duodenal crypt cells that give rise to the epithelial cells of the villi. TfR2 plays a role in whole body iron homeostasis, but the mechanisms of regulation have not been elucidated.

Cells endocytose transferrin receptor-transferrin-iron complexes. In endosomes, $Fe^{3+}$ is released and reduced to $Fe^{2+}$, which is transported to the cytosol (via a divalent metal transporter, DMT1; see Section 2). The transferrin receptor-transferrin complex is moved back to the cell surface, and transferrin is released into the blood.

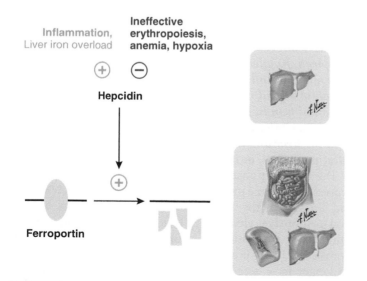

Inflammation,
Liver iron overload

Ineffective
erythropoiesis,
anemia, hypoxia

⊕    ⊖

**Hepcidin**

⊕

**Ferroportin**

**Fig. 15.6** **Hepcidin secretion from the liver controls iron transport.**

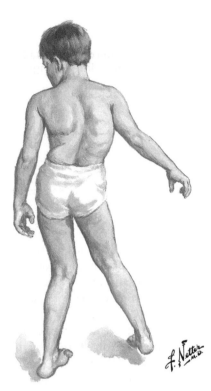

**Fig. 15.7** **A child who has Friedreich ataxia.** The ataxia leads to a wide gait. The patient also has scoliosis. Later, the patient will likely use a wheelchair.

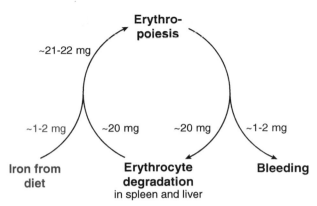

**Fig. 15.8** **Major iron turnover in the normal human body.** Numbers refer only to iron, not its salts.

## 5. IRON IN MITOCHONDRIA

*Mitochondria use iron to produce heme and iron-sulfur clusters. Patients who have the neurodegenerative disease Friedreich ataxia carry a trinucleotide repeat expansion in the frataxin gene that greatly reduces the expression of frataxin, a protein that plays a role in iron homeostasis in mitochondria.*

DMT1 in the outer mitochondrial membrane and **mitoferrins** in the inner mitochondrial membrane transport iron from the cytosol to the mitochondrial matrix for the production of heme and iron-sulfur clusters. The final steps of **heme** synthesis take place inside mitochondria (see Chapter 14). Heme can be exported from mitochondria and used for the production of hemoglobin, myoglobin, and cytochromes (see Chapter 14). **Iron-sulfur clusters** (2Fe-2S and 4Fe-4S) are part of the active site of the **iron-sulfur proteins**, including some complexes of oxidative phosphorylation and an enzyme of the citric acid cycle (see Section 1 and Chapters 22 and 23). **Frataxin** seems to be a chaperone that helps incorporate iron into iron-sulfur proteins. Mitochondria also store iron inside ferritin.

Patients who have **Friedreich ataxia** (Fig. 15.7) are homozygous (or compound heterozygous) for a mutant frataxin gene. Almost 1% of the population is heterozygous for a pathogenic frataxin allele. Friedreich ataxia has an incidence of about 1:50,000. Pathogenic frataxin alleles contain an expanded **trinucleotide repeat** in intron 1 that leads to reduced transcription of the frataxin gene, which in turn leads to a reduced amount of frataxin protein. Affected patients have muscle weakness, ataxia, and impaired vision, hearing, and speech. The onset of symptoms usually occurs between the ages of 5 and 40 years. Most patients die of dysfunction of the heart (e.g., cardiomyopathy and arrhythmia).

## 6. DAILY FLOW OF IRON

*Iron is chiefly needed for the biosynthesis of new red blood cells. Iron from ineffective erythropoiesis and old red blood cells is recycled and normally provides ~95% of the iron for new red blood cells. We lose iron chiefly by bleeding into the lumen of the intestine or uterus.*

Healthy adults need iron principally for **erythropoiesis**. Every day, 1% of the red blood cells are removed and replaced by new red blood cells. The synthesis of heme for hemoglobin in new red blood cells requires 21 to 22 mg of iron per day (see Fig. 15.8). When old red blood cells are degraded in the bone marrow, spleen, or liver, almost all of their iron is recycled; this yields ~20 mg iron per day. A small amount of iron is lost daily in sweat or blood into the lumen of the intestine (2-4 mL/day) or uterus (~30 mL/menstrual period); the iron contained in this blood cannot be recaptured (in contrast, iron is recovered from bleeding into an internal space, such as muscle or the retroperitoneal space). Hence, erythropoiesis must derive the remaining 1 to 2 mg of iron per day from the diet (see Section 2) or from iron stores (in ferritin or hemosiderin; see Section 1). The liver experiences some turnover of **cytochromes** and their heme, but the near-complete recycling of iron covers the needs of de novo synthesis. **Myoglobin** in muscle contains high levels of heme-iron, but it turns over so slowly that it does not contribute appreciably to the daily turnover of iron.

There are two pathways for the recovery of iron from red blood cells at the end of their lives. In healthy persons, about 90% of red blood cells are degraded by macrophages in the spleen or Kupffer cells in the liver. The remaining ~10% of the red blood cells lyse within the blood stream; there, **haptoglobin** (synthesized and secreted by hepatocytes) binds free hemoglobin, and **hemopexin** (also synthesized and secreted by hepatocytes) binds free heme. Macrophages in the spleen

**Table 15.1** **Required Daily Iron Intake**

| Patient Group | Required Daily Net Absorption of Iron (mg) | Required Approximate Daily Dietary Iron Intake (mg) | |
|---|---|---|---|
| | | Patients Who Eat Meat | Vegetarians |
| Postmenopausal women, men | ~1.0 | ~8 | ~15 |
| Women in reproductive years | ~1.5 | ~18 | ~30 |
| Pregnant women | ~2.5 | ~27 | ~50 |

and Kupffer cells in the liver endocytose *haptoglobin-hemoglobin* complexes; hepatocytes endocytose *hemopexin-heme* complexes. After dissociation of these complexes in the lysosomes, haptoglobin and hemopexin are released back into the blood for reuse.

To make up for losses, healthy men and postmenopausal women need to absorb ~1 mg of iron per day from their **diet** (intestinal uptake is described in Section 2 and Fig. 15.5); menstruating or lactating women need to absorb ~1.5 mg per day; and pregnant women need to absorb ~2.5 mg of iron per day (Table 15.1). Most vitamin preparations for expectant mothers provide sufficient iron, but if a pregnant woman becomes anemic, additional iron is given. **Vegetarians** (who consume little heme) need about 80% more iron in their diet than do omnivores.

The iron cost of **pregnancy** is about 1,000 mg of iron, which is equal to about 25% of the normal body iron content. About one-quarter of this iron is transferred to the fetus via the placenta; about another quarter is eventually lost with the placenta and bleeding during a normal vaginal delivery, and about half goes into an expanded red blood cell mass from which the iron is reused after the delivery. Subsequent **lactation** costs ~0.5 mg iron per day.

When needed (e.g., after a major loss of blood), ferritin and hemosiderin iron stores in the body can liberate as much as ~40 mg of iron per day for erythropoiesis.

There is no regulated process of iron excretion.

## 7. INTERPRETATION OF LABORATORY DATA RELATED TO IRON

*Serum iron, total iron-binding capacity, and serum ferritin are commonly measured to assess a patient's iron status.*

The **total iron-binding capacity** (TIBC) of a patient's serum (often reported in µg/dL) is a measure of the maximal amount of iron that can be bound by transferrin. It is therefore a functional measure of the concentration of transferrin in the serum. The TIBC is increased in iron deficiency (see below) and in pregnancy, and is decreased in iron overload.

Most iron in blood plasma (reported as **serum iron** in µg/dL) is bound to transferrin. Measurements of the TIBC and serum iron allow one to calculate the **transferrin saturation** (serum iron/TIBC, expressed as a percentage). The

normal transferrin saturation is 20% to 50% (i.e., $Fe^{3+}$ occupies 20% to 50% of the iron-binding sites on transferrin; the 2:1 stoichiometry for $Fe^{3+}$: transferrin does not matter in this calculation). The transferrin saturation is decreased in iron deficiency; it is increased in iron overload or acute iron poisoning (see below).

The amount of **ferritin** in the human body is approximately proportional to the body's **iron stores**. An iron-responsive element in ferritin mRNA (see Section 3) regulates ferritin biosynthesis according to need. A small amount of ferritin is normally secreted into the plasma, and additional ferritin can be released into the blood when tissue cells are damaged. The liver removes ferritin from the blood. Even in persons with an iron overload, much of the serum ferritin is apoferritin, which contains no iron. Overall, only ~0.01% of all ferritin is circulating in the blood, and the serum concentration of ferritin reflects the size of the body's iron stores. Normal serum ferritin levels in men are ~100 µg/L and in premenopausal women ~40 µg/L. Elevated serum ferritin levels occur in persons with inflammation or iron overload (see below).

## 8. IRON DEFICIENCY

*Patients become iron deficient mostly through excessive bleeding (i.e., if bleeding amounts to more than ~9 mL per day) and through pregnancy, occasionally also as a consequence of bariatric surgery, chronic infection, or chronic inflammation. Persons with advanced iron deficiency develop anemia due to decreased synthesis of heme and hemoglobin as well as ineffective erythropoiesis. Iron-deficiency anemia is associated with an elevated TIBC, elevated transferrin saturation, elevated red cell distribution width (anisocytosis), decreased mean corpuscular volume (MCV), and decreased mean corpuscular hemoglobin concentration (MCHC). Iron deficiency is treated with oral iron supplements (e.g., ferrous sulfate) or with special parenteral iron preparations.*

### 8.1. Iron-Deficiency Anemia

Worldwide, iron deficiency (Fig. 15.9) is the most common cause of **anemia**. Folate deficiency is another common cause of anemia (see Chapters 36 and 37). Iron deficiency leads to diminished heme synthesis (see Chapter 14) in reticulocytes

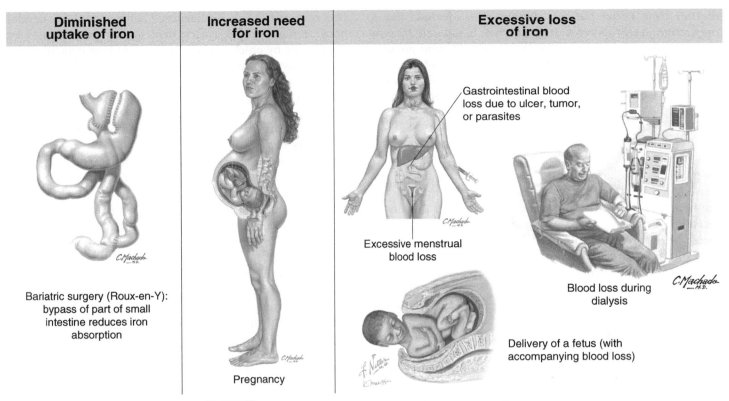

| **Diminished uptake of iron** | **Increased need for iron** | **Excessive loss of iron** |
|---|---|---|

Bariatric surgery (Roux-en-Y): bypass of part of small intestine reduces iron absorption

Pregnancy

Gastrointestinal blood loss due to ulcer, tumor, or parasites

Excessive menstrual blood loss

Blood loss during dialysis

Delivery of a fetus (with accompanying blood loss)

**Fig. 15.9** **Common causes of iron-deficiency anemia.**

and their precursors, which decreases hemoglobin production and the rate of erythropoiesis, causing anemia. Women are more likely to be iron deficient than men due to lower food intake and higher iron losses associated with pregnancy, lactation, and menstruation. Excessive **gastrointestinal** or **menstrual blood loss** is the most common cause of iron-deficiency anemia in the Western world. Excessive gastrointestinal blood loss may be due to **ulcers**, **tumors**, **infection** with hookworms (which suck blood in the intestine), infection with *Schistosoma* (which causes bleeding), or several other intestinal diseases. Patients on **hemodialysis** lose blood during the dialysis procedure and often also have reduced intestinal iron absorption. Patients who have had **bariatric surgery** (a treatment for obesity) often develop iron deficiency because dietary iron bypasses the duodenum, the principal site of iron absorption in the small intestine. Similarly, patients who use a **proton pump inhibitor** to inhibit acidification of stomach contents have compromised iron absorption, such that they are often unable to take up sufficient iron if they have recurrent, increased losses of blood (e.g., heavy periods or blood donations).

Iron deficiency leads to a gradual depletion of iron in brain and muscle, and finally in the red bone marrow. Depletion of iron from the brain can lead to fatigue. Anemia is a late consequence of iron deficiency and also leads to fatigue.

Iron-deficiency anemia is associated with low blood hemoglobin and low hematocrit, abnormally small (microcytic) red blood cells (i.e., low MCV; see Chapter 16), hypochromic red blood cells (i.e., low MCHC), low mean red blood cell hemoglobin content (i.e., low MCH), increased red cell distribution width (anisocytosis, a measure of the size heterogeneity of red blood cells), low transferrin saturation (less than ~16%), low serum ferritin (less than ~12 μg/L), and increased free red blood cell protoporphyrin (protoporphyrin + $Fe^{2+}$ → heme; see Chapter 14).

Iron deficiency can be treated with **oral iron** supplements or **parenteral iron** preparations. In the latter preparations, the toxicity of iron is reduced by complexing the iron with gluconate, dextran, sucrose, or another carbohydrate.

## 8.2. Anemia of Inflammation

Anemia of inflammation is a result of a chronic inhibition of iron transport by inflammation. As described in Section 3, chronic inflammation increases the secretion of **hepcidin**, which in turn inhibits iron release into the bloodstream from macrophages in the spleen, Kupffer cells in the liver, and epithelial cells in the intestine. The resulting lower concentration of iron in the blood is less hospitable to bacteria. Chronic inflammation, via long-term lowering of serum iron (see Section 8.1.), leads to anemia.

## 9. IRON OVERLOAD

*In iron-overloaded cells, iron participates in generating reactive radicals. Overt symptoms occur when total body iron stores are about 10 times the normal amount. Excess iron accumulates in the liver, heart, certain endocrine cells, skin, joints, and sometimes also in the central nervous system. Patients with hereditary hemochromatosis absorb too much dietary iron. Other patients develop iron overload due to ineffective erythropoiesis, frequent red blood cell transfusions, or excessive treatment with intravenous iron preparations. Acute iron poisoning from excess intake of iron pills is seen chiefly in small children. Iron overload is treated by phlebotomy or with an iron chelator, depending on the etiology.*

## 9.1. General Comments on Iron Overload

In patients who have iron overload, iron accumulates predominantly in the liver, pancreas, anterior pituitary, and (sometimes) the heart. Most of the excess iron is stored inside ferritin or hemosiderin. Severe systemic iron overload is associated with **cirrhosis**, **impaired insulin secretion, hypogonadism**, and **cardiomyopathy**. Some patients also develop a distinctive type of arthropathy and a hyperpigmentation of the skin (either brownish or grayish). Liver iron overload also greatly increases the risk of developing primary **liver cancer**. Men are much more likely to have iron overload than women. In men, higher testosterone levels reduce hepcidin secretion and thus increase iron absorption. Additionally, women, unlike men, lose extra iron with menstruation and pregnancy.

Iron overload should be diagnosed before symptoms develop because most of the concomitant pathologic processes are irreversible by phlebotomy as a means of iron depletion.

Overt symptoms of systemic iron overload develop when the body contains ~15 to 40 g of iron instead of the normal 2 to 4 g. As patients with an iron overload develop excessive ferritin iron stores and associated liver damage, laboratory assays reveal increasing serum concentrations of **ferritin** and **liver enzymes**.

Iron overload may be toxic due to increased levels of free iron. Free iron is toxic, because $Fe^{2+}$ and $Fe^{3+}$ may generate highly reactive **radicals** (e.g., $Fe^{2+} + H_2O_2 \rightarrow Fe^{3+} + OH^- + \bullet OH$; see Chapter 21). The radicals may react with proteins, lipids, and DNA in mitochondria and other subcellular structures, thus damaging them (see Section 9.6). For instance, $\bullet OH$, the hydroxyl radical, may react with polyunsaturated fatty acids and create an avalanche of lipid peroxyl radicals (see Chapter 21).

Possible causes of iron overload are briefly explained in Table 15.2. The three major causes of iron overload are **hemochromatosis** (increased iron absorption), **frequent transfusion of erythrocytes**, and **ineffective erythropoiesis** (e.g., β-thalassemia major). **Excessive intravenous (IV) iron** and

**Table 15.2    Causes of Iron Overload**

| Cause | Explanations |
|---|---|
| **Excessive uptake of iron from diet** | |
| Ineffective erythropoiesis<br>Hemolytic anemia<br>Chronic hypoxia | Hepcidin release is inhibited even when the liver is overloaded with iron (see Section 3). Hence, intestinal epithelial cells can release too much iron into the bloodstream. |
| Excessive dietary iron | When the diet contains >100 mg iron/day, the body's controls do not sufficiently reduce intestinal iron uptake. |
| Hemochromatosis | Hereditary excessive uptake of iron from the diet as a consequence of inadequate hepcidin synthesis and secretion or as a result of hepcidin-unresponsive ferroportin. |
| Adult onset | Due to mutant HFE protein or mutant TfR2 transferrin receptors (which participate in iron sensing), or due to mutant ferroportin (which exports iron from cells). |
| Juvenile onset | Symptoms at 10 to 30 years of age. Caused by mutant hepcidin or mutant hemojuvelin. Hemojuvelin is required for a regulated increase in transcription of the hepcidin gene. |
| **Frequent blood transfusions** | Heme iron in transfused blood bypasses the controls on the intestinal iron uptake. One unit of packed RBCs (volume is up to 250 mL) contains up to **250 mg** iron (i.e., up to 250 days' worth of normal intestinal iron uptake).<br>Patients with severe hemolytic anemia, such as β-thalassemia major (see Chapter 17), are at greatest risk. Making matters worse in these patients, chronic anemia (by reducing hepcidin secretion) also increases iron uptake from the diet.<br>(Note: Transfusions that replace erythrocytes lost during surgery are not harmful because they only replace lost erythrocytes and thus iron. Nonetheless, risks for infectious and noninfectious adverse events occur with every unit of transfused erythrocytes.) |
| **Excessive infusion of iron** | This is an iatrogenic disease due to excess iron given to anemic patients along with erythropoietin, such as to patients who receive regular hemodialysis. |

chronic excessive uptake of iron from oral supplements are uncommon causes of iron overload.

## 9.2. Hemochromatosis

**Hemochromatosis** is a genetic condition of increased iron absorption that can result in an iron overload. Causes for hemochromatosis are listed in Table 15.2. Most patients with hemochromatosis take up only milligram amounts of excessive iron each day so that the common type of hemochromatosis (HFE hemochromatosis) typically manifests in 40- to 60-year-olds. A subgroup of patients with hemochromatosis, patients who have **juvenile hemochromatosis**, take up even larger amounts of dietary iron and therefore have an earlier onset of disease (as early as the first decade of life).

Since a patient with hemochromatosis releases too much iron into the blood, both the serum **iron** concentration and the **transferrin saturation** are already increased in the presymptomatic stage of the disease. The regulation of tissue iron uptake via the transferrin receptor 1 (TfR1) does not prevent the excessive uptake of iron from the blood into tissues. The liver, in particular, acts as a sink for excess iron, probably because it expresses the TfR2 transferrin receptor, which takes up transferrin-bound iron even when intracellular iron stores are already large.

The most common form of hemochromatosis is due to homozygosity for a missense mutation in the **HFE** gene. The mutant HFE protein fails to stimulate **hepcidin** synthesis and secretion adequately, leading to the excessive transfer of dietary iron from the intestine into the blood and organs in the body (Fig. 15.10). Most patients are of Northwest-European origin. Although there are many different *HFE* mutations, most (~85%) patients with *HFE* hemochromatosis are homozygous for a **C282Y** mutation in the *HFE* gene; a minority (~15%) is compound heterozygous for an **H63D** and a C282Y mutation, and ~2% are homozygous for H63D.

Some 5% to 10% of *all* European and U.S. whites are heterozygous for the C282Y mutation, and about 0.1% to 0.4% (i.e., up to 1 in 250) are homozygous. Heterozygosity for C282Y in the absence of H63D is usually benign. Although almost all homozygotes for the C282Y *HFE* allele accumulate too much iron, only 20% to 50% of these patients develop organ damage. Gender, alcohol consumption, iron intake, and genes other than *HFE* appear to modify the expression of the disease.

About 2% of Western European whites are homozygous for HFE H63D, and another 2% are compound heterozygous for C282Y and H63D. These persons rarely exhibit an iron overload. If they do develop an iron overload, they usually have concomitant alcoholic liver disease, nonalcoholic fatty liver, or chronic hepatitis (especially hepatitis C). It is thought that the combination of these HFE genotypes and one of these liver conditions leads to decreased hepcidin secretion and therefore increased iron absorption.

Persons can be tested for the C282Y and the H63D mutations as a means of diagnosing the hemochromatosis risk before iron overload and associated symptoms occur.

**Mutant HFE protein**

Insufficient production and secretion of hepcidin

Excessive transfer of iron to the blood

Elevated serum iron and transferrin saturation

Excessive transfer of iron to various organs, damaging them:

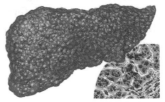

Damage recognizable by elevated **liver enzymes** in blood. **Cirrhosis** may develop. There is an increased risk of **liver cancer**.

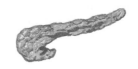

The pancreas becomes fibrotic and atrophic. **Insulin secretion** becomes impaired, causing diabetes.

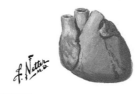

In the heart, contraction and signal transmission are impaired, causing **cardiomyopathy**.

**Fig. 15.10** **Abnormal regulation of iron metabolism in hereditary *HFE* hemochromatosis.**

The most common form of **juvenile hemochromatosis** is due to mutations in the gene (*HJV*) that encodes **hemojuvelin**. The disease is inherited in autosomal recessive fashion. Like mutant HFE protein, mutant hemojuvelin does not permit adequate stimulation of hepcidin synthesis, which in turn leads to the excessive transfer of dietary iron from the intestine into the blood.

With the exception of patients who have anemia, hereditary hemochromatosis is usually treated with weekly **phlebotomy**. At each session, ~500 mL of blood is removed, the erythrocytes of which contain 200 to 250 mg of heme iron. Progress is followed by monitoring serum ferritin.

## 9.3. Iron Overload With Blood Transfusions

Patients who need frequent **erythrocyte transfusions** due to insufficient erythropoiesis often develop a secondary iron overload. For instance, patients who have β-thalassemia major need regular transfusions of erythrocytes to survive. Patients who have sickle cell anemia occasionally also need packed red blood cell transfusions. As senescent transfused cells are degraded, all of their iron is recovered, stored, and sometimes reused. In patients with β-thalassemia major, iron accumulation from transfusions and excessive absorption from the diet (stimulated by ineffective erythropoiesis) is so large that it presents a major challenge for treatment. In patients who have iron overload due to blood transfusions, the iron is removed by **chelation** therapy (see Section 9.4).

## 9.4. Iron Chelation Therapy

Three major drugs are used to chelate (i.e., bind) iron and excrete a drug-iron complex. **Desferrioxamine (deferoxamine)** is usually given intravenously, often overnight and via a small battery-driven pump. **Deferasirox** and **deferiprone** are administered orally. All three drugs bind $Fe^{3+}$ in blood plasma, and the resulting complex is excreted via the urine and/or the bile and feces.

## 9.5. Hemosiderosis and Siderosis

The term **hemosiderosis** is used to describe pathologic amounts of **hemosiderin** in cells. Hereditary and secondary hemochromatosis are associated with hemosiderosis of the liver, heart, and pancreas. **Pulmonary hemosiderosis** is due to iron accumulation in macrophages from chronic local bleeding, a disease that is very different from the hemochromatoses described above.

The term **siderosis** is used for a disease that results from the **inhalation** of pathogenic amounts of iron fumes or iron dust, commonly by welders or miners. **Siderosis** is uncommon and usually benign.

## 9.6. Acute Iron Poisoning

Clinically apparent, acute iron poisoning occurs with the intake of greater than 20 mg of Fe/kg body weight. Iron poisoning is the most common cause of lethal poisoning in children under the age of 6 years. As little as 550 mg iron can be fatal to a small child. Supplements and chewable multivitamin preparations are the usual sources of iron. A single tablet of ferrous sulfate often contains ~60 mg iron. A high luminal concentration of iron damages the gastrointestinal mucosa.

Symptoms of systemic toxicity occur when the total serum iron exceeds the iron-binding capacity of transferrin (i.e., above a serum iron of about 300 µg/dL). A high serum iron concentration (usually more than 500 µg/mL) may be associated with metabolic acidosis, cardiovascular collapse, coma, and liver failure.

Treatment of iron poisoning often involves gut decontamination and chelation of iron in blood with intravenous **desferrioxamine**.

## SUMMARY

- In healthy human beings, red blood cells contain the body's largest store of iron (~2.4 g, in the form of heme-iron). Additional iron (~1.4 g) is found in the liver, spleen, and muscle as heme-iron or as iron stored inside macrophages as ferritin or hemosiderin.

- Most iron is needed for the synthesis of heme by reticulocytes and their precursors. When red blood cells lyse in the circulation or when they are degraded, macrophages in the spleen and Kupffer cells in the liver recover the iron from the heme. This iron is shuttled back to cells that actively synthesize heme.

- There are no regulated means of iron excretion; iron is lost mainly through bleeding.

- Men need to absorb ~1 mg iron per day, menstruating or lactating women ~1.5 mg iron per day, and pregnant women ~2.5 mg iron per day to maintain a normal iron balance. The iron content of the daily diet needs to be 10 to 20 times larger than the daily need.

- Iron is absorbed mostly in the duodenum and jejunum and stored temporarily in the cytosol in a ferritin complex. From there, iron is released into the bloodstream through the iron transporter ferroportin, unless the hormone hepcidin inhibits this transport by inducing the degradation of ferroportin.

- The liver secretes hepcidin in response to inflammation and high liver iron stores. Hepcidin inhibits the release of iron not only from intestinal epithelial cells, but also from Kupffer cells, macrophages in the spleen, and macrophages in the bone marrow.

- Ineffective erythropoiesis, anemia, and anoxia inhibit hepcidin release. These conditions favor the absorption of iron from the diet.

- In blood plasma, iron is bound to transferrin. Peripheral cells endocytose the transferrin-iron complex via specific surface transferrin receptors, retrieve the iron, and release transferrin back into the circulation.

- Determinations of the total iron-binding capacity of serum, the iron content of serum, and the concentration of ferritin in serum allow assessment of the iron status of a patient.

- Iron deficiency causes anemia through inadequate heme and hemoglobin synthesis. Iron deficiency is most often caused by gastrointestinal or menstrual bleeding but can also be caused by excessive blood donation. Patients with chronic inflammation secrete too much hepcidin and thus release too little iron from the intestine, liver, and spleen; eventually, this leads to anemia.

- Hemochromatosis is a hereditary condition of excessive iron absorption that sometimes leads to iron accumulation in the liver, pituitary, pancreas, and the heart. Hereditary hemochromatosis is usually associated with abnormally low concentrations of circulating hepcidin. Most often, *HFE* is mutated. Normal HFE protein plays a role in stimulating hepcidin synthesis and secretion in response to elevated liver iron stores. Abnormally low concentrations of circulating hepcidin may also be the result of chronic ineffective erythropoiesis, anemia, or hypoxia.

■ Iron overload can be secondary to frequent erythrocyte transfusions that are needed to treat diverse types of chronic anemia.

■ Large, excessive amounts of supplemental iron, especially in small children, damage the gastrointestinal mucosa and increase serum iron to levels that exceed the iron-binding capacity of transferrin. Unbound iron then damages the vasculature, brain, and liver, which may be lethal.

## FURTHER READING

■ Barton JC. Hemochromatosis and iron overload: from bench to clinic. *Am J Med Sci.* 2013;346(5):403-412.

■ Chang TP-Y, Rangan C. Iron poisoning: a literature-based review of epidemiology, diagnosis, and management. *Pediatr Emerg Care.* 2011;27:978-985.

■ Crownover BK, Covey CJ. Hereditary hemochromatosis. *Am Fam Physician.* 2013;87:183-190.

■ Ganz T, Nemeth E. Hepcidin and iron homeostasis. *Biochim Biophys Acta.* 2012;1823:1434-1443.

# Review Questions

1. A 52-year-old woman presents with arthritis in her hands. Her serum ferritin is 510 µg/L (normal, 15-200 µg/L), her serum iron is 180 µg/dL (normal, 50-170 µg/dL), and her total iron-binding capacity is 240 µg/dL (normal, 220-420 µg/dL). Further testing reveals that she is homozygous for the C282Y mutation of the *HFE* gene. Radiographs of her hands are consistent with an abnormality of iron homeostasis as the cause of arthritis. Which of the following would be the most appropriate treatment for this patient?

    **A.** IV deferoxamine (= desferrioxamine)
    **B.** IV iron dextran
    **C.** phlebotomy
    **D.** Oral deferasirox
    **E.** Oral iron sulfate

2. A 49-year-old woman presents with hypermenorrhea (menorrhagia; excessive menstrual flow). Her past history is significant for gastric bypass surgery three years prior. Laboratory analysis of a blood sample reveals the following:

    ■ Hemoglobin (g/dL): 7.8
    ■ MCV (fL): 67
    ■ Serum iron (µg/dL): 20 (normal, 50-170)
    ■ Total iron-binding capacity (µg/dL), 400 (normal, 220-420)
    ■ Serum ferritin (ng/mL): 20 (normal, 12-150)
    ■ Serum folate (ng/mL): 10 (normal, 2.5-20)
    ■ Serum cobalamin ($B_{12}$; pg/mL): 650 (normal, 200-900)

    Which of the following is the most likely explanation for the abnormal laboratory findings?

    **A.** Excessive dietary iron intake
    **B.** Folate deficiency
    **C.** Hemochromatosis
    **D.** Iron deficiency
    **E.** Pernicious anemia

3. Serum hepcidin is not yet measured in routine clinical care, but it is measured for research purposes. Serum from patients with which one of the following diseases shows the highest concentration of hepcidin?

    **A.** Untreated juvenile hemochromatosis
    **B.** Inflammation
    **C.** Treated *HFE* hemochromatosis
    **D.** Iron-deficiency anemia

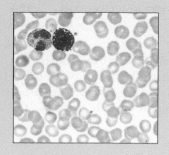

# Chapter 16

# Erythropoiesis, Hemoglobin Function, and the Complete Blood Count

## SYNOPSIS

■ Erythropoiesis is the production of new red blood cells (erythrocytes). Erythrocytes are made in the bone marrow under the regulation of the hormone erythropoietin, which is secreted from the kidneys, depending on the local concentration of oxygen.

■ Hemoglobin inside erythrocytes carries oxygen from the lungs to peripheral cells. The binding of oxygen to hemoglobin is regulated by pH, the concentration of carbon dioxide, and the concentration of 2,3-bisphosphoglycerate inside red blood cells.

■ Blood loss and diseases that affect the lungs, kidneys, bone marrow, heart, or erythrocytes, may affect oxygen delivery to tissues and the production of red blood cells (Fig. 16.1).

■ Important information regarding a patient's health status can be derived from the complete blood count (CBC) and the fraction of immature erythrocytes. The quality of tissue oxygenation can also be judged by the color of a patient's skin.

## LEARNING OBJECTIVES

*For mastery of this topic, you should be able to do the following:*

■ Describe erythropoiesis and its regulation, and list commonly measured laboratory values that provide insight into this process.

■ List treatment options to increase the rate of erythropoiesis in an anemic patient.

■ Explain how hemoglobin binds oxygen in the lungs and how it delivers oxygen to tissues, thereby paying attention to pH, partial $CO_2$ pressure, and 2,3-bisphosphoglycerate.

■ Explain how oxygen is delivered from the mother to the fetus, taking into account the structural differences between adult and fetal hemoglobin and $O_2$ binding affinity.

■ Compare and contrast the structure and the $O_2$ binding properties of hemoglobin and methemoglobin. Identify means to lower a patient's elevated fraction of methemoglobin.

■ Explain the deleterious effects of CO on hemoglobin function. Describe how an increase in environmental CO can lead to tissue hypoxia.

■ Identify the effects of smoking on blood and hemoglobin. List smoking-induced changes in typical blood laboratory values.

■ Explain the role of amyl nitrite and sodium nitrite in the treatment of cyanide poisoning.

■ Use a patient's skin color to infer an abnormality in the fraction of deoxyhemoglobin in the patient's blood.

## 1. ERYTHROPOIESIS

*Under the influence of growth factors (e.g., erythropoietin), stem cells in the bone marrow give rise to erythroblasts that lose their nuclei to become reticulocytes. The reticulocytes are released into the bloodstream where they continue to synthesize hemoglobin until they lose their RNA, mitochondria, and endoplasmic reticulum to become mature red blood cells. The kidneys secrete erythropoietin depending on the renal*

*oxygen concentration. Renal oxygen sensing involves the oxygen-dependent hydroxylation of hypoxia-inducible factors (HIFs) that regulate transcription. With certain patients, exogenous recombinant erythropoietin effectively stimulates erythropoiesis, so that these patients do not need blood transfusions.*

### 1.1. Location of Erythropoiesis

Except during embryonic and early fetal life, the **bone marrow** produces virtually all red blood cells (Fig. 16.2). In young children, all bones produce red blood cells. In normal adults, erythropoiesis (the production of erythrocytes) is restricted to the axial skeleton and the proximal ends of the humeri and femora. Adult patients with a markedly increased rate of erythropoiesis have an increased amount of bone marrow and also produce red blood cells in additional bones. Children with an increased rate of erythropoiesis may develop **bone deformities,** such as tower skull and frontal bossing.

### 1.2. Major Stages in Erythropoiesis

Stem cells divide asymmetrically (one daughter cell remains a stem cell, the other becomes partially differentiated), and their offspring eventually divide symmetrically to produce erythroblasts (Fig. 16.3). **Hematopoietic stem cells** in the bone marrow (through asymmetric division) give rise to **progenitor cells**, which can circulate in the blood and populate new sites in the bone marrow. The original progenitor cells can give rise to progenitor cells that have a more restricted cell fate. Erythroid progenitor cells eventually give rise to **proerythroblasts**, which in turn give rise to **erythroblasts** (i.e., **normoblasts**).

Erythroblasts begin synthesizing **hemoglobin**. Over a period of a few days, erythroblasts become smaller and lose their nucleus to become marrow **reticulocytes**, which are released into the bloodstream. In the bloodstream, a reticulocyte synthesizes about one-third of the final amount of hemoglobin of a mature red blood cell (globin mRNAs are synthesized 2 to 3 days earlier, before enucleation; proteins bind specifically to the 3′-untranslated region of α- and β-globin mRNA and thereby protect the RNA from degradation; see also Chapter 6). After ~1 day in the circulation, reticulocytes lose their mRNA, endoplasmic reticulum, and mitochondria, and the reticulocytes become **mature erythrocytes**. A mature red blood cell stays in circulation for about 120 days. Then, macrophages in the spleen or liver degrade it (for the degradation of heme, see Chapter 14; for the reuse of iron, see Chapter 15).

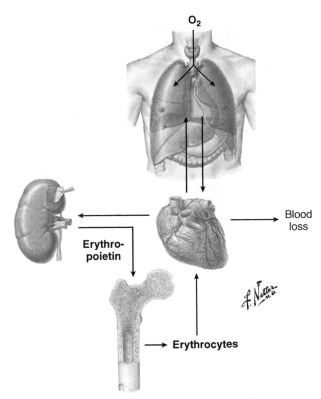

**Fig. 16.1** **Factors that influence oxygen transport in the human body.**

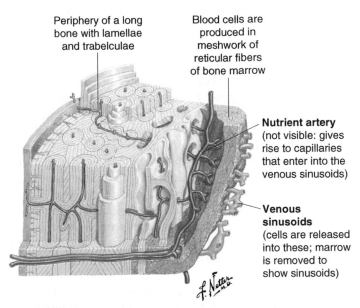

**Fig. 16.2** **Architecture of bone and bone marrow.**

Periphery of a long bone with lamellae and trabelculae

Blood cells are produced in meshwork of reticular fibers of bone marrow

**Nutrient artery**
(not visible: gives rise to capillaries that enter into the venous sinusoids)

**Venous sinusoids**
(cells are released into these; marrow is removed to show sinusoids)

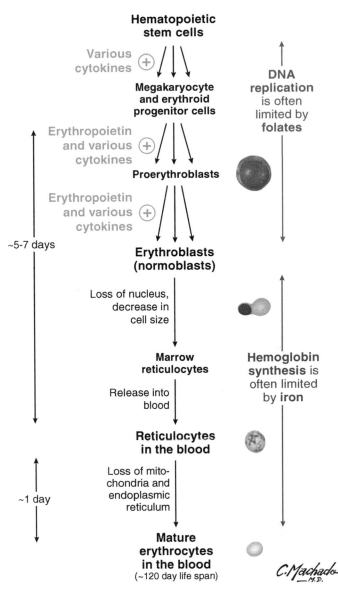

**Fig. 16.3** **Erythropoiesis in bone marrow.**

In most patients, supplements of a folate and iron lead to a modest increase in hematocrit. Folates are required for adequate DNA replication in dividing cells (see Fig. 16.3 and Chapters 36 and 37). Iron is required for heme synthesis (see Chapters 14 and 15). In patients with a pronounced deficiency of either folates or iron, red blood cell precursors die at an abnormally high rate.

## 1.3. Role of Erythropoietin in the Control of Red Blood Cell Production

Red blood cell production is controlled by a large number of cytokines, among them **erythropoietin**, granulocyte-macrophage colony-stimulating factor (GM-CSF), and insulin-like growth factor 1 (IGF-1). Cytokines are an ill-defined, large family of proteins that control cell growth and differentiation. In contrast to hormones, cytokines are not secreted by a discrete gland (e.g., the pancreas), but by a number of cells in the body. Erythropoietin is the cytokine that usually exerts the greatest control over the rate of red blood cell production.

Cells in the cortex and outer medulla of the **kidneys** (Fig. 16.4) synthesize erythropoietin and release it into the bloodstream. These cells are in a somewhat oxygen-poor region with an oxygen concentration that is rarely affected by physiological changes in blood flow. Erythropoietin is secreted from endothelial cells in capillaries around tubules and/or

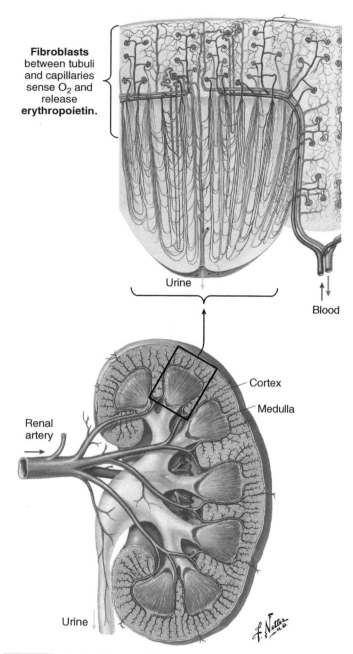

**Fibroblasts** between tubuli and capillaries sense $O_2$ and release **erythropoietin.**

Urine

Blood

Renal artery

Cortex

Medulla

Urine

**Fig. 16.4** **Peritubular cells in the kidneys secrete erythropoietin into the bloodstream in an oxygen-dependent fashion.**

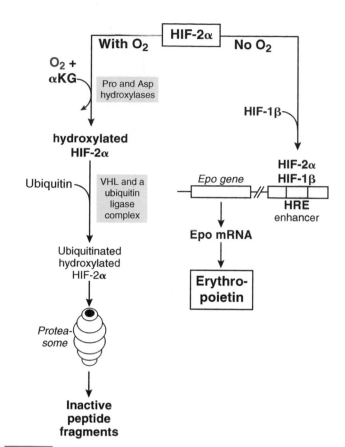

**Fig. 16.5** **Role of hypoxia-inducible factor (HIF) and von Hippel-Lindau factor (VHL) in the $O_2$-dependent regulation of transcription of the erythropoietin (Epo) gene.** HRE, hypoxia-response element.

fibroblasts between capillaries and tubules. The rate of erythropoietin secretion depends on the concentration of **oxygen** in these peritubular cells (see below). In patients with severe hypoxia (a condition of insufficient oxygen in tissues), the **liver** also synthesizes and releases some erythropoietin.

## 1.4. Oxygen-Dependent Secretion of Erythropoietin

Oxygen sensing in the kidneys and other cells involves the $O_2$-dependent modification of HIF-1α, HIF-2α, or HIF-3α transcription factors. **HIF** stands for **hypoxia-inducible factor.** HIF-α factors are constantly synthesized in the

cytoplasm (Fig. 16.5). HIF-2α regulates the transcription of the erythropoietin gene. In the *absence* of **oxygen**, HIF-2α moves into the nucleus, binds to HIF-1β, and stimulates transcription of the erythropoietin gene. In the *presence* of a normal concentration of oxygen, almost all HIF-2α is *destroyed* in a pathway that involves hydroxylation by an **$O_2$-dependent prolyl hydroxylase** or **asparaginyl hydroxylase** and ubiquitination by a protein complex that includes the **von Hippel-Lindau factor** (**VHL**). Mutant, nonfunctional VHL favors tumorigenesis, as does the inhibition of prolyl hydroxylases by the citric acid cycle intermediates **succinate** and **fumarate**, and of asparaginyl hydroxylases by **citrate** or **oxaloacetate** (see Chapter 22).

Besides a role in regulating the transcription of the erythropoietin gene in the kidneys, HIF-1α and HIF-2α modify the transcription of more than 1000 other genes in a variety of organs. Increased HIF-dependent transcription favors anaerobic glycolysis and angiogenesis, for example. HIF dimers mainly work through a **hypoxia-response element** (**HRE**) in the promoter or enhancer region of a target gene.

## 1.5. Clinical Uses of Recombinant Erythropoietin

Recombinant erythropoietin can be injected into a patient to stimulate erythropoiesis; this therapy decreases the need for

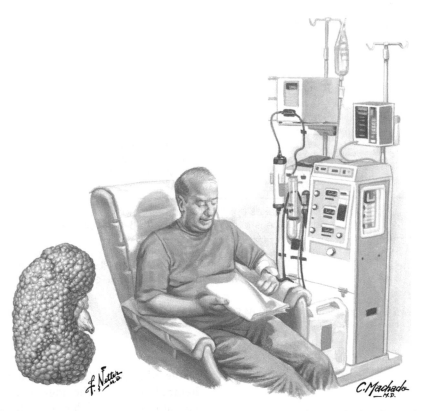

**Fig. 16.6** Erythropoietin can greatly reduce the need for blood transfusion in patients with late-stage chronic glomerulonephritis.

blood transfusions. Patients who have lost most of their **kidney function** and receive dialysis (Fig. 16.6) no longer secrete enough erythropoietin and become deficient in red blood cells (by itself, the liver does not synthesize sufficient erythropoietin). These patients are often treated with injections of **recombinant erythropoietin**, which is isolated from cultured mammalian cells that express the human erythropoietin gene. Erythropoietin can also be used to reduce the need for blood transfusion in other clinical settings, such as radiation therapy or chemotherapy for cancer.

## 2. PROTEIN COMPOSITION OF HEMOGLOBIN

*The normal hemoglobins are tetramers of two different types of globins. Each globin binds heme as a prosthetic group. The most commonly encountered normal hemoglobins are hemoglobin A (composition: $\alpha_2\beta_2$) and hemoglobin F (composition: $\alpha_2\gamma_2$).*

There are several types of **hemoglobin**, each with a different **globin** composition. All types of hemoglobin contain four globins per molecule of hemoglobin (Fig. 16.7). Globins are 142- to 147-amino acid proteins. Each globin molecule has a hydrophobic pocket that binds one **heme** molecule (see Chapter 14) noncovalently. Globins constrain the reactivity of heme so that the heme-$Fe^{2+}$ atom can reversibly bind $O_2$. Globins and heme are synthesized during the approximately week-long differentiation of erythroblasts into erythrocytes (see Fig. 16.3). Mature red blood cells cannot synthesize

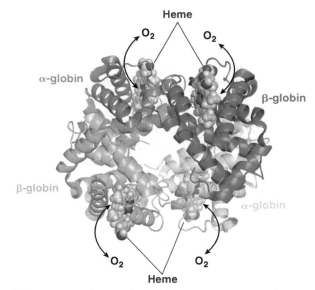

**Fig. 16.7** **X-ray crystallographic structure of deoxygenated hemoglobin A.** Heme atoms are shown as spheres. Based on Protein Data Bank file 1HBB. (From Kavanaugh JS, Rogers PH, Case DA, Arnone A. High-resolution x-ray study of deoxyhemoglobin Rothschild 37 beta Trp—Arg: a mutation that creates an intersubunit chloride-binding site. *Biochemistry.* 1992;31:4111-4121.)

globins. There are four clinically important types of globin, all derived from different genes: $\alpha$, $\beta$, $\gamma$, and $\delta$. There are two genes for $\alpha$-globin, two genes for $\gamma$-globin, and there is one gene each for $\beta$- and $\delta$-globin. All normal hemoglobins of newborns and adults consist of two $\alpha$-globins that are paired

**Table 16.1**    **Hemoglobins in Normal Blood**

| Name | Globin Composition | Comments |
|---|---|---|
| Hemoglobin **A** (HbA) | $\alpha_2\beta_2$ | Usually makes up ~**96%** of the hemoglobin in an adult and ~25% of the hemoglobin of a newborn (these numbers include HbA$_{1c}$; see below). |
| Hemoglobin **A$_{1c}$** (HbA$_{1c}$) | $\alpha_2\beta_2$ (glycated) | HbA$_{1c}$ is **glycated** HbA. The glycation (a reaction of glucose with the N-terminal valine of β-globin) is a slow, nonenzymatic reaction (see Section 8.3 in Chapter 39). Its rate depends on the concentration of **glucose** in the blood. HbA$_{1c}$ usually makes up about 5% of the hemoglobin in an adult. Patients with **diabetes** usually have an elevated HbA$_{1c}$, while patients who lose their red blood cells prematurely have a decreased HbA$_{1c}$. |
| Hemoglobin **A$_2$** (HbA$_2$) | $\alpha_2\delta_2$ | Usually makes up 2%–3% of the hemoglobin in an adult. A higher percentage is found in patients with **β-thalassemia**. |
| Hemoglobin **F** (HbF) | $\alpha_2\gamma_2$ | Usually makes up ~**75%** of the hemoglobin in a **newborn** (at term). Inside red blood cells, it has a higher affinity for $O_2$ than HbA. This helps the fetus extract oxygen from the mother's blood. HbF makes up ~1% of the hemoglobin in a healthy adult. |

The hemoglobins in this table have a molecular weight of about 64,500.
The abnormal hemoglobins C, E, H, and S are discussed in Chapter 16.

with two β-, γ-, or δ-globins. Table 16.1 lists these normal hemoglobins.

## 3. OXYGEN BINDING BY HEMOGLOBIN AND MYOGLOBIN

*Each hemoglobin molecule can bind up to four molecules of oxygen. In the lungs, hemoglobin is almost saturated with oxygen. In peripheral tissues at rest, hemoglobin releases about one-fourth of its oxygen. Hemoglobin releases much more oxygen in tissues that have a low concentration of oxygen, a low pH, or a high concentration of $CO_2$. On a time scale of days, changes in the concentration of bisphosphoglycerate inside red blood cells adjust the affinity of hemoglobin for oxygen. Myoglobin stores $O_2$ inside muscle cells.*

### 3.1. Cooperative Binding of $O_2$ to Hemoglobin

Hemoglobin carries oxygen from an environment of relatively high concentration (i.e., the alveoli, or the placenta) to an environment of an intermediate concentration (i.e., the capillaries of the tissues). Oxygen has a relatively low solubility in water. Thanks to the presence of hemoglobin inside red blood cells, whole blood may contain ~70 times more oxygen than blood plasma. Oxygen ($O_2$) moves across cells and cell membranes by simple passive diffusion (i.e., without a transporter). The high surface/volume ratio of the disk shape of red blood cells facilitates the equilibration of solutes between the cytosol and the extracellular space.

Although the terms oxidation and oxygenation sound similar, they have very different meanings. **Oxidation** refers to a change in redox state. Oxidation of hemoglobin usually refers to the process of oxidizing heme-$Fe^{2+}$ to heme-$Fe^{3+}$, forming methemoglobin (see Section 5.2). **Oxygenation** refers

to the addition of $O_2$; oxygenated hemoglobin is called **oxyhemoglobin**. In oxyhemoglobin, $O_2$ reversibly binds to heme-$Fe^{2+}$ atoms in hemoglobin. Each hemoglobin can bind up to four molecules of $O_2$ (one $O_2$ per heme; see Fig. 16.7). The release of $O_2$ from a molecule is called **deoxygenation**; deoxygenated hemoglobin is called **deoxyhemoglobin**.

As 1, 2, or 3 molecules of $O_2$ bind to hemoglobin, conformational changes in the protein facilitate binding of a subsequent molecule of $O_2$. The process by which occupation of one binding site affects the ligand affinity of a neighboring binding site is referred to as **cooperativity**. For proteins with cooperativity toward the binding of a ligand (e.g., hemoglobin and $O_2$), a graph of the ligand concentration versus the fraction of liganded protein is S shaped (Fig. 16.8). For enzymes with a cooperativity toward a substrate, a curve of substrate concentration versus enzyme activity is likewise S shaped (see Fig. 10.4).

Hemoglobin is oxygenated in the capillary bed of the alveoli (Fig. 16.9). In humidified air at sea level and 37°C, the **partial pressure of oxygen**, the p$O_2$, is ~150 mm Hg (or 150 torr, see Fig. 16.8; the total air pressure is ~760 mm Hg; the p$O_2$ can be thought of as a concentration of $O_2$). In the alveolar gas space, the concentration of $O_2$ is ~100 mm Hg; it is lower than that of humidified air due to the competition between blood that removes $O_2$ and ventilation that adds $O_2$.

The **P$_{50}$** value of hemoglobin for $O_2$ is the partial pressure of oxygen (p$O_2$), at which hemoglobin is half-maximally saturated with oxygen (see Fig. 16.8). As red blood cells move between tissues, the P$_{50}$ changes in response to differences in temperature and the concentrations of $H^+$ and $CO_2$ (see Section 3.2). A low P$_{50}$ enhances $O_2$ loading in the lungs, while a high P$_{50}$ enhances $O_2$ unloading in the tissues. (In a matter of days, the concentration of 2,3-bisphosphoglycerate also regulates the P$_{50}$; see Section 3.3.)

The p$O_2$ of heavily exercising muscle is about 25 mm Hg.

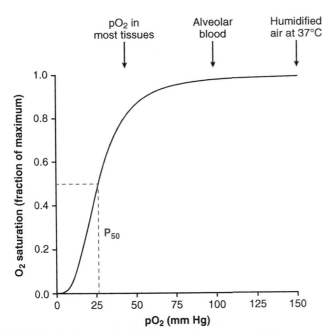

**Fig. 16.8** **Cooperative binding of $O_2$ to hemoglobin near sea level.** The curve is representative of the conditions in the pulmonary venous effluent blood. The $P_{50}$ value of hemoglobin for oxygen binding is the $pO_2$ at which hemoglobin is half-maximally saturated with $O_2$. 1 mm Hg = 1 torr.

## 3.2. Short-Term Regulation of the $O_2$ Affinity of Hemoglobin

In a time frame of microseconds, the affinity of hemoglobin for $O_2$ is regulated by temperature, the concentration of hydrogen ions, and the concentration of $CO_2$. An increase in any of these parameters favors unloading of $O_2$ from oxyhemoglobin (Fig. 16.10).

A 4°F (2°C) increase in **temperature** (e.g., in exercising muscle or during illness) increases the $P_{50}$ by ~15%, thus promoting the release of oxygen.

As blood flows through tissues, the **pH** drops, which decreases the binding of $O_2$ to hemoglobin (see Fig. 16.10). All tissues produce acids such as $H_2CO_3$ (from $CO_2$, which is mostly produced by the citric acid cycle; see Chapter 22) and lactic acid (mostly from anaerobic glycolysis; see Chapter 19). In the extended fasting state, the liver also releases significant quantities of ketone bodies (i.e., acids) into the blood (see Chapter 27). When tissues release acids into the blood, the acids dissociate to form $H^+$. As the pH of blood decreases (i.e., as the concentration of $H^+$ increases), certain amino acid residues on hemoglobin (e.g., the side chain of His-146 on β-globin and the amino terminus of α-globin) become protonated, and the affinity of hemoglobin for oxygen decreases. This effect is called the **Bohr effect**.

The increased concentration of **$CO_2$** in the peripheral circulation lowers the affinity of hemoglobin for $O_2$. $CO_2$ can reversibly carboxylate the N-terminus of β-globin (and less frequently of α-globin) to form **carbamino-hemoglobin** (globin-$NH_3^+$ + $CO_2$ ↔ globin-NH-$COO^-$ + $2H^+$). The $H^+$

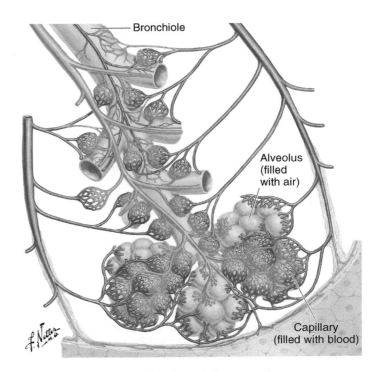

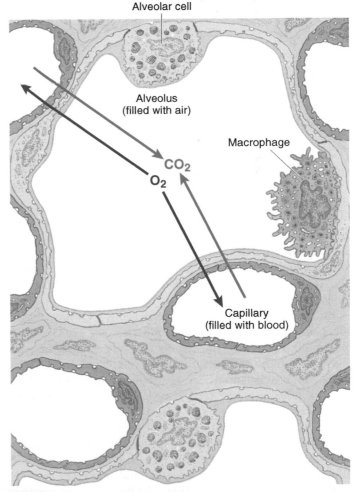

**Fig. 16.9** **Passive diffusion of $O_2$ and $CO_2$ between the alveoli and the capillaries in the lungs.** Arrows indicate the normal direction of net diffusion of $O_2$ and $CO_2$.

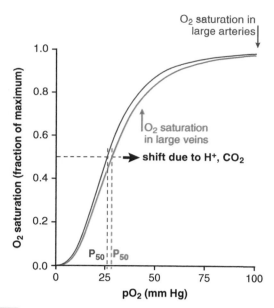

**Fig. 16.10** **Relationship between the $pO_2$ and the oxygen saturation of hemoglobin A in a healthy patient at sea level.** The drop in $pO_2$ and the increase in $P_{50}$ occur in the capillaries. In a healthy person at rest, hemoglobin loses about one-fourth of its oxygen as red blood cells pass through the capillaries of peripheral tissues.

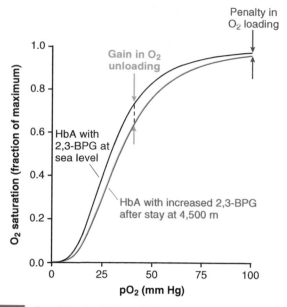

**Fig. 16.11** **An altitude-induced increase in the concentration of 2,3-bisphosphoglycerate (2,3-BPG) decreases the affinity of hemoglobin for $O_2$.** Data are based on changing elevation from 0 to 4,500 m for 5 days and assuming a Hill coefficient of 2.9.

release by this carboxylation reaction contributes to the Bohr effect. Carboxylation decreases the affinity of hemoglobin for $O_2$ (see Fig. 16.10). Conversely, in the lungs, the oxygenation of hemoglobin decreases the affinity of hemoglobin for $CO_2$ (i.e., the N-terminus of β-globin is harder to carboxylate). This effect is called the **Haldane effect**.

Of all the $CO_2$ transported from the tissues back to the lungs, only ~15% is transported via carboxylated hemoglobin, while ~85% of the $CO_2$ is transported as $CO_2$, $H_2CO_3$, and $HCO_3^-$ in solution.

The Bohr effect (pH) and the Haldane effect ($CO_2$) cause a lowering of the affinity of hemoglobin for $O_2$ in the peripheral tissues compared with the lungs (i.e., the $P_{50}$ of hemoglobin for $O_2$ is higher in the peripheral tissues than in the lungs; see Fig. 16.10). This favors the loading of $O_2$ in the lungs and unloading of $O_2$ in the tissues.

In a patient who is at rest, the pH and $CO_2$ have a small effect on $O_2$-unloading in the capillaries (see Fig. 16.10). In maximally exercising muscle on the other hand, or when blood flow to a tissue is impaired severely, pH and $CO_2$ can cause a more substantial decrease in the affinity of hemoglobin for $O_2$. Under extreme circumstances, almost all $O_2$ dissociates from hemoglobin.

$H^+$, $CO_2$, and 2,3-bisphosphoglycerate (see below) each affect the affinity of hemoglobin for $O_2$ via a site that is different from the $O_2$ binding site; such effects are called **allosteric effects**. Other proteins and enzymes are also subject to allosteric effects (see Chapter 10). Cooperativity usually implies the presence of allosteric effects (e.g., as one globin subunit in deoxyhemoglobin binds $O_2$, it undergoes a change of conformation that is transmitted to other globins).

## 3.3. Long-Term Regulation of the $O_2$ Affinity of Hemoglobin

The concentration of **2,3-bisphosphoglycerate (2,3-BPG)** optimizes the $O_2$ affinity of hemoglobin in the long run (i.e., in a matter of days). This is important because inefficient $O_2$ loading or unloading leads to an increase in the total mass of red blood cells, the viscosity of blood, cardiac work output, and the risk of thrombosis. 2,3-BPG is produced from 1,3-BPG, a metabolite in glycolysis (see Chapter 19). 2,3-BPG binds into a cavity between the amino termini of the β-globins of hemoglobin and thereby lowers the affinity of hemoglobin for oxygen. 2,3-BPG has a much greater affinity for deoxyhemoglobin than for oxyhemoglobin.

Persons who live at a high **altitude** have a higher concentration of 2,3-BPG in their red blood cells than people who live at sea level; the increased concentration of 2,3-BPG in red blood cells improves $O_2$ delivery. While the $pO_2$ of humidified air at sea level is ~150 mm Hg, it is only ~100 mm Hg at an elevation of 3,000 m (~10,000 ft). As is evident from Fig. 16.11, a 2,3-BPG-induced change in $pO_2$ has a greater effect on hemoglobin oxygenation in the steep portion of the curve than in the flat portion. Such a change affects $O_2$ *unloading* more than $O_2$ loading. In addition, increased ventilation at higher elevations makes up for decreased $O_2$ loading in the lungs. Upon changing altitude, it takes ~20 hours for a half-maximal change in the $P_{50}$ of hemoglobin for $O_2$ to occur. The trade-off for altitude-induced deoxygenation of hemoglobin is a decreased oxygen reserve in blood.

An *increase* in the concentration of 2,3-BPG inside red blood cells (and a corresponding decrease in the oxygen affinity of hemoglobin) is also seen in patients with **hypoxia** and in patients with (usually partial) **blocks in glycolysis** distal to

1,3-BPG and 2,3-BPG (e.g., pyruvate kinase deficiency; see Chapter 19).

A *decrease* in the concentration of 2,3-BPG inside red blood cells (and a corresponding increase in the oxygen affinity of hemoglobin) is observed in patients with a **low blood pH** (e.g., lactic acidosis or ketoacidosis), in patients with (usually partial) **blocks in glycolysis** proximal to 1,3-BPG and 2,3-BPG (e.g., **hypophosphatemia),** and in patients with 2,3-BPG mutase deficiency (rare; see Chapter 19).

**Chronic mountain sickness** is characterized by a low oxygen saturation of hemoglobin, high hematocrit, hypertrophy of the right side of the heart, and pulmonary hypertension. The disease develops over a period of years of living at high altitude (usually greater than 3,000 m or 9,800 ft above sea level). The disease has a prevalence of up to 15% in the South American highlands. Affected patients have less than about 85% oxygen saturation of hemoglobin in the arterial blood. The hypoxia drives erythropoiesis so that patients have more than about 20 g hemoglobin/dL blood (equal to a hematocrit of >60%). The hypoxia also increases the output of the heart, blood pressure in the lungs, and the rate of breathing. Long-term treatment involves moving to a lower altitude.

**Acute mountain sickness** is seen in persons who move to a higher altitude and shortly afterward complain of fatigue, headache, and nausea.

**High-altitude pulmonary edema** is accompanied by excess fluid around the lungs, which reduces a person's ability to breathe. The edema progressively worsens the condition. If present, pulmonary edema usually develops after a 1- to a 4-day stay at more than about 2,500 m (8,200 ft) above sea level. The arterial oxygen saturation is often around 50% to 75%. Treatment involves immediate descent to a lower altitude. Administration of pure oxygen also helps. Without treatment, the affected person may die within hours.

**High-altitude cerebral edema** is accompanied by excess fluid in the brain, impairing brain function. High-altitude cerebral edema occurs in a similar setting as high-altitude pulmonary edema, is treated in a similar fashion, and is equally dangerous.

### 3.4. Maternal-Fetal Exchange of $O_2$

In the placenta, maternal blood oxygenates the fetal blood, which has a considerably lower oxygen concentration than the maternal blood. In the presence of physiological concentrations of 2,3-BPG, the $P_{50}$ for HbF is about 25% lower than the $P_{50}$ for HbA. While the mother's blood in the placental vein has a $pO_2$ of ~40 mm Hg, the fetus' blood in the umbilical vein (i.e., oxygenated blood exiting from the placenta) has a $pO_2$ of ~35 mm Hg. The fetus' blood in the umbilical artery (i.e., blood returning to the placenta for oxygenation) has a $pO_2$ of ~20 mm Hg.

### 3.5. Binding of $O_2$ to Myoglobin

Myoglobin is a heme-containing protein the size of a single globin subunit of hemoglobin. Each molecule of myoglobin can reversibly bind one molecule of $O_2$; the $P_{50}$ is ~4 mm Hg. Myoglobin shows no cooperativity in binding $O_2$. The affinity of myoglobin for $O_2$ is not influenced by 2,3-BPG. Myoglobin may have a role in storing $O_2$. It is found chiefly in the cytoplasm of cardiac and skeletal muscle.

## 4. TRANSPORT AND BUFFERING FUNCTION OF $CO_2$ AND $HCO_3^-$ IN BLOOD

### $CO_2$ and bicarbonate form the major pH buffer in blood.

In peripheral tissues, carbon dioxide ($CO_2$) passively diffuses across the plasma membrane bilayer into erythrocytes, and bicarbonate ($HCO_3^-$) enters erythrocytes via an anion exchanger (Fig. 16.12). As mentioned above, most of the $CO_2$ produced by tissues is carried back to the lungs as bicarbonate ions dissolved in water. A small fraction of the $CO_2$ binds to hemoglobin and allosterically decreases its affinity for oxygen. The plasma membrane of red blood cells contains an anion exchanger, band 3, that exchanges $HCO_3^-$ for chloride ($Cl^-$) across the lipid bilayer; this transporter can move $HCO_3^-$ in either direction.

The drug **acetazolamide** inhibits carbonic anhydrase in several tissues. The drug is used in the treatment of a variety of diseases, such as high-altitude sickness, glaucoma, and congestive heart failure. In the kidneys, acetazolamide leads to decreased excretion of protons and an increased loss of $HCO_3^-$; as a consequence, the pH of blood decreases.

$CO_2$ and $HCO_3^-$ form the major pH buffer in blood plasma and red blood cells. In water, $CO_2$ is spontaneously hydrated to carbonic acid according to the reaction $CO_2 + H_2O \leftrightarrow H_2CO_3$. At equilibrium, there is much more $CO_2$ than $H_2CO_3$. Inside red blood cells, **carbonic anhydrase** catalyzes this reversible hydration of $CO_2$ and thereby shortens the time needed to establish equilibrium. $H_2CO_3$ spontaneously dissociates: $H_2CO_3 \leftrightarrow HCO_3^- + H^+$. The combination of these two reactions, the system $CO_2 + H_2O \leftrightarrow H_2CO_3 \leftrightarrow HCO_3^- + H^+$,

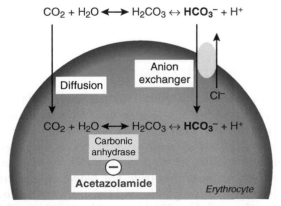

**Fig. 16.12** **Transport of $CO_2$ and $HCO_3^-$ across the red blood cell plasma membrane in the peripheral capillary bed.** In the lungs, the flux is reversed.

forms the major pH buffer of blood. The pH is determined by the ratio of the concentrations of $HCO_3^-$ and $CO_2$ according to the **Henderson-Hasselbalch** equation:

$$pH = pK_{CO2} + \log([HCO_3^-]/[CO_2])$$

$pK_{CO2}$ is about 6.1 at 37°C. As an example, at pH 7.1, the term $\log[(HCO_3^-)/(CO_2)]$ equals 1; hence, there is 10 times more $HCO_3^-$ than $CO_2$.

Analyses of blood for **blood gasses** are most often carried out with arterial blood at 37°C. The following parameters are often measured: pH, $pO_2$ (partial pressure of $O_2$), $pCO_2$ (partial pressure of $CO_2$), the concentration of $HCO_3^-$, and saturation of hemoglobin with oxygen ($SaO_2$ for arterial blood, $SvO_2$ for venous blood). Approximate normal values for these parameters in arterial blood are pH, 7.35 to 7.45; $pO_2$, 75 to 105 mm Hg; $pCO_2$, 33 to 45 mm Hg; and concentration of $HCO_3^-$, 22 to 28 mEq/L. The saturation of hemoglobin with oxygen decreases with altitude; $SaO_2$ is usually greater than 90%. If the $pO_2$ of peripheral blood is abnormally low, the patient has **hypoxia**.

If the pH of the blood is abnormally low, the patient has an **acidemia**; if the pH is abnormally high, the patient has an **alkalemia**.

Patients who have a **metabolic acidosis** have a low blood pH and low concentrations of $HCO_3^-$ and $CO_2$ in the blood. Tissues of these patients release $H^+$ into the blood at an abnormally high rate. The $H^+$ may stem, for instance, from the release of lactic acid or the ketone bodies acetoacetic acid and β-hydroxybutyric acid (see Chapter 27). In the blood, the concentration of $HCO_3^-$ becomes low because $HCO_3^-$ is consumed by buffering $H^+$ ($HCO_3^- + H^+ \rightarrow H_2CO_3 \rightarrow CO_2$). The low pH stimulates breathing and concomitant exhaling of $CO_2$ to a lower than normal blood $pCO_2$. This is an attempt to normalize the pH by defending the ratio $[HCO_3^-]/[CO_2]$ of the above Henderson-Hasselbalch equation. At a lower rate than the lungs, the kidneys can also rid the blood of acid by deprotonating $H_2CO_3$, excreting $H^+$ as part of $NH_4^+$, and returning $HCO_3^-$ to the blood (see Chapter 35); however, in metabolic acidosis, the rate of renal $HCO_3^-$ production is much smaller than the rate of $HCO_3^-$ consumption by buffering.

# 5. CARBON MONOXYHEMOGLOBIN AND METHEMOGLOBIN

*Carbon monoxide is a poisonous gas that binds tightly to hemoglobin and impairs oxygen delivery. Other chemicals, such as oxidizing drugs or the vasodilator nitric oxide (NO), can oxidize the heme iron in hemoglobin, generating methemoglobin, which is not suitable for tissue oxygenation either. An enzyme inside red blood cells reduces the heme-iron of methemoglobin and thus restores hemoglobin. Since methemoglobin binds cyanide, methemoglobin is sometimes generated pharmacologically in patients who have cyanide poisoning.*

## 5.1. Carbon Monoxyhemoglobin

Carbon monoxide (CO) binds to heme-$Fe^{2+}$ in hemoglobin with ~200-fold greater affinity than $O_2$ (i.e., at 0.1% CO and 20% $O_2$, CO and $O_2$ bind to hemoglobin about equally well). CO stems from incomplete combustion of carbon-containing substances; it is odorless and colorless. Hemoglobin with CO bound to all four heme irons is called **carbon monoxyhemoglobin** (hemoglobin with less than 3 CO is called **partial** carbon monoxy-hemoglobin or **hetero**-carbon monoxy-hemoglobin). Carbon monoxy-hemoglobin is also called **carboxy-hemoglobin**. Partial carbon monoxy-hemoglobin has an abnormally high affinity for $O_2$ such that it cannot be used for physiological oxygen delivery.

Elevated amounts of CO bound to hemoglobin are found in patients who smoke or are otherwise exposed to elevated concentrations of CO. **Smoking** 20 cigarettes per day leads to a mean CO saturation of hemoglobin of ~7% before bedtime; the CO saturation decreases to ~2% to 3% by waking. In a **pregnant** woman who is a heavy smoker, fetal and maternal blood contain the same amounts of carbon monoxy-hemoglobin because CO diffuses from the maternal blood across the placenta to the fetal blood.

**Carbon monoxide poisoning** decreases a patient's capacity for $O_2$ delivery to the tissues. In nonsmokers, a carbon monoxy-hemoglobin fraction of greater than 3% to 4% indicates CO poisoning; in smokers, the threshold is about 10%. To favor the binding of $O_2$ to heme in place of CO, CO-poisoned patients are treated with pure $O_2$ at normal pressure or in a pressure chamber (commonly at about three times the normal pressure). CO is physiologically produced in the human body and functions as a signaling molecule. CO signaling pathways contribute to the pathology of carbon monoxide poisoning in a yet poorly understood fashion. In the United States about 3% of CO-poisoned patients who get to a hospital die from the poisoning.

## 5.2. Oxidation of Hemoglobin to Methemoglobin

In oxygenated hemoglobin, the heme-$Fe^{2+}$ (with $O_2$ bound to it) can be oxidized to the $Fe^{3+}$ state, producing oxidized hemoglobin, which can no longer be used for the delivery of oxygen. Hemoglobin with four heme-$Fe^{3+}$ is called **methemoglobin**, while hemoglobin with 1 to 3 heme-$Fe^{3+}$ is called **partial** methemoglobin, or **hetero**-methemoglobin. Oxygenated hemoglobin auto-oxidizes to generate partial methemoglobin and superoxide ($O_2\bullet$) at a rate of ~3%/day. Like partial carbon monoxy-hemoglobin (see Section 5.1), partial methemoglobin has an abnormally high affinity for $O_2$ such that it cannot be used for $O_2$ delivery to tissues. The heme-$Fe^{3+}$ in methemoglobin cannot bind $O_2$.

**NO** is a short-lived gas that is mainly produced in endothelial cells, neurons, and neutrophils, from which it can diffuse to adjacent cells. In blood vessels, NO inhibits platelet activation and relaxes smooth muscle. To regulate blood flow in the arterioles, endothelial cells synthesize NO in response to shear stress. To this end, **NO synthase** catalyzes the reaction

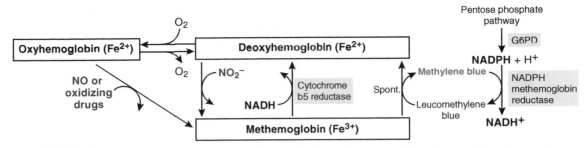

**Fig. 16.13** **Causes and treatment of acquired methemoglobinemia.** G6PD, glucose-6-phosphate dehydrogenase; NADH, reduced nicotinamide adenine dinucleotide; NADPH, NADH phosphate; NO, nitric oxide.

arginine + 2 NADPH + 2 H$^+$ + 2 O$_2$ → citrulline + NO + 2 NADP$^+$ + 2 H$_2$O. NO signals in two major ways: (1) NO reacts with **heme-iron**, for instance in soluble guanylyl cyclase, which in turn produces cyclic guanosine monophosphate (cGMP) that activates protein kinase G; and (2) NO also reacts with the –SH group of cysteine residues, forming an S-nitrosothiol (-SNO) in a process called **S-nitrosylation** that modifies the properties of a protein.

**Erythrocytes** participate in both the production and removal of NO. These processes are incompletely understood. On one hand, deoxyhemoglobin converts circulating nitrite (NO$_2^-$) to NO. This reaction likely plays a role in producing NO-induced vasodilation during local hypoxia. On the other hand, deoxyhemoglobin also binds NO to form S-nitroso-hemoglobin (SNO-hemoglobin), which acts as a relatively long-lived reservoir of NO. Furthermore, oxyhemoglobin can oxidize NO to nitrate (NO$_3^-$), thereby producing partial **methemoglobin** (see Fig. 16.13).

**Methemoglobinemia** is often due to an ingested toxin (e.g., **nitrite**) or due to **oxidizing drugs** (e.g., uricases, benzocaine, lidocaine, metabolites of prilocaine, EMLA cream, sulfonamides, primaquine, dapsone, or nitrofurantoin). Methemoglobinemia can also be due to an unstable variant hemoglobin (e.g., **hemoglobin M**) and, less frequently, due to a **deficiency of cytochrome b5 reductase** (Fig. 16.13).

A methemoglobinemia-induced **cyanosis** due to impaired oxygen delivery is seen when more than ~20% of all heme-iron is heme-Fe$^{3+}$. A fraction of more than 70% heme-Fe$^{3+}$ is usually fatal.

Red blood cells contain the enzyme **cytochrome b5 reductase** (also called **methemoglobin reductase**; see Fig. 16.13), which uses NADH produced in glycolysis to reduce the heme-Fe$^{3+}$ of methemoglobin to heme-Fe$^{2+}$, thereby restoring hemoglobin. Normal human blood contains less than 3% methemoglobin.

**Methylene blue** helps convert methemoglobin to deoxyhemoglobin (see Fig. 16.13). This process uses NADPH and NADPH methemoglobin reductase, an enzyme that normally plays little role in methemoglobin reduction. NADPH stems from the oxidative branch of the pentose phosphate pathway (see Chapter 21). Methylene blue is ineffective in patients who have a severe **glucose 6-phosphate dehydrogenase deficiency** (see Chapter 21) because they cannot provide NADPH at an adequate rate.

**Cyanide**-poisoned patients can be given **amyl nitrite** (via inspired air) and/or **sodium nitrite** (by vein) to produce about 10% to 30% **methemoglobin**, which traps cyanide (CN$^-$). Induction of methemoglobinemia is contraindicated in patients who also have carbon monoxide poisoning (see Section 5.1). Other methods of treatment involve binding cyanide with hydroxocobalamin and facilitating the removal of cyanide with thiosulfate (see Section 1.3 in Chapter 23). The toxicity of cyanide is primarily due to its inhibition of complex IV of oxidative phosphorylation (see Chapter 23). Methemoglobin has a higher affinity for cyanide than does complex IV. The temporary binding of cyanide by methemoglobin buys the patient time to react cyanide with thiosulfate, producing thiocyanate, which is excreted in the urine. The half-life of cyanide in plasma is 20 to 60 min.

## 6. CLINICALLY IMPORTANT LABORATORY DATA ON RED BLOOD CELLS

*Laboratory analyses of blood to determine the volume and number of red blood cells, the concentration of hemoglobin, and the number of reticulocytes provide essential data on a patient's state of health.*

A **complete blood count** (**CBC**) refers to the following set of parameters that are measured in a blood sample: hematocrit, hemoglobin, red blood cell count, mean corpuscular volume, mean corpuscular hemoglobin, mean corpuscular hemoglobin concentration, red blood cell distribution width, white blood cell count, and platelet count. A CBC is one of the most frequently performed blood tests. A **reticulocyte count** must be requested separately. A request for a CBC with a **differential count** of white blood cells also includes counts for lymphocytes, monocytes, neutrophils, eosinophils, and basophils.

In modern clinical laboratories, CBCs are performed on automated machines that use a combination of spectrophotometry (to measure hemoglobin), antibody staining (to identify platelets), flow cytometry (to count cells and infer sizes), and/or impedance measurements when a cell passes through an aperture (to count cells and infer sizes). Abnormal values are often investigated with additional less-automated methods.

The **hematocrit** is the ratio of the volume of packed (as in a centrifuge) red blood cells/volume of blood (Fig. 16.14). It

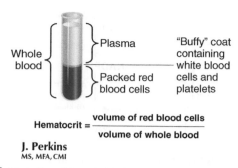

$$\text{Hematocrit} = \frac{\text{volume of red blood cells}}{\text{volume of whole blood}}$$

J. Perkins
MS, MFA, CMI

**Fig. 16.14** **Relationship of the hematocrit to the packed red blood cell fraction of centrifuged blood.**

is typically reported as a percentage, and in people living close to sea level, it is usually about 45% (typical normal ranges are 36%–46% in women and 41%–53% in men). In well-equipped laboratories, the hematocrit is no longer measured but estimated from other values.

**Blood plasma** is the fluid that surrounds red blood cells, white blood cells, and platelets; blood **serum** is the fluid that can be recovered from coagulated, centrifuged blood. Compared with plasma, serum is devoid of proteins that form a clot.

The concentration of **hemoglobin** in whole blood (g/dL) is usually about 15 g/dL in patients living close to sea level (typical normal ranges are 12.0–16.0 g/dL in women and 13.5–17.5 g/dL in men).

In practice, hematocrit and hemoglobin concentration are well correlated. As a rule of thumb, the numerical value of the hematocrit (%) is three times larger than the numerical value of hemoglobin (g/dL). For example, at a hemoglobin concentration of 10 g/dL, a hematocrit of 30% is expected.

**Transfusion** of one unit of packed red blood cells into a patient who does not actively bleed increases the concentration of hemoglobin in whole blood by ~1 g/L and the hematocrit by ~3 to 4 percentage points (e.g., from 15% to ~18%–19%).

The **red blood cell count** is the number of red blood cells per μL (mm³) of blood. In patients living close to sea level, the red blood cell count is usually about 5 million/μL (typical normal ranges are 3.5–5.5 million/μL in women and 4.3–5.9 million/μL in men).

A patient with an abnormally *low* hematocrit, concentration of hemoglobin in the blood, or number of red blood cells per microliter of blood is said to have **anemia**. In most markedly anemic patients all three of these parameters are abnormally low. Anemia is caused by insufficient red blood cell production, premature loss of red blood cells, or a combination of these processes.

An abnormally *high* hematocrit, hemoglobin concentration in the blood, or number of red blood cells per microliter of blood often indicates that the patient is **dehydrated** (this would go along with elevated blood urea nitrogen; see Chapter 35) or a heavy **smoker** (carbon monoxide in smoke binds to hemoglobin and decreases its capacity for $O_2$ transport; hence, more red blood cells are needed for adequate oxygenation of tissues; see Section 5.1). More rarely, it is due to excessive

synthesis of red blood cells, in which case it is a true **polycythemia** (also called **erythrocytosis**). A true *primary* polycythemia is due to an inherited or acquired defect in the stem cells that give rise to red blood cells. A *secondary* polycythemia is due to an elevated concentration of circulating cytokines (most often erythropoietin in response to renal hypoxia). Healthy persons who have normally adjusted to living at **high altitude** have an increased concentration of hemoglobin, hematocrit, and red blood cell count compared with persons living at sea level; obviously, a different, elevation- or location-appropriate set of reference values must be used for these patients.

The mean volume of individual red blood cells is called the **mean corpuscular volume (MCV)**. The MCV is normally 80 to 100 fL (1 fL = $10^{-15}$ L ≅ 1 μm³). If the MCV is abnormally high, the red blood cells are said to be **macrocytic**. This is usually due to a problem with **DNA replication** and cell proliferation (see Fig. 16.3 and Chapter 37). If the MCV is abnormally low, the red blood cells are said to be **microcytic**. This is usually due to a problem with **hemoglobin synthesis** (this includes iron deficiency; see also Fig. 16.3 and Chapters 15 and 17).

The mean amount of hemoglobin inside red blood cells is called the **mean corpuscular hemoglobin (MCH)**. The MCH is normally 25 to 35 pg.

The mean concentration of hemoglobin inside red blood cells is called the **mean corpuscular hemoglobin concentration (MCHC)**. The MCHC is usually about 31 to 36 g/dL. Erythrocytes with a normal MCHC are **normochromic**, those with an abnormally low MCHC are **hypochromic**, and those with an abnormally high MCHC are **hyperchromic**. A severe impairment of hemoglobin synthesis (e.g., in thalassemia [see Chapter 17] or iron deficiency [see Chapter 15]) leads to both microcytosis (low MCV) and hypochromia (low MCHC). A severe impairment of DNA synthesis often leads to macrocytosis and hypochromia.

The **red blood cell distribution width (RDW)** is a measure of the variation in red blood cell size. Under normal circumstances, the distribution of red blood cell size is nearly Gaussian, and the RDW is about 13%. An elevated RDW indicates abnormal variation in the size of red blood cells and is referred to as **anisocytosis**. An increased RDW is observed, for instance, in iron deficiency (see Chapter 15) and in folate deficiency (see Chapter 36).

The **platelet count** indicates the number of platelets per microliter (μL or mm³) of blood. The normal range is 150,000 to 400,000/μL.

The white blood cell count is the number of white blood cells per microliter of blood. It is usually about 7,000/μL. An abnormally low white blood cell count is referred to as **leukopenia**; it can be due to stem cell disorders, chemotherapy, radiation therapy, or a decreased life span in the bloodstream. An abnormally high white blood cell count is referred to as **leukocytosis**; it is a classic sign of infection or leukemia.

The **white blood cell differential** is an account of the fraction (%) of different types of white blood cells: lymphocytes, monocytes, neutrophils, basophils, and eosinophils.

The percentage of **reticulocytes** in the whole blood is a clinically useful indicator of red blood cell production. Reticulocytes can be discerned from mature red blood cells by their RNA content. In flow cytometers, reticulocytes are identified after staining of nucleic acids with a fluorescent dye. Normally, reticulocytes make up 0.5% to 1.5% of all circulating red blood cells. An abnormally high reticulocyte count usually indicates a compensatory increase in hematopoiesis due to the premature loss of red blood cells.

## 7. COLOR OF HEMOGLOBINS

*The color of a patient's skin reflects the ligands and oxidation state of heme-iron in hemoglobin. With a pulse oximeter, one can measure a patient's pulse rate as well as the apparent $O_2$ saturation of hemoglobin.*

### 7.1. Effect of Hemoglobin on Skin Color

The color of heme in blood capillaries near the surface affects the color of the skin; assessment of skin color is part of the physical examination of a patient. The oxidation state and ligand of the heme-iron in hemoglobin affect the absorption spectrum of hemoglobin. In sunlight, oxygenated hemoglobin looks red, whereas deoxygenated hemoglobin looks dark purplish red. Patients with excessively oxygenated hemoglobin (i.e., patients who do not unload $O_2$ normally, such as from increased affinity of hemoglobin for $O_2$) have a **ruddy** appearance. Patients with poorly oxygenated blood (e.g., patients with heart and lung disease) look **cyanotic** (Fig. 16.15).

Patients with lethal **carbon monoxide** (CO) poisoning may have a **cherry-red** appearance because carbon monoxyhemoglobin (i.e., hemoglobin with CO bound to it) has a cherry-red color. However, most patients who present with carbon monoxide poisoning have lower carboxyhemoglobin concentrations and do not have a cherry-red appearance.

In patients with **cyanide** poisoning, venous blood looks unusually red because cyanide primarily inhibits oxygen consumption by mitochondria, which in turn leaves capillary blood well oxygenated.

Although **methemoglobin** (i.e., oxidized hemoglobin, $Fe^{3+}$) imparts a brownish color to drawn blood, patients with more than about 15% methemoglobin have a cyanotic appearance due to increased oxygen unloading from normal hemoglobin (Fig. 16.16).

### 7.2. Pulse Oximeter

In intensive care, respiratory care, surgical wards, and obstetric wards, the **pulse rate** and the degree of **oxygenation of hemoglobin** of patients are often monitored noninvasively with a two-wavelength or multiwavelength pulse oximeter. Red and infrared light, which travel well through tissues, are shone through the nail bed of a finger or toe or through the earlobe, and transmitted light is analyzed. Reflected light can

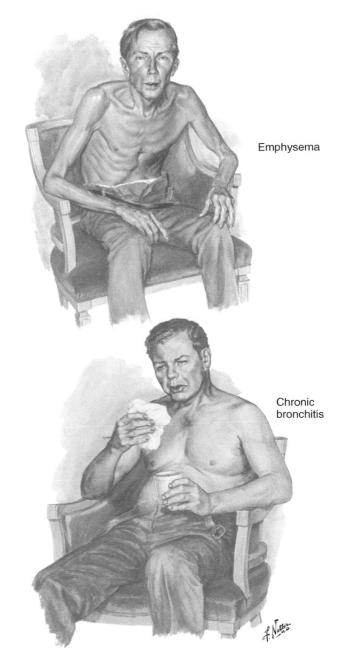

Emphysema

Chronic bronchitis

**Fig. 16.15** **Oxygen saturation of blood affects skin color.** Extremes of men who have chronic obstructive pulmonary disease (COPD). Most COPD is induced by smoking. Emphysema is characterized by pursed-lip breathing, which keeps the bronchi from collapsing. Chronic bronchitis is characterized by inadequate oxygen saturation of blood in the lungs, leading to secondary heart failure, which exacerbates hypoxia.

also be measured (e.g., from the forehead, or from the cheek of a fetus during labor and delivery).

Oscillations in the amount of transmitted or reflected light of different wavelengths are used to calculate the pulse rate and the $O_2$ saturation of hemoglobin. For a pulse oximeter to work, the volume of the arterial bed of the tissue must oscillate with the heartbeat (Fig. 16.17). The ratio of the pulsatile portions of red and infrared light depends on the state of

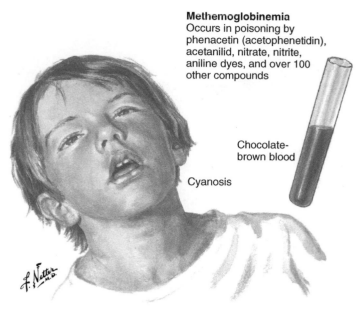

**Methemoglobinemia**
Occurs in poisoning by phenacetin (acetophenetidin), acetanilid, nitrate, nitrite, aniline dyes, and over 100 other compounds

Chocolate-brown blood

Cyanosis

Fig. 16.16    **Methemoglobinemia.**

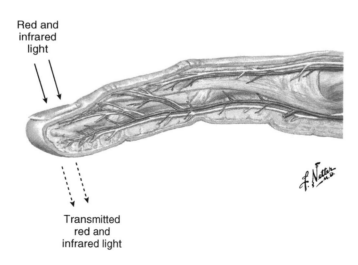

Red and infrared light

Transmitted red and infrared light

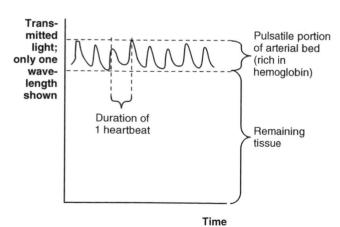

Trans-mitted light; only one wave-length shown

Duration of 1 heartbeat

Pulsatile portion of arterial bed (rich in hemoglobin)

Remaining tissue

Time

Fig. 16.17    **Principle of pulse oximetry with a measurement of transmitted red and infrared light.**

oxygenation of hemoglobin (the nonpulsatile portion of the signal is not analyzed). The pulse oximeter compares actual measurements to reference measurements that were made on volunteers who simultaneously had arterial blood drawn and analyzed in a laboratory by a different setup. A two-wavelength pulse oximeter with a probe is calibrated to provide a readout of apparent oxygen saturation of normal hemoglobin; this readout may be wrong in the presence of **methemoglobin** or **carbon monoxy-hemoglobin**. Multiwavelength pulse oximeters can be constructed so that they show the concentrations of oxygenated hemoglobin, carbon monoxy-hemoglobin, and methemoglobin).

## SUMMARY

■ Under the control of erythropoietin from the kidneys, stem cells in the bone marrow give rise to erythroblasts. Over the course of ~1 week, erythroblasts differentiate into reticulocytes, which are released into the bloodstream. For ~1 day, the reticulocytes continue to synthesize hemoglobin. Then, they lose the last of their mitochondria, endoplasmic reticulum, and mRNA, and thus become mature erythrocytes. The lifetime of a mature erythrocyte in the bloodstream is ~120 days.

■ In a healthy patient, the reticulocytes make up ~1% of all red blood cells.

■ The transcription of the erythropoietin gene and many other genes is regulated by the HIF/hydroxylase/VHL system in an oxygen-dependent fashion. Patients who have a major loss of kidney function no longer secrete sufficient erythropoietin and are commonly treated with recombinant erythropoietin.

■ The most common fetal hemoglobin is hemoglobin F, which has an $\alpha_2\gamma_2$ globin composition. The most common adult hemoglobin is hemoglobin A, which has an $\alpha_2\beta_2$ subunit composition. $HbA_{1c}$ is glycated hemoglobin A. The fraction of $HbA_{1c}$ is indicative of the average concentration of glucose in the blood, which is of clinical interest in patients who have diabetes.

■ Hemoglobin cooperatively binds $O_2$, and this process is allosterically regulated by $H^+$, $CO_2$, and 2,3-BPG. Hemoglobin releases $O_2$ in tissue capillaries as a consequence of a lower local $pO_2$ and pH, and a higher $pCO_2$. 2,3-BPG regulates the affinity of hemoglobin for $O_2$ from day to day. The concentration of 2,3-BPG increases with altitude and decreases when hypophosphatemia develops.

■ Under physiological conditions, hemoglobin F has a higher affinity for $O_2$ than does hemoglobin A; this facilitates $O_2$ delivery from the mother to her fetus.

■ $CO_2$ and $HCO_3^-$ form the major pH buffer of blood. Most of the $CO_2$ produced in tissues is carried back to the lungs as $HCO_3^-$ dissolved in erythrocyte cytosol and blood plasma. The remainder (~15%) of the $CO_2$ produced in tissues binds to the N-terminus of $\beta$-globin and thus lowers the affinity of hemoglobin for $O_2$, which increases $O_2$ delivery to the tissues.

- The ratio of $[HCO_3^-]/[CO_2]$ determines the pH of blood, and the pH of blood is a major regulator of breathing. Patients with a metabolic acidosis neutralize excess $H^+$ with $HCO_3^-$, forming $CO_2$, which they give off through the lungs. The process leads to blood with a low concentration of $HCO_3^-$ and a low $pCO_2$.
- Carbon monoxide (CO), which is poisonous, binds to heme-$Fe^{2+}$ of hemoglobin with greater affinity than $O_2$ and increases the oxygen affinity of the remaining globin-hemes in the same hemoglobin molecule. As a result, carbon monoxyhemoglobin and partial carbon monoxyhemoglobin cannot be used for $O_2$ delivery. Hemoglobin in the blood of smokers contains a few percent of carbon monoxyhemoglobin. CO crosses the placenta and impairs $O_2$ delivery in the fetus.
- NO is an endogenous vasodilator and platelet inhibitor. Hemoglobin can produce, store, and remove NO. NO, and oxidizing drugs can oxidize hemoglobin to methemoglobin or partial methemoglobin ($\geq 1$ heme-$Fe^{2+}$ is heme-$Fe^{3+}$). These methemoglobins cannot be used for physiological $O_2$ delivery. Cytochrome b5 reductase normally keeps methemoglobin at less than 3% of all hemoglobin. Cyanide-poisoned patients are sometimes treated with a nitrite to produce methemoglobin, which binds cyanide.
- Patients who have unintended methemoglobinemia (e.g., due to ingestion of a nitrite or an oxidizing agent) can be treated with methylene blue. Methylene blue gets reduced to leucomethylene blue by an enzyme that uses NADPH. Leucomethylene blue in turn spontaneously reduces heme-$Fe^{3+}$ in methemoglobin to heme-$Fe^{2+}$. Methylene blue is ineffective in patients who have a severe G6PD deficiency.
- Analysis of a patient's blood often includes determinations of hematocrit, hemoglobin concentration, red blood cell count, reticulocyte count, and mean corpuscular volume. Anemia is characterized by a lack of red blood cells and hemoglobin. An excess of red blood cells and hemoglobin is often caused by dehydration, heavy smoking, or a malignancy. Microcytic and macrocytic red blood cells, respectively, are cells with an abnormally small and an abnormally large mean corpuscular volume. Hypochromic and hyperchromic red blood cells, respectively, are cells with an abnormally low and an abnormally high mean corpuscular hemoglobin concentration. Microcytosis and hypochromia usually occur together as a result of a problem with hemoglobin synthesis. Macrocytosis is generally due to a problem with DNA replication. Micro- and macrocytosis are often accompanied by anemia.
- Deoxygenated and oxygenated hemoglobin, methemoglobin, and carbon monoxy-hemoglobin have different colors. Patients with a markedly increased fraction of deoxygenated hemoglobin look cyanotic. In pulse oximetry, variations in the amount of light passing through a pulsating arterial bed (e.g., fingernail, toenail, or earlobe) are used to estimate the pulse rate and the arterial $O_2$ saturation of blood. With a two-wavelength pulse oximeter, the presence of abnormal hemoglobins or hemoglobin ligands may lead to an erroneous readout.

## FURTHER READING

- Grocott MP, et al. Arterial blood gases and oxygen content in climbers on Mount Everest. *N Engl J Med.* 2009;360: 140-149.
- Haase VH. Regulation of erythropoiesis by hypoxia-inducible factors. *Blood Rev.* 2013;27:41-53.
- Hampson NB, Piantadosi CA, Thom SR, Weaver LK. Practice Recommendations in the diagnosis, management, and prevention of carbon monoxide poisoning. *Am J Respir Crit Care Med.* 2012;186:1095-1101.
- Hsia CC. Mechanisms of disease: respiratory function of hemoglobin. *N Engl J Med.* 1998;338:239-248.
- Law MR, Morris JK, Watt HC, Wald NJ. The dose-response relationship between cigarette consumption, biochemical markers and risk of lung cancer. *Br J Cancer.* 1997; 75(11):1690-1693.
- Roueche B. Eleven blue men. In: Roueche B, ed. *The Medical Detectives.* New York: Penguin Books; 1988. This article describes a case of nitrite poisoning.

# Review Questions

1. A 12-year-old boy has a mutant HIF-$2\alpha$ (hypoxia inducible factor-$2\alpha$) that is only poorly hydroxylated and therefore has an unusually long lifetime. This mutation is expected to have which one of the following effects?

   **A.** Decreased tissue oxygenation (hypoxia)
   **B.** High hematocrit
   **C.** Low MCV
   **D.** Low reticulocyte count

2. In the emergency department, a 36-year-old male patient who was rescued from a fire in an industrial plant receives amyl nitrite by a mask. Which one of the following conditions is this patient most likely receiving treatment for?

   **A.** Carbon monoxide poisoning
   **B.** Cyanide poisoning
   **C.** Hypoxia
   **D.** Methemoglobinemia

3. Which one of the options below correctly describes effects on the $P_{50}$ of hemoglobin for oxygen inside red blood cells?

| Option | Effect of a Decrease in pH | Effect of an Increase in $pCO_2$ | Effect of an Increased Concentration of 2,3-BPG |
|---|---|---|---|
| A. | $P_{50}$ decreases | $P_{50}$ decreases | $P_{50}$ decreases |
| B. | $P_{50}$ decreases | $P_{50}$ increases | $P_{50}$ increases |
| C. | $P_{50}$ increases | $P_{50}$ decreases | $P_{50}$ decreases |
| D. | $P_{50}$ increases | $P_{50}$ increases | $P_{50}$ increases |

4. A woman who used to live at sea level moved to a place 6,000 ft above sea level, where the air pressure is only 80% of that at sea level. After 1 week of residence at 6,000 ft, a blood sample was taken from the woman, and the $O_2$ saturation of hemoglobin (in intact red blood cells) was measured as a function of the partial pressure of oxygen. Which one of the curves at right most likely represents the data for this woman's red blood cells? (The solid curve is the reference for sea level.)

A. A
B. B
C. C
D. D

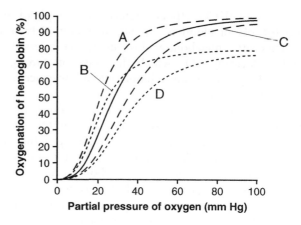

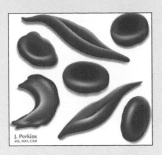

## Chapter 17 Hemoglobinopathies

### SYNOPSIS

- Hemoglobinopathies are caused by heritable mutations that affect the expression of globins, the amino acid sequence of globins, or both.
- More than 5% of the world's population are carriers of hemoglobin disorders. These are predominantly found among patients with geographic ancestry in areas in which malaria has been endemic.
- The most common hemoglobinopathies are hemoglobin H disease, β-thalassemia, sickle cell anemia, hemoglobin C disease, and hemoglobin E disease. The most severe symptoms are experienced by those with β-thalassemia major (who require frequent blood transfusions and iron chelation therapy), and those with sickle cell anemia (who experience acute painful episodes and organ failure as a result of local hypoxia).

### LEARNING OBJECTIVES

*For mastery of this topic, you should be able to do the following:*
- Compare and contrast the genetic basis of the common forms of α- and β-thalassemia.
- Compare and contrast the pathology and major complications of a patient who has hemoglobin H disease and a patient who has β-thalassemia major (considering, in particular, circulating bilirubin, the need for blood transfusions, and the risk of hemochromatosis).
- Describe the pathogenesis of sickle cell anemia, paying special attention to patient age.
- Compare and contrast the major complications of sickle cell anemia and β-thalassemia major.
- Identify the causes and inheritance patterns of α-thalassemia trait, hemoglobin H disease, hemoglobin Barts hydrops fetalis syndrome, β-thalassemia, sickle cell trait, and sickle cell anemia, along with other forms of sickle cell disease.
- Compare and contrast the hemoglobin composition in the blood of a healthy adult and a healthy baby in the months after birth.
- Use laboratory data on hemoglobin composition to determine whether a patient has β-thalassemia minor, β-thalassemia major, sickle cell trait, sickle cell anemia, sickle cell hemoglobin C disease, hemoglobin C disease, or hemoglobin E disease.

## 1. LINK BETWEEN MALARIA AND SOME HEMOGLOBINOPATHIES

*The most common hemoglobinopathies are found in populations that have been exposed to malaria for an extended period.*

**Malaria** is the result of an infection with the protozoans *Plasmodium vivax*, *P. malariae*, *P. ovale*, or *P. falciparum*, all of which are transmitted by mosquitoes. The parasites initially develop in the liver. Then they invade red blood cells and multiply within them. As parasite-laden red blood cells lyse, they release toxins that lead to fever and inflammation of multiple tissues. Malaria may be accompanied by anemia, coma, and death.

Hemoglobins C, E, and S, as well as the impaired synthesis of α- and β-globin, are predominantly found in populations from geographic areas in which malaria has been endemic for generations. Patients who are heterozygous for α-thalassemia or sickle cell anemia (described below) are less likely to develop *severe* malaria than patients who are homozygous for normal hemoglobin. Furthermore, patients who are homozygous for hemoglobin C have a greatly reduced risk of developing malaria (Fig. 17.1).

## 2. THALASSEMIAS

*The most common thalassemias are the result of impaired production of the normal adult hemoglobin (HbA) and the noxious effects of excess α- or β-globins. A decreased number of α-globin alleles (usually due to large-scale deletions) is the cause of most cases of α-thalassemia trait, hemoglobin H disease, and hemoglobin Barts hydrops fetalis syndrome. β-Thalassemia is usually due to point mutations in the β-globin gene or its promoter.*

### 2.1. General Comments About the Thalassemias

The most common thalassemias are characterized by an impaired synthesis of normal α- or β-globin with concomitant aggregation of excess β-, γ-, or α-globin. When the synthesis of α- or β-globin is compromised or absent, most of the excess globins of the complementary type (α, β, or γ) are destroyed. However, some of these excess globins form **homotetramers** ($\alpha_4$, $\beta_4$, or $\gamma_4$), which are useless as $O_2$ carriers and impair red blood cell production and survival. Precipitated, aggregated, and modified globin homotetramers may be visible by light microscopy as **inclusions** in red blood cells.

Impaired globin synthesis leads to **microcytosis** and **anemia** (see Chapter 16). The less efficient globin synthesis is, the more pronounced is the microcytosis of the red blood cells. The anemia leads to a compensatory expansion of the erythropoietic bone marrow, which may even lead to skeletal abnormalities. However, the expanded bone marrow cannot fully compensate for the anemia.

The terms **thalassemia minor** and **thalassemia major** describe the clinical severity of a thalassemia and stem from a time when the molecular defects were unknown. Typically, patients with thalassemia minor are asymptomatic but have

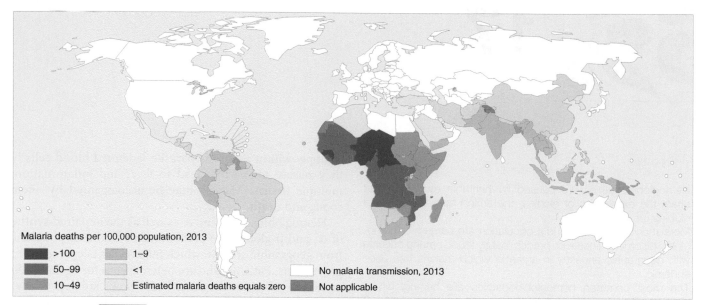

**Fig. 17.1  Malaria deaths in countries with ongoing transmission of the disease in 2013.**
Note that in the past, malaria was also endemic in the Mediterranean basin. (From *World Malaria Report 2014.* World Health Organization, Geneva, Switzerland; p. 37. Available at http://www.alma2015.org/sites/default/files/reference-document/world_malaria_report_2014.pdf.)

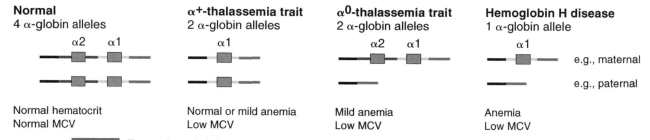

**Fig. 17.2  Examples of deletions of α-globin genes in common forms of α-thalassemia.** The diagram shows maternal and paternal chromosomes, each of which normally carries two α-globin genes (α1 and α2). Shaded boxes denote genes, and colored lines represent the DNA that flanks these genes. Deletions are typically larger than the affected gene itself (not to scale). There is some variation in the borders of the deletions.

microcytic red blood cells. Patients with thalassemia major are symptomatic and anemic, and their red blood cells have pronounced microcytosis.

## 2.2. α-Thalassemia Trait, Hemoglobin H Disease, and Hemoglobin Barts Hydrops Fetalis Syndrome

α-Thalassemia trait, hemoglobin H disease, and hemoglobin Barts hydrops fetalis syndrome develop in response to an insufficient production of α-globin; patients with these disorders have, respectively, only 2, 1, and 0 functional α-globin alleles instead of the normal 4.

There are **two different α-globin genes** (α1 and α2; Fig. 17.2); both genes encode the same α-globin amino acid sequence. The two α-globin genes are next to each other on chromosome 16. Normally, the α2 globin gene gives rise to ~70% of all α-globin. Most people have four α-globin alleles (genotype αα/αα; the α2 gene is written to the left

of the α1 gene; the slash separates the two homologous chromosomes).

In most cases, loss of function of one or more α-globin alleles is due to **large deletions** involving one or both α-globin genes. In the shorthand for a genotype, a deletion of a single α-globin allele is denoted with a dash (e.g., αα/α–). The common deletions may have arisen from misalignment of chromatids at meiosis (α1 aligning with α2), followed by crossover, resulting in a deletion of one α-globin gene on one chromatid (whereby the sister chromatid gains one α-globin gene).

Patients with only three functional α-globin genes (genotypes –α/αα or α–/αα) are **silent carriers** of α-thalassemia. Their red blood cell indices are in the normal range.

Patients with only two functional α-globin genes (genotypes –α/–α, –α/α–, α–/α–, α–/–α, or ––/αα) have **α-thalassemia trait** (also called **α-thalassemia minor**; see Fig. 17.2). Most of these patients are asymptomatic, but their red blood cells are **microcytic** (mean corpuscular volume

[MCV] ~70 fL; normal erythrocytes have an MCV of 80–100 fL; see Chapter 16). Mild anemia may be present. Patients with the haplotypes α– and –α are sometimes said to have a form of **α+-thalassemia**, while patients with a haplotype of – – are said to have a form of **α0-+thalassemia**. With β-thalassemia, the superscripts are used differently (see below). Patients with α+-thalassemia produce more α-globin than patients with α0-thalassemia.

Patients with only one functional α-globin gene (genotypes – –/–α or – –/α–) have **hemoglobin H disease** (see Fig. 17.2). Hemoglobin H consists of **β4 globin tetramers**, which arise from β-globin that was synthesized in excess of α-globin, but escaped intracellular degradation. As red blood cells age in the bloodstream, hemoglobin H forms aggregates (inclusions) that can be seen under a light microscope after staining with brilliant cresyl blue. The spleen removes red blood cells with hemoglobin H aggregates before the cells are 120 days old. The red blood cells of patients with hemoglobin H disease are **microcytic** (MCV: ~65 fL) and **hypochromic** (mean corpuscular hemoglobin concentration [MCHC] is low). The patients are **anemic**, mostly because their red blood cells are removed prematurely from the bloodstream (this is accompanied by splenomegaly). A concomitant compensatory bone marrow expansion may cause skeletal changes, typically in the skull. Most patients do not require chronic blood transfusions.

In the absence of α-globin genes (not shown), **hemoglobin Barts hydrops fetalis** syndrome develops, which usually results in fetal or perinatal death. Hydrops is an abnormal accumulation of fluid in at least two compartments of the fetus. A fetus with hemoglobin Barts hydrops fetalis poses a substantial risk to the mother's life, and early detection is important.

In contrast to the above, there are also **point mutations** in the α-globin gene that can lead to a severe form of hemoglobin H disease. These mutations are sometimes referred to as **nondeletional variants**. The most common of these is **Constant Spring** in the α2-globin gene (α$^{CS}$), which is due to a point mutation in the stop codon that results in a 9-amino acid extension at the C-terminus. Most affected patients have the genotype – –/α$^{CS}$–, and this disorder is often referred to as **hemoglobin Constant Spring (HCS) disease**. α-Globin$^{CS}$ is unstable, and patients have ongoing mild hemolytic anemia. During illness with high fever, affected patients may develop life-threatening anemia.

## 2.3. β-Thalassemia

**β-Thalassemia** is caused by inadequate production or function of **β-globins**. There is only one β-globin gene. A wide variety of **mutations** can give rise to β-thalassemia. Most of these involve one or a few bases in the promoter of the β-globin gene or in the β-globin gene itself that leads to altered RNA synthesis or processing, altered mRNA stability, altered protein sequence, altered hemoglobin stability, or a combination of these. Examples are shown in Fig. 17.3. The shorthand **β0** denotes a **lack of expression** of β-globin, **β+** indicates a **reduced expression**, and **β** denotes a **normal** expression. (The "0" and "+" terminology of β-thalassemia is different from the one used for α-thalassemia; see Section 2.2.)

Patients with **β-thalassemia minor** are usually asymptomatic, although mild anemia may occur, especially during **pregnancy**. These patients have the genotype **β/β+** or **β/β0**. The patients' red blood cells are microcytic (MCV <75 fL; normal

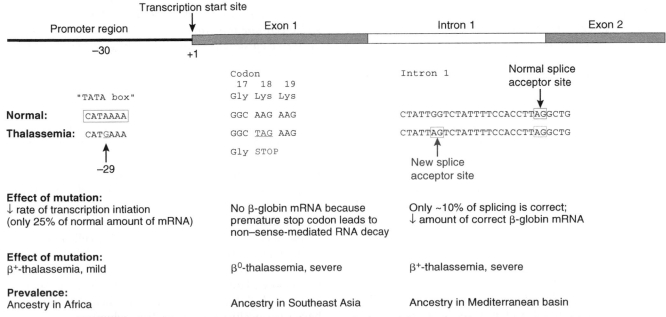

**Fig. 17.3** **Examples of mutations that cause β-thalassemia.** Three commonly observed alleles and the population in which they commonly occur are shown. The phenotype applies to patients who are homozygous for the given mutation. The β-globin gene contains two introns and three exons; the normal stop codon is in exon 3. The structure of the gene is not drawn to scale.

erythrocytes have an MCV of 80 to 100 fL) and hypochromic, but this is often compensated by an increased red blood cell count.

By definition, patients with **β-thalassemia intermedia** have symptomatic anemia but maintain a hemoglobin concentration of greater than 6 to 7 g/dL blood (i.e., about half the normal value or more) without transfusions. These patients have the genotype $\beta^+/\beta^+$ or $\beta^+/\beta^0$. The MCV is about 50 to 75 fL and the MCH about 16 to 24 pg.

Patients with **β-thalassemia major** chronically require **blood transfusions**. These patients have the genotype $\beta^0/\beta^0$ or, occasionally, $\beta^+/\beta^0$ or $\beta^+/\beta^+$. Untransfused patients show a massive expansion of the erythropoietic bone marrow, and even the liver and spleen may produce red blood cells. $\alpha_4$ **Globin tetramers** accumulate, precipitate, give rise to noxious products, and thus lead to the premature destruction of red blood cell precursors in the bone marrow (i.e., **ineffective erythropoiesis**) and of mature red blood cells in the bloodstream. When red blood cells of these patients are stained with methyl violet, aggregates of $\alpha_4$ globin tetramers are visible by light microscopy. The red blood cells of patients with β-thalassemia major contain an increased fraction of **hemoglobin F** ($\alpha_2\gamma_2$ globin subunit structure) and **hemoglobin A$_2$** ($\alpha_2\delta_2$ globin subunit structure). Due to a high rate of destruction of hemoglobin-containing immature and mature red blood cells, untransfused patients with β-thalassemia major are jaundiced (see Chapter 14), and their liver and spleen are enlarged. The MCV is less than 70 fL and the MCH less than 20 pg.

Patients with β-thalassemia major are at risk for complications such as folate deficiency, gout, iron overload, and gallstones. **Folate deficiency** develops as a result of the high rate of erythropoiesis and the concomitant need for nucleotides (see Chapter 37). **Gout** results from the high rate of destruction of purine nucleotides in immature and mature red blood cells (see Chapter 38). **Iron overload** is a consequence of transfusions of red blood cells and excessive iron uptake from the intestine (stimulated by ineffective erythropoiesis and anemia; see Chapter 15). Overload occurs particularly in the liver, heart, and endocrine glands. Excess iron can be removed by chelation therapy, often with nightly intravenous desferrioxamine. Prevention of organ damage due to iron overload is currently the most challenging part of managing β-thalassemia major. Black pigment **gallstones** form in large part due to the precipitation of calcium salts of bilirubin monoglucuronide, which is formed at an elevated rate when red blood cell precursors are destroyed. (β-Thalassemia intermedia and other hemolytic anemias are also associated with an increased incidence of gallstones.)

Because β-globin is a part of adult hemoglobin A but not the fetal hemoglobin F, β-thalassemia becomes clinically apparent only around **6 months of age** (Fig. 17.4; a similar time course is seen with **sickle cell anemia**, a disease due to the production of a mutant β-globin; see Section 3).

Parents who both have β-thalassemia minor (genotypes $\beta/\beta^+$ or $\beta/\beta^0$) may produce **offspring** with β-thalassemia major (genotypes $\beta^0/\beta^0$, $\beta^+/\beta^0$, or $\beta^+/\beta^+$).

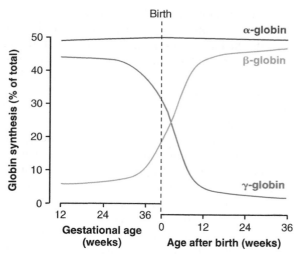

**Fig. 17.4** **Globin synthesis during normal fetal and postnatal development.** The globin composition of blood lags temporally due to the ~120-day life span of mature red blood cells. (Modified from Wood WG. Haemoglobin synthesis during human fetal development. *Br Med Bull.* 1976;32:282.)

The β-thalassemia allele has a geographic distribution akin to past endemic malaria (see Fig. 17.1), but among these areas, it is least common in Africa.

**Carriers** for β-thalassemia can often be detected based on an elevated fraction of HbA$_2$ (Table 17.2).

## 3. SICKLE CELL ANEMIA AND HEMOGLOBIN S

*Sickle cell anemia is caused by homozygosity for the mutant $\beta^S$-globin allele. Deoxygenated sickle cell hemoglobin ($\alpha_2\beta^S_2$) polymerizes, changes the shape of red blood cells, and alters the properties of red blood cell membranes. Patients with sickle cell anemia suffer from recurrent acute painful vaso-occlusive episodes, anemia, and progressive organ failure.*

### 3.1. Cause and the Genetics of Sickle Cell Anemia

Sickle cell anemia is due to a hereditary presence of sickle hemoglobin associated with acute painful vaso-occlusive episodes and subsequent organ damage (see Section 3.3). **Sickle hemoglobin (hemoglobin S)** has an $\alpha_2\beta^S_2$ composition; $\beta^S$-**globin** is β-globin in which the negatively charged amino acid Glu at residue 6 is replaced by the uncharged, hydrophobic amino acid Val. Patients who are homozygous for the $\beta^S$-globin allele (genotype $\beta^S/\beta^S$) have **sickle cell anemia.** Patients who are heterozygous for the $\beta^S$-globin allele (genotype $\beta/\beta^S$) have **sickle cell trait**, which is associated with few symptoms (see below). However, patients who have one $\beta^S$-globin allele and one β-globin allele for another hemoglobinopathy may have vaso-occlusive episodes (see below).

**Sickle cell trait** offers carriers some protection against *Plasmodium falciparum* **malaria.** However, patients with sickle cell anemia have no such protection.

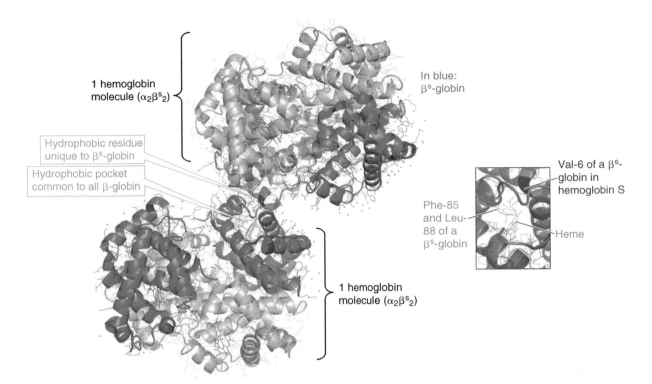

1 hemoglobin molecule ($\alpha_2\beta^S_2$)

Hydrophobic residue unique to $\beta^S$-globin

Hydrophobic pocket common to all $\beta$-globin

In blue: $\beta^S$-globin

Val-6 of a $\beta^S$-globin in hemoglobin S

Phe-85 and Leu-88 of a $\beta^S$-globin

Heme

1 hemoglobin molecule ($\alpha_2\beta^S_2$)

**Fig. 17.5** **Model of a human deoxyhemoglobin S dimer and mechanism of polymerization.** Two hemoglobin molecules are shown, each with 2 $\alpha$- and 2 $\beta^S$-globins. Although both $\beta^S$-globins in a hemoglobin S molecule have a Val as the sixth residue (shown in red), Val of only one $\beta^S$-globin per hemoglobin molecule binds into a hydrophobic pocket on a $\beta$-globin of a neighboring hemoglobin molecule. The hydrophobic pocket consists of Phe-85, Leu-88, and heme. (Based on Protein Data Bank [www.rcsb.org] file 2HBS by DJ Harrington DJ, Adachi K, Royer WE Jr. The high resolution crystal structure of deoxyhemoglobin S. *J Mol Biol.* 1997;272:398-407.)

In general, the sickle cell mutation is common in populations that have been exposed to malaria for many generations. Sickle cell anemia is most prevalent in patients with ancestry in **Africa**, and less so in the **Mediterranean** region or **India**. In the **United States**, about 10% of African Americans have sickle cell trait, and about 0.2% have sickle cell anemia. Genes outside the $\beta$-globin locus influence the course of sickle cell anemia (an example is increased expression of fetal hemoglobin; see Section 3.3).

Affected children do not develop symptoms of sickle cell anemia until 2 to 4 months of age. This time frame is due to the normal increase in expression of the $\beta$-globin gene, the normal decrease in expression of the $\gamma$-globin genes around the time of birth (see Fig. 17.4), and the life span of red blood cells. **Newborns** can be **screened** for sickle cell anemia by analyzing their hemoglobin by electrophoresis, isoelectric focusing, or high-pressure liquid chromatography; by analyzing their DNA; or by a combination of these techniques (see Section 6).

## 3.2. Polymerization of Deoxyhemoglobin S

When deoxygenated hemoglobin S polymerizes, the mutant Val6 residue of $\beta^S$-globin binds into a hydrophobic pocket of another hemoglobin molecule. The hydrophobic pocket is formed by heme and the hydrophobic sidechains of Phe85 and Leu88 of a $\beta$-globin (Figs. 17.5 and 17.6). This hydrophobic pocket is present for instance in normal $\beta$-globin, in $\beta^S$-globin, and in $\beta^C$-globin (see Section 4). For polymerization into multimers, a single $\beta^S$-globin chain per hemoglobin is sufficient. Hence, deoxygenated $\alpha_2\beta^S_2$, $\alpha_2\beta\beta^S$, and $\alpha_2\beta^C\beta^S$ tetramers can all polymerize.

The polymerization of hemoglobin S has a **lag time** (delay time) that changes considerably with even a **small change in the concentration** of deoxyhemoglobin S. The lag time depends on the concentration of deoxyhemoglobin S approximately to the **power** of 30. Normally, red blood cells spend less than about 4 seconds in the capillary bed, which is not sufficient for appreciable polymerization. When deoxygenated sickle cells stay in a capillary for a considerably longer time, they may sickle and occlude the microcirculation, causing a vaso-occlusive episode.

In patients with sickle cell anemia, a low affinity of hemoglobin S for oxygen and impaired lung function both favor the deoxygenation of hemoglobin S and thus contribute to polymerization. Damage to the **lungs** is probably due to repeated episodes of vaso-occlusion because red blood cells normally reside in the capillary bed of the alveoli for several seconds. As a result, many patients have an **arterial oxygen saturation** of less than 85% to 90%, which further contributes to sickling.

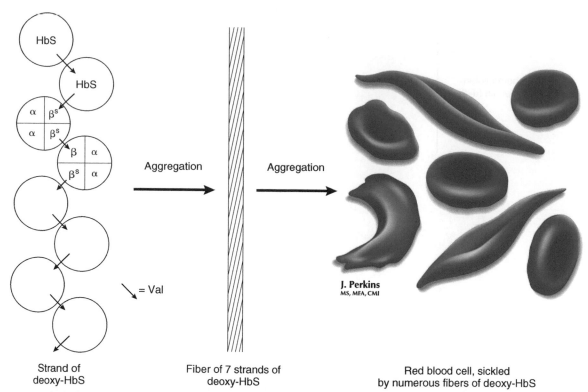

Strand of
deoxy-HbS

Fiber of 7 strands of
deoxy-HbS

Red blood cell, sickled
by numerous fibers of deoxy-HbS

J. Perkins
MS, MFA, CMI

= Val

**Fig. 17.6** **Polymerization of deoxyhemoglobin S.** Both hemoglobin S (subunit composition $\alpha_2\beta^S_2$) and hybrid hemoglobin of the type $\alpha_2\beta\beta^S$ can polymerize as shown in Fig. 17.5, thereby forming a strand. Seven such strands can be twisted into a fiber, and the fibers in turn can aggregate into large structures that distort and damage red blood cells.

## 3.3. Vaso-Occlusive Episodes in Sickle Cell Anemia

**Vaso-occlusive episodes** are caused by red blood cells occluding the microcirculation, which in turn gives rise to local hypoxia. These episodes may be extremely painful and last hours to weeks. Temporary vaso-occlusion may also be debilitating because of damage to the lungs, heart, bones, joints, kidneys, spleen, and brain.

Hemoglobin S alters the properties of red blood cells and the luminal lining of blood vessels (i.e., the endothelium). The $Fe^{2+}$ in the hemes in hemoglobin S is oxidized to $Fe^{3+}$ at a higher rate than in hemoglobin A, and heme dissociates more rapidly from hemoglobin S than from hemoglobin A. Both of these abnormalities give rise to increased **oxidative damage** (see Chapter 21). Oxidative damage and the effects of polymerization of deoxyhemoglobin S alter the **properties of red blood cells**. Compared with normal red blood cells, the red blood cells of patients with sickle cell anemia (1) become more dehydrated with age, (2) stick more to the blood vessel endothelium, (3) increase the viscosity of blood, (4) are less deformable, (5) are more likely to initiate vaso-occlusion (in turn causing infarction), and (6) have a decreased life span (causing **anemia**). In patients with sickle cell anemia, as much as 30% of all red blood cells hemolyze in the bloodstream rather than in the spleen and liver (in unaffected patients, only ~10% of the red blood cells lyse in the bloodstream). Not all hemoglobin S lost into blood plasma can sufficiently be removed by **haptoglobin** (a protein in blood plasma that binds hemoglobin and carries it to the liver; see Chapter 14); remaining hemoglobin S may thus scavenge the vasodilator **nitric oxide** (NO) prematurely (see Chapter 16), thereby contributing to vaso-occlusion.

Several factors influence the incidence of vaso-occlusive episodes; among them are **temperature** and the concentrations of **hemoglobin F** and hemoglobin S. Extremes of both high and low temperature increase the likelihood of acute painful episodes. Thus an increase in temperature decreases the oxygen affinity and also favors the polymerization of hemoglobin S, whereas a decrease in temperature leads to a decrease in blood flow through peripheral tissues and thus to greater deoxygenation of hemoglobin S. **Infection**, besides affecting body temperature, often increases the adhesion of red blood cells to the endothelium. **Exertion** and **anemia** both lead to greater deoxygenation of hemoglobin, and **dehydration** increases the concentration of hemoglobin S inside red blood cells. These conditions favor the polymerization of deoxyhemoglobin S. Patients with a high fraction of hemoglobin F ($\alpha_2\gamma_2$) and F cells (red blood cells that contain about 20% HbF) often have fewer vaso-occlusive episodes because hybrid hemoglobin $\alpha_2\beta^S\gamma$ delays and inhibits polymerization and because a lower concentration of hemoglobin S prolongs the lag time for polymerization.

The chemotherapeutic drug and inhibitor of nucleotide reductase **hydroxyurea** (see Chapter 37) increases the fractions of hemoglobin F and F cells. Some patients with frequent vaso-occlusive episodes respond favorably to treatment with hydroxyurea.

Sickle cell anemia is a **chronic hemolytic anemia**. In patients with sickle cell anemia, red blood cells have a shortened life span that can be as low as 10 to 25 days (the normal life span of red blood cells is ~120 days). At a few years of age, children with sickle cell anemia tend to lose much of the function of their spleen to sickle cell–induced infarction, a process called **autosplenectomy**. In patients without a functioning spleen, the liver removes red blood cells. Functionally asplenic children have decreased immunity and therefore routinely receive prophylactic treatment with **vaccines** and **antibiotics**.

Patients with sickle cell anemia eventually show damage to various organs. Children are at a high risk of cerebrovascular infarcts. Adults commonly suffer from **acute chest syndrome**, which is due in part to infarction of lung tissue and bone. Chronic damage to the lungs leads to pulmonary hypertension. Kidney damage stems from infarcts that occur in the peritubular capillaries, presumably due to the physiologically especially low pH and $pO_2$ in the renal medulla. As a result, patients with sickle cell anemia may experience **hematuria**, and they usually cannot concentrate urine normally when stressed by water deprivation (i.e., they have **hyposthenuria**).

Patients with **sickle cell trait** (genotype $\beta/\beta^S$) are usually free of obvious vaso-occlusive acute painful episodes because the concentration of deoxyhemoglobin S and the duration of the deoxygenated state of hemoglobin S do not permit polymerization. However, with pronounced hypoxia, the red blood cells of patients with sickle cell trait do sickle. In fact, most patients with sickle cell trait have kidney damage as they have hyposthenuria and experience hematuria at one time or another. Furthermore, heat illness and death during high-intensity exercise in a hot environment are much more common in patients who have sickle cell trait than in the general population.

Patients who have **sickle-$\beta^0$-thalassemia** have a sickle cell disease that resembles sickle cell anemia. If there is some expression of a β-globin with normal function (as in **sickle-$\beta^+$-thalassemia**), the severity of the symptoms is reduced.

## 4. HEMOGLOBIN C, HEMOGLOBIN SC, AND HEMOGLOBIN E DISEASE

*Patients with hemoglobin C, SC, or E disease produce mutant β-globins. Patients with hemoglobin C or E disease may have mild anemia. Patients with hemoglobin SC disease can have vaso-occlusive acute painful episodes, similar to patients with sickle cell anemia. Patients who are heterozygous for both hemoglobin E and β-thalassemia may be severely anemic.*

**Hemoglobin C** shortens the life span of red blood cells, but in the absence of other pathogenic hemoglobins, hemoglobin C causes only mild disease. Hemoglobin C has an $\alpha_2\beta^C_2$ composition, where $\beta^C$-globin is β-globin in which Glu (negatively charged) in residue 6 is replaced by Lys (positively charged; in

$\beta^S$-globin the same residue is replaced by Val). Hemoglobin C forms intracellular aggregates and crystals that lead to the premature removal of red blood cells. Patients with the genotype $\beta/\beta^C$ have **hemoglobin C trait** and are asymptomatic. Patients with the genotype $\beta^C/\beta^C$ have **hemoglobin C disease**; they show microcytosis, mild hemolysis, mild anemia, and moderate splenomegaly (a response to an increased rate of red blood cell degradation). Hemoglobin C in the red blood cells of patients with hemoglobin C disease has a decreased affinity for $O_2$. This leads to the release of a larger fraction of bound $O_2$ and thus ensures normal tissue oxygenation despite mild anemia.

The red blood cells of patients with **hemoglobin SC disease** (i.e., sickle cell hemoglobin C disease) can **sickle in vivo**, causing **vaso-occlusive acute painful episodes**. These patients have the genotype $\beta^C/\beta^S$ and produce some β-globins with a Glu6Lys and others with a Glu6Val amino acid substitution. Red blood cells from patients with hemoglobin SC disease contain a higher fraction of HbS than red blood cells from patients with sickle cell trait (genotype $\beta/\beta^S$). Patients with hemoglobin SC disease have less severe and fewer painful vaso-occlusive episodes than patients with sickle cell anemia (genotype $\beta^S/\beta^S$).

**Hemoglobin E** has an $\alpha_2\beta^E_2$ composition; $\beta^E$-globin is β-globin in which Glu (negatively charged) in residue 26 is replaced by Lys (positively charged). Hemoglobin E has normal oxygen transport properties. About half of the $\beta^E$-globin RNA is **spliced** to an mRNA that is destroyed via **nonsense-mediated RNA decay** (see Chapter 7). Homozygotes and heterozygotes for hemoglobin E are both asymptomatic, but they have microcytosis (MCV: 55 to 65 fL; normal MCV: 80 to 100 fL) and hypochromia. Homozygotes may also have mild anemia. The $\beta^E$-globin allele is common among patients with Southeast Asian ancestry (allele frequency up to 15%). Patients with a $\beta^E/\beta^+$ or $\beta^E/\beta^0$ genotype (i.e., heterozygotes for both **β-thalassemia** and hemoglobin E) can have symptoms that range from mild anemia to severe anemia that needs to be treated with blood transfusions.

## 5. SUMMARY OF THE CAUSES AND MANIFESTATIONS OF THE MOST COMMON HEMOGLOBINOPATHIES

See Table 17.1.

## 6. HEMOGLOBIN ANALYSIS FOR THE DIAGNOSIS OF HEMOGLOBIN DISORDERS

*Electrophoresis, isoelectric focusing, and/or chromatography are often used to characterize and quantify hemoglobin species in a patient's red blood cells. Interpretation of these data is up to the health care provider.*

Analyses of hemoglobin species are often performed as part of newborn screening, follow-up of abnormal laboratory results, or genetic counseling, as well as before

**Table 17.1**   **Causes and Manifestations of the Most Common Hemoglobinopathies**

| Disease | Genotype (Molecular Cause of Disease) | Clinical Observations |
|---|---|---|
| **α-Thalassemia** | | |
| Silent carrier | $\alpha\alpha/\alpha-$ or $\alpha\alpha/-\alpha$ (impaired synthesis) | None or mild microcytosis (asymptomatic) |
| Trait/minor | $\alpha-/\alpha-$, $\alpha-/-\alpha$, $-\alpha/-\alpha$, $-\alpha/\alpha-$, or $--/\alpha\alpha$ (impaired synthesis) | Microcytosis (asymptomatic) |
| Hemoglobin H disease | $--/-\alpha$ or $--/\alpha-$ (impaired synthesis of α-globin; excess β-globin) | Anemia, microcytosis, skeletal changes |
| Hb Barts hydrops fetalis | $--/--$ (no α-globin synthesis; excess γ- and β-globin) | Hydrops fetalis, perinatal death |
| **β-Thalassemia** | | |
| Minor | $\beta/\beta^+$ or $\beta/\beta^0$ (impaired synthesis) | Microcytosis, hypochromia, increased red blood cell count (asymptomatic) |
| Major | $\beta^0/\beta^0$ or $\beta^+/\beta^0$ or $\beta^+/\beta^+$ (impaired synthesis; excess α-globin) | Anemia after ~6 mo of age, microcytosis, ineffective erythropoiesis, skeletal changes |
| Sickle cell trait | $\beta/\beta^S$ (Glu6Val; impaired synthesis) | Hematuria, hyposthenuria |
| Sickle cell anemia | $\beta^S/\beta^S$ (Glu6Val; impaired synthesis; sickling and impaired survival of red blood cells) | Anemia starting at 2–4 mo of age, vaso-occlusive episodes, skeletal changes, autosplenectomy, organ failure, hematuria, hyposthenuria |
| Hemoglobin C disease | $\beta^C/\beta^C$ (Glu6Lys; impaired synthesis; impaired stability of red blood cells) | Microcytosis, mild anemia, mild hemolysis, moderate splenomegaly |
| Hemoglobin SC disease | $\beta^S/\beta^C$ (Glu6Val and Glu6Lys; impaired synthesis; sickling and impaired survival of red blood cells) | Anemia, vaso-occlusive episodes, splenomegaly or autosplenectomy |
| Hemoglobin E disease | $\beta^E/\beta^E$ (Glu26Lys; impaired synthesis) | Microcytosis, mild anemia, hypochromia (asymptomatic) |
| Hemoglobin E/β-thalassemia | $\beta^E/\beta^+$ or $\beta^E/\beta^0$ ($\beta^E$: Glu26Lys with impaired synthesis, $\beta^0$: impaired synthesis) | Microcytosis, anemia, hypochromia |

medical interventions that present increased risk to patients who have a hemoglobinopathy or carry an allele for a hemoglobinopathy.

The **hemoglobin composition** in red blood cells is currently determined by electrophoresis, isoelectric focusing, or high-pressure liquid chromatography, and final diagnoses of hemoglobinopathies increasingly rely on analyzing globin mRNA in the red blood cell fraction and/or DNA in the white blood cell fraction of a blood sample. For most lab assays, the same volume of red blood cells is used for each patient, regardless of **hematocrit**. The results of the electrophoresis are reported for each hemoglobin as a **fraction of all hemoglobins** present in the sample (e.g., 96% HbA); these results are independent of the hematocrit. Sometimes, blood samples from **family members** are analyzed as part of a final diagnosis of a hemoglobinopathy (e.g., homozygosity for HbS vs. compound heterozygosity for HbS and $\beta^0$-thalassemia).

Results of hemoglobin analyses are typically reported as idealized fractions of hemoglobins rather than as fractions of individual globins. Commonly reported hemoglobins are A, $A_2$, C, E, F, S, and Barts. Physiologically, additional forms of hemoglobin exist. For instance, the red blood cells of patients who have sickle cell trait contain not only pure hemoglobin A and S, but also hemoglobin with the composition $\alpha_2\beta^S\beta$. If an analysis method cannot distinguish certain hemoglobins, these are reported in aggregation (e.g., hemoglobin $A_2$ + C + E after electrophoresis on cellulose acetate at pH ~8.5; see Table 17.2).

## SUMMARY

■ Patients who produce either α- or β-globin at an abnormally low rate and patients who are heterozygous for

## Table 17.2   Typical Results of Hemoglobin Analyses

| Hemoglobin Disease | HbA ($\alpha_2\beta_2$) | HbA$_2$ ($\alpha_2\delta_2$) | HbF ($\alpha_2\gamma_2$) | Other Hemoglobins |
|---|---|---|---|---|
| Normal newborn | ~20% | <1% | ~80% | |
| Normal adult | ~96% | ~2.5% | <1% | |
| $\alpha^0$-Thalassemia minor | ~Normal | ~Normal | ~Normal | At birth: ~6% Hb Barts ($\gamma_4$) |
| Hemoglobin H disease | ~80% (adult) | <2%* | ~10% | At birth: ~35% Hb Barts ($\gamma_4$)*<br>Adult: ~9% HbH ($\beta_4$)* |
| Hb Barts hydrops fetalis | 0% | 0% | 0% | ~80% Hb Barts ($\gamma_4$)*, ~20% embryonic Hb, ~0% HbH ($\beta_4$) |
| $\beta^0$-Thalassemia carrier | ~93% | >3.5%* | ~2% | |
| $\beta^0$-Thalassemia major | 0%* | >3.5%* | ~96%* | |
| Sickle cell trait | ~60% | ~Normal | ~1% | ~40% HbS |
| Sickle cell anemia | 0%* | ~Normal | ~5% | ~90% HbS* |
| Hemoglobin C disease | 0%* | ~Normal | ~1% | ~95% HbC* |
| Hemoglobin E disease | 0%* | ~Normal | ~1% | ~95% HbE* |

*These abnormal values are of special diagnostic value.

hemoglobin C, E, or S are more likely to survive malaria than patients who produce normal amounts of hemoglobin A.

- Thalassemia typically results from the deficient production of α- or β-globin. Patients with thalassemia major are anemic, and their red blood cells are microcytic. The red blood cells contain noxious homotetramers of excess complementary globins, such as $\alpha_4$, $\beta_4$, or $\gamma_4$, often as part of inclusions.

- Humans have two α-globin genes. Patients with three or two normal α-globin alleles are usually asymptomatic. Patients with only one normal α-globin allele have hemoglobin H disease. Hemoglobin H disease is apparent at birth by the presence of hemoglobin Barts ($\gamma_4$) and later in life by the presence of hemoglobin H ($\beta_4$). Patients with hemoglobin H disease are anemic and have microcytic erythrocytes of decreased life span. Patients who have only one $\alpha^{CS}$ allele (carrying a point mutation) have a particularly severe form of the disease called hemoglobin HCS disease. A complete deficiency of functioning α-globin genes leads to hemoglobin Barts hydrops fetalis and death before or shortly after birth; furthermore, it threatens the mother's health.

- Patients with β-thalassemia minor have one normal and one abnormal β-globin allele. Their red blood cells are microcytic and hypochromic, yet the patients usually remain asymptomatic. Patients with β-thalassemia major have no normal β-globin allele, and they have pronounced anemia (more severe than patients with hemoglobin H disease). The anemia is due to ineffective erythropoiesis

and decreased survival of circulating red blood cells ($\alpha_4$ is noxious). The anemia develops around 6 months of age. Patients with β-thalassemia major depend on blood transfusions, and they need chelation therapy to remove excess iron from their body, which they acquire both enterally and via blood transfusions.

- Patients with sickle cell anemia are homozygous for $\beta^S$-globin (Glu6Val substitution). Deoxyhemoglobin S can polymerize and damage red blood cells. Erythrocytes from patients with sickle cell anemia adhere excessively to the vascular endothelium, and the spleen or liver removes them long before they are 120 days old. The polymerization of deoxyhemoglobin S has a lag time so that polymerization takes place only during a minority of oxygenation/deoxygenation cycles. Patients with sickle cell anemia suffer from occasional and potentially life-threatening acute painful episodes, which are the result of local vaso-occlusion. Due to the extreme concentration dependence of the polymerization reaction, both a small decrease in the concentration of deoxyhemoglobin S and an increase in the fraction of hemoglobin F (induced by treatment with hydroxyurea) can drastically decrease the incidence of vaso-occlusive crises. The red blood cells of patients with sickle cell trait do not sickle under physiological conditions.

- $\beta^C$-globin is Glu6Lys- and $\beta^E$-globin is Glu26Lys-substituted β-globin. Patients who are homozygous for $\beta^C$-globin have hemoglobin C disease and mild hemolytic anemia due to aggregation and crystallization of hemoglobin C that shortens the life span of red blood cells. Patients with hemoglobin SC disease have symptoms that are intermediate between sickle cell trait and sickle cell anemia. Patients with hemoglobin E disease are homozygous for $\beta^E$-globin. They have microcytic red blood cells and mild anemia due to an impaired production of $\beta^E$-globin mRNA, which in turn impairs globin synthesis.

■ Hemoglobin analyses provide clues to hemoglobinopathies. If an adult patient has mostly hemoglobin F, the patient may have $\beta^0$-thalassemia, and family members with an elevated fraction of hemoglobin $A_2$ may be $\beta^0$-thalassemia carriers. The presence of hemoglobin Barts at birth and hemoglobin H after that are characteristic of hemoglobin H disease. If hemoglobin C, E, or S account for the majority of the hemoglobin in a patient's red blood cells, the patient likely has hemoglobin C disease, hemoglobin E disease, or sickle cell anemia, respectively.

## FURTHER READING

■ Piel FB, Weatherall DJ. The $\alpha$-thalassemias. *N Engl J Med.* 2014;371:1908-1916.
■ Quinn CT. Sickle cell disease in childhood; from newborn screening through transition to adult medical care. *Pediatr Clin N Am.* 2013;60:1363-1381.
■ Bynum WF. Mosquitoes bite more than once. *Science.* 2002;295:47-48. (An entertaining account of how Dr. Ross found *Plasmodium* in mosquitoes and won a Nobel Prize.)

# Review Questions

1. A woman and a man consider having children. The woman has hemoglobin H disease. The man has $\alpha^0$-thalassemia trait. What is the risk that their child will have the genotype for hemoglobin H disease?

   A. 0%
   B. 12.5%
   C. 25%
   D. 50%
   E. 100%

2. On her first visit to an obstetrician, a 33-year-old pregnant patient is screened for hemoglobin disorders. Hemoglobin electrophoresis yields the following result: HbA: 93%, HbS: 0%, HbF: 2%, HbA$_2$+HbC+HbE: 5% (normal: 2.5%). The patient's hemoglobin is 11.2 g/dL and the MCV is 70 fL. The patient's total iron-binding capacity is normal. She has no history of recent bleeding or blood donation. Based on these laboratory values and her history, the most likely diagnosis is which of the following?

   A. $\beta$-thalassemia minor
   B. Hemoglobin C trait
   C. Hemoglobin E trait
   D. Hemoglobin SC disease
   E. Sickle cell trait

3. Preoperative screening of a 45-year-old African-American woman for sickle cell disease reveals the following: 60% HbA, 2.5% HbA$_2$+HbC, 1% HbF, 36% HbS. This patient most likely has which of the following?

   A. $\beta^+$-thalassemia
   B. Diabetes
   C. Sickle cell anemia
   D. Sickle cell trait
   E. Sickle cell-hemoglobin C disease

4. A woman and a man consider having children. The woman has $\alpha^0$-thalassemia trait, and the man has $\alpha^+$-thalassemia trait. What is the risk that their child will have hemoglobin H disease?

   A. 0%
   B. 25%
   C. 50%
   D. 100%

5. A patient who has sickle cell disease could have which one of the following genotypes?

   A. $\beta$-globin (normal)/$\beta$-globin$^0$
   B. $\beta$-globin (normal)/$\beta$-globin$^S$
   C. $\beta$-globin$^C$/$\beta$-globin$^C$
   D. $\beta$-globin$^C$/$\beta$-globin$^S$

6. A patient with which one of the following sets of laboratory data is most likely to have a hemoglobinopathy?

   A. Direct bilirubin/total bilirubin = 25%, normal ferritin
   B. ↓ Serum iron, ↓ MCV, ↓ hemoglobin
   C. ↑ Red blood cell count, ↑ hematocrit, normal bilirubin
   D. ↑ Total bilirubin, ↑ serum lactate dehydrogenase (LDH), ↓ MCV
   E. ↑ Total bilirubin, ↑ serum lactate dehydrogenase (LDH), ↑ MCHC

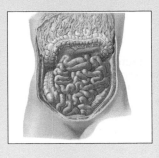

# Chapter 18

# Carbohydrate Transport, Carbohydrate Malabsorption, and Lactose Intolerance

## SYNOPSIS

- Carbohydrates in the form of monosaccharides, disaccharides, and starches make up a large portion of our diet.
- The pancreas secretes amylase into the intestine. The outer surface of the microvilli of intestinal epithelial cells contains disaccharidases. Together, these enzymes degrade starches and disaccharides into monosaccharides, principally glucose, galactose, and fructose.
- Intestinal epithelial cells take up monosaccharides and then release them into the bloodstream.
- If intestinal digestive enzymes have reduced activity, or if monosaccharides are not properly taken up, carbohydrates reach the colon. There, bacteria degrade the carbohydrates to acids and to gases that may cause flatulence and abdominal pain.
- Certain dietary carbohydrates cannot be digested by humans. An enzyme supplement can aid in digestion and thus lessen the adverse effects of metabolism by bacteria.
- Lactose malabsorption is common among adults and is usually due to the normal hereditary inactivation of the expression of lactase after the first few years of life.
- A variety of transporters facilitate the recovery of monosaccharides from the glomerular filtrate and the uptake of monosaccharides from the blood into peripheral cells. In adipose tissue and skeletal muscle, insulin regulates monosaccharide transport.
- Inhibitors of renal glucose transporters and intestinal carbohydrate-degrading enzymes are used in the treatment of diabetes.

## LEARNING OBJECTIVES

*For mastery of this topic, you should be able to do the following:*
- Describe the digestion of dietary starch and disaccharides and list transporters for monosaccharides, paying attention to tissue location.
- Interpret biopsy reports about disaccharidase activities.
- Explain the symptoms of lactose restriction (also called lactose intolerance, lactase deficiency, or hypolactasia) and describe an appropriate strategy for the prevention of symptoms.
- Describe the function and use of α-galactosidase (Beano).
- Describe the functions and uses of lactulose and sorbitol.
- Compare and contrast the characteristics of glucose transporters.
- Describe the effect of SGLT2 inhibitors on plasma glucose concentrations.
- Describe the effects of α-glucosidase inhibitors on carbohydrate digestion and list carbohydrates that can be absorbed even in the presence of an α-glucosidase inhibitor.

## 1. CLASSIFICATION OF CARBOHYDRATES

*The most important dietary carbohydrates are glucose, fructose, and di-, oligo-, and polysaccharides that are made up of glucose, fructose, and galactose. Fiber contains carbohy-drates that cannot be digested by human enzymes in the small intestine.*

**Carbohydrates** were originally defined as compounds of the summary chemical formula $C_n(H_2O)_n$, but now the term also includes their derivatives, even if they have a slightly different formula. The physiologically important carbohydrates are mono-, di-, oligo-, and polysaccharides. **Saccharide** is an ill-defined term that derives from the Latin saccharum (meaning sugar) and refers to carbohydrates that resemble chemically the sugars found in food (Fig. 18.1). **Monosaccharides** typically have five to seven carbon atoms; pentoses contain five carbons, hexoses six, and heptoses seven. The most common monosaccharide is glucose ($C_6H_{12}O_6$). **Disaccharides** consist of two monosaccharides that are joined by a glycosidic bond (e.g., sucrose). **Oligosaccharides** typically consist of 3 to 10 monosaccharides (e.g., maltotriose). **Polysaccharides** consist of more than 10 monosaccharides (e.g., **glycogen**, which serves as an energy store in humans and animals; see Chapter 24). **Starches** are polysaccharides that serve as energy stores in plants; they consist of amylose and amylopectin.

In di-, oligo-, and polysaccharides, the monosaccharides are typically joined by glycosidic bonds that contain oxygen; such bonds are called **O-glycosidic** bonds. **N-Glycosidic** linkages, by contrast, contain nitrogen; these bonds are found in nucleotides, linking the ribose and the base (see Chapters 1, 37, and 38).

The quantitatively most important sugars in the diet are glucose, galactose, and fructose. **Glucose** makes up the majority of dietary carbohydrates. Glucose is found as a monosaccharide in honey and fruits, as part of the disaccharides sucrose (table sugar) and lactose (milk sugar), and as the constituent of the glucose polymers amylose, amylopectin, and glycogen (see Fig. 18.1 and Chapter 24). **Galactose** is found almost exclusively in milk products as part of lactose (see Chapter 20). **Fructose** is found chiefly in dietary sucrose, in biochemically made high-fructose corn syrup, and as a monosaccharide in honey and many fruits (see Table 20.1).

Glucose and galactose exist in solution as mixtures of their **α- and β-anomers**, which differ in the orientation of their –H and –OH groups at carbon number 1 (C-1) relative to the sugar ring structure. Since the sugar ring opens and closes frequently between the ring oxygen and C-1, α-anomers of these monosaccharides can rapidly become β-anomers and vice versa. One can indicate this rapid anomerization by writing "H, OH" next to a squiggly line that emanates from the anomeric carbon; examples are given in Fig. 18.1 with lactose, maltotriose, and maltose. The clinically used term **dextrose** refers to crystals of α-glucose. Once dextrose is

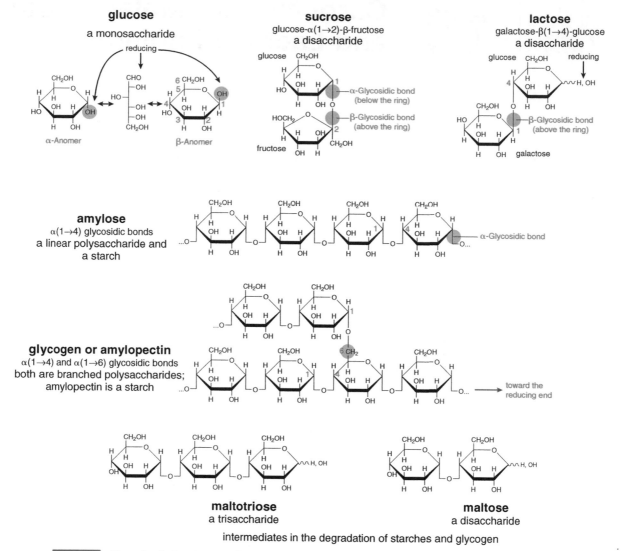

**Fig. 18.1** **Chemical structures of common dietary carbohydrates.** The branches of amylopectin are ~25 residues long. Glycogen usually has shorter branches and a larger molecular weight than amylopectin. Amylose, amylopectin, and glycogen typically contain a hundred to many thousands of glucose residues. Blue numbers indicate the chemical numbering of carbon atoms.

dissolved in water, some $\alpha$-glucose rapidly isomerizes to $\beta$-glucose, so that comparable amounts of $\alpha$- and $\beta$-glucose are present in solution.

**Reducing sugars** in stools are sometimes measured in the diagnostic evaluation of diarrhea. Reducing sugars have an aldehyde carbon (–CH=O) available for a redox reaction with $Cu^{2+}$ or $Ag^+$ in Fehling or Benedict solution, respectively. Glucose, lactose, galactose, and fructose are reducing sugars. When the aldehydes of glucose, galactose, or fructose are part of a glycosidic bond, they are no longer reducing. Hence, sucrose is not a reducing sugar. Starches contain only a single, terminal monosaccharide that is reducing, which pales compared with a large number of nonreducing glycosidic bonds (see Fig. 18.1).

The term **fiber** encompasses polysaccharides (see Section 4 below) and **lignins** (polymers containing various methoxyphenols) that cannot be digested by human enzymes. Fiber is made by plants. **Soluble fiber** dissolves in water and forms a gel that slows the rate of digestion and the absorption of starch. Soluble fiber consists of **pectic substances** (branched polysaccharides rich in a derivative of galactose) and **gums**, which are found in fruits, legumes, and oats. Bacteria in the colon degrade soluble fiber to various short-chain acids and gases. **Insoluble fiber** does not dissolve in water and is poorly degraded by intestinal bacteria. Insoluble fiber is typically found in the outer layers of grains (i.e., in "**bran**") and consists mostly of lignins and the polysaccharides **cellulose** and **hemicellulose**. Insoluble fiber increases the bulk of feces.

## 2. DIGESTION OF POLYSACCHARIDES AND DISACCHARIDES IN THE SMALL INTESTINE

*The pancreas secretes amylase into the duodenum. Amylase partially hydrolyzes starches and glycogen. The outer surface of small-intestinal epithelial cells contains disaccharidases that hydrolyze disaccharides, as well as branch points in polysaccharides. The main disaccharidases of the small intestine are lactase-glycosylceramidase, sucrase-isomaltase, maltase-glucoamylase, and trehalase.*

## 2.1. Structure of the Small Intestine

The small intestine consists of the duodenum, jejunum, and ileum. The duodenum and jejunum, but less so the ileum, contain many **folds** (plicae; Fig. 18.2). The folds and the remainder of the intestinal wall are covered by numerous 1-mm-long **villi**. The villi are fingerlike projections with central blood capillaries and a surface made up of many

**Microvilli**

Absorptive epithelial cell

**Villus**

**Fold (plica)**

**Crypt**

Absorptive epithelial cell

Goblet cell (secretes mucins)

Proliferating transit-amplifying cells

Paneth cells and stem cells

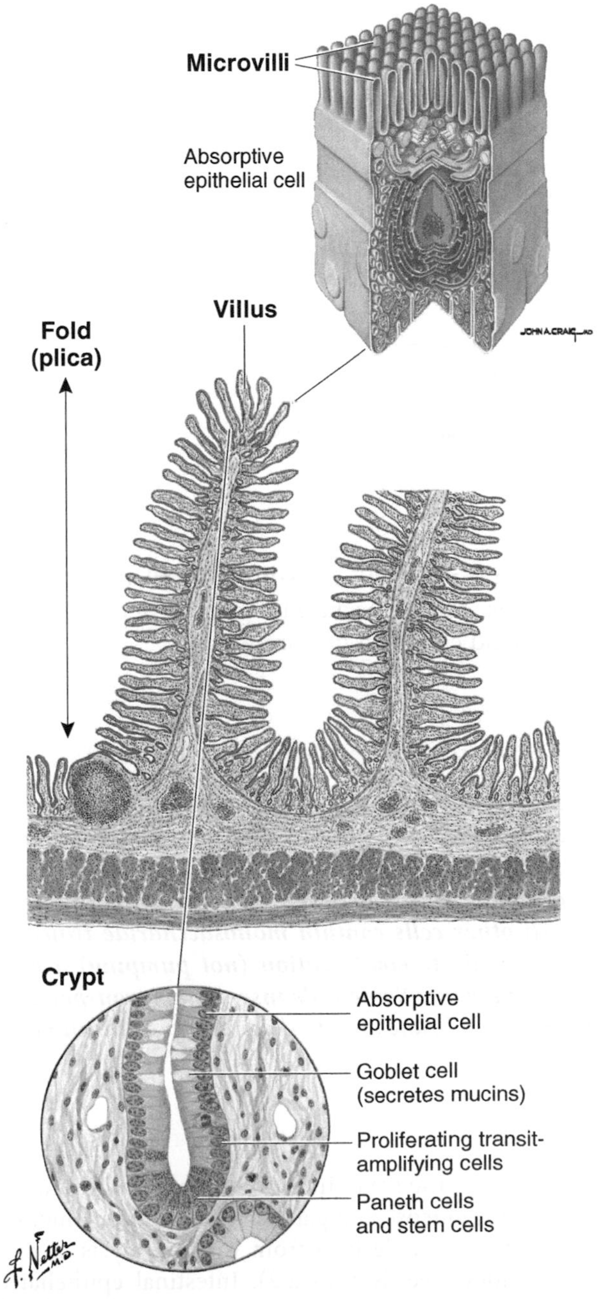

**Fig. 18.2** **Structure of the jejunum.** The structures of the duodenum and ileum are similar, except that there are fewer folds.

absorptive epithelial cells. Each absorptive epithelial cell has a plasma membrane that forms numerous **microvilli** (there are ~200 million microvilli per square centimeter of villus). As a result, the small intestine has a surface area of about 200 m². The wells at the base of (and between) the villi are called **crypts**. **Stem cells** near the bottom of a crypt give rise to absorptive **epithelial cells** that migrate to the tip of the villus; there, epithelial cells are shed approximately 2 to 3 days after their creation. **Goblet cells**, which migrate like absorptive cells, secrete mucins that give rise to **mucus** that covers the intestinal epithelium. **Paneth cells** at the base of the crypts play a role in immune surveillance and in maintaining the stem cells.

## 2.2. Hydrolysis of Polysaccharides and Disaccharides to Monosaccharides

Carbohydrates account for 30% to 60% of the typical human caloric intake. A good portion of this carbohydrate is starch. An adult thus consumes the equivalent of about 200 to 450 g of glucose per day.

The small intestine contains polysaccharidases and disaccharidases that degrade dietary carbohydrates (Fig. 18.3). In the lumen of the intestine, polysaccharides in food particles are first degraded by **amylase**. Some of the amylase is derived from saliva (where it degrades amylose on teeth, the tongue, and the rest of the mouth, but plays only a minor role in the overall digestion of starch). Most of the amylase is secreted by the pancreas. Amylase degrades amylose and the linear portions of amylopectin mostly to **maltose** and **maltotriose**. In this way, amylopectin gives rise to **limit dextrins**, which are glucose polymers with linear portions of at most 10 monosaccharides. **Maltase-glucoamylase** and **sucrase-isomaltase** hydrolyze glucose residues near the branch points of limit dextrins, and isomaltase then hydrolyzes $\alpha(1\rightarrow6)$-linked residues. Mono-, di-, and oligosaccharides diffuse through the layer of mucus that covers the intestinal epithelium. In this way, they reach disaccharidases that are anchored to the luminal surface of intestinal epithelial cells. Some of the starch and glycogen escapes complete digestion in the small intestine and is degraded by **bacteria** in the ileum and colon (see Section 4 below). Normally, few bacteria colonize the stomach, duodenum, and jejunum.

Intestinal microvilli contain four different **disaccharidase complexes** (Fig. 18.4), which are encoded by four different genes and contain seven different hydrolytic enzyme activities, as described below. Each complex is derived from a single protein, protrudes into the intestinal lumen, and is anchored in the membrane of a microvillus (most often, the anchor consists of a membrane-spanning stretch of hydrophobic amino acids). Proteases, secreted from the pancreas into the lumen of the intestine, gradually degrade the disaccharidases. As a result, the disaccharidases have a mean lifetime of approximately 7 hours, and their activity changes up to two fold over the course of a day. Data on disaccharidase activities in biopsy material therefore must be interpreted accordingly.

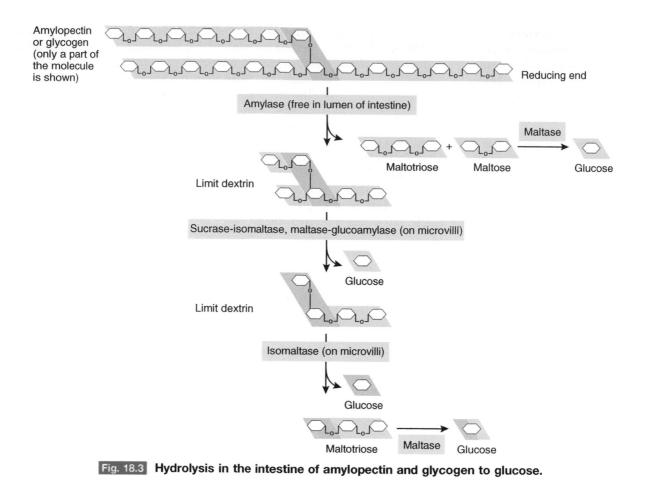

**Fig. 18.3** **Hydrolysis in the intestine of amylopectin and glycogen to glucose.**

The **sucrase** subunit of sucrase-isomaltase (see Fig. 18.4) hydrolyzes **sucrose** (see Fig. 18.1) into glucose and fructose; the isomaltase subunit hydrolyzes $\alpha(1\rightarrow6)$-glycosidic bonds that form the branch points in **limit dextrins**, which arise from the degradation of the branched polysaccharides amylopectin and glycogen (see Fig. 18.3). Sucrase-isomaltase also accounts for about 80% of the **maltose**-hydrolyzing activity in the intestine.

The **maltase** subunit of maltase-glucoamylase (see Fig. 18.4) hydrolyzes maltose (see Fig. 18.1) to glucose, while the **glucoamylase** subunit hydrolyzes $\alpha(1\rightarrow4)$-glycosidic bonds in **starch** to glucose. Maltase accounts for about 20% of the maltose-hydrolyzing activity in the intestine. Compared with amylase, glucoamylase prefers shorter polyglucose chains; furthermore, while amylase produces only maltose and maltotriose, glucoamylase produces only glucose. In addition, glucoamylase works at the end of a polyglucose chain, whereas amylase functions better at internal sites.

The **lactase** domain of lactase-glycosylceramidase (see Fig. 18.4) catalyzes the hydrolysis of **lactose** (see Fig. 18.1) to galactose and glucose, while the glycosylceramidase domain catalyzes the hydrolysis of a **glucosylceramide** to glucose and ceramide (ceramides contain two fatty acids; see Chapter 11). Lactase-glycosylceramidase is chiefly expressed in infancy (see Section 5 below).

**Trehalase** (see Fig. 18.4) hydrolyzes trehalose to glucose. **Trehalose** is the disaccharide glucose-$\alpha(1\rightarrow\alpha1)$-glucose, which is found chiefly in mushrooms.

## 3. TRANSPORT OF MONOSACCHARIDES

*Sodium-driven transporters for glucose and galactose pump glucose and galactose into intestinal epithelial cells and cells of the kidney tubules. Other transport proteins then facilitate equilibration of sugars between these epithelial cells and the blood. All other cells contain monosaccharide transporters that only facilitate equilibration (not pumping) across the plasma membrane. Some cells insert these transporters into the plasma membrane only in the presence of insulin or upon exercise.*

### 3.1. Intestinal Monosaccharide Transport

The microvilli of the small intestine contain a sodium-driven transporter for glucose and galactose (Fig. 18.5). Glucose and galactose are chiefly derived from the hydrolysis of di- and polysaccharides (see Section 2.2). Intestinal epithelial cells, like other cells in the body, contain a relatively *low* concentration of Na$^+$, while the intestinal lumen contains a much *higher*

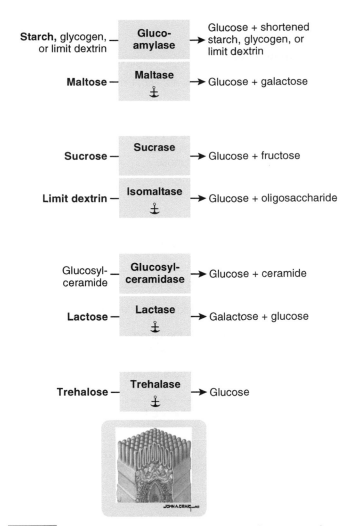

Starch, glycogen, or limit dextrin — **Gluco-amylase** → Glucose + shortened starch, glycogen, or limit dextrin

Maltose — **Maltase** → Glucose + galactose

Sucrose — **Sucrase** → Glucose + fructose

Limit dextrin — **Isomaltase** → Glucose + oligosaccharide

Glucosyl-ceramide — **Glucosyl-ceramidase** → Glucose + ceramide

Lactose — **Lactase** → Galactose + glucose

Trehalose — **Trehalase** → Glucose

**Fig. 18.4** **Disaccharidases of the small intestine are anchored to the microvilli.** Close stacking of enzyme names indicates tight binding of two enzymes; the anchoring unit is labeled.

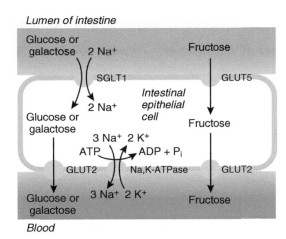

*Lumen of intestine*

*Blood*

**Fig. 18.5** **Transport of glucose, galactose, and fructose from the intestinal lumen to the bloodstream.**

concentration of $Na^+$ (the $Na^+$ in the intestinal lumen derives mostly from the fluid that is secreted by the exocrine pancreas). The inward-directed concentration gradient for $Na^+$ drives the uptake of glucose and galactose through the **Na:glucose cotransporter (SGLT1)**. This transporter has a 2 $Na^+$:1 monosaccharide stoichiometry, which allows virtually complete uptake of glucose and galactose from the intestinal lumen. The Na:glucose cotransporter transports either glucose or galactose.

The transport of glucose into the intestine tends to collapse the transmembrane $Na^+$ gradient; however, the basolateral membrane contains a **$Na^+$, $K^+$-ATPase**, which pumps $Na^+$ out of the cell into the extracellular space, from where it enters the bloodstream ($Na^+$ returns to the intestinal lumen via the pancreas; $K^+$ leaves the cell via $K^+$-channels).

The basolateral membrane of small-intestinal epithelial cells contains a transporter (**GLUT-2**) that facilitates the equilibration of **glucose** and **galactose** between the epithelial cells and the blood. Thus, whenever the concentration of glucose or galactose is higher in the intestinal epithelial cells than in

the blood, glucose or galactose show a net movement from the absorptive cells into the blood. Conversely, when the blood contains a higher concentration of glucose or galactose, these monosaccharides move from the blood into intestinal epithelial cells.

The small-intestinal epithelial cells also contain a transporter (**GLUT-5**) that facilitates the flow of **fructose** from the intestinal lumen into epithelial cells. Efflux of fructose from intestinal epithelial cells and uptake into other cells largely occurs via GLUT-2 transporters. The liver removes fructose from the blood and phosphorylates it, thereby acting as a sink for fructose (see Chapter 20).

### 3.2. Monosaccharide Transport in Tissues Other Than the Intestine

Different glucose transporters move glucose and galactose between the blood and peripheral cells (Table 18.1). Some of these transporters are in the cell membrane at all times, as in red blood cells or hepatocytes. Others are stored intracellularly and move into the plasma membrane only when the concentration of **insulin** is elevated; this is the case in adipose tissue and skeletal muscle. In skeletal muscle, contraction also causes plasma membrane insertion of these glucose transporters (for more details, see Chapters 19, 24, 25, and 26). In a variety of tissues, **hypoxia** can induce the expression, plasma membrane insertion, and activity of yet other passive glucose transporters.

The **GLUT glucose transporters** bind glucose on one side of the membrane, undergo a **conformational change**, and then release glucose on the other side of the membrane (Fig. 18.6). Thus, the substrate-binding site is alternately accessible from the inside and outside of a cell. Since these are passive transporters that facilitate diffusion, transport occurs from the side with the higher to the side with the lower glucose concentration. Section 2.2 of Chapter 11 contains a general discussion and classification of transport proteins in membranes.

**Table 18.1** **Glucose Transporters in Human Tissues**

| Category of Transporter | Tissue Location | Specific Transporter, Comments |
|---|---|---|
| Na+-driven pump | Intestinal epithelium (luminal side) | SGLT1 accepts glucose and galactose and is a 2 Na$^+$:1 monosaccharide cotransporter. |
| | Kidney tubules | SGLT2 accepts glucose (not galactose) and is a 1 Na$^+$:1 monosaccharide cotransporter; it moves the bulk of filtered glucose. SGLT1 moves the remainder of the filtered glucose. |
| Facilitated diffusion, not insulin-regulated | Erythrocytes | GLUT-1 facilitates uptake of glucose into erythrocytes for energy generation. |
| | Liver | GLUT-2 allows the liver to take up glucose in the fed state and release it in the fasting state. |
| | Intestinal epithelium | GLUT-2 equilibrates glucose between the basolateral side of epithelial cells and the blood. |
| | Kidneys | GLUT-1 and GLUT-2 equilibrate glucose with the blood. |
| | Islet β-cells | GLUT-2 equilibrates extracellular and intracellular glucose, which facilitates intracellular glucose sensing. |
| | Brain | GLUT-1 and GLUT-3 allow neurons and glial cells to take up glucose for energy generation. |
| Facilitated diffusion, insulin-sensitive | Adipocytes | GLUT-4 is active postprandially to transport glucose for deposition of fatty acids as triglycerides. |
| | Muscle (skeletal and cardiac) | GLUT-4 is active during muscle contraction and also postprandially to provide glucose for contraction and glycogen synthesis. |

The glucose transporters **GLUT-1**, **GLUT-3**, and **GLUT-4** also transport **dehydroascorbic acid**. Many animals, but not humans, can derive **L-ascorbic acid** (**vitamin C**) from glucose. L-ascorbate is an important redox cofactor with a variety of functions. It plays a role in reducing $Fe^{3+}$ in the lumen of the intestine to $Fe^{2+}$ that is then taken up (see Section 2 in Chapter 15). It is a required cofactor for the hydroxylation of proline residues in collagen to form hydroxyproline (see Section 1.2 in Chapter 12) and in the synthesis of norepinephrine in the nervous system (see Fig. 35.14). L-ascorbate also functions as an antioxidant throughout the body (see Section 2.3 in Chapter 21), but it is present at an especially high concentration in the brain. When L-ascorbate donates two electrons, it becomes dehydroascorbate. While dehydroascorbate is transported by GLUTs, L-ascorbate is mostly transported by the **Na$^+$-dependent vitamin C transporters 1 and 2**.

## 4. BACTERIAL METABOLISM OF UNDIGESTED CARBOHYDRATES THAT REACH THE COLON

*Bacteria in the distal ileum and the colon degrade some of the unabsorbed carbohydrates. This degradation may give rise to borborygmi, abdominal pain, and flatus. Hydrogen gas in exhaled air is a convenient diagnostic measure of bacterial metabolism following oral carbohydrate intake.*

The **intestinal flora** plays important roles in carbohydrate digestion and the conservation of water and electrolytes. Bacteria colonize the colon and distal ileum in large numbers, and adults excrete more than 50 g of microorganisms per day. Bacteria in the colon degrade carbohydrates to diverse products, such as **hydrogen** ($H_2$), methane, acetic acid, butyric acid, and propionic acid, which are taken up into the bloodstream or leave the intestine with feces. Indeed, oxidation of butyric acid is the principal source of energy in epithelial cells of the colon. When bacteria in the colon have been decimated

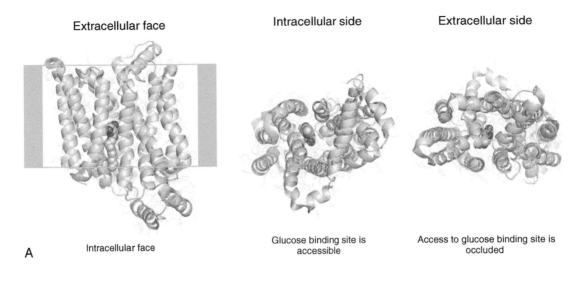

Extracellular face

Intracellular side

Extracellular side

A    Intracellular face

Glucose binding site is
accessible

Access to glucose binding site is
occluded

**Concept model for transport**

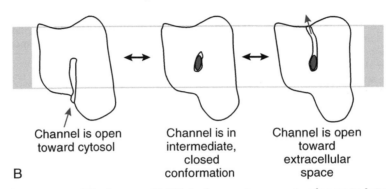

Channel is open
toward cytosol

Channel is in
intermediate,
closed
conformation

Channel is open
toward
extracellular
space

B

**Fig. 18.6** **Crystal structure of the human GLUT-1 glucose transporter (open to intracellular side).** The structure contains a glucose analog with a 9-carbon alkyl chain. (Data from Protein Data Bank [www.rcsb.org] file 4PYP and Deng D, Xu C, Sun P, et al. Crystal structure of the human glucose transporter GLUT1. *Nature.* 2014;510:121-125.)

(e.g., by **antibiotics**), or when the metabolic capacity of the normal intestinal flora is overwhelmed by unabsorbed carbohydrates, the remaining osmotically active nutrients may attract enough water to cause **diarrhea**, with the attendant loss of water and electrolytes. Per each mole of unabsorbed, osmotically active carbohydrate, the stools contain about 3.5 L of water (for instance, 1 g of lactose in the colon pulls with it about 10 g of water). Therefore, osmotically active, poorly degradable carbohydrates, such as insoluble **fiber** (see Section 1), are useful as **stool softeners.**

A **hydrogen breath test** following a carbohydrate load is often used in the diagnosis of carbohydrate malabsorption (Fig. 18.7). When bacteria digest carbohydrates in the colon, they produce gases, including $H_2$. $H_2$ diffuses to the blood, and, upon reaching the lungs, some of it is exhaled. The more carbohydrates the bacteria digest, the more $H_2$ is found in exhaled air. $H_2$ in a patient's breath is often measured before and at several time points 0.5 to 8 hours after the administration of a test sugar (e.g., lactose, fructose, xylose; often 25 to 50 g in an otherwise healthy adult). Patients differ in their gut microflora; as a result, up to 20% of patients fail to exhale

significant $H_2$ from undigested carbohydrate. However, such patients can be given **lactulose** (galactose-$\beta(1{\rightarrow}4)$-fructose), a sugar that is digested only by bacteria, to test for a proper $H_2$ response. Lactulose is also used as a laxative.

A hydrogen breath test after oral **lactulose** or **glucose** is also used to evaluate patients for **small-intestinal bacterial overgrowth**. An affected patient exhales an abnormally large amount of $H_2$. Glucose shows lower sensitivity than lactulose because the proximal small intestine absorbs glucose before it reaches the distal portion.

If the **stool pH** of a patient with diarrhea is below 5.6, the patient most likely has pure **carbohydrate malabsorption** (see Section 5). When excessive quantities of carbohydrates (at least about 50 g) reach the colon, the bacteria in the colon produce more acids (e.g., acetic acid, propionic acid, and butyric acid) from these carbohydrates than the colon can absorb, and the acids then lower the pH of feces to an abnormally low value.

Some carbohydrates are normally only *partially* digested by human enzymes in the small intestine. Thus, normally, 5% to 20% of **starch** (especially amylose) escapes degradation by

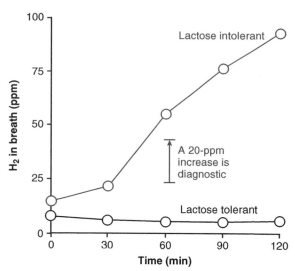

**Fig. 18.7** **Approximate mean H$_2$ in breath during a lactose breath hydrogen test.** Patients were classified by lactase nonpersistence genotype. (Based on data from Waud JP, Matthews SB, Campbell AK. Measurement of breath hydrogen and methane, together with lactase genotype, defines the current best practice for investigation of lactose sensitivity. *Ann Clin Biochem.* 2008;45:50-58 and Nagy D, Bogacsi-Szabo E, Varkonyi A, et al. Prevalence of adult-type hypolactasia as diagnosed with genetic and lactose hydrogen breath tests in Hungarians. *Eur J Clin Nutr.* 2009;63:909-912.)

Figure labels: H$_2$ in breath (ppm); Lactose intolerant; A 20-ppm increase is diagnostic; Lactose tolerant; Time (min)

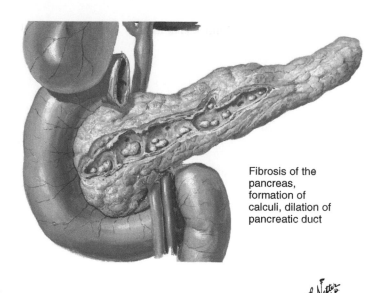

Fibrosis of the pancreas, formation of calculi, dilation of pancreatic duct

**Fig. 18.8** **Chronic pancreatitis.** The disease is commonly due to long-term excessive consumption of alcohol, but it can also be due to a mutation in the chloride transporter CFTR or the protease trypsinogen.

amylase and disaccharidases. Similarly, **fructose**, when present in sufficient quantity, can escape intestinal uptake and lead to abdominal pain and diarrhea. This frequently happens with children who drink large volumes of apple juice.

Some carbohydrates cannot be digested by *human* enzymes in the small intestine, whereas *bacteria* in the ileum and colon can digest them. Since humans do not produce α-galactosidase, they cannot degrade dietary α-galactosides, the major ones being raffinose and stachyose. **Raffinose** (galactose-α(1→6)-glucose-α(1→2)-β-fructose) and **stachyose** ("galactose-elongated raffinose" (i.e., galactose-α(1→6)-galactose-α(1→6)-glucose-α(1→2)-β-fructose) are both found in legumes (e.g., beans) and to a lesser extent in vegetables of the *Brassica* genus (e.g., cabbage, Brussels sprouts, and broccoli). Bacteria in the colon do possess α-galactosidase and degrade these oligosaccharides. Oral **α-galactosidase** (**Beano**) cleaves dietary raffinose and stachyose into galactose and sucrose while in the small intestine; Beano can thus prevent abdominal discomfort after the ingestion of raffinose or stachyose. Human enzymes also fail to degrade **sorbitol**, a reduced derivative of glucose. Sorbitol is quite abundant in prunes, and somewhat less abundant in pear juice and apple juice. Sorbitol is the most frequently used sugar in "sugarless" chewing gum. Sorbitol can be used as an **excipient**, an inactive substance that acts as a carrier of an active substance in a tablet. Intestinal bacteria do degrade sorbitol, and these bacteria can produce gas.

Most **insoluble fiber** (i.e., cellulose, lignins) *cannot* be digested by either human enzymes or bacteria in the human intestine. The nature of insoluble fiber is described in Section 1.

## 5. CARBOHYDRATE MALABSORPTION

*Carbohydrate malabsorption occurs when dietary carbohydrate is not adequately digested either by the patient's pancreatic and small-intestinal enzymes or by bacteria in the colon and distal ileum. Carbohydrate malabsorption is usually due to pancreatic insufficiency, diminished functional capacity of the small intestine to degrade and transport carbohydrates, or an inadequate bacterial flora.*

### 5.1. General Comments

Inadequate digestion of carbohydrates can be the cause of inadequate growth in young children.

Oral sugar **tolerance tests** provide information about the overall digestive capacity of the intestine. Such tests are less invasive and often more meaningful than measurements of disaccharidase activities in biopsies of the jejunal or duodenal epithelium. The oral load is usually 2 g/kg of body weight, not to exceed 50 g total. Oral sugar tolerance tests may include measurements of sugar in blood or feces (see Section 1); alternatively, bacterial metabolites may be measured in blood (e.g., acetate), feces (e.g., lactate), or exhaled air (e.g., hydrogen gas; see Section 4).

As a rule, sugars are absent from the stools. If sugars are found in the stools, the patient has carbohydrate malabsorption.

### 5.2. Pancreatic Insufficiency

Patients with severe pancreatic insufficiency due to **pancreatitis** (Fig. 18.8), pancreatic **cancer**, or **cystic fibrosis** have significantly decreased small-intestinal carbohydrate absorption.

As pancreatic insufficiency develops, digestion of lipids and proteins is impaired before the digestion of starch and glycogen. Oral pancreatic enzymes can make up for the abnormality.

## 5.3. Diminished Capacity of the Small Intestine to Degrade Carbohydrates

The most common problem of carbohydrate absorption is **lactose intolerance** (also called **lactose restriction, lactase deficiency**, and **hypolactasia**), which affects most of the world's **adults**. The exceptions are people from ethnic groups in which the keeping of cattle and the consumption of unfermented milk is or was common (i.e., parts of Africa, Asia, and Europe). These latter adults express sufficient lactase to handle about 50 to 100 g of lactose per day (the amount contained in about 0.8 to 1.7 L of milk). Lactase persistence is inherited in an autosomal dominant fashion. In people with nonpersistence, consumption of as little as 3 g lactose/day may be more than the small-intestinal lactase can handle and may lead to excessive production of gas by bacteria in the colon (see Fig. 18.7). The patient then experiences any of the following: bloating, borborygmi (i.e., rumbling in the intestine from moving gas and fluid), abdominal pain, flatulence, and diarrhea (Fig. 18.9). Patients with poor lactose tolerance should either avoid consuming more lactose than their lactase can handle, or they should take **oral lactase** (drops or pills). Lactose amounts to approximately 6% of the weight of milk (regardless of the fat content), 4% of ice cream, 4% of cheese, and 2% of yogurt. Some milk products are treated with lactase to reduce their lactose content.

The **diagnosis of lactose intolerance** may involve an oral lactose tolerance test (50 g of lactose in water by mouth with repeated measurement of $H_2$ in exhaled air [Fig. 18.7] or measurement of the concentration of glucose in blood).

**Premature babies** are often lactose intolerant because cells of the small intestine fully express lactase only late in the third trimester of pregnancy, but **congenital lactase deficiency** is rare. Premature babies and babies with congenital lactase deficiency are both treated with an appropriate low-lactose diet.

Infection of the upper small intestine with the pathogenic protozoan *Giardia lamblia* is very common. The infection leads to villus atrophy and consequent symptoms of malabsorption.

The decimation of absorptive epithelial enterocytes by cancer **chemotherapy**, protein **malnutrition**, or **bacterial toxins** also leads to carbohydrate malabsorption.

**Celiac disease** (also called celiac sprue or gluten-sensitive enteropathy) is an autoimmune disease that is characterized by chronic inflammation of the small-intestinal mucosa, atrophy of intestinal villi, and malabsorption. In Europe and North America, celiac disease affects about 1% of the population. In affected patients, inflammation occurs in response to the consumption of **gliadin** proteins (which are part of **gluten**) present in wheat, rye, and barley. The inflammation leads to a loss of epithelial cells and a concomitant loss of digestive and absorptive capacity.

In the treatment of type 2 diabetes, **acarbose**, an analog of polysaccharides, is sometimes used to inhibit amylase and intestinal disaccharidases; acarbose thus induces mild carbohydrate malabsorption. Acarbose inhibits α-glucosidases, such as amylase, maltase, and sucrase; it does not inhibit β-glucosidases (e.g., lactase). Flatulence and diarrhea are side effects of acarbose.

**Short bowel syndrome** occurs in patients who have less than 50% of the normal length of small bowel. In these

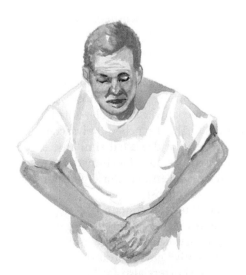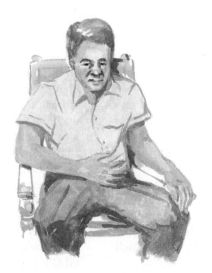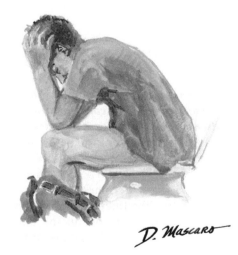

**Fig. 18.9** **Adverse effects of lactose in lactose-intolerant patients.** The same symptoms apply to other components of the diet that elicit extensive gas production by bacteria and/or result in osmotically active compounds in the colon.

patients, absorption of carbohydrates in the small intestine is significantly reduced, while bacterial fermentation is increased.

**Trehalase deficiency** causes diarrhea after the consumption of mushrooms, but the link between cause and effect is often not recognized. Affected patients should abstain from consuming the offending sugar. Among most populations, trehalase deficiency is probably uncommon.

**Congenital sucrase-isomaltase deficiency** affects about 0.1% of the population in Europe and the United States and roughly 5% of the Inuit in the arctic regions of Greenland, Canada, and Alaska. The deficiency first manifests in infants when they ingest sucrose with formula or other food (note that many formulas are free of sucrose). The final diagnosis relies on sucrase-isomaltase activity in biopsy material. There are many different sucrase-isomaltase mutations. Almost all patients with sucrase-isomaltase deficiency lack sucrase activity but this can be of limited clinical consequence because maltase-glucoamylase splits $\alpha(1{\rightarrow}4)$-glycosidic bonds. Some patients have no loss in isomaltase activity, whereas others have complete loss of it, which greatly impairs degradation of amylopectins [i.e., $\alpha(1{\rightarrow}6)$-branched starches]. Some 5% of the U.S. population is heterozygous for sucrase-isomaltase deficiency, and some of these patients therefore have a reduced capacity for carbohydrate digestion. Treatment of any sucrase-isomaltase deficiency involves the restriction of starch and/or sucrose intake to a tolerable level.

**Glucose-galactose malabsorption** is due to a deficiency in the **Na$^+$-driven glucose transporter** (**SGLT1**) in the intestine. This rare deficiency becomes apparent shortly after the first feeding. Lactose in milk is hydrolyzed to galactose and glucose, which reach the colon and cause massive diarrhea. Treatment is difficult because patients must not consume appreciable quantities of any carbohydrates that contain glucose or galactose. Patients can absorb fructose, but the consumption of a large amount of fructose is unhealthy (see Chapter 20). The transporter deficiency affects the kidney tubules to a lesser degree because the tubules also express the SGLT2 Na-driven glucose transporter (see Table 18.1).

## 6. SGLT INHIBITORS: DRUGS THAT INHIBIT Na$^+$-COUPLED GLUCOSE TRANSPORT

*Drugs that inhibit Na$^+$-coupled glucose uptake in the kidneys are used to lower the concentration of glucose in the blood of patients who have type 2 diabetes.*

Without treatment, patients who have **diabetes** have chronically elevated concentrations of glucose in the blood. Long-term, chronic hyperglycemia leads to damage of the retina, kidneys, peripheral nerves, and other systems (see Chapter 39). Treatment of diabetes is aimed at lowering the concentration of glucose in the blood towards the normal value. The treatment should not induce hypoglycemia, which is acutely dangerous.

Inhibition of the Na$^+$-coupled glucose transporter **SGLT2** by one of the **gliflozin** drugs lowers blood glucose in type 2 diabetic patients by preventing the uptake of some of the filtered glucose in the kidneys. The kidneys use two types of glucose transporter to recover glucose from the glomerular filtrate, SGLT2 and SGLT1. SGLT2 transporters in the proximal *convoluted* tubules have a 1:1 stoichiometry for Na$^+$ and glucose and they normally transport most of the filtered glucose. Then, cells in the proximal *straight* tubule use SGLT1 transporters with a 2 Na$^+$:1 glucose stoichiometry to take up essentially all remaining glucose. In the kidneys, SGLT1 transporters have a lower transport capacity than the SGLT2 transporters. Near-complete inhibition of SGLT2 by a gliflozin leaves all of the glucose transport to the SGLT1 transporters, which exceeds their capacity and thus results in a ~35% loss of filtered glucose. This ongoing loss of glucose into the urine leads to a lowering of blood glucose by about 10 mg/dL. Currently, FDA-approved inhibitors are **canagliflozin, dapagliflozin,** and **empagliflozin.**

## SUMMARY

- The most common dietary carbohydrates are the monosaccharides glucose, galactose, and fructose; the disaccharides lactose, and sucrose; and the polysaccharides starch and glycogen. Lactose consists of glucose and galactose, while sucrose consists of glucose and fructose. The starches consist of variable mixtures of the linear polysaccharide amylose and the branched polysaccharide amylopectin; the structure of glycogen resembles that of amylopectin. Glucose, galactose, fructose, and lactose are reducing sugars.

- Fiber consists of oligosaccharides, polysaccharides, and lignins that cannot be digested by human enzymes; however, bacteria in the gut can degrade part of this fiber.

- The walls and folds of the small intestine are covered with villi of ~1 mm length. The surface of the villi contains absorptive cells that are continually renewed. The plasma membrane of these absorptive cells forms numerous microvilli, to which disaccharidases are anchored. The microvilli and disaccharidases are covered by mucus, through which di- and oligosaccharides diffuse much faster than do large polysaccharides.

- In the small intestine, amylase degrades the linear polysaccharide amylose to maltotriose and maltose. Sucrase-isomaltase and maltase-glucoamylase hydrolyze maltotriose and maltose to glucose. The branched polysaccharides amylopectin and glycogen are degraded similarly, except that branched oligosaccharides, so-called limit dextrins, are also formed. Sucrase-isomaltase and maltase-glucoamylase hydrolyze limit dextrins to glucose.

- Microvilli of the small intestine contain Na$^+$-dependent glucose transporters (SGLTs) that pump glucose or galactose into intestinal epithelial cells. Glucose and galactose leave these cells via facilitative glucose transporters of the GLUT family. GLUT transporters also facilitate the entry of glucose and galactose into peripheral cells. SGLT and GLUT transporters also participate in the recovery of glucose from blood filtrate in the kidneys.

■ Gliflozin inhibitors of SGLTs induce glucosuria and are used in the treatment of type 2 diabetes.

■ Fructose diffuses through facilitative transporters in the absorptive epithelial cells into the bloodstream.

■ The colon and the terminal ileum contain bacteria that degrade unabsorbed carbohydrates to acids and gasses that are either taken up into the bloodstream or leave the intestine via feces or flatus. Since humans do not digest 10% to 25% of dietary starch, bacteria degrade it. Bacteria also degrade some of the dietary fiber (most of it soluble), and most of the dietary sorbitol, lactulose, raffinose, and stachyose, which human enzymes cannot degrade. Saccharides that are osmotically active and at most only partially degraded by bacteria are effective as stool softeners.

■ Carbohydrate malabsorption occurs as a consequence of inadequate secretion of amylase from the pancreas, inadequate disaccharidase activity, or inadequate uptake of monosaccharides. Laboratory data that are indicative of carbohydrate malabsorption are increased breath hydrogen, blood lactate, or fecal acetate after a carbohydrate load, or a pH of feces lower than 5.6. The release of pancreatic amylase may be compromised by pancreatitis, pancreatic cancer, or cystic fibrosis. The absorptive capacity of the intestinal epithelium may be diminished by inflammatory bowel disease, infection, protein malnutrition, or a hereditary deficiency of a disaccharidase or a monosaccharide transporter.

## FURTHER READING

■ Barker N. Adult intestinal stem cells: critical drivers of epithelial homeostasis and regeneration. *Nat Rev Mol Cell Biol.* 2014;15:19-33.

■ Berry AJ. Pancreatic enzyme replacement therapy during pancreatic insufficiency. *Nutr Clin Pract.* 2014;29:312-321.

■ Hammer HF, Hammer J. Diarrhea caused by carbohydrate malabsorption. *Gastroenterol Clin North Am.* 2012;41: 611-627.

■ Mueckler M, Thorens B. The SLC2 (GLUT) family of membrane transporters. *Mol Aspects Med.* 2013;34:121-138.

# Review Questions

1. A patient has symptoms of lactase deficiency. A hydrogen breath test during an oral 50 g lactose load is negative, even though the patient has symptoms of malabsorption. To determine whether there is a problem with the hydrogen breath test, the test should be repeated with which of the following?

   A. Antibiotics
   B. Fructose
   C. Galactose
   D. Glucose
   E. Lactulose

2. In response to a large mixed meal, the number of glucose transporters in the plasma membrane increases most markedly in which one of the following cell types?

   A. Adipocyte
   B. Hepatocyte
   C. Intestinal epithelial cell
   D. Neuron
   E. Red blood cell

3. A patient who has diabetes routinely takes acarbose, an inhibitor of intestinal α-glucosidases. One day, he accidentally also injects too much insulin and becomes mildly hypoglycemic. Which one of the following carbohydrates should he consume to increase the concentration of glucose in his blood as quickly as possible?

   A. Amylose
   B. Lactose
   C. Maltose
   D. Stachyose
   E. Sucrose

4. Abnormally low lactase activity was found in biopsied material from the small intestine of a 2-month old, ill baby who had persistent severe vomiting and diarrhea. The baby had been breastfed. The low lactase activity could be due to which of the following?

   A. Congenital isomaltase deficiency
   B. Deficiency of the intestinal fructose transporter
   C. Insufficient secretion of amylase
   D. Protein malnutrition

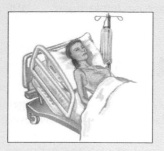

# Chapter 19

# Glycolysis and Its Regulation by Hormones and Hypoxia

## SYNOPSIS

- Glycolysis is the process of converting glucose to pyruvate. All cells can perform glycolysis.
- Red blood cells and the glial cells of the brain always depend on glycolysis for adenosine triphosphate (ATP) production; most other cells can produce sufficient ATP from other fuels.
- As you will see in Chapters 22 and 23, mitochondria can metabolize pyruvate to $CO_2$ and water by the combination of the citric acid cycle and oxidative phosphorylation (Fig. 19.1); this yields a much larger amount of ATP than does glycolysis alone.
- If pyruvate is not metabolized in mitochondria, it is reduced to lactate, which is released into the blood. This happens, for instance, in red blood cells, contracting fast-twitch muscle cells, and hypoxic cells.
- Adenosine monophosphate (AMP) stimulates glycolysis, while ATP feedback inhibits it. As a result, glycolysis tends to maintain a constant, relatively high concentration of ATP. Furthermore, ATP that is produced in the combination of citric acid cycle and oxidative phosphorylation attenuates the flux in glycolysis.
- In some cells, glycolysis is regulated by hormones (e.g., insulin, glucagon, and epinephrine).
- If mitochondrial ATP production is impaired (e.g., due to local hypoxia), glycolysis speeds up and produces lactic acid. The human body cannot handle the acid load that results from persistent anoxia in *all* organs; the resulting acidosis is fatal.
- Flux in glycolysis is impaired during hypophosphatemia, which is a complication of parenteral nutrition, chronic alcohol abuse, or diabetic ketoacidosis.
- Heritable deficiencies of enzymes of glycolysis are quite rare. In red blood cells, they give rise to hemolytic anemia.

## LEARNING OBJECTIVES

*For mastery of this topic, you should be able to do the following*:
- Describe the overall purpose of glycolysis, its reactants and products, its cellular location, and its tissue distribution.
- Describe the roles of hexokinase or glucokinase, phosphofructokinase-1 (PFK-1), and pyruvate kinase in glycolysis, thereby paying attention to the compounds that regulate the activity of these enzymes.
- Describe the roles of AMP, ATP, fructose 1,6-bisphosphate, and fructose 2,6-bisphosphate in the regulation of glycolysis.
- Explain how and in which tissues insulin, glucagon, and epinephrine can regulate flux in glycolysis.
- Compare and contrast aerobic and anaerobic glycolysis regarding the tissues and conditions in which they occur. Describe the reactants and products of these two processes.
- Describe the purpose of the reaction catalyzed by lactate dehydrogenase, its reactants, and products, cellular and tissue location. Interpret the findings of an elevated concentration of lactate dehydrogenase in blood plasma.
- Describe the role and fate of cytosolic NADH produced in glycolysis.
- Predict changes in the rate of ATP synthesis and the concentrations of intermediates of glycolysis when there is a deficiency of an enzyme of glycolysis (e.g., diminished activity of glyceraldehyde phosphate dehydrogenase, or pyruvate kinase deficiency).
- Describe the cause, signs, and treatment of pellagra.
- Describe the role and production of 2,3-bisphosphoglycerate in red blood cells, and list the factors that influence its concentration.
- Interpret/explain the reason for a strong positron emission tomography (PET) scan signal from tissue that is exposed to radioactively labeled fluorodeoxyglucose.

## 1. CHEMICAL REACTIONS OF GLYCOLYSIS

*Glycolysis produces two molecules of pyruvate per molecule of glucose.*

**Glucose transporters** move glucose between the extracellular and the intracellular space (see Section 3 in Chapter 18 and Table 18.1). Glycolysis takes place in the cytosol.

The reactions of glycolysis are shown in Fig. 19.2. The **net reaction** of glycolysis is:

$$\text{Glucose} + 2\,\text{ADP} + 2\,\text{phosphate} + 2\,\text{NAD}^+$$
$$\rightarrow 2\,\text{pyruvate} + 2\,\text{ATP} + 2\,\text{NADH} + 2\,\text{H}^+ + 2\,\text{H}_2\text{O}$$

All cells are capable of glycolysis. As detailed in Section 4, several intermediates and products of glycolysis constitute a starting or end point for other metabolic pathways (see Fig. 19.11).

There are no plasma membrane transporters for the *phosphorylated* intermediates of glycolysis, and the lipid bilayer does not allow them to pass through.

Enzymes that catalyze irreversible reactions are regulated as described in Sections 3 and 5 below. Enzymes that catalyze reversible reactions are not regulated.

Glycolysis by itself yields a modest amount of **ATP** (see Fig. 19.2). Early in the pathway, ATP is consumed, but ATP is later produced such that the return is greater than the initial investment. The conversion of glucose to pyruvate yields two ATP and 2 NADH. In *anaerobic* glycolysis, explained in Section 2, the net gain is two ATP, while in *aerobic* glycolysis, the gain is about 5 to 7 ATP because NADH can also give rise to ATP (see Section 2 and Chapter 23).

In glycolysis, **NAD$^+$** serves as an electron acceptor (i.e., as an oxidizing agent; see Figs. 19.2 and 19.3). NAD$^+$ is an abbreviation of nicotinamide adenine dinucleotide. The pyridine ring of NAD$^+$ is the electron acceptor. The nitrogen of the pyridine ring is positively charged, and hence it

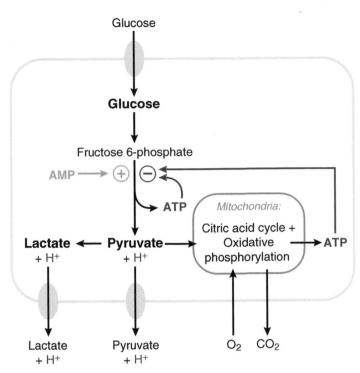

**Fig. 19.1** **Overview of cellular ATP production and its effect on glycolysis.**

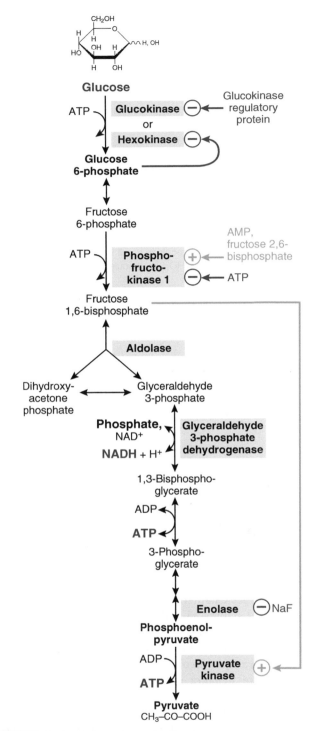

**Fig. 19.2** **Reactions of glycolysis.** NaF is used clinically to inhibit glycolysis in blood samples.

is commonplace to write this species as $NAD^+$; however, at physiologic pH, $NAD^+$ is in fact negatively charged because it carries two negative charges on its phosphate groups. With the incorporation of *one proton* and *two electrons*, $NAD^+$ is reduced to **NADH**. Many biochemical reactions produce two electrons and *two* $H^+$, and the partial redox reaction is then $NAD^+ + 2H^+ + 2e^- \rightarrow NADH + H^+$.

NAD$^+$ and NADH play a major role in various other metabolic pathways that are linked to ATP generation. Besides glycolysis, NADH is also produced in the citric acid cycle (see Chapter 22), fatty acid oxidation (see Chapter 27), and ketone body oxidation (see Chapter 27). NADH is oxidized to $NAD^+$ chiefly in oxidative phosphorylation (see Chapter 23), a process that is responsible for most of the ATP production in cells that contain respiring mitochondria.

The type of ATP synthesis that occurs in glycolysis is called **substrate level phosphorylation** as opposed to *oxidative* phosphorylation, which occurs in mitochondria (see Chapter 23). In glycolysis, a substrate with a "high-energy" phosphate bond phosphorylates ADP to generate ATP. In oxidative phosphorylation, reduced compounds (e.g., NADH) are oxidized and thereby generate an electrochemical $H^+$ gradient that drives the phosphorylation of ADP to ATP.

$NAD^+$ and NADH (as well as $NADP^+$ and NADPH; see Chapter 21) are synthesized from **niacin mononucleotide** (Fig. 19.4). Niacin mononucleotide, in turn, is derived either from **niacin (vitamin B$_3$, nicotinic acid)** in the diet or the degradation of the amino acid **tryptophan** (see Fig. 35.16). Most humans produce about half of their niacin mononucleotide from nicotinic acid in the diet and derive the remainder from the degradation of tryptophan.

If tryptophan and niacin intake are abnormally low, **pellagra** develops (see Fig. 19.5). Pellagra is associated with dementia, dermatitis, and diarrhea (often called the "three D's"; at times, a fourth "D" is added for death). Pellagra due to *inadequate nutrition* is endemic in parts of Africa and Asia; in developed nations, it is now seen mostly in patients with an intestinal disease, **Hartnup disease** (which affects the uptake of tryptophan; see Chapter 34), chronic **alcoholism**, or **anorexia** nervosa.

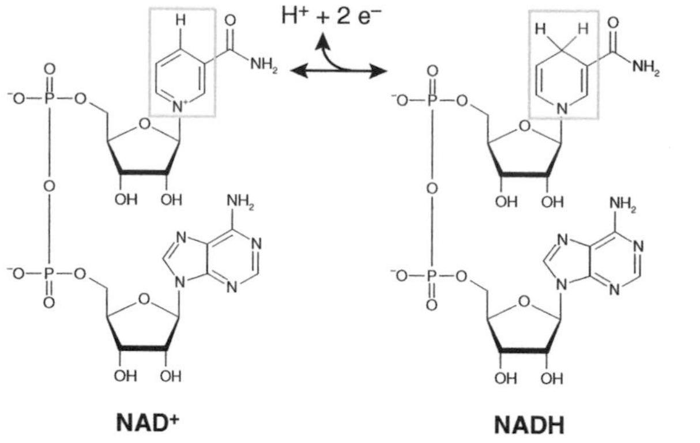

$$H^+ + 2\,e^-$$

**NAD⁺**                    **NADH**

**Fig. 19.3** **Structures of NAD⁺ and NADH.** The yellow boxes highlight the pyridine ring, which can gain or lose electrons. As NAD⁺ is reduced to NADH, another molecule in a cell is oxidized (e.g., in glycolysis, an aldehyde group, –CHO, is oxidized to a carboxyl group, –COOH).

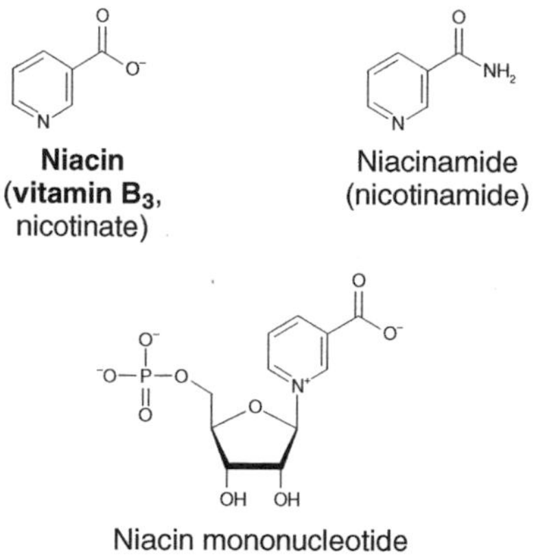

**Niacin**
**(vitamin B₃,**
nicotinate)

Niacinamide
(nicotinamide)

Niacin mononucleotide

**Fig. 19.4** **Structures of precursors of NAD⁺.**

Insufficient conversion of tryptophan to niacin mononucleotide occurs in patients who have a deficiency of **vitamin B₂** (**riboflavin**; see Chapter 22) or **vitamin B₆** (**pyridoxine**; see Section 2.3 in Chapter 35 and Section 9 in Chapter 36), and in patients taking medications long term, such as **isoniazid**, **5-fluorouracil**, **6-mercaptopurine**, **phenobarbital**, **azathioprine**, or **chloramphenicol**.

Treatment of pellagra involves extra doses of **niacin** or nicotinamide.

Unrelated to pellagra, in patients with dyslipidemia, niacin in very large doses is sometimes used to increase the fraction of HDL particles.

## 2. AEROBIC VERSUS ANAEROBIC GLYCOLYSIS

*Glycolysis can be carried out either in aerobic or anaerobic fashion. In anaerobic glycolysis, reducing power from NADH is transferred to pyruvate, producing lactate that is released into the blood as lactic acid. The advantage of anaerobic glycolysis is that it allows ATP to be produced in the absence of oxygen; its disadvantage is that it produces lactic acid, which may cause life-threatening acidosis. In aerobic*

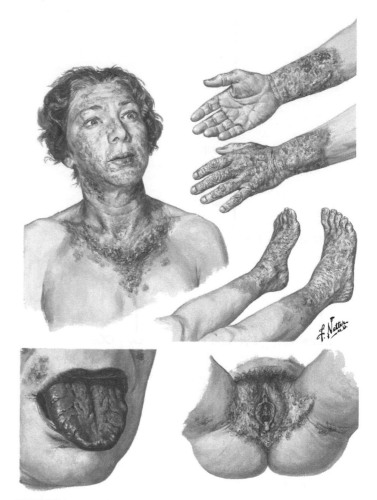

**Fig. 19.5** **Lesions that are typical of pellagra.** Most patients show erythema on the backs of their hands and feet, sometimes in a glove-and-stocking fashion. Lesions on the face and around the neck ("Casal's necklace") are also common. About one-third of patients with pellagra show cheilitis, angular stomatitis, and glossitis. Perineal lesions are common. Women are more readily affected because estrogen inhibits tryptophan degradation to niacin mononucleotide.

*glycolysis, the reducing power from NADH is ultimately transferred to the O₂ inside mitochondria. The advantage of aerobic glycolysis (working together with the citric acid cycle and oxidative phosphorylation) is that for each glucose molecule it yields about 15 times more ATP than does anaerobic glycolysis.*

### 2.1. Production of NADH in Glycolysis

In glycolysis, the oxidation of glyceraldehyde 3-phosphate to 1,3-bisphosphoglycerate consumes NAD⁺ and produces NADH + H⁺ (see Fig. 19.2). The supply of NAD⁺ is small compared with the rate of this reaction. Hence, NADH has to be recycled to NAD⁺; otherwise, glycolysis rapidly comes to a standstill. NADH can be oxidized to NAD⁺ in three different ways (Figs. 19.6 and 19.7): (1) via the reduction of pyruvate to lactate; (2) via the glycerol-phosphate shuttle; or (3) via the malate-aspartate shuttle. Production of lactate works in the

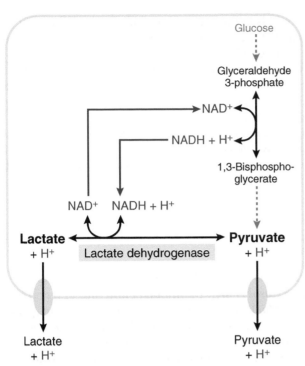

**Fig. 19.6** In anaerobic glycolysis, NADH reduces pyruvate to lactate.

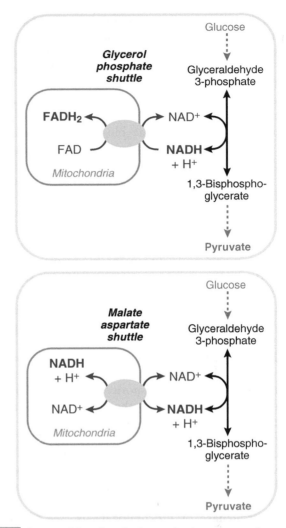

**Fig. 19.7** In aerobic glycolysis, reducing power from NADH is transferred into mitochondria via the glycerolphosphate shuttle (top) or the malate-aspartate shuttle (bottom). The shuttles are depicted in a simplified manner. There is no transmembrane transport of NAD+ or NADH.

absence of oxygen and is an integral part of *anaerobic* glycolysis (see Section 2.2). The shuttles require the *presence* of oxygen and functioning mitochondria and permit *aerobic* glycolysis (see Section 2.3).

## 2.2. Cells Performing Anaerobic Glycolysis Release Lactic Acid

Anaerobic glycolysis does not require oxygen, and it occurs in cells that have no or few functioning mitochondria (e.g., in red blood cells, contracting fast-twitch muscle fibers, and in all hypoxic cells). NADH reduces pyruvate to lactate, catalyzed by lactate dehydrogenase (LDH; see Fig. 19.6). Lactate leaves the cell through a **monocarboxylic acid transporter, MCT**, as lactic acid (MCT transporters also transport pyruvic acid, the ketone bodies acetoacetic acid and β-hydroxybutyric acid [see Section 5 in Chapter 27], and acetic acid).

Anaerobic glycolysis results in the net phosphorylation of 2 moles of ADP to ATP per mole of glucose metabolized. The cell eventually hydrolyzes the ATP to ADP and phosphate. If ATP hydrolysis and anaerobic glycolysis are combined, the net result is

$$\text{glucose} \rightarrow 2\,\text{lactate}^- + 2\,\text{H}^+ \ or$$

$$\text{glucose} \rightarrow 2\,\text{lactic acid}$$

Since the pK of lactic acid is about 4, most of the lactic acid in the cytosol and blood plasma dissociates into lactate⁻ and H⁺. From the above equation it is apparent that a cell that performs anaerobic glycolysis releases lactic acid into its environment.

Tissues that depend on anaerobic glycolysis are red blood cells; the lens of the eye (there are no blood vessels and little ATP is needed; glucose and lactic acid diffuse between the lens, the vitreous body, and the aqueous humor); the renal medulla (a tissue that maintains a countercurrent transport gradient, and the cells involved in this are too far from blood vessels to allow proper oxygenation); glial cells of the brain (see Section 5.2) contracting fast-twitch muscles; contracting slow-twitch muscles that exceed their aerobic capacity; and any hypoxic tissue. When these cells release lactate into the bloodstream, other cells (e.g., in the liver, heart, or skeletal muscle) take it up and metabolize it. Cells in the skin epithelium produce lactic acid and release it to the surface as a bacteriostatic agent.

Patients who produce too much lactic acid or do not adequately remove lactic acid from the blood can develop **lactic acidosis**, which may be life-threatening. Lactic acidosis is characterized by an abnormally high concentration of lactic acid (i.e., lactate) and an abnormally low pH in blood.

Causes of lactic acidosis are compromised oxidative phosphorylation (e.g., due to hypoxia), or an inadequate removal of lactate and pyruvate due to severe alcohol intoxication (see Section 3.1 in Chapter 30), pyruvate dehydrogenase deficiency (see Section 5.6 in Chapter 22), or a block in gluconeogenesis (see Section 4.1 in Chapter 25). A low blood pH is neurotoxic.

When lactic acid enters the blood and dissociates into lactate$^-$ and H$^+$, it acidifies the blood; conversely, when lactic acid leaves the blood, it alkalinizes it. A lactic acid–induced shift to a lower pH is buffered by bicarbonate, $HCO_3^-$, which binds H$^+$ and thereby becomes carbonic acid ($H_2CO_3$), which in turn dissociates into water and $CO_2$. Driven by a lowered blood pH, the affected person exhales extra $CO_2$ into the environment. These processes lead to a low concentration of bicarbonate and $CO_2$ in the blood plasma (the pH of blood depends on the ratio $[HCO_3^-]/[CO_2]$; see Section 4 in Chapter 16; in acidosis, the ratio is too small). The kidneys can also neutralize acid (see Chapter 35), but their capacity is much smaller than the $CO_2$-removing capacity of the lungs.

The **lactate/pyruvate ratio** in blood plasma is sometimes used to pinpoint the cause of lactic acidosis in a patient. Since the monocarboxylic acid transporters equilibrate both lactic acid and pyruvic acid across the plasma membrane, the lactate/pyruvate ratio in the blood reflects on the ratio of NADH/NAD$^+$ in the cytosol (it is not the same, but proportional to it). The lactate/pyruvate ratio is *increased* in patients who have tissue **hypoxia** or a problem in the **electron transport** chain (see Chapter 23). The lactate/pyruvate ratio is *normal* in acidotic patients who have a defect in **pyruvate dehydrogenase** or **gluconeogenesis** (see Chapters 22 and 25).

## 2.3. Aerobic Glycolysis: Cells Produce ATP From the Reducing Power of NADH

In aerobic glycolysis, NADH from glycolysis is oxidized to NAD$^+$, and the reducing power from NADH is then transferred into the mitochondria by one of the shuttles described below. The *outer* mitochondrial membrane is permeable to small molecules, including NAD$^+$ and NADH. However, NAD$^+$ and NADH cannot cross the *inner* mitochondrial membrane (or the plasma membrane) because they are both hydrophilic, charged molecules, and there are no transporters for them.

The **glycerol phosphate shuttle** transfers the reducing power *unidirectionally* from the cytosolic NADH to intramitochondrial FAD, thereby generating FADH$_2$ inside the mitochondria (see Fig. 19.7). The structures of FAD and FADH$_2$ are shown in Fig. 22.5.

The **malate-aspartate shuttle** transfers reducing power *bidirectionally* between NADH in the cytosol and NADH in the mitochondria (see Fig. 19.7). This shuttle can thus generate NADH in the mitochondria or the cytosol. Export of reducing equivalents from the mitochondria through the malate-aspartate shuttle is required for gluconeogenesis from

amino acids in the liver and the kidneys (see Chapter 25) and for some of the production of NADPH for fatty acid synthesis (see Chapter 27).

Inside the mitochondria, **oxidative phosphorylation** oxidizes NADH to NAD$^+$ and FADH$_2$ to FAD, thereby generating ATP (see Chapter 23). In cells with oxygenated mitochondria, pyruvate can be oxidized to $CO_2$ in the citric acid cycle (see Chapter 22); this yields additional NADH, FADH$_2$, and ATP. In this way, the complete oxidation of glucose to $CO_2$ yields about 15 times more ATP than does anaerobic glycolysis from glucose to lactate.

## 3. BASIC MECHANISMS IN THE REGULATION OF GLYCOLYSIS

*Glycolysis is regulated such that the concentration of ATP in the cytosol is high (millimolar) and that of free AMP low (nanomolar). In some cells, glycolysis is the principal means of ATP production; in others it has only a backup role. In most normal cells, the activities of hexokinase (or glucokinase), phosphofructokinase 1, and pyruvate kinase are the key determinants of flux through glycolysis. The activity of these enzymes is regulated by AMP, ATP, fructose phosphates, or the degree of phosphorylation of the enzyme.*

### 3.1. Overview

The regulation of glucose use varies appreciably from tissue to tissue. In adipose tissue and the hypoglycemic brain, glucose transport limits glucose use. In red blood cells and glycolytic (fast-twitch) muscle, ATP consumption is usually the limiting factor. In the liver, the concentrations of insulin and glucagon are the master controllers. In all cells, hypoxia activates glycolysis via an abnormally high concentration of AMP. In chronically hypoxic cells, there is also increased synthesis of enzymes of glycolysis.

### 3.2. Introduction to Insulin, Glucagon, Epinephrine, and Norepinephrine

Insulin, glucagon, epinephrine, and norepinephrine are among the many hormones that affect the rate of glycolysis in a tissue-specific manner. The release of these hormones into the bloodstream is covered in Chapter 26. A brief overview of this material is provided here, sufficient to understand the regulation of glycolysis. Pancreatic islet β-cells secrete **insulin** into the blood in response to an elevated concentration of glucose (e.g., after a carbohydrate meal). Islet α-cells secrete **glucagon** when the concentration of glucose is low. Chromaffin cells in the medulla of the adrenal glands secrete **epinephrine** and **norepinephrine** in response to sympathetic input from splanchnic nerves. These nerves in turn fire in response to exercise or hypoglycemia.

Insulin, glucagon, epinephrine, and norepinephrine are water-soluble hormones that cannot cross plasma membranes;

they bind to plasma membrane receptors that transmit a signal to the cytosol (see Chapters 26 and 33). Insulin stimulates glucose use and storage, whereas glucagon promotes endogenous glucose production. Epinephrine and norepinephrine promote glucose use by the heart.

### 3.3. Introduction to AMP-Dependent Protein Kinase

**AMP-dependent protein kinase** (**AMPK**) is an important energy sensor inside cells. **AMP** and **ADP** activate AMPK, whereas ATP inhibits it. Several kinases and phosphatases further modulate AMPK activity.

When AMPK is active, it phosphorylates enzymes so as to modify cell growth, proliferation, the production of new mitochondria, and flux in metabolism. In metabolism, high AMPK activity leads to increased ATP production via glycolysis and fatty acid oxidation, and to reduced use of ATP due to inhibition of the synthesis of fatty acids, triglycerides, cholesterol, and proteins. (Further details are provided in Chapters 8, 25, 27, and 39.) Indirect activation of AMPK activity with **metformin** has proven very successful in the treatment of **diabetes** (see Chapter 39). Metformin is sometimes also used to treat **polycystic ovary syndrome** (see Chapter 26).

### 3.4. Regulation of Glucose Transport

There are several types of glucose transporters (see Table 18.1 and Section 3.2 in Chapter 18). After synthesis, glucose transporters of most types are inserted into the plasma membrane and remain there. Transporters of the **GLUT-4** subtype, however, frequently move between intracellular storage vesicles and the plasma membrane. When the concentration of **insulin** is low, the GLUT-4 transporters are mostly stored intracellularly. When the concentration of insulin is high, the storage vesicles fuse with the plasma membrane and the GLUT-4 transporters are incorporated into the plasma membrane; this increases the capacity for glucose uptake. (Details of the signal transduction mechanism for insulin are provided in Chapter 26.) GLUT-4 transporters are predominantly found in adipose tissue and muscle. In muscle, besides insulin, exercise also leads to the insertion of GLUT-4 transporters into the plasma membrane. This effect is at least in part mediated by AMPK. Muscle can thus store glucose as glycogen after exercise and after a meal, and it can use glucose from the blood during exercise.

### 3.5. Regulation of Hexokinase and Glucokinase Activities

Humans have three hexokinases with a relatively low $K_m$ for glucose (i.e., they are half-maximally saturated by <0.2 mM glucose; Fig. 19.8). Humans also produce **glucokinase** (also called type IV hexokinase), which has a comparatively high $S_{0.5}$ for glucose (it is half-maximally active at ~5 mM glucose).

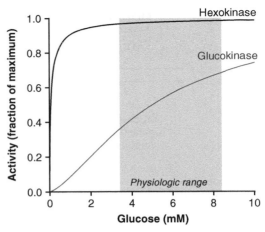

**Fig. 19.8** **Difference in the kinetic behavior between hexokinases (types I to III) and glucokinase (hexokinase type IV).** Five mM glucose corresponds to 90 mg glucose/dL.

Almost all cells contain a low-$K_m$ **hexokinase**, and unless glucose transport is limiting, these enzymes are nearly saturated with glucose even during hypoglycemia (see Fig. 19.8). Glucose 6-phosphate, the product of the hexokinase-catalyzed reaction, *inhibits* hexokinase; this is variably called *product* inhibition or *feedback* inhibition. By itself, the product inhibition ensures that the concentration of glucose 6-phosphate is held constant.

**Glucokinase** is found only in the liver and in glucose-sensing cells of the pancreas, jejunal enterocytes, and hypothalamus. The activity of glucokinase changes markedly between hypo- and hyperglycemia because glucokinase has a low affinity for glucose, shows cooperativity toward glucose, and is not inhibited by glucose 6-phosphate. In the liver, the activity of glucokinase is further regulated by a **glucokinase regulatory protein** (GKRP) that responds to dietary fructose; details are provided in Section 5.6. The role of glucokinase in glucose-sensing inside pancreatic β-cells is described in Chapter 26.

### 3.6. Regulation of Phosphofructokinase 1

Glucose-6-phosphate is not only an intermediate of glycolysis; it is also an intermediate in the synthesis and degradation of glycogen (see Chapter 24) and one of the starting points for the pentose phosphate shunt pathway (see Chapter 21). The phosphorylation of fructose 6-phosphate to fructose 1,6-bisphosphate is thus the first irreversible reaction that commits a metabolite to glycolysis. This reaction is catalyzed by **phosphofructokinase 1** (**PFK1**); this enzyme usually exerts the greatest control over glycolysis (pancreatic islet β-cells are an exception; see Chapter 26).

There are several isoenzymes for PFK1; **AMP** *stimulates* all of them, and **ATP** *inhibits* them. Since **adenylate kinase** maintains the equilibrium 2 ADP ↔ AMP + ATP, an elevated concentration of AMP is an indicator of poor phosphorylation of ADP and AMP. In some tissues, **citrate** (from the citric acid cycle; see Chapter 22) also inhibits PFK1.

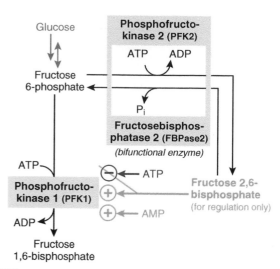

**Fig. 19.9** Regulation of phosphofructokinase 1 by fructose 2,6-bisphosphate.

The regulatory sugar phosphate **fructose 2,6-bisphosphate** markedly increases the activity of PFK1 and thereby abrogates the inhibitory effect of ATP. Fructose 2,6-bisphosphate is synthesized from fructose 6-phosphate by the bifunctional enzyme **phosphofructokinase 2/fructose bisphosphatase 2 (=6-phosphofructo-2-kinase/fructose 2,6-bisphosphatase, PFK2/FBPase 2;** Fig. 19.9). There are four isoenzymes, the activity of which is regulated by signaling pathways that respond, for example, to cellular stress, hypoxia, AMP, insulin, glucagon, or epinephrine. Fructose 2,6-bisphosphate can stimulate glycolysis beyond the flux that would be needed to produce ATP from glucose. Intermediates and products of glycolysis can thus be used for other metabolic pathways.

### 3.7. Regulation of Pyruvate Kinase

In all cells, the rate of the pyruvate kinase–catalyzed reaction is regulated allosterically by the concentration of **fructose 1,6-bisphosphate** so that the concentration of intermediates in glycolysis stays approximately constant, regardless of flux (Figs. 19.2 and 19.10). This ensures that intermediates are available for other pathways (Fig. 19.11). The activation of pyruvate kinase by fructose 1,6-bisphosphate is an example of feed-forward activation. All reactions between fructose 1,6-bisphosphate and phosphoenolpyruvate are reversible (i.e., they proceed according to the concentrations of reactants and products). If one reactant piles up, all reactants of upstream *reversible* reactions also pile up. Therefore, if the pyruvate kinase–catalyzed reaction proceeds at too low a rate, the concentration of fructose 1,6-bisphosphate rises, which in turn increases the activity of pyruvate kinase, thus forming a regulatory loop.

When certain cells in the liver and kidneys carry out **gluconeogenesis** (see Chapter 25), hormone-induced phosphorylation inactivates pyruvate kinase.

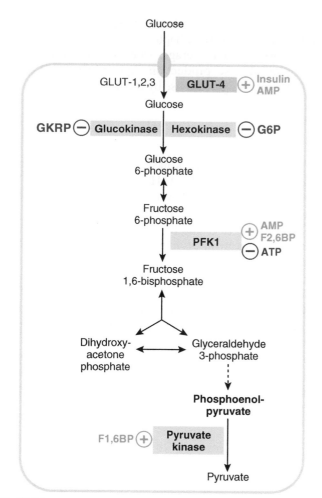

**Fig. 19.10** Summary of mechanisms that can regulate flux through glycolysis.

### 3.8. Summary of the Regulation of Flux in Glycolysis

Fig. 19.10 summarizes mechanisms that can regulate flux through glycolysis.

## 4. INTERACTIONS OF GLYCOLYSIS WITH OTHER PATHWAYS

*Intermediates of glycolysis feed into multiple other pathways or derive metabolites from them. The main pathways are glycogen metabolism, the pentose phosphate shunt pathway, the citric acid cycle, and amino acid metabolism.*

Fig. 19.11 shows the connections between glycolysis and other metabolic pathways. **Glycogen** synthesis and degradation are described in Chapter 24. The degradation of **galactose** and **fructose** is described in Chapter 20. The **pentose phosphate shunt** pathway is explained in Chapter 21. The production of **2,3-bisphosphoglycerate** is detailed in Section 5.1 below. Chapters 22 and 23, respectively, are devoted to the **citric acid cycle** and **oxidative phosphorylation**. **Fatty acid synthesis** from **citrate** is described in Chapter 27, while **triglyceride synthesis** is presented in Chapter 28. The conversion of lactate or alanine to pyruvate and the use of pyruvate and glycerol for

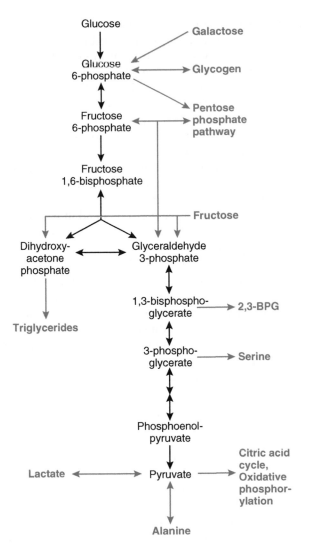

**Fig. 19.11** **Overview of glycolysis and its links with other pathways.**

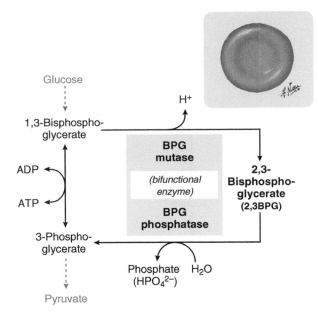

**Fig. 19.12** **Production of 2,3-bisphosphoglycerate in red blood cells.**

the synthesis of glucose (i.e., gluconeogenesis) are described in Chapter 25.

## 5. TISSUE-SPECIFIC REGULATION OF GLYCOLYSIS

*Glycolysis is a central pathway of metabolism and crucial for a cell's survival. Accordingly, regulation of glycolysis is extraordinarily complex; however, it is yet incompletely understood. This section provides an introduction to the regulation of glycolysis in the context of key metabolic processes in red blood cells, brain, adipose tissue, heart, skeletal muscle, and the liver.*

### 5.1. Regulation of Glycolysis in Red Blood Cells

In red blood cells, glycolysis is the only pathway that generates ATP. GLUT-1 glucose transporters are always in the plasma membrane and equilibrate intracellular and extracellular

glucose. Hexokinase produces a near-constant concentration of glucose 6-phosphate, which is needed both for glycolysis and for the production of NADPH (used to repair oxidative damage; see Chapter 21). PFK1 regulates flux through glycolysis based on the concentrations of AMP and ATP. Fructose 1,6-bisphosphate feed-forward activates pyruvate kinase. This activation ensures that the concentrations of the intermediates between fructose 1,6-bisphosphate and phosphoenolpyruvate are near constant, which is important for the production of 2,3-bisphosphoglycerate, a regulator of the oxygen affinity of hemoglobin (see below). In mature red blood cells, which do not contain mitochondria, lactate is the end product of glycolysis. In contrast, **reticulocytes** (which still synthesize hemoglobin; see Chapter 16) contain mitochondria that can oxidize some of the pyruvate to $CO_2$.

Red blood cells use **2,3-bisphosphoglycerate** (2,3-BPG) to adjust the affinity of hemoglobin for $O_2$ (see Chapter 16). 2,3-BPG is produced from 1,3-bisphosphoglycerate (1,3-BPG) and later metabolized to 3-phosphoglycerate by a single, bifunctional enzyme, bisphosphoglycerate mutase/bisphosphoglycerate phosphatase (Fig. 19.12). The balance of the mutase and the phosphatase activities of this enzyme determines the concentration of 2,3-BPG. During hypoxia or at higher altitude, the concentration of 2,3-BPG is increased. However, at a molecular level, the regulation of the BPG mutase/BPG phosphatase is not understood. In erythrocytes, about one of every four 1,3-BPG molecules takes the 2,3-BPG "detour"; hence, these cells gain only about 1.5 mol ATP per mol glucose metabolized. When the concentration of 1,3-BPG is abnormal due to a problem in glycolysis, the concentration of 2,3-BPG is typically also abnormal. **Hereditary, deficient BPG mutase activity** (a very rare disease) is associated with high hematocrit, a fine illustration of the need for 2,3-BPG to optimize the oxygen affinity of hemoglobin.

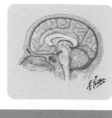

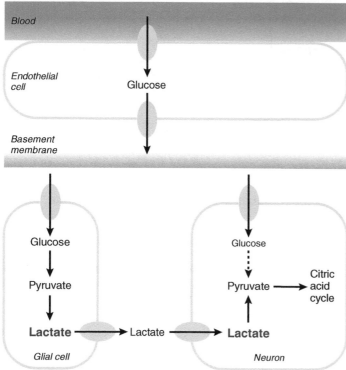

**Fig. 19.13** **Supply of fuel to the brain.** Endothelial cells form the walls of blood vessels. The blood vessel walls are enveloped by a basement membrane that consists largely of extracellular matrix proteins (see Chapter 12). The basement membrane forms a filter, through which small molecules can pass. Glial cells convert glucose to lactate and "feed" the lactate to neurons. Neurons oxidize lactate via the citric acid cycle (see Chapter 22) to $CO_2$.

## 5.2. Regulation of Glycolysis in the Brain

The concentration of glucose in brain tissue is considerably lower than in the cerebrospinal fluid or in the blood. Endothelial cells that line the walls of blood vessels in the brain contain glucose transporters that transport glucose from the blood to the extracellular space (Fig. 19.13). From there, glucose diffuses through the basement membrane (a meshwork of extracellular matrix proteins that envelopes the blood vessels) to the extracellular space near glial cells and neurons. The concentration of glucose in cerebrospinal fluid (obtained by lumbar puncture) is ~55% that in serum. However, at a plasma glucose concentration of 90 mg/dL or more, the concentration of glucose in the brain tissue (measured by magnetic resonance imaging [MRI]) is only about 30% of that in blood plasma. Furthermore, when the plasma glucose concentration is only about 40 mg/dL, there is essentially no more free glucose in brain tissue.

**Glial cells** take up glucose from the extracellular space and convert it to lactate, which they release for the benefit of neurons (see Fig. 19.13). Glial cells tend to neurons by regulating their growth and properties, feeding them, insulating their axons, or recycling their neurotransmitters. Neurons take up lactate, oxidize it in the citric acid cycle (see Chapter 22), and obtain energy from oxidative phosphorylation (see Chapter 23). In addition, neurons also directly take up a small amount of glucose, which then enters into the pathway sequence glycolysis–citric acid cycle/oxidative phosphorylation to produce $CO_2$ and $H_2O$.

To a limited extent, the brain can use **lactate** and **ketone bodies** in place of glucose. Lactate uptake from the blood can replace only a small fraction of the glucose that the brain normally uses. However, the brain of an adult who fasts for 8 days can cover about 75% of its energy needs with ketone bodies. In adults, ketone body production is normally low and increases substantially only after 1 to 2 days of fasting. Thus, after an overnight fast, the brain covers only about 5% of its energy needs with the oxidation of ketone bodies. Newborns and young children produce ketone bodies in response to fasting much sooner than adults. For instance, both children who are a few months old and fast for ~8 hours and newborns produce and consume ketone bodies at a rate (relative to body weight) that adults achieve only after more than 48 hours of fasting.

In a normoglycemic or hyperglycemic person, **hexokinase** provides a near-constant concentration of glucose 6-phosphate. A very small amount of glucose 6-phosphate is used for the synthesis of glycogen as an emergency fuel reserve (see Chapter 24). PFK1 activity is the chief determinant of glycolytic flux; the cytosolic concentrations of **AMP**, ATP, and **fructose 2,6-bisphosphate** (much more so in glial cells than in neurons) determine the activity of PFK1. Fructose 2,6-bisphosphate, produced by phosphofructokinase 2, provides glial cells with an override of the ATP inhibition of glycolysis so that these cells can release lactate for the benefit of neurons.

During **hypoglycemia** (an abnormally low concentration of glucose in the blood), the brain can no longer take up an adequate amount of glucose and therefore loses function. Hypoglycemia most frequently occurs after the accidental administration of excess **insulin** or oral **hypoglycemic agents** that stimulate insulin secretion despite the hypoglycemia (see Chapter 39); less frequently it is due to an inherited abnormality of carbohydrate or lipid metabolism that comes to the fore in the fasting state (see Chapters 24, 25, and 27). If the concentration of glucose in the blood falls to 20 to 35 mg/dL, stupor and coma set in, and eventually brain electrical activity disappears. With severe hypoglycemia of less than 25 mg glucose/dL in the blood plasma, glial cells cannot produce enough lactate for neurons (see Fig. 19.13), the concentration of ATP inside neurons drops precipitously, neurotransmitters flood the extracellular space, dendrites swell, and necrosis sets in.

## 5.3. Regulation of Glycolysis in Adipocytes

When the concentration of insulin is elevated after a mixed meal, adipocytes increase their glucose uptake and deposit fatty acids as triglycerides (see Chapter 28). An elevated concentration of **insulin** leads to translocation of GLUT-4 glucose transporters from intracellular storage vesicles to the plasma membrane; at the same time, the lipoprotein lipase activity in the blood vessels of the adipose tissue increases, which brings about an influx of fatty acids (see Chapter 28). Via glycolysis and a side reaction to it, glucose is converted to **glycerol 3-phosphate**, which is esterified with fatty acids to form triglycerides (see Figs. 19.11, 28.2, and 28.5).

In the fasting state, adipocytes produce most of their energy from sources other than glucose (i.e., endogenous and exogenous triglycerides, as well as exogenous ketone bodies).

## 5.4. Regulation of Glycolysis in Heart Muscle

ATP use of the heart is very high. The heart can use fatty acids, glucose, lactate, and ketone bodies for ATP production.

At rest, in the fasting state, or after a high-fat/low-carbohydrate meal, the heart uses almost no glucose and produces its ATP mostly from the β-oxidation of fatty acids (see Chapter 27). Under these conditions, the heart also uses some lactate and ketone bodies.

The heart substantially increases its use of glucose after a high-carbohydrate meal, during exercise or a high workload, and during hypoxia, whereby insulin, epinephrine, AMP, and AMP-dependent protein kinase are key regulators. **Insulin** and active **AMP-dependent protein kinase (AMPK)** can each induce the insertion of **GLUT4 glucose transporters** into the cardiomyocyte plasma membrane. **AMP** directly activates PFK1, the main rate-limiting enzyme of glycolysis. AMP also activates AMPK. Insulin, **epinephrine**, and AMPK each increase **phosphofructokinase 2** activity, which leads to an increase in the concentration of fructose 2,6-bisphosphate, which in turn activates PFK1.

While **insulin** increases glucose use by the heart, it decreases **fatty acid** use. The mechanisms for increased glucose use are described above. Fatty acid use is decreased by an insulin-induced increase in the concentration of malonyl-CoA, which inhibits the transport of fatty acids from the cytosol into the mitochondria (see Chapter 27).

**Hypoxia** increases glucose use in the heart, as it does in all tissues. Hypoxia slows ATP production via oxidative phosphorylation, which leads to an increased concentration of AMP, which in turn increases the uptake and use of glucose, in part via AMPK (see above).

During a **high workload**, the heart increases its glucose use and decreases its fatty acid use because ATP production from glucose requires less **oxygen** than ATP production from fatty acids. The complete oxidation of glucose via glycolysis, conversion of all pyruvate to acetyl-CoA, the oxidation of acetyl-CoA in the citric acid cycle, and oxidation of all NADH and FADH$_2$ in oxidative phosphorylation with concomitant production of ATP yields about 2.7 ATP per single O-atom used. In contrast, the activation of a C-16 fatty acid and complete oxidation via β-oxidation, the citric acid cycle, and oxidative phosphorylation yields only about 2.4 ATP per O-atom used.

## 5.5. Regulation of Glycolysis in Skeletal Muscle

Muscle consists of fibers of several types that differ in their use of oxygen for glucose metabolism. Some fibers perform mostly *anaerobic* glycolysis, others mostly *aerobic* glycolysis with oxidation of most substrates to $CO_2$. The gastrocnemius muscle (Fig. 19.14), for instance, contains mostly fibers that perform anaerobic glycolysis. The soleus muscle, on the other hand, contains mostly fibers that oxidize substrates to $CO_2$. Both muscles extend the foot; the gastrocnemius is used mainly for high-force, short-duration activities, and the soleus is used mainly for maintaining posture.

**Glycolytic fibers** are fast-twitch fibers that contain only a few mitochondria; they can contract and deliver full force in

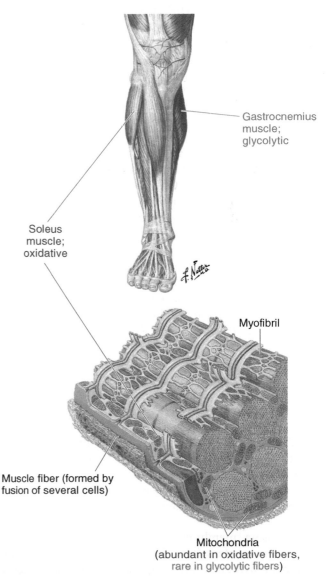

Gastrocnemius muscle; glycolytic

Soleus muscle; oxidative

Myofibril

Muscle fiber (formed by fusion of several cells)

Mitochondria (abundant in oxidative fibers, rare in glycolytic fibers)

**Fig. 19.14** **Anterior view of the muscles of the left leg (superficial dissection).**

less than 0.1 second because all components for anaerobic glycolysis are present (if insufficient glucose is available, endogenous glycogen can be degraded to glucose 6-phosphate; see Chapter 24). The drawback of glycolytic fibers is that they produce and release lactic acid; if all muscle fibers performed only anaerobic glycolysis during exercise, the human body could not remove enough lactic acid from the blood to prevent life-threatening acidosis.

**Oxidative fibers** (the majority of fibers in the soleus muscle) are slow-twitch fibers that have abundant mitochondria and continuously need to import oxygen; however, increased oxygen delivery depends on an increase in blood flow. Even though these fibers can contract within a fraction of a second, blood flow typically takes a few minutes to become maximal. This is a reason for athletes to warm up before a competition. Besides glucose, oxidative fibers also use fatty acids and ketone bodies for energy generation. When oxygen is limiting, oxidative fibers can also perform anaerobic glycolysis.

Successful **sprinters** typically rely on muscles that perform appreciable anaerobic glycolysis, while **marathon runners** rely on muscle fibers that oxidize substrates to $CO_2$ and produce very little lactic acid.

During **contraction**, glycolytic and oxidative skeletal muscle fibers use glucose from the blood and also glucose 6-phosphate from the degradation of **glycogen** (see Chapter 24). Glucose and glucose 6-phosphate undergo glycolysis to pyruvate. When most of the glycogen is used up, or when the **intracellular pH** is low, **muscle fatigue** sets in.

In response to exercise or insulin, the main glucose transporter in skeletal muscle, GLUT-4, moves from intracellular vesicles to the plasma membrane. Exercise increases the concentration of AMP, which in turn activates PFK1 and **AMPK** (see Section 3). AMPK favors the translocation of GLUT-4 to the plasma membrane.

In the **recovery** phase, the glycogen stores are built up again; this happens both after exercise has ended and even more so after a meal when an elevated concentration of insulin causes the translocation of GLUT-4 to the plasma membrane and activates glycogen synthase (see Chapter 24).

## 5.6. Regulation of Glycolysis in the Liver

After a meal, the liver oxidizes glucose (see Chapters 22 and 23), stores glucose as glycogen (see Chapter 24), and converts a small amount of glucose into triglycerides (see Chapters 27 and 28). In the fasting state, the liver degrades glycogen to glucose (see Chapter 24); converts lactate, many amino acids, and glycerol into glucose (see Chapter 25); and turns fatty acids into ketone bodies (see Chapter 27), whereby it releases glucose and ketone bodies for the benefit of other tissues.

The plasma membrane of hepatocytes always contains **glucose transporters** (GLUT-2). The liver *takes up* glucose after a carbohydrate-containing meal and *releases* glucose in the fasting state. Although hormones do not regulate the membrane insertion of glucose transporters in the liver, they regulate glucose metabolism, which in turn affects the direction and rate of glucose transport across the hepatocyte plasma membrane.

In contrast to other tissues, the liver expresses **glucokinase** and a **GKRP**. Glucose 6-phosphate does not inhibit glucokinase. However, GKRP binds to glucokinase, inhibits it, and induces its translocation to the nucleus. In the fasting state, glucokinase is largely sequestered in the nucleus; this process is modestly enhanced by the high concentration of fructose 6-phosphate that is typical of the glucose-producing liver in the fasting state (see also Chapters 24 and 25). Conversely, **glucose** influx from the diet into hepatocytes leads to a partial release of glucokinase from GKRP in the nucleus, followed by transport into the cytosol. As a result, glucose-phosphorylating activity in intact hepatocytes shows an even greater dependence on blood glucose than does glucokinase alone (see Fig. 19.8). Fructose 1-phosphate, which is present only when dietary **fructose** or **sorbitol** are absorbed (see Chapter 20), further enhances the release of glucokinase from GKRP.

Since glycolysis and gluconeogenesis have essentially the same intermediates and use the same enzymes for the reversible steps, it is important that enzymes that catalyze the irreversible steps in glycolysis are inactivated during **gluconeogenesis**. Similarly, enzymes that catalyze irreversible steps in gluconeogenesis need to be inactivated during glycolysis. To this end, glucokinase activity is regulated as described above by GKRP, PFK1 activity is regulated by fructose 2,6-bisphosphate, and pyruvate kinase is regulated by phosphorylation/dephosphorylation (see Chapter 25).

AMP, ATP, and **fructose 2,6-bisphosphate** allosterically control the activity of PFK1. The regulation of PFK1 (and thus glycolysis) by AMP and ATP ensures adequate ATP production. *After a meal*, when the concentration of **insulin** is relatively high, protein phosphatase 2C, which is part of the insulin signaling network (see Chapter 26), dephosphorylates the bifunctional enzyme PFK2/FBPase 2 and thereby activates its phosphofructokinase 2 domain (see Fig. 19.9). This leads to an increase in the concentration of fructose 2,6-bisphosphate, which in turn activates PFK1. Activation of PFK1 by fructose 2,6-bisphosphate overrides the inhibition of PFK1 by ATP. As a result, although the concentration of ATP is high, glycolysis can proceed at a high rate and its intermediates and products can be used for the synthesis of fatty acids and triglycerides (see Chapters 27 and 28). In the *fasting* state or during vigorous, prolonged *exercise*, **glucagon** and **epinephrine** activate protein kinase A (see Chapters 26 and 33), which phosphorylates PFK2/FBPase 2 and thereby activates its fructosebisphosphatase 2 domain (see Fig. 19.9). This leads to the degradation of the regulatory sugar fructose 2,6-bisphosphate. Without fructose 2,6-bisphosphate bound to it, PFK1 is readily inhibited by ATP. This ATP stems from mitochondria that oxidize fatty acids. The resulting low PFK1 activity means that glucose enters glycolysis only sparingly.

The activity of **pyruvate kinase** is regulated not only by a feed-forward activation from **fructose 1,6-bisphosphate** but also by inhibition from **glucagon**- or **epinephrine**-induced phosphorylation. This signaling pathway is described in detail in Chapters 24 and 26. When gluconeogenesis is active, the inactivation of pyruvate kinase prevents a vicious cycle between phosphoenolpyruvate and pyruvate. In the fed state, **insulin** antagonizes the effects of glucagon and epinephrine.

## 6. COMMON LABORATORY METHODS AND ASSAYS

### 6.1. Preservation of Metabolites in Blood Samples

For lab assays (e.g., of blood glucose and lactate), **blood collection tubes** often contain sodium **fluoride** (NaF) to inhibit **enolase**, the enzyme that converts 2-phosphoglycerate to phosphoenolpyruvate (see Fig. 19.2). Inhibition of any step in glycolysis leads to the inhibition of the entire pathway (see Chapter 10).

### 6.2. Plasma or Serum Lactate Dehydrogenase

It is common to measure the activity of **LDH** in blood plasma of patients. On an ongoing basis, damaged cells leak this enzyme into the blood. All tissues have the same concentration of LDH, and cells normally contain a greater than 500-fold higher concentration of LDH than blood plasma. The liver eliminates LDH from blood plasma. There are several isozymes of LDH in plasma, and they have plasma half-lives of several hours to several days. Most of the LDH in blood plasma derives from red blood cells and platelets. Even a slight amount of hemolysis increases the concentration of LDH in the plasma.

An elevated LDH by itself does not provide any information on which tissue is damaged. It is uncommon for liver disease to be the cause of an elevated LDH. If blood tests of aspartate aminotransferase, alanine aminotransferase, creatine kinase, hemoglobin, bilirubin, or reticulocyte count are not sufficiently diagnostic, electrophoresis for LDH isoenzyme distribution can help narrow down the tissue source of LDH.

### 6.3. 2-Fluoro-Deoxyglucose Positron Emission Tomographic Scans

Radioactive 2-[18]F-deoxyglucose (FDG) together with positron emission tomography (PET) scanning is used to assess glucose metabolism in tissues. FDG contains a fluorine atom in place of the hydroxyl group found in glucose. FDG enters cells through glucose transporters. Inside cells, FDG mixes with glucose. Hexokinase phosphorylates glucose in proportion to the rate of glycolysis since hexokinase is designed to maintain a constant concentration of glucose 6-phosphate. Hexokinase can phosphorylate FDG to FDG 6-phosphate, and it does so in proportion to glucose. In most tissues FDG 6-phosphate is not appreciably metabolized further or degraded. Hence, FDG (used at an appropriately small dose) accumulates at a rate that is proportional to the rate of glycolysis.

FDG-PET scans are primarily used for imaging tumors and the brain. Tumors and active regions of the brain take up FDG at an especially high rate (see Fig. 8.19). FDG-PET scans help locate metastases and help diagnose certain dementias.

## 7. DISEASES THAT INVOLVE AN ABNORMAL FLUX IN GLYCOLYSIS

*An elevated concentration of lactate in the blood is most often the result of tissue hypoxia that increases the rate of anaerobic glycolysis. Hypophosphatemia impairs glycolysis (and with it ATP production) in a wide variety of tissues. Hypophosphatemia is most commonly seen in patients who get too little phosphate or waste too much of it in the kidneys. Hereditary deficiencies of enzymes of glycolysis are uncommon and usually affect predominantly the red blood cells, leading to premature hemolysis. The most common disease is pyruvate kinase deficiency.*

### 7.1. Lactate Accumulation

The concentration of lactate in the blood is a function of both tissue lactate production and lactate consumption. Compared with daily lactate production, the amount of lactate that circulates in the blood is very small (<1/1000). Hence, even a relatively small change in production or consumption can have a sizable effect on the plasma concentration of lactate.

**Hyperlactatemia** is a condition of an abnormally high concentration of lactate in the blood, which is typically defined as greater than 2 mM lactate (normal reference value: 0.5 to 1.5 mM).

**Lactic acidosis** develops when lactate production exceeds consumption such that the pH in the blood drops and the concentrations of both bicarbonate and $CO_2$ become abnormally low (due to buffering and increased ventilation; see Chapter 16). Lactic acidosis is typically seen when the blood lactate concentration is 4 mM or greater.

The term **anion gap** refers to the difference between measured serum or plasma concentrations of the cations $Na^+$ and $K^+$ ($K^+$ is often omitted) and the anions $Cl^-$ and $HCO_3^-$. Blood contains other cations and anions that are not usually measured. Blood must always have the same number of positive and negative ions. The anion gap is therefore an indicator of the concentration of "unmeasured" ions, which often means anions such as lactate or formate (see Chapter 36) or acetoacetate and β-hydroxybutyrate (see Chapter 27). A patient who has a lactic acidosis may thus have an increased anion gap.

Lactate production increases when a tissue experiences **hypoxia** that forces it to decrease ATP production from oxidative phosphorylation and increase ATP production via anaerobic glycolysis (see Section 2.2).

**Shock** is a condition of tissue hypoperfusion that leads to tissue hypoxia and hyperlactatemia. Early on, the shock is reversible, but later it leads to multi-organ failure and death. Shock can have a variety of causes. **Hypovolemic (hemorrhagic) shock**, for instance, is a consequence of massive blood loss. It is accompanied by vasoconstriction and the redistribution of blood flow away from the skin, kidneys, and gastrointestinal tract. **Septic shock** is due to severe sepsis from a severe infection that leads to vasodilation, an increase in microvascular permeability, and leukocyte accumulation in tissues that are remote from the primary site of infection. Patients with septic shock may have tissue hypoperfusion with consequent injuries to their lungs and kidneys, and sometimes also their liver.

Besides the abovementioned disorders, hyperlactatemia may also be caused by near-maximal **exercise**, a grand mal **seizure**, metabolism of **ethanol** (see Chapter 30), or any impairment of **mitochondrial ATP production**.

## 7.2. Effect of Hypophosphatemia on Glycolysis

In health care, standard laboratory methods report the concentration of **phosphorus** (P) in the serum. Phosphorus is not present in the blood in elemental form, but mostly as free phosphate (mostly as $HPO_4^{2-}$). The reported phosphorus is normal at about 3.0 to 4.5 mg P/dL ($\cong$1.0 to 1.5 mM phosphate). The term **hypophosphatemia** refers to an abnormally low concentration of phosphate in the blood, and this is evident from an abnormally low reported serum phosphorus.

Hypophosphatemia impairs flux in glycolysis by reducing the activity of **glyceraldehyde 3-phosphate dehydrogenase**, which converts glyceraldehyde 3-phosphate to 1,3-bisphosphoglycerate (see Fig. 19.2). In tissues with mitochondria, hypophosphatemia also impairs ATP production by **oxidative phosphorylation** (see Chapter 23). **Tissue oxygenation** suffers because red blood cells contain less **2,3-bisphosphoglycerate** to facilitate the dissociation of $O_2$ from hemoglobin.

Hypophosphatemia progressively impairs the function of red blood cells, white blood cells, glial cells, skeletal muscle, and heart muscle. Phosphate-deficient red blood cells hemolyze prematurely. Diminished leukocyte function can lead to sepsis. When serum phosphorus falls below about 1 mg P/dL, the patient may stop breathing, have seizures, and show cardiac arrhythmias.

To make up for losses, humans need to take in about 0.7 g of phosphorus per day. Even though total body stores amount to 500 g or more of "phosphorus," phosphate cannot be sufficiently mobilized to cover a deficit in intake of a few days.

Hypophosphatemia is most commonly observed in connection with parenteral nutrition, malnourishment, chronic alcohol abuse, diabetic ketoacidosis, sepsis, respiratory alkalosis, or primary hyperparathyroidism (Fig. 19.15). The need for phosphate was first recognized when **parenteral nutrition** was developed. Patients who receive parenteral nutrition after

**Refeeding in patient with anorexia or malnutrition:**

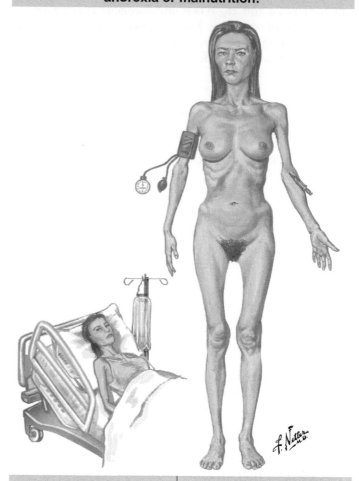

**Alcohol addiction:**

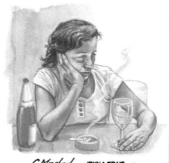

**Hyperparathyroidism:**

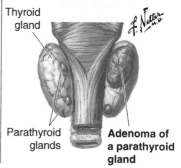

Thyroid gland

Parathyroid glands

**Adenoma of a parathyroid gland**

**Fig. 19.15**  Some causes of hypophosphatemia.

a period of severe **fasting** (e.g., due to **anorexia**) or **malnutrition** need extra phosphate in the infusate to avoid developing hypophosphatemia as part of **refeeding syndrome**, which also includes other electrolyte abnormalities. Patients who chronically abuse **alcohol** take in little phosphate, and their kidneys lose an excessive amount of phosphate. Prolonged **acidosis** (e.g., **diabetic ketoacidosis**) leads to the loss of phosphate from tissues and the body. Normalization of metabolism is often accompanied by increased tissue uptake of phosphate, which can lead to hypophosphatemia. In **sepsis**, hypophosphatemia develops early and is a predictor of patient survival. Though persistent hypophosphatemia itself can lead to sepsis, most patients develop sepsis for other reasons. Patients who have **respiratory alkalosis** due to mechanical hyperventilation shift phosphate from the blood into the tissues. **Parathyroid hormone** inhibits the recovery of filtered phosphate in the kidneys. Patients with **hyperparathyroidism** become hypophosphatemic because they tend to lose too much phosphate. Hyperparathyroidism is most often due to an adenoma of a parathyroid gland.

Patients with significant symptoms and severe hypophosphatemia are treated with an *intravenous infusion* of a solution containing phosphate. Moderate hypophosphatemia is often treated with an *oral* phosphate salt.

## 7.3. Hemolytic Anemias Due to Hereditary Deficiencies of Enzymes of Glycolysis

Hemolytic anemia can have many causes, such as a problem with hemoglobin, as in sickle cell anemia or thalassemia (see Chapter 17), a problem with handling oxidative stress, as in G6PD deficiency (see Chapter 21), or a problem with an enzyme in glycolysis, as discussed below. Since mature red blood cells cannot synthesize enzymes, red blood cells are more readily affected by unstable mutant proteins than other cells that can still synthesize proteins.

**Pyruvate kinase deficiency** is the most common deficiency of a red blood cell enzyme of glycolysis. It has a worldwide distribution and shows a recessive pattern of inheritance. About 1% of all people are carriers, and about 1 : 10,000 are affected by the disease. In the United States, the disease is particularly common among the Amish. Red blood cell pyruvate kinase deficiency (with <30% of the normal activity remaining) is accompanied by nonspherocytic hemolytic anemia, usually with persistent hyperbilirubinemia, high reticulocyte count, a tendency to accumulate excessive amounts of iron (presumably due to ineffective erythropoiesis and hypoxia; see Chapter 15), and an increased incidence of gallstones (due to the increased excretion of bilirubin glucuronides; see Chapter 14). The pyruvate kinase deficiency is commonly due to a decreased affinity of the enzyme for the activator fructose 1,6-bisphosphate, and it always reduces ATP production in red blood cells so that processes such as ion pumping and maintenance of cell shape are compromised. The pyruvate kinase deficiency also causes an accumulation of all intermediates between fructose 1,6-bisphosphate and phosphoenolpyruvate (including 1,3-bisphosphoglycerate); as a result, the concentration of 2,3-bisphosphoglycerate also rises; this, in turn, lowers the oxygen affinity of hemoglobin inside red blood cells (see Chapter 16). At low altitude, this latter effect is beneficial because it improves oxygen delivery in these anemic patients; the drawback is a smaller $O_2$ reserve in circulating red blood cells.

Pyruvate kinase in red blood cells and liver derives from the same gene, though each tissue uses a different promoter and with that a different first exon. Even if the mutation is in a common exon (i.e., exons $\geq 3$), a red blood cell pyruvate kinase deficiency does not affect glucose metabolism in the liver in a clinically relevant fashion.

For a detailed history of a patient with pyruvate kinase deficiency, see Bowman and Procopio in the Further Reading section.

Deficiencies of **other enzymes of glycolysis** are known, but they are very rare.

## SUMMARY

- Glycolysis produces pyruvate from glucose. Tissues without mitochondria or cells without adequate oxygen perform anaerobic glycolysis. In anaerobic glycolysis, pyruvate is converted to lactic acid, which is released into the bloodstream.
- Cells that have well-oxygenated mitochondria can perform aerobic glycolysis; thereby pyruvate enters the citric acid cycle.
- Pellagra is characterized by diarrhea, dermatitis, and dementia. The disease is due to a deficiency of the vitamin niacin, which is needed for the synthesis of $NAD^+$, NADH, $NADP^+$, and NADPH. Some niacin can be made in the body by degradation of excess tryptophan. Pellagra is due to inadequate nutrition or drugs that interfere with $NAD^+$ production from tryptophan.
- Hypoglycemia primarily leads to an impairment of the central nervous system. Glial cells normally produce lactate for the benefit of neurons; during hypoglycemia, glial cell lactate production is insufficient, and neurons become short of ATP. Severe hypoglycemia (plasma glucose <20 mg/dL in an adult) leads to permanent damage of neurons and is often lethal.
- Hypophosphatemia is a common complication of parenteral nutrition, long-standing acidosis, ketoacidosis, chronic alcohol abuse, sepsis, or renal failure. Hypophosphatemia inhibits the glyceraldehyde 3-phosphate dehydrogenase–catalyzed reaction in glycolysis. This leads primarily to the hemolysis of red blood cells, to decreased production of 2,3-bisphosphoglycerate and thus increased oxygen affinity of hemoglobin, and to impaired brain function due to decreased glycolysis and ATP production; the latter is also due to decreased oxygen delivery from red blood cells. Severe hypophosphatemia can be fatal.
- Hereditary deficiencies of enzymes of glycolysis are uncommon. Among them, a deficiency of the pyruvate kinase that is expressed in red blood cells (and also in the liver) is the most common; it leads to chronic hemolytic anemia with hyperbilirubinemia, and patients are at an increased risk of hemochromatosis and gallstones. However, glycolysis in the liver is not affected in a clinically recognizable manner.

## FURTHER READING

- Bowman HS, Procopio F. Hereditary non-spherocytic hemolytic anemia of the pyruvate-kinase–deficient type.

*Ann Intern Med.* 1963;567-591. This paper contains detailed descriptions of five individual cases.

■ Kraut AM. *Goldberger's War; The Life and Work of a Public Health Crusader.* New York: Hill and Wand; 2003:313 Goldberger found that pellagra is due to a nutritional deficiency rather than due to infection. This is an easily readable and interesting account of what it meant to be a physician in the U.S. Public Health Service at the beginning of the twentieth century.

■ Languren G, Montiel T, Julio-Amilpas A, Massieu L. Neuronal damage and cognitive impairment associated with hypoglycemia: an integrated review. *Neurochem Int.* 2013;63:331-343.

■ Mehanna HM, Moledina J, Travis J. Refeeding syndrome: what it is, and how to prevent and treat it. *BMJ.* 2008; 336:1495-1498.

# Review Questions

1. In the fed state (but not in the fasting state), fat cells have to make dihydroxyacetone phosphate to esterify fatty acids and deposit them as triglycerides in an intracellular droplet. Insulin-dependent activation of which one of the following enzymes allows fat cells to produce dihydroxyacetone phosphate from glucose even at a low concentration of AMP?

   A. 2,3-bisphosphoglycerate (2,3-BPG) mutase
   B. Aldolase
   C. Enolase
   D. Glyceraldehyde 3-phosphate dehydrogenase
   E. Lactate dehydrogenase
   F. Phosphofructokinase 1 (PFK1)
   G. Pyruvate kinase

2. A 2-year-old Amish girl has a hereditary pyruvate kinase deficiency, such that her red blood cells show only 5% of the normal pyruvate kinase activity. The patient's erythrocytes have a decreased lifespan, and her skin chronically has a yellow tinge. Which one of the following effects on red blood cells is also characteristic of this disorder?

   A. In glycolysis, about 20 times more ATP is generated in the step 3-phosphoglycerate → 2-phosphoglycerate than in the step phosphoenolpyruvate → pyruvate.
   B. Instead of lactate, erythrocytes release phosphoenolpyruvate into the blood.
   C. The concentration of 2,3-bisphosphoglycerate (2,3-BPG) is abnormally high.
   D. The concentration of all intermediates between fructose 1,6-bisphosphate and phosphoenolpyruvate is abnormally low.

3. Below is a schematic diagram of a part of glycolysis. Which arrow correctly identifies a hypophosphatemia-induced change in the concentration of an intermediate of glycolysis?

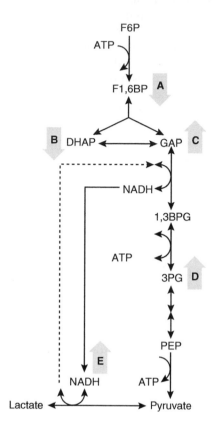

   A. A
   B. B
   C. C
   D. D
   E. E

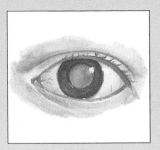

## Chapter 20

# Fructose and Galactose Metabolism: Hereditary Fructose Intolerance and Galactosemia

## SYNOPSIS

- Fructose is a monosaccharide. The main sources of dietary fructose are table sugar, industrially prepared high-fructose corn syrup, and fruits. In the Western world, the daily per capita consumption of fructose is about 50 g/day; without sweeteners, it would be about 8 g/day.
- Dietary fructose enters the bloodstream via fructose transporters in intestinal epithelial cells. The liver and the kidneys phosphorylate fructose and thus act as a fructose sink. Phosphorylated fructose is cleaved, and the products enter glycolysis in the liver and kidneys.
- Hereditary fructose intolerance is due to a deficiency of aldolase B, the enzyme that cleaves phosphorylated fructose. The prevalence of hereditary fructose intolerance is about 1 in 20,000. Many affected patients have not been diagnosed. Hence, patients should not be infused with fructose or sorbitol (which is converted to fructose). If a patient with this deficiency regularly consumes fructose, the function of the liver and kidneys becomes severely compromised.
- Galactose is also a monosaccharide. Lactose (milk sugar) is the main dietary source of galactose. Galactose is absorbed via glucose transporters and is degraded in most tissues. The degradation products of galactose enter glycolysis.
- Galactosemia is due to a hereditary inadequate degradation of galactose. Most often, galactosemia is due to a deficiency of galactose 1-phosphate uridyltransferase. In affected infants, the consumption of milk leads to an acutely toxic state with jaundice, hepatomegaly, and vomiting. Treatment involves the elimination of most galactose from the diet.

## LEARNING OBJECTIVES

*For mastery of this topic, you should be able to do the following:*
- List the foods that are rich in fructose.
- Outline the normal metabolism of dietary fructose.
- Describe the molecular basis of hereditary fructose intolerance.
- Explain the pathogenesis of organ damage in patients who have hereditary fructose intolerance and who consume an amount of fructose in their diet that is typical of the unaffected population.
- Explain renal Fanconi syndrome and describe its effects on kidney function.
- Describe the polyol pathway, paying attention to conditions that activate it.
- List the foods that are rich in galactose.
- Identify the molecular cause of classic galactosemia.
- Explain the pathogenesis of organ damage in patients who have classic galactosemia.
- Compare and contrast hereditary fructose intolerance and classic galactosemia with regard to cause, pattern of inheritance, pathogenesis, age of onset of symptoms, and treatment.

## 1. NORMAL METABOLISM OF FRUCTOSE

*Fructose is a constituent of sweeteners, fruits, and vegetables. It is metabolized chiefly in the liver and kidneys. Fructokinase and aldolase B catalyze the first two steps of fructose degradation.*

### 1.1. Sources of Fructose

**Fructose** is a 6-carbon sugar that is a natural part of the human diet. Fructose (Fig. 20.1) is also called **fruit sugar**. Like glucose, fructose is a reducing sugar. The largest amounts of fructose are usually consumed with sweeteners, such as high-fructose corn syrup, sucrose (table sugar; see Fig. 18.1), honey, and maple syrup. Table 20.1 provides a list of the fructose content of various foods and beverages. The main calorie-containing sweeteners—sucrose, high-fructose corn syrup, and honey—consist of roughly equal amounts of glucose and fructose.

In developed nations, the per capita fructose consumption is about 50 g/day (total carbohydrate consumption is about 400 to 500 g/day); without added sweeteners, fructose consumption would only be near 8 g/day (equivalent to <2% of all calories). Adverse effects of a high fructose intake are discussed in Section 3.4. The World Health Organization recommends that less than 10% of all calories come from honey, syrups, fruit juices, or mono- and disaccharides that are *added* to foods. At a total intake of 2000 kcal/day, less than 50 g of added sweeteners should be consumed; this translates to less than 25 g of fructose.

### 1.2. Uptake of Fructose

The microvilli of small-intestinal epithelial cells contain a **fructose transporter** (GLUT-5) that facilitates the movement of fructose down a concentration gradient and into the cells (see Fig. 18.5). GLUT-2 glucose transporters in the basolateral membrane of intestinal epithelial cells allow further equilibration of fructose with the extracellular space and blood. From there, fructose enters the liver and, to a lesser degree, the kidneys and the intestine via the same transporters. These organs act as sinks for fructose because they trap fructose by phosphorylation (see Section 1.3 and Fig. 20.2).

### 1.3. Metabolism of Dietary Fructose

Fructose metabolism is normally limited by aldolase B activity, and fructose metabolites enter glycolysis. Fig. 20.2 shows

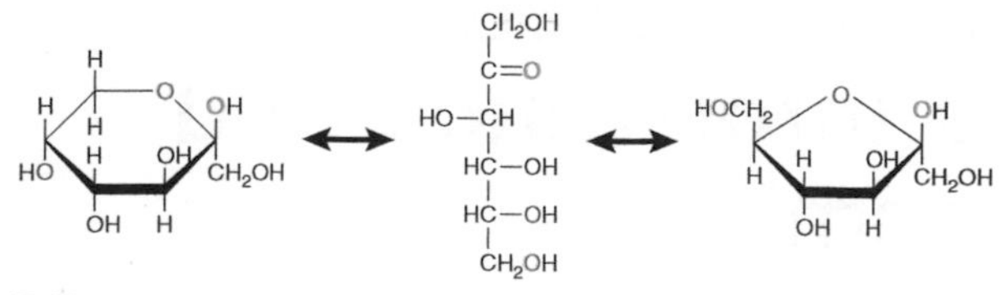

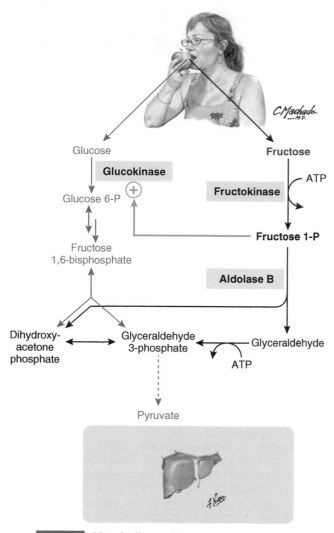

β-D-Fructopyranose
(most prevalent)

Intermediate
open form

β-D-Fructofuranose

**Fig. 20.1**   Structure of D-fructose.

**Table 20.1**   **Sugar Content of Various Foods**

| | Content in g/100 g Food | | |
|---|---|---|---|
| | Total Carbohydrate | Fructose | Galactose |
| White sugar | 100 | 51 | 0 |
| Honey | 82 | 43 | 0 |
| High-fructose corn syrup, HFCS-42 | 71 | 30 | 0 |
| High-fructose corn syrup, HFCS-55 | 77 | 42 | 0 |
| Cola (with HFCS) | 10 | 5 | 0 |
| Apple | 13 | 8 | 0 |
| Cooked carrot | 7 | 2 | 0 |
| Boiled white potato | 18 | 0 | 0 |
| Cooked white rice | 28 | 0 | 0 |
| Whole cow's milk | 5 | 0 | 3 |
| Plain yogurt | 6 | 0 | 3 |

**Fig. 20.2**   **Metabolism of fructose in the liver.**

the metabolism of fructose in detail. **Fructokinase** (also called **ketohexokinase**) has a much higher rate of flux than **aldolase B**; as a consequence, fructose 1-phosphate transiently accumulates. In the liver, fructose 1-phosphate serves as a signal for the influx of dietary carbohydrate, and it activates glucokinase (see Sections 3.5 and 5.6 in Chapter 19); as a result, dietary *fructose* helps clear dietary *glucose* from the blood.

Humans have three aldolase isoenzymes (A, B, and C); all of them function in glycolysis and gluconeogenesis (see Chapter 25), but only aldolase B can cleave fructose 1-phosphate. Fructokinase and aldolase B are expressed mainly in the liver, kidneys, and intestine.

## 2. POLYOL PATHWAY AND ITS ROLE IN DISEASE

*In the polyol pathway, glucose is reduced to sorbitol, which in turn is oxidized to fructose. In patients with chronic hyperglycemia, increased production of sorbitol and fructose from glucose contributes to cataract formation and small-vessel disease that brings about retinopathy, nephropathy, and peripheral neuropathy.*

The **polyol pathway** consists of the two steps: glucose → sorbitol → fructose (Fig. 20.3), and it is present in a wide variety of cells. Sorbitol is a sugar alcohol. Aldose reductase, the rate-limiting enzyme of the polyol pathway, has a very low affinity for glucose ($K_m \geq 50$ mM). Thus, the flux in the pathway is markedly increased during hyperglycemia.

In the medulla of the **kidney**, hypertonicity stimulates the synthesis of aldose reductase, and sorbitol helps to maintain the intracellular osmotic pressure. In other cells, aldose reductase may detoxify various aldehydes. In the male reproductive tract, the polyol pathway produces fructose as a fuel for sperm (see below).

A large amount of natural **sorbitol** is found in dried prunes (15 g/100 g); decreased amounts are found in other fruits (0.1 to 2.5 g/100 g). Sorbitol is also found in some pills, chewing gums (sorbitol does not promote caries), jams, baked goods, and ice creams. The liver converts dietary sorbitol to fructose, which it degrades.

On U.S. food labels, sorbitol is considered to be a carbohydrate, not a sugar. Consequently, foods with added sorbitol may carry the label "no sugar added."

In diabetic patients who have chronic **hyperglycemia**, activity in the polyol pathway is thought to contribute to lens cataracts, peripheral **neuropathy**, **retinopathy**, and **nephropathy** (Fig. 20.4). Increased aldose reductase activity lowers the concentration of NADPH and thus also lowers the concentration of reduced glutathione (Fig. 20.5). This in turn may permit the presence of increased amounts of reactive oxygen species, which then inflict damage to various cell components (see Chapter 21). In addition, sorbitol may accumulate in tissues that have low sorbitol dehydrogenase activity. This may damage cells through osmotic effects and contribute to neuropathy, retinopathy, and the formation of cataracts. Diabetes-related complications are discussed further in Chapter 39.

In the evaluation of **infertility**, **fructose** is often measured in the ejaculate. About 90% of the fructose in the ejaculate is derived from the **seminal vesicles** (Fig. 20.6), which synthesize fructose via the polyol pathway. The concentration of fructose in semen (normally more than about 7 mM when measured 1 hour after ejaculation) thus serves as an indicator of the function of the seminal vesicles. In the absence of fructose, sperm have a much shortened lifespan.

## 3. ABNORMAL FRUCTOSE ABSORPTION AND METABOLISM

*The most significant heritable disease of fructose metabolism is a deficiency of aldolase B, which causes hereditary*

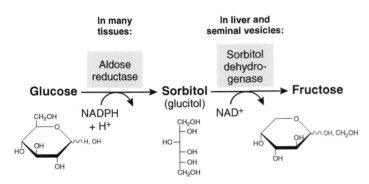

**Fig. 20.3** **The polyol pathway.** Aldose reductase also reduces galactose, producing galactitol (see Fig. 20-9).

**Normal retina:**

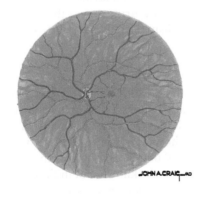

**Peripheral neuropathy:**

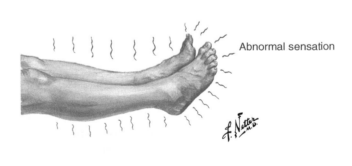

Abnormal sensation

**Proliferative diabetic retinopathy:**

Hemorrhage

Distention

Exudates

Infarction

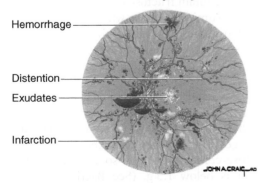

**Diabetic nephropathy:**

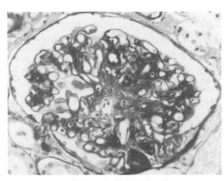

Thickened basement membrane of glomeruli

**Fig. 20.4** **Complications of diabetes due in part to increased flux through the polyol pathway.**

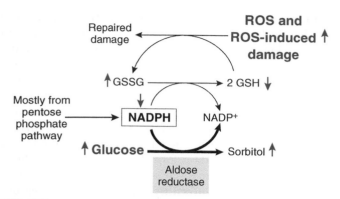

**Fig. 20.5** Hyperglycemia-induced increase in flux through the polyol pathway causes increased reactive oxygen species (ROS) and ROS-induced damage. GSH, glutathione; GSSG, oxidized glutathione.

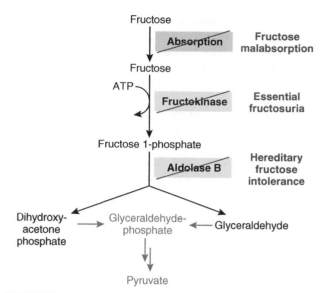

**Fig. 20.7** Sites of problems with fructose metabolism.

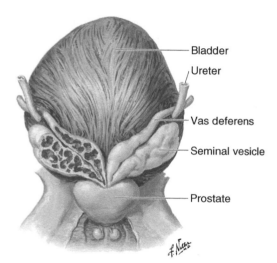

**Fig. 20.6** Most of the fructose in semen stems from fructose secreted by the bilateral seminal vesicles.

*fructose intolerance (HFI). If affected patients consume fructose, their liver and kidneys suffer from a depletion of intracellular adenosine triphosphate (ATP) and phosphate and thus fail to perform their regular functions; this can be lethal.*

## 3.1. Fructose Malabsorption

All humans suffer from intestinal discomfort if they consume more fructose than they can absorb. Normally, the small intestine can absorb ~15 g or more of fructose from a pure fructose solution. If fructose reaches the colon, it may give rise to abdominal discomfort (from gas produced by bacteria) and diarrhea (from osmosis; see Chapter 18).

Patients who have fructose malabsorption (Fig. 20.7) have intestinal discomfort after a relatively low dose of fructose. Malabsorption is often determined by a hydrogen breath test (see Section 4 in Chapter 18). There is no agreed-upon definition for fructose malabsorption, and it is not clear why certain patients can tolerate only a small amount of fructose.

## 3.2. Fructosuria

Fructosuria is a very rare and harmless disease that is due to the absence of **fructokinase** (see Fig. 20.7). Affected patients do not efficiently phosphorylate fructose; as a result, dietary fructose remains in the bloodstream for several hours. Fructose is lost from the bloodstream by filtration in the kidneys and excretion with urine (hence the name fructosuria), as well as by metabolism (details are poorly known).

## 3.3. Hereditary Fructose Intolerance

Patients with HFI have an **aldolase B deficiency** and become extremely ill when they consume even an average amount of fructose. Aldolase B cleaves fructose 1-phosphate (see Fig. 20.7). HFI shows autosomal recessive inheritance and affects about 1 in 20,000 people. More than 60 mutations in the aldolase B gene are known, but in Europe and North America, about 75% of affected patients are homozygous or compound heterozygous for the mutations A149P and A174D. The first symptoms usually appear in infants with the introduction of fructose-containing foods (see Table 20.1). Some soy-based infant formulas contain fructose in the form of sucrose. Most babies start consuming fructose when they start eating solid foods. Affected babies experience abdominal pain within a few minutes of fructose consumption, which is accompanied by nausea, vomiting, and hypoglycemia. Affected children who chronically ingest fructose have retarded growth and may incur irreversible or even lethal damage to their liver and kidneys. Since there is associated discomfort, fructose-intolerant children learn to avoid the most offending foods; however, for good health, they must knowingly exclude additional fructose-containing foods so that the daily fructose consumption is below 1.5 g. (See Baerlocher et al. in the Further Reading section for individual histories of several patients with HFI.)

If a patient with HFI consumes fructose, the liver, kidneys, and intestine accumulate fructose 1-phosphate to a high concentration (up to about 10 mM; Fig. 20.8). In the process, cytosolic ATP is used. Furthermore, phosphate is temporarily locked up in fructose 1-phosphate, leading to a severe

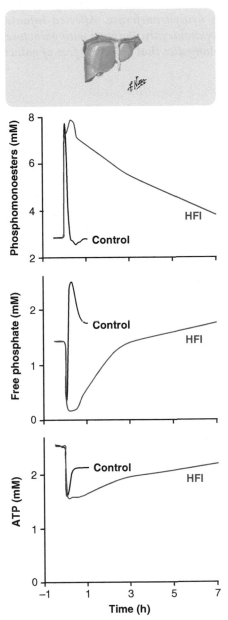

**Fig. 20.8** **Effect of intravenous fructose on phosphate-containing compounds in the liver.** Magnetic resonance imaging studies of three healthy volunteers and one volunteer with hereditary fructose intolerance were performed. After an overnight fast, patients were infused with 0.2 g of fructose/kg body weight (~30% of average daily Western consumption). The change in the phosphomonoester concentration is mostly due to fructose 1-phosphate. Note that even in the controls, the concentration of adenosine triphosphate (ATP) did not recover to its original value. (Modified from Boesiger P, Buchli R, Meier D, Steinmann B, Gitzelmann R. Changes of liver metabolite concentrations in adults with disorders of fructose metabolism after intravenous fructose by 31P magnetic resonance spectroscopy. *Pediatr Res.* 1994;36:436-440.)

deficit in cytoplasmic phosphate. The release of phosphate from hydroxyapatite in the mitochondria and the uptake of phosphate from the blood are too slow to maintain a near-normal cytoplasmic concentration of phosphate. As a result of the cell-wide phosphate deficiency, insufficient ADP is phosphorylated to ATP. Under these circumstances, ADP and AMP are degraded to urate, which is released into the blood (see Chapter 38). Marked depletion of ATP in the kidneys and liver causes failure of these organs. In the kidneys, the proximal tubules fail to take up electrolytes from the glomerular filtrate, a condition called renal **Fanconi syndrome**. The liver no longer secretes adequate amounts of clotting factors, and patients may show petechiae. Patients also have fructose-induced hypoglycemia, which is incompletely understood. The hypoglycemia may be due to excessive activation of glucokinase in the liver (see Chapter 19) and the inhibition of glycogenolysis and gluconeogenesis (see Chapters 24 and 25). Glycogenolysis is impaired by the low concentration of phosphate and gluconeogenesis by the low concentration of ATP.

In patients with HFI who do not consume fructose, glycolysis and gluconeogenesis in the liver and kidneys are not significantly impaired because these tissues also express aldolase A and because aldolase B has residual activity toward its substrates in glycolysis and gluconeogenesis.

### 3.4. Concerns About High Fructose Consumption in the General Population

A small amount of fructose is part of the traditional human diet, appears to serve as an indicator of the influx of carbohydrate from the diet (see Chapter 19), and improves glucose tolerance. However, a high consumption of fructose, typically from fructose-containing sweeteners, may have adverse effects. Fructose consumption of 100 g/day or more is associated with **hypertriglyceridemia** and often with **hypercholesterolemia**. The following mechanism has been suggested as a cause of the hypertriglyceridemia (see Figs. 19.11 and 20.2). Given the normal abundance of enzymes of fructose metabolism and glycolysis, and because of a difference in control, fructose metabolism can feed trioses into glycolysis at a greater rate than can occur with glucose. Then, pyruvate and citrate are also produced at a higher rate, fatty acyl-CoA are synthesized at a higher rate, and fatty acyl-CoA are readily esterified with glycerol 3-phosphate, thereby giving rise to triglycerides.

High fructose intake is also associated with **gout** (see Section 4 in Chapter 38). A high intake of **fructose** from sucrose, high-fructose corn syrup, fruit juices, or fruit can lead to an accumulation of AMP in the liver and kidneys. AMP is then degraded into urate, which can lead to hyperuricemia, a precondition for gout.

Approximately 1 in 70 persons is a carrier for HFI and has decreased aldolase B activity and thus an impaired capacity to metabolize fructose 1-phosphate. Whether an average rate of fructose consumption is particularly harmful to this population remains to be determined. The data on ATP shown in

Fig. 20.8 raise the possibility that the current high fructose consumption is detrimental even to the general population.

For healthy persons, the benefits of consuming fruit are thought to outweigh the potential adverse effects of fructose in the fruit.

### 3.5. Problems With the Use of Fructose or Sorbitol in Medicine

In most countries the intravenous administration of fructose or sorbitol is restricted. As is evident from Fig. 20.8 and Sections 3.3 and 3.4, infusion of fructose can pose serious threats to the liver of patients with normal or compromised aldolase B activity. Sorbitol is metabolized to fructose (see Section 2) and is therefore equally troublesome. Many patients with HFI do not know that they are fructose intolerant; a significant infusion of fructose could be lethal to such a patient.

## 4.  NORMAL METABOLISM OF GALACTOSE

*A large number of tissues degrade galactose to glucose 6-phosphate.*

The principal dietary source of galactose is the disaccharide **lactose** (see Fig. 18.1) from milk products (see Table 20.1). The structure of galactose is shown in Fig. 20.9. Galactose is a reducing sugar.

In the small intestine, **lactase** cleaves lactose into glucose and galactose (see Chapter 18). Galactose moves from the lumen of the intestine into absorptive epithelial cells via the same $Na^+$-driven glucose transporters (SGLT1) as does dietary glucose (see Fig. 18.5). Then, via glucose transporters, galactose is released into the bloodstream and taken up from the blood by other tissues.

All cells can metabolize galactose and feed the products into glycolysis, glycogen synthesis, or gluconeogenesis (see Fig. 20.9). The pathway from galactose to glucose 1-phosphate

is also called the **Leloir pathway**. Glycogen synthesis is discussed in Chapter 24. Gluconeogenesis is active in the fasting state and decreases in the fed state (see Chapter 25).

## 5. GALACTOSEMIA

*Classic galactosemia is due to a deficiency of galactose 1-phosphate uridyltransferase. Affected infants show cataracts and hepatomegaly. Patients with galactosemia need to follow a lifelong diet that is largely free of galactose.*

### 5.1. Classical Galactosemia

Classical galactosemia is due to a deficiency of **galactose 1-phosphate uridyltransferase** (see Fig. 20.9), which leads to increased concentrations of galactose 1-phosphate, galactose, and galactitol. Since most tissues (including red blood cells) normally metabolize galactose, damage in patients with galactosemia affects *many* tissues. Galactose 1-phosphate accumulates inside cells and temporarily traps **phosphate** (this is comparable to the accumulation of fructose 1-phosphate in patients with HFI; see Fig. 20.8). As a result, phosphorylation of ADP to ATP is impaired, which leads to cell damage. Furthermore, since the phosphorylation of galactose to galactose 1-phosphate is a reversible reaction, a galactose 1-phosphate uridyltransferase deficiency also leads to an elevated concentration of galactose. Galactose then activates aldose reductase from the polyol pathway, which generates **galactitol** (the $K_m$ of aldose reductase for galactose is ~15 mM; see Section 2). Galactitol is not a substrate of sorbitol dehydrogenase, the second enzyme of the polyol pathway. Galactitol, once formed, cannot be degraded; it is lost into the blood, filtered in the glomeruli, and not recovered from kidney tubules; thus it is excreted in the urine. Tissue damage may be due to a combination of osmotic effects of galactitol that alter intracellular signaling and free radical damage due to depletion of NADPH from the formation of galactitol (see Fig. 20.9). Finally, a

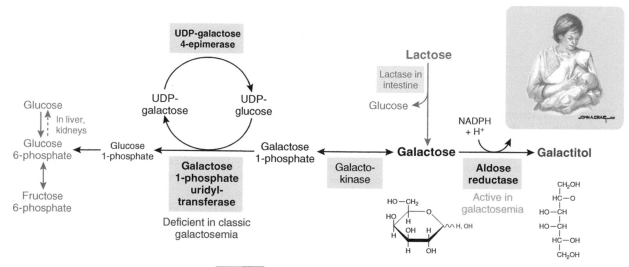

**Fig. 20.9**  **Metabolism of galactose.**

deficiency of galactose 1-phosphate uridyltransferase might also alter glycosylation of proteins (see Chapter 7).

In Europe and North America, the **incidence** of classical galactosemia is on the order of 1 in 35,000, with appreciable variation between countries. The disease is inherited in an autosomal **recessive** fashion.

Although well over 200 **mutations** in galactose 1-phosphate uridyltransferase are known, only a handful of mutations are common among affected patients. The mutation S135L is common among individuals with African ancestry, while Q188R is common among individuals with European ancestry. The severity of the disease can be correlated with certain mutations. DNA-based prenatal diagnosis is possible.

Classical galactosemia is usually evident after a few days of milk ingestion by a newborn, who may then exhibit symptoms of jaundice, hepatomegaly, vomiting, diarrhea, and Fanconi syndrome (Fig. 20.10). Some newborns also develop sepsis or coagulation defects. The urine of affected newborns tests positive for a reducing substance (galactose; see Section 1 in Chapter 18) and tests negative for glucose. Fanconi syndrome is due to a low concentration of ATP in the kidneys, as in patients with HFI after fructose ingestion (see Section 3.3). Galactosemia may also be detected by a newborn screening test.

**Treatment** of galactosemia involves greatly reducing dietary galactose intake by stopping breastfeeding or milk-based formula and feeding newborns a soy-based formula that has a low galactose content. Without treatment, patients become severely intellectually impaired. Dairy products (containing the disaccharide lactose or the monosaccharide galactose) are excluded from the diet. The degradation of glycoproteins and glycolipids in the body itself generates a significant amount of galactose, which is tolerated so that the complete exclusion of dietary galactose is unnecessary. Hence, patients who have classic galactosemia can consume fruits and vegetables, even if they contain small amounts of galactose (up to ~0.3 g galactose/100 g food). The success of treatment can be followed with measurements of the concentration of galactose 1-phosphate in red blood cells.

Treatment with a galactose-restricted diet is lifesaving and prevents severe mental impairment, but treated patients still face major problems with **mentation**, reproduction, and eyesight. About 80% of children with galactosemia have a full-scale IQ score of less than 90 (the test is designed for a maximum of 160 and a mean of 100 in the population at large). Affected children are likely to have problems with speech. Virtually all females develop **hypergonadotrophic hypogonadism** in their teens (i.e., an impaired response of the gonads to gonadotropins with subsequent hypertrophy of the gonadotropin-secreting anterior pituitary gland). Some of these women are sterile due to atrophy of the ovaries. About 10% of patients who have galactosemia develop **cataracts** at an early age; this is treatable with surgery. Some of the long-term problems seen in patients with galactosemia may be a consequence of in utero exposure to galactose.

## 5.2. Nonclassical Galactosemia

Patients with nonclassical galactosemia have a deficiency of **galactokinase** or **uridine diphosphate (UDP)-galactose/ UDP-glucose 4-epimerase**. Patients with a galactokinase deficiency primarily develop cataracts due to a persistently elevated concentration of galactose in the blood and the consequent formation of galactitol in the lenses. These patients do not show damage to liver, kidneys, and brain that is typical of classical galactosemia. Patients with a very rare, generalized epimerase deficiency have symptoms that are similar to those of patients with classical galactosemia.

## 6. LACTOSE SYNTHESIS IN THE LACTATING BREAST

*The lactating breast synthesizes lactose from glucose and galactose. Most of the lactose is derived from glucose in the blood. Lactose is the principal osmolyte of milk and thus plays a role in determining milk volume.*

Fig. 20.11 shows the pathway of lactose synthesis in the lactating mammary gland.

The synthesis of lactose depends on the presence of **lactose synthase**, which is a complex of soluble **α-lactalbumin** and a membrane-anchored **galactosyl transferase** in the Golgi apparatus. Most cells express a small amount of galactosyl transferase for the purpose of protein glycosylation in which the enzyme transfers galactose to glucose that is covalently linked to the side chain amino group of a protein (see Chapter 7). Several weeks before pregnancy term and throughout lactation, the mammary gland expresses vastly increased amounts of galactosyl transferase. Late in pregnancy, the mammary glands also express α-lactalbumin, and there is a further

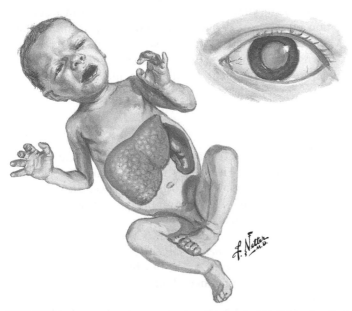

**Fig. 20.10** **Galactosemia often manifests itself within the first few days of life.** Cataracts are occasionally seen at birth but generally develop only later.

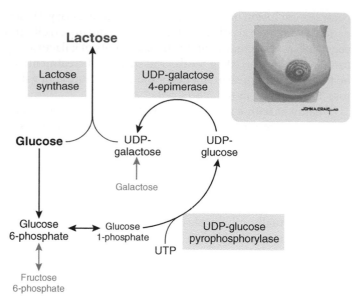

**Lactose**

Lactose synthase

UDP-galactose 4-epimerase

**Glucose**

UDP-galactose

UDP-glucose

Galactose

Glucose 6-phosphate

Glucose 1-phosphate

UDP-glucose pyrophosphorylase

UTP

Fructose 6-phosphate

**Fig. 20.11** **Synthesis of lactose from glucose in the lactating breast.** All cells can carry out the above reactions except the lactose synthase–catalyzed reaction. Only the mammary gland produces lactose synthase, and it does so only during the third trimester of pregnancy and during lactation. Cells use uridine diphosphate (UDP)-glucose for the synthesis of glycogen (see Chapter 24) and UDP-galactose for glycosylation of proteins (see Chapter 7). UTP, uridine triphosphate.

marked increase around the time of delivery. α-Lactalbumin binds glucose and forms a complex with galactosyl transferase such that glucose (instead of protein-linked glucose) becomes the favored acceptor of galactose, thus forming lactose.

In the lactating breast, in the *fed* state, all of the glucose and about 70% of the galactose in lactose are derived from glucose in the blood. After a 1-day *fast*, about 70% of the glucose and about 50% of the galactose are derived from glucose in the blood. It is unclear which processes contribute the remaining glucose and galactose. Gluconeogenesis, the process of glucose synthesis from nonglucose precursors that normally occurs in the liver and kidneys (see Chapter 25), might also be active in the lactating mammary gland. Galactose can serve as a precursor for lactose synthesis if the lactating woman consumes a large amount of galactose (typically as lactose from dairy products; see Figs. 20.9 and 20.11).

α-Lactalbumin and lactose are both secreted into milk. Milk contains about 7 g of lactose/dL (i.e., about 70 times more carbohydrate on a weight basis than is found in blood plasma). Milk also contains about 1 to 2 g of protein/ dL, of which about 0.2 to 0.3 g/dL is α-lactalbumin. Since lactose is the main osmolyte of milk, it determines milk volume.

## SUMMARY

- Fructose is present in many sweeteners as well as fruits and vegetables. The liver, kidneys, and intestinal mucosa degrade fructose to intermediates of glycolysis (or gluconeogenesis). In the liver, one intermediate, fructose

1-phosphate, activates glucokinase and thus serves as an indicator of the influx of carbohydrate from the diet.

- The polyol pathway converts glucose to sorbitol and fructose, thereby consuming NADPH. In hyperglycemic patients, increased flux through this pathway is responsible for some of the damage to the lenses and small blood vessels in the retina, glomeruli, and peripheral nerves. In patients with classic galactosemia and a consequently elevated concentration of galactose in tissues, the production of galactitol by the polyol pathway gives rise to lens cataracts.

- Hereditary fructose intolerance (HFI) has an incidence of about 1 in 20,000. The disease is due to a deficiency of aldolase B. Upon consumption of fructose, this leads to an accumulation of fructose 1-phosphate in the liver and the kidneys. This, in turn, is accompanied by a severe drop in intracellular phosphate, as well as a drop in intracellular ATP, that impairs the function of the liver and kidneys. Affected patients must exclude fructose-containing sweeteners, fruits, and many vegetables from their diet.

- Many patients have undiagnosed HFI, and carriers for the disease (about 1% of the population) also show a mild impairment of fructose metabolism. Most countries restrict the intravenous infusion of fructose or its precursor, sorbitol.

- Due to the extensive use of fructose-containing sweeteners, per capita fructose consumption in developed nations is several times higher than it used to be in antiquity. High fructose consumption is associated with hyperlipidemia and gout.

- Galactose is present predominantly in lactose in milk products. Most tissues degrade galactose to glucose 6-phosphate, which enters glycolysis or gluconeogenesis.

- Patients who have classical galactosemia are deficient in galactose 1-phosphate uridyltransferase. After the consumption of galactose, the deficiency leads to an accumulation of galactose 1-phosphate and a drop in intracellular phosphate and ATP. After consuming milk, affected newborns vomit, and they develop hepatomegaly and Fanconi syndrome. Treatment involves the lifelong exclusion of most dietary galactose.

## FURTHER READING

- Baerlocher K, Gitzelmann R, Steinmann B, Gitzelmann-Cumarasamy N. Hereditary fructose intolerance in early childhood: a major diagnostic challenge. *Helv Paediatr Acta*. 1978;33:465-487. This report contains a survey of 20 symptomatic patients.

- Berry GT. Galactosemia: when is it a newborn screening emergency? *Mol Genet Metab*. 2012;106:7-11.

- Bouteldja N, Timson DJ. The biochemical basis of hereditary fructose intolerance. *J Inherit Metab Dis*. 2010;33: 105-112.

- Coss KP, Doran PP, Owoeye C, et al. Classical galactosaemia in Ireland: incidence, complications and outcomes of treatment. *J Inherit Metab Dis*. 2013;36:21-27.

■ Galactosemia Foundation: http://www.galactosemia.org. This website has information about the galactose content of a wide range of foods; click on "Galactosemia," then "Diet Resources" and "Galactose Contents in Food."

■ Hennermann JB, Schadewaldt P, Vetter B, Shin YS, Mönch E, Klein J. Features and outcome of galactokinase deficiency in children diagnosed by newborn screening. *J Inherit Metab Dis.* 2011;34:399-407.

■ Jones HF, Butler RN, Brooks DA. Intestinal fructose transport and malabsorption in humans. *Am J Physiol Gastrointest Liver Physiol.* 2011;300:G202-G206.

■ Lobitz S, Velleuer E. Guido Fanconi (1892-1979): a jack of all trades. *Nat Rev Cancer.* 2006;6:893-898.

■ Van Calcar SC, Bernstein LE, Rohr FJ, Scaman CH, Yannicelli S, Berry GT. A re-evaluation of life-long severe galactose restriction for the nutrition management of classic galactosemia. *Mol Genet Metab.* 2014;112:191-197.

# Review Questions

1. Newborns who have galactosemia due to a galactose 1-phosphate uridyltransferase deficiency and who are breastfed during their first three weeks of life usually develop liver dysfunction, bleeding, hyperbilirubinemia (too much bilirubin in the blood), abnormalities of ion transport in the kidney tubules, diarrhea, and vomiting. They also tend to become septic. These pathologic events are most likely due to which of the following?

   A. Bacterial metabolism of lactose to various gases and acids
   B. Impaired ATP production in various tissues
   C. Impaired uptake of glucose and galactose in the intestine
   D. Protein malnutrition, which leads to decreased synthesis of clotting factors

2. Common to HFI and galactosemia is that consumption of the offending sugar:

   A. is followed by metabolism of the sugar in liver, kidneys, muscle, heart and brain.
   B. leads to an increase in the concentration of $HCO_3^-$ in blood plasma.
   C. lowers the concentration of phosphate inside hepatocytes.
   D. normally occurs during the first few days of life.

3. A patient with a deficiency of aldolase B is expected to suffer from nausea the most after consuming 20 g of which of the following carbohydrates?

   A. Amylopectin
   B. Galactose
   C. Glucose
   D. Lactose
   E. Sucrose

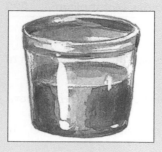

# Chapter
# 21
# Pentose Phosphate Pathway, Oxidative Stress, and Glucose 6-Phosphate Dehydrogenase Deficiency

## SYNOPSIS

- The pentose phosphate pathway branches off glycolysis and can feed back into glycolysis, albeit at a different point of the pathway. All cells are capable of the pentose phosphate pathway.
- The pentose phosphate pathway provides 5-carbon sugars for biosyntheses and reducing power (in the form of reduced nicotinamide adenine dinucleotide phosphate [NADPH]) for repair processes and biosyntheses.
- Cells with mitochondria can also make NADPH via another pathway.
- Reactive oxygen species (ROS) damage DNA, lipids, and proteins. Antioxidants (e.g., vitamin E, vitamin C, and glutathione) react with ROS or play a role in repairing ROS-induced damage.
- Some of the patients whose ancestors are from areas in which malaria has been endemic have a decreased activity of glucose 6-phosphate dehydrogenase (G6PD); their pentose phosphate pathway can therefore produce NADPH only at a decreased rate. Reduced NADPH production impairs the repair of oxidative damage in red blood cells. As a result, red blood cells may lyse in the bloodstream. Hence, affected patients must avoid oxidizing drugs.

## LEARNING OBJECTIVES

*For mastery of this topic, you should be able to do the following:*
- Describe the overall purpose of the pentose phosphate pathway as well as its reactants, products, and cellular location.
- Describe the role of reduced glutathione (GSH) in the body and the contribution of NADPH to its formation.
- Compare and contrast the production and removal of radicals, taking into account the roles of vitamin E, vitamin C, and glutathione.
- Describe an episode of drug-induced hemolytic anemia in a patient who has G6PD deficiency, and list key drugs that might be contraindicated in this patient.
- Select laboratory tests to diagnose G6PD deficiency.
- Predict the results of a complete blood count in a person who has a G6PD deficiency and just passed a hemolytic crisis.

## 1. STEPS OF THE PENTOSE PHOSPHATE PATHWAY

*The pentose phosphate pathway can be divided into an oxidative branch and a nonoxidative branch. The oxidative branch produces NADPH. The nonoxidative branch produces predominantly ribose 5-phosphate, which is used for the synthesis of nucleotides.*

### 1.1. General Comments

The pentose phosphate pathway is also called **pentose phosphate shunt**, **hexose monophosphate shunt**, or **6-phosphogluconate pathway**.

Fig. 21.1 shows a condensed version of the pentose phosphate pathway with its connections to glycolysis. Detailed versions of the two major branches of the pathway are shown in Figs. 21.3 and 21.4. The oxidative branch can proceed in only one direction, whereas the nonoxidative branch can proceed in two directions.

The pentose phosphate pathway is found in the cytosol of all cells, and it produces NADPH and ribose 5-phosphate. **NADPH** is used to maintain a reducing environment, synthesize fatty acids and steroids, and eliminate highly damaging oxidative radicals and peroxides. **Ribose 5-phosphate** is used in the de novo synthesis of purine and pyrimidine nucleotides as well as in the salvage of purine nucleotides (see Chapters 37 and 38).

Flux in the pentose phosphate pathway differs among tissues and varies over time. In red blood cells and brain, about 5% to 7% of all glucose 6-phosphate metabolism occurs via the pentose phosphate shunt. In the brain, the pentose phosphate pathway is about three times more active in patients who have a traumatic brain injury than in healthy persons. In the normal heart, the flux of glucose 6-phosphate through the pentose phosphate pathway is only about 1% of the flux through glycolysis.

### 1.2. Oxidative Branch

The oxidative branch of the pentose phosphate pathway produces **NADPH**, the structure of which is shown in Fig. 21.2. The oxidized form of NADPH is written as NADP$^+$ to indicate that a nitrogen at the business end of the molecule carries a positive charge, analogous to conventions about NAD$^+$ (see Fig. 19.3 and Section 1 of Chapter 19). NADPH differs from NADH in a phosphate group. Most enzymes distinguish between NADPH and NADH; in metabolism, these reducing agents function essentially independent of each other. In most cells, the ratio of NADPH/NADP$^+$ is about 100, whereas the ratio of NADH/NAD$^+$ is only about 0.01. This makes NADPH a stronger reducing agent than NADH.

In the oxidative branch of the pentose phosphate pathway, **glucose 6-phosphate dehydrogenase** (G6PD) and 6-phosphogluconate dehydrogenase each give rise to NADPH (Fig. 21.3). The reactions in the oxidative branch are

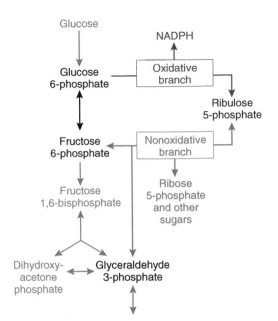

**Fig. 21.1** **The core elements of the pentose phosphate pathway and its interface with glycolysis.**

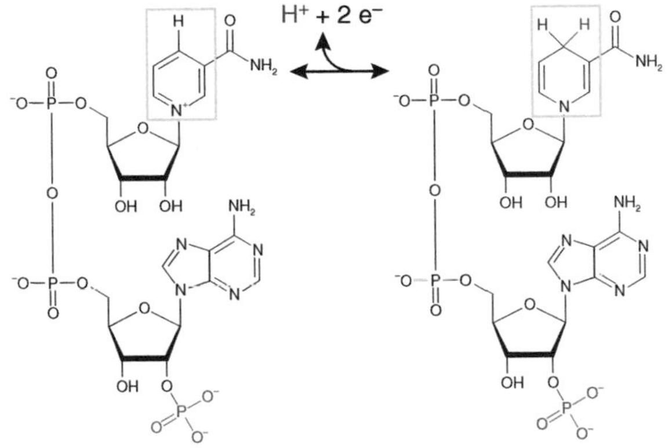

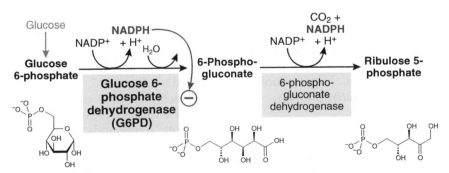

irreversible and start with glucose 6-phosphate from the glycolytic pathway. The first enzyme, G6PD, is the rate-limiting enzyme. It is controlled by product inhibition from NADPH and by the depletion of the substrate NADP$^+$. In the liver, enzyme expression is also enhanced after a carbohydrate-rich meal (this helps with NADPH production when turning carbohydrates into fatty acids; see Chapter 27). The second enzyme, 6-phosphogluconate dehydrogenase, gives rise to the sugar end product of the oxidative branch, ribulose 5-phosphate. The activity of 6-phosphogluconate dehydrogenase is not regulated. The net reaction of the oxidative branch is:

$$Glucose\ 6\text{-phosphate} + H_2O + 2\ NADP^+$$
$$\rightarrow ribulose\ 5\text{-phosphate} + CO_2 + 2\ NADPH + 2\ H^+$$

As described in Section 3, a hereditary deficiency of G6PD can lead to hemolytic anemia.

## 1.3. Nonoxidative Branch

The nonoxidative branch of the pentose phosphate pathway produces sugar phosphates, principally ribose 5-phosphate, which is used for the production of nucleotides. A simplified scheme is shown in Fig. 21.4. All reactions are reversible, and there is no regulation of the activity of the enzymes in this branch. Hence, the concentrations of sugar phosphates in the nonoxidative branch of the pentose phosphate pathway depend on the concentrations of fructose 6-phosphate and glyceraldehyde 3-phosphate in glycolysis.

The net reaction for the conversion of ribulose 5-phosphate to intermediates of glycolysis via the pentose phosphate pathway is:

$$3\ ribulose\ 5\text{-phosphate}$$
$$\rightarrow 2\ fructose\ 6\text{-phosphate} + glyceraldehyde\ 3\text{-phosphate}$$

**Transketolase activity** inside red blood cells is used to estimate the **thiamine** reserves in the body. Patients who have thiamine deficiency have abnormally low transketolase

**Fig. 21.2** **NADP$^+$ and its reduced form, NADPH.** Compared with NADH and NAD$^+$, NADPH and NADP$^+$ have a phosphate group (bottom, red) in place of a hydroxyl group.

**Fig. 21.3** **The oxidative branch of the pentose phosphate pathway produces NADPH.** When there is little need for the production of NADPH, G6PD activity is limited by a low concentration of NADP$^+$ and by product inhibition from NADPH.

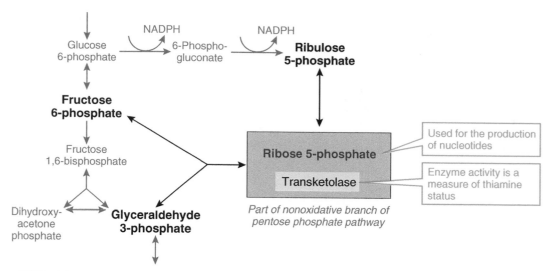

Fig. 21.4 **Fig. 21.4** **The nonoxidative branch of the pentose phosphate pathway produces mainly ribose 5-phosphate.** The reactions and stoichiometry of the nonoxidative branch are very complex and are thus depicted in a simplified version as a gray box and two connecting reactions. The nonoxidative branch includes several enzymes, including transketolase.

activity. However, low transketolase activity plays no role in the pathologic effects of thiamine deficiency. Thiamine deficiency is described in Section 5.2.2 of Chapter 22.

## 1.4. Independent Versus Joint Operation of the Branches

The oxidative and the nonoxidative branches of the pentose pathway can operate independently or jointly. The oxidative branch is unidirectional, and the nonoxidative pathway is bidirectional. When a cell needs only NADPH, it runs the oxidative branch and the nonoxidative branch from ribulose 5-phosphate to intermediates of glycolysis. When a cell needs only ribose 5-phosphate, it uses only the nonoxidative branch, starting with fructose 6-phosphate and glyceraldehyde 3-phosphate in glycolysis. When a cell needs both NADPH and ribose 5-phosphate, it uses the oxidative branch, followed by the conversion of ribulose 5-phosphate to ribose 5-phosphate via the nonoxidative branch.

## 2. PROCESSES THAT USE NADPH INSIDE CELLS

*NADPH is used in biosyntheses and the defense against ROS and radicals inside cells. NADPH, together with antioxidants (e.g., vitamins C and E) and enzymes, helps reduce the amount of free radicals and repair oxidative damage.*

### 2.1. Use of NADPH in Biosynthetic Pathways

The liver, and to a lesser degree, the adipose tissue, uses NADPH to synthesize fatty acids from carbohydrates. Besides NADPH from the pentose phosphate pathway, the liver also uses NADPH produced by malate dehydrogenase (decarbox-

**Glutathione (GSH, reduced glutathione)**
γ-glutamyl-cysteinyl-glycine

**Oxidized glutathione (GSSG, glutathione disulfide)**
Bis(γ-glutamyl-cysteinyl-glycine) disulfide

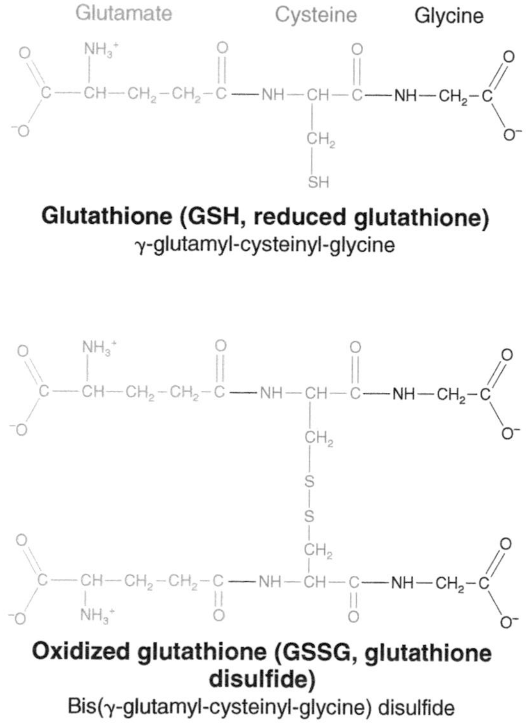

**Fig. 21.5** Reduced and oxidized forms of glutathione.

ylating). This and the de novo synthesis of fatty acids are detailed in Chapter 27.

Cytochrome P450 enzymes use NADPH to produce steroids (see Chapter 31) or to detoxify various drugs and other xenobiotic compounds.

### 2.2. NADPH Reduces Oxidized Glutathione

**Glutathione** is a reducing agent inside cells. The structure of glutathione is shown in Fig. 21.5. Glutathione consists of the tripeptide γGlu-Cys-Gly. Glutathione is synthesized by two enzymes (i.e., not by the mechanism of mRNA translation). The side chain of the Cys is the business end of glutathione. Reduced glutathione is commonly written as **GSH** (the SH stands for the thiol group in the Cys side chain). Two molecules of GSH can become oxidized to the homodimer oxidized glutathione (**GSSG**) by forming a disulfide bridge between the Cys side chains of two GSH molecules (see Fig. 21.5).

**Glutathione reductase** uses NADPH to reduce GSSG to GSH. Inside healthy cells, the concentration of GSH far exceeds that of GSSG. Thus, cells maintain large reservoirs of both NADPH and GSH.

## 2.3. Removal of ROS and Repair of ROS-Induced Damage

**ROS** are highly reactive oxygen-containing molecules, such as the **superoxide anion radical** ($\bullet O_2^-$), the **hydroxyl radical** ($\bullet OH$), **organic peroxides** (ROOH), and **hydrogen peroxide** (HOOH, $H_2O_2$). The extreme reactivity of radicals is due to the presence of an unpaired electron (denoted by the dot).

ROS-induced damage to DNA, proteins, and lipids contributes significantly to pathologic processes. Damage to DNA that is not properly repaired (see Chapter 2) can lead to genetic changes that result in **cancer**. Damage to proteins, particularly those with long half-lives, such as collagen, elastin, and crystallin (a protein of the eye lens), leads to changes associated with **aging**. Damage to lipids is a significant contributor to **atherosclerosis**.

Some ROS are formed intentionally and are important to the function of peroxisomes and the normal immune response, whereas other ROS are produced in undesired side reactions. About 1% of the oxygen consumed by the body is converted to ROS, mostly as an unintentional byproduct of **oxidative phosphorylation** (Fig. 21.6; see Chapter 23). Free **iron** considerably enhances the undesired formation of ROS via the Haber-Weiss and Fenton reactions (see Chapter 15). Neutrophils generate hypochlorous acid (HOCl) to kill pathogens.

Superoxide anions ($\bullet O_2^-$) derive chiefly from oxidative phosphorylation and cytochrome P450 enzymes (see Fig. 21.6). The **superoxide anion** is a weak radical, but in the presence of iron it gives rise to highly reactive **hydroxyl radicals** ($\bullet OH$). $\bullet OH$ is one of the most aggressive radicals; it diffuses only 5 to 10 times its diameter until it reacts. $\bullet OH$ can react with guanine in DNA (forming 8-oxo-guanine; see Section 1 in Chapter 2), hydroxylate phenylalanine and tyrosine in proteins, and give rise to lipid radicals. Oxidative damage to lipids leads to a self-propagating cycle of damage (Fig. 21.7).

Glutathione peroxidase, which removes $H_2O_2$ and lipid peroxides, contains **selenium** (Se) in **selenocysteine** that is part of the catalytic site (see Chapter 9). Adequate Se in the diet has a cancer-preventive effect, perhaps through reduced free radical damage to DNA.

We acquire **Se** mainly from cereals and animals. The amount of Se in cereal foods depends on the amount of Se in the soil. For instance, wheat from the United States is high in Se, whereas wheat from unfortified soils in the United Kingdom and Finland is low in Se.

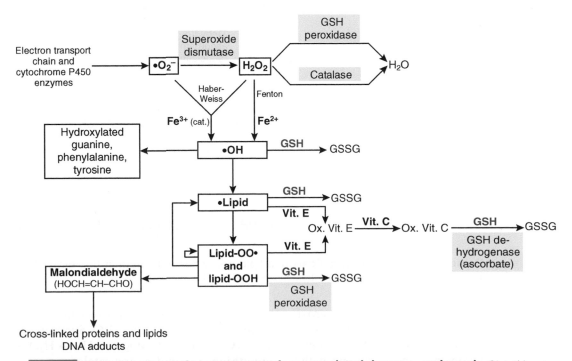

**Fig. 21.6** **Overview of reactive oxygen species, associated damage, and repair.** Glutathione (GSH), vitamin E, and vitamin C are involved in removing radicals. Maintenance of an adequate concentration of GSH requires an adequate supply of NADPH from the pentose phosphate shunt.

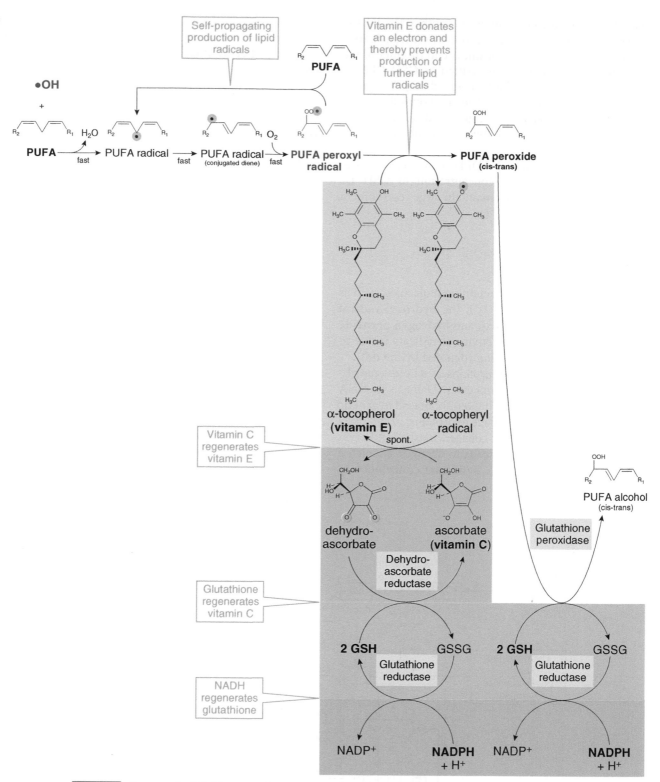

**Fig. 21.7** **Removal of lipid peroxyl radicals and lipid peroxides with vitamin E, vitamin C, glutathione, and NADPH.** *PUFA,* polyunsaturated fatty acid (see Chapter 27).

When **Se deficiency** develops, glutathione peroxidase activity is first to dwindle. Se-deficient patients have decreased antioxidant defenses and increased susceptibility to infection, cancer, myopathy, and cardiomyopathy. Susceptibility to infection increases further with vitamin E deficiency.

The body's defense against oxidative damage rests in part on removing ROS (see Fig. 21.6). **Superoxide dismutase** converts $\bullet O_2^-$ to $H_2O_2$ ($2\ \bullet O_2^- + 2\ H^+ \rightarrow H_2O_2 + O_2$), and both **glutathione peroxidase** and **catalase** remove $H_2O_2$ ($2\ GSH + H_2O_2 \rightarrow GSSG + 2\ H_2O$; $2\ H_2O_2 \rightarrow 2\ H_2O + O_2$). Together with the maintenance of an environment of a low concentration of free **iron**, this minimizes the production of •OH. •OH cannot be effectively removed by an enzyme because it reacts before it could diffuse to an enzyme. •OH and the lipid radicals it gives rise to are removed to some degree by **glutathione**, which is ubiquitous. Glutathione also removes lipid radicals (2 GSH + 2 •lipid → GSSG + 2 lipid). Fig. 21.7 shows how the fat-soluble **vitamin E**, ascorbate, glutathione, and NADPH work together in a chain to react with various lipid radicals.

Degradation of cyclized lipid peroxyl radicals yields **malondialdehyde**, which in turn **crosslinks proteins** and/or **lipids** (see Fig. 21.6). In clinical research, the concentration of circulating malondialdehyde is sometimes used as a measure of oxidative damage.

The terms **antioxidant** and **free radical scavengers** are used synonymously for compounds that react with oxidants by donating at least one H with its one electron. Antioxidants are frequently divided into fat-soluble and water-soluble compounds. The major **fat-soluble antioxidants** in the human body are:

- **Vitamin E.**
- **Carotenes,** including **vitamin A, β-carotene** (in carrots, pumpkins), and **lycopene** (in tomatoes).
- **Coenzyme QH2 (ubiquinol)** is found in all membranes, reacts with ROS, and thereby protects unsaturated fatty acids in membranes. Ubiquinol is also part of the electron transport chain (see Chapter 23) in the inner mitochondrial membrane.
- **Dihydrolipoic acid** is active both in the cytosol and in membranes. Lipoic acid (see Fig. 22.5) is sometimes used in the treatment of painful diabetic neuropathy. Cells reduce exogenous lipoic acid to the antioxidant dihydrolipoic acid. The R(+) enantiomer of lipoic acid also serves as a reversibly reduced prosthetic group of pyruvate dehydrogenase, α-ketoglutarate dehydrogenase, and branched-chain ketoacid dehydrogenase.
- **Bilirubin** is a degradation product of heme that circulates in blood as part of its transport from the spleen to the liver (see Chapter 14).

The major **water-soluble** antioxidants include:

- **Ascorbate**
- **Glutathione**
- **Uric acid,** which preferentially reacts with peroxynitrite, the product of a reaction between superoxide anion and nitric oxide

Finally, the body's defense against oxidative damage also includes the repair of damage to DNA and proteins. DNA **base excision repair** repairs 8-oxo-guanine in DNA (see Section 1 in Chapter 2), which is the predominant DNA base damage inflicted by ROS (from •OH, reacting with guanine). The concentration of 8-oxo-guanine can be used as a measure of a cell's stress. Damage to proteins from ROS and hypochlorous acid affects mostly cysteine and methionine residues; this can lead to the formation of cysteine disulfides and methionine

sulfoxide, for example. Thioredoxin- or glutaredoxin-dependent enzymes reduce disulfide bonds (–S–S–). Methionine sulfoxide reductase reduces methionine sulfoxide. Other types of damage often remain unrepaired and are dealt with by the ongoing degradation of proteins and concurrent synthesis of new proteins.

## 3. GLUCOSE 6-PHOSPHATE DEHYDROGENASE DEFICIENCY

*A deficiency of G6PD is a common X-linked disorder that is prevalent in populations originating from certain regions where malaria has been, or still is, endemic. It is marked by an increased incidence of neonatal jaundice and then, throughout life, by susceptibility to hemolysis after oxidative stress.*

Deficiency of G6PD (see Section 1) is very common in populations originating from parts of the world where malaria has been or still is endemic (i.e., equatorial Africa, Middle East, Mediterranean, and Southeast Asia; see Fig. 17.1). The reason for this finding is that G6PD-deficient persons are less likely to have severe malaria. About 5% to 25% of people from the above populations have one of the variant alleles with low G6PD activity. The gene is located on the X chromosome; males are more frequently symptomatic than females. Low G6PD activity limits production of NADPH and maintenance of GSH (glutathione), thereby impairing the defense against oxidative stress (see Section 2). A total lack of the enzyme is lethal.

When G6PD-deficient erythrocytes experience excessive oxidative damage due to impaired defense against ROS, they hemolyze in the bloodstream (**intravascular hemolysis**) and give rise to **hematuria**. In unaffected persons, only a small number of red blood cells normally lyse in the bloodstream, and most erythrocytes are instead cleared by the spleen and liver (see Chapter 14). In G6PD-deficient persons, the hemolysis is more extensive than normal and can lead to anemia and jaundice. Some patients with severe disease require a transfusion of fresh red blood cells. Often, **Heinz bodies** (aggregates of damaged globin) accumulate inside red blood cells of G6PD-deficient individuals who experience increased oxidative stress. Heinz bodies are detected by microscopic observation of a stained blood smear. The hemolysis resolves once the oxidizing substance that triggered the attack is removed.

About 140 mutations in the G6PD gene are known, which explains in part the variation in patient response to oxidative stress. A variant called **G6PD A–** is common in people whose origin is in Africa. The variant entails two point mutations that lead to the amino acid substitutions Val68Met and Asn126Asp. **G6PD Mediterranean** is common in people from the Mediterranean, the Middle East, and India; it entails a point mutation that leads to a Ser188Phe substitution. The large majority of G6PD variants affects the **stability** of the G6PD protein. These variants have minimal effect on cells that continuously synthesize new G6PD. However, the instability of G6PD

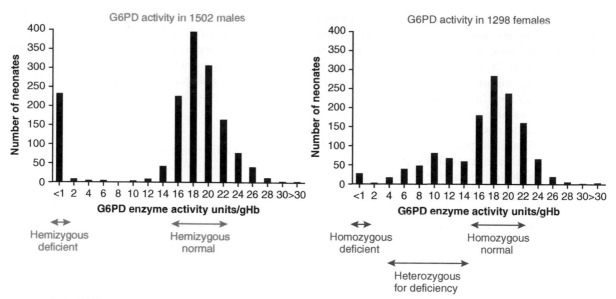

**Fig. 21.8** **G6PD activity in male and female newborns.** G6PD activity was measured in newborns of Sephardic Jewish ethnicity, a group in which G6PD deficiency is common. Blue and red arrows indicate approximate ranges. (Modified from Algur N, Avraham I, Hammerman C, Kaplan M. Quantitative neonatal glucose-6-phosphate dehydrogenase screening: distribution, reference values, and classification by phenotype. *J Pediatr.* 2012;161:197-200.)

affects red blood cells, which cannot synthesize new G6PD molecules (mature erythrocytes do not have DNA, RNA, or ribosomes). Severe G6PD deficiency can also impair the function of peripheral nerves, perhaps due to loss of G6PD activity during transport in axons.

Since **females** show patchy, random **X-inactivation**, heterozygous females show a broad range of approximately intermediate G6PD activity that eludes easy classification (Fig. 21.8).

G6PD-deficient newborns are at increased risk for **neonatal jaundice** (see Chapter 14) and its complications. Severe hyperbilirubinemia leads to brain damage. Many cases of severe neonatal hyperbilirubinemia are due to a G6PD deficiency. Hence, all newborns who are at risk of G6PD deficiency due to parental carrier status or ethnic background should have their bilirubin levels monitored closely.

Erythrocytes of G6PD-deficient individuals may hemolyze during an **infection**, such as during pneumonia, hepatitis B, or symptomatic infection with cytomegalovirus (a herpes virus).

After ingestion of **fava beans** (also called broad beans), erythrocytes of G6PD-deficient persons may hemolyze. Fava beans (from the plant *Vicia faba*) contain vicine, which is an oxidizing agent. Hemolysis precipitated by fava beans has been known since antiquity and has been referred to as **favism**.

**Oxidative drugs** that predictably cause hemolysis in patients with at least mild G6PD deficiency are **primaquine** and **dapsone** (used as antimalarials), **methylene blue** (used to treat methemoglobinemia), **phenazopyridine** (used as an analgesic and antipyretic), and the $H_2O_2$-producing **uricases,** such as rasburicase and pegloticase (used mostly in the treatment of tumor lysis syndrome and in gout that cannot be treated with other drugs). Severe hemolysis can lead to acute

**Table 21.1** **WHO Classification of G6PD Deficiency**

| Class | Hemolysis | G6PD Activity, % of Normal |
|---|---|---|
| I | Chronic | <10 |
| II | Only with infection or drugs | <10 |
| III | Only with infection or drugs | 10–60 |

kidney injury. In a setting of mild hemolysis, an oxidative drug is sometimes continued because the number of susceptible older erythrocytes abates with time. Hence, some oxidizing drugs are given only to at-risk patients who have been screened for a G6PD deficiency, whereas others are given without pre-screening but are discontinued at the first sign of significant hemolysis.

Information on drug sensitivity often refers to the World Health Organization's **classification** (Table 21.1).

Testing for G6PD deficiency involves measuring the activity of G6PD in red blood cells or assessing the presence of variant G6PD alleles. A semiquantitative **fluorescence spot test** measures NADPH fluorescence in red blood cells. It is positive for patients who have less than about 20% of the normal G6PD activity. A **quantitative test of G6PD activity** measures NADPH production by G6PD from NADP and glucose 6-phosphate, using a red blood cell hemolysate. G6PD activity is reported relative to the number of red blood cells (i.e., the red blood cell count) or the hemoglobin concentration in blood. The presence of a significant amount of white blood cells can increase measured G6PD activity and thereby mask a G6PD deficiency in red blood cells. Lab results can also be misinterpreted if there is an unusual fraction of red blood cells with good G6PD activity, such as after old red blood cells have undergone hemolysis, after transfusion of normal red blood cells, or after the entry of a wave of new reticulocytes into the blood. For this reason, the most reliable measurements of G6PD activity are made well after hemolytic crises and transfusions. **DNA-based methods** currently often detect only a limited number of frequently occurring mutations. DNA-based assays can be performed regardless of hemolytic crisis. DNA-based methods can also identify heterozygous females much more reliably than a quantitative test of G6PD activity would (see Fig. 21.8).

A very small proportion of G6PD-deficient individuals have a severe deficiency that causes **chronic nonspherocytic hemolytic anemia** and may eventually also give rise to damage to peripheral nerves.

## SUMMARY

- The pentose phosphate pathway provides pentoses and/or reducing power in the form of NADPH.
- In erythrocytes, the pentose phosphate pathway is the only pathway that generates NADPH.
- In the presence of iron, superoxide anions and $H_2O_2$ give rise to highly reactive hydroxyl radicals that attack DNA, proteins, and lipids. Resulting lipid radicals can self-propagate and thus give rise to an avalanche of lipid radicals.
- Enzymes remove superoxide anions and $H_2O_2$. GSH reacts with hydroxyl radicals and thus removes them. Vitamin E, vitamin C, and reduced glutathione play a role in removing lipid and lipid peroxyl radicals. NADPH reduces oxidized glutathione.
- G6PD-deficient patients produce NADPH at a reduced rate and are prone to hemolytic attacks due to infections and/or oxidizing agents (e.g., drugs or fava beans).
- G6PD deficiency is X-linked. The deficiency is most common among people whose ancestors are from areas in which malaria is or was endemic.

## FURTHER READING

- Dahl J-U, Gray MJ, Jakob U. Protein quality control under oxidative stress conditions. *J Mol Biol.* 2015;427:1549-1563.
- Luzzatto L, Seneca E. G6PD deficiency: a classic example of pharmacogenetics with on-going clinical implications. *Br J Haematol.* 2014;164:469-480.

# Review Questions

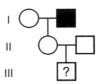

1. In the above pedigree of G6PD deficiency, I-2 has a moderate G6PD deficiency. I-1 and II-2 have no family history of G6PD deficiency, and G6PD deficiency is generally rare in people of their ethnic background. What is the likelihood that III-1 will have a G6PD deficiency?

   A. 0%
   B. 12.5%
   C. 25%
   D. 50%
   E. 100%

2. A 25-year-old man returning from a country with endemic malaria was given primaquine for prevention of malaria. Shortly after starting the drug, he presented with dark urine. Which of the following effects did primaquine have on his red blood cells?

   A. It damaged the cells by acting as a free radical scavenger or antioxidant.
   B. It exerted more oxidative stress on his red blood cells than the cells could handle.
   C. It inhibited G6PD and therefore led to an increase in the concentration of oxidized glutathione.
   D. It irreversibly reduced oxidized glutathione to GSH.
   E. It required more flux in the sugar phosphate branch of the pentose phosphate shunt pathway than the maximal flux that was available.

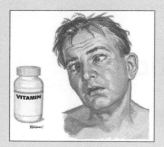

# Chapter 22

# Citric Acid Cycle and Thiamine Deficiency

## SYNOPSIS

- The citric acid cycle occurs in the mitochondria. It chiefly oxidizes acetyl-coenzyme A (acetyl-CoA) to $CO_2$, thereby generating reduced nicotinamide adenine dinucleotide (NADH), reduced flavin adenine dinucleotide ($FADH_2$), and guanosine triphosphate (GTP) (Fig. 22.1). Acetyl-CoA is derived from either the oxidative decarboxylation of pyruvate or the degradation of fatty acids or ketone bodies. Other compounds that enter the citric acid cycle are derived primarily from amino acids (see Chapter 25).
- Intermediates of the citric acid cycle serve as precursors for gluconeogenesis and the biosynthesis of fatty acids, heme, and various amino acids (see Chapters 14, 25, 27, 34, and 35).
- Pyruvate not only generates acetyl-CoA for the citric acid cycle, it also gives rise to oxaloacetate, which helps maintain the concentration of all other intermediates of the citric acid cycle.
- NADH and $FADH_2$ generated in the citric acid cycle are fed into oxidative phosphorylation for the production of adenosine triphosphate (ATP; see Chapter 23). When the use of NADH by oxidative phosphorylation slows, the citric acid cycle also slows, because an elevated concentration of NADH inhibits the citric acid cycle.
- The enzymes and reactions that link pyruvate to the citric acid cycle, and some of the enzymes and reactions of the citric acid cycle itself, require vitamins. Deficiencies of thiamine, riboflavin, niacin, and biotin are clinically important.
- A portion of gliomas (brain tumors), acute myelogenous leukemias, tumors in the cavity or on the surface of bone, and melanomas contain a mutant isocitrate dehydrogenase that generates an abnormal, tumorigenic metabolite.
- Patients who are heterozygous for a deficiency of succinate dehydrogenase or fumarase (two enzymes of the citric acid cycle) are at an increased risk of developing certain tumors, such as pheochromocytomas, paragangliomas, renal cell carcinoma, and fibroids.

## LEARNING OBJECTIVES

*For mastery of this topic, you should be able to do the following:*
- Describe the overall purpose of the pyruvate dehydrogenase (PDH) complex as well as its reactants and products, cellular location, and tissue distribution.
- Describe the regulation of PDH and the conditions that must be met for pyruvate to be oxidized to acetyl-CoA and for acetyl-CoA to be fed into the citric acid cycle.
- Describe the overall purpose of the citric acid cycle as well as its reactants and products, cellular location, and tissue distribution.
- Explain how metabolite concentrations in the citric acid cycle are maintained.
- Describe in broad strokes how reducing equivalents produced in the oxidative decarboxylation of pyruvate and in the citric acid cycle give rise to ATP.

- Describe the regulation of flux through the citric acid cycle vis-à-vis the flux through glycolysis, the electron transport chain, and oxidative phosphorylation.
- Describe the clinical result of severe thiamine deficiency, and connect the symptoms to the biochemical role of thiamine in the PDH complex and the citric acid cycle.
- Explain the rationale for providing thiamine along with glucose to patients who have hypoglycemia and/or alcohol intoxication.
- Describe the role of biotin in mitochondrial metabolism.
- Explain what a biotinidase deficiency is and how it is treated.
- Provide a credible scenario for tumorigenesis in cells that contain no or minimal activity of succinate dehydrogenase (SDH) or fumarase (i.e., fumarate hydratase [FH]). Do the same for cells that express a mutant isocitrate dehydrogenase (IDH) that produces 2-hydroxo-glutarate.

## 1. MITOCHONDRIA CONVERT PYRUVATE TO ACETYL-COA

*Transport proteins move pyruvate into mitochondria. There, the PDH complex (a large multienzyme complex) converts pyruvate to acetyl-CoA. The conversion of pyruvate to acetyl-CoA requires thiamine (vitamin $B_1$) and riboflavin (vitamin $B_2$).*

**Pyruvate** stems from glycolysis, lactate, or alanine (see Chapters 19, 25, 34, and 35). Mitochondria take up pyruvate via a transporter in the inner mitochondrial membrane (the outer membrane of the mitochondria is permeable to small molecules such as pyruvate; Fig. 22.2).

The **PDH complex** oxidatively and irreversibly decarboxylates pyruvate and thereby forms acetyl-CoA (see Fig. 22.2). CoA is an abbreviation for **coenzyme A**, the structure of which is shown in Fig. 22.3. The synthesis of coenzyme A requires **pantothenic acid** (**vitamin $B_5$**). Pantothenic acid deficiency in humans is not well described.

The PDH complex is a huge complex of proteins. It consists of many copies of E1 (PDH), E2 (dihydrolipoyl acetyltransferase), and E3 (dihydrolipoyl dehydrogenase). The complex also contains an E3-binding protein (protein X, dihydrolipoyl dehydrogenase-binding protein) that binds to both E2 and E3, and two types of regulatory enzymes, PDH kinase, and PDH phosphatase.

The E1, E2, and E3 subunits of the PDH complex contain prosthetic groups. Thus, the E1 subunits contain **thiamine pyrophosphate**, which is derived from **thiamine (vitamin $B_1$**; Fig. 22.4). We consume thiamine mainly with cereals, and the consequences of its deficiency are well known and serious (see Section 5). The E2 subunits contain **lipoic acid**. Lipoic acid is

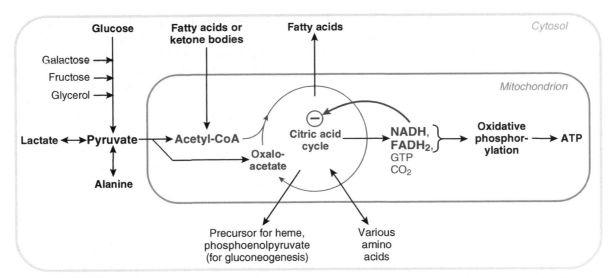

**Fig. 22.1** **Overview of the metabolites that feed into the citric acid cycle or are derived from it.**

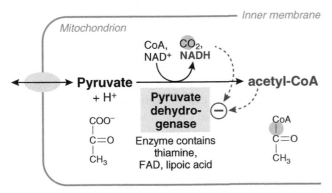

**Fig. 22.2** **Uptake of pyruvate into mitochondria and oxidative decarboxylation of pyruvate to acetyl-coenzyme A (CoA).** The structure of CoA is shown in Fig. 22.3. FAD, flavin adenine dinucleotide.

**Thiamine pyrophosphate**

Reacts with C of keto-group of R-CO-COO⁻, then facilitates removal of -COO⁻ to liberate $CO_2$

**Lipoic acid**

Attaches to side chain of a lysine residue of the dehydrogenase

Accepts an intermediate from thiamine pyrophosphate and oxidizes it

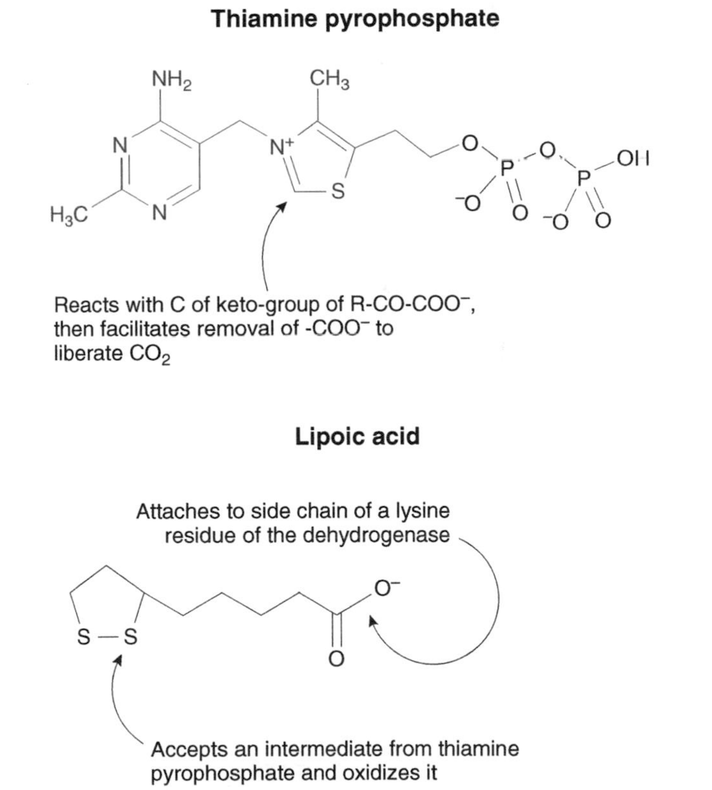

**Fig. 22.4** **Structures of thiamine pyrophosphate and lipoic acid.** Thiamine pyrophosphate is produced from thiamine (vitamin B₁) with the help of thiamine pyrophosphate synthetase and ATP. Both thiamine pyrophosphate and lipoic acid are tightly bound to the pyruvate dehydrogenase complex, the α-ketoglutarate dehydrogenase complex (see Section 2), and the branched-chain ketoacid dehydrogenase complex (see Chapter 35).

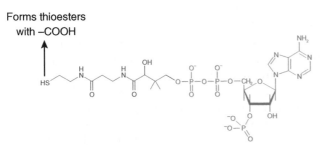

**Forms thioesters with –COOH**

**Pantothenic acid (vitamin B₅)**    3'-Phosphorylated ADP

**Fig. 22.3** **Structure of coenzyme A.** Coenzyme A, a thiol, forms thioesters with carboxylic acids such as acetate, propionate, acetoacetic acid (a ketone body), and fatty acids; thus, coenzyme A "carries" acyl groups (i.e., it carries R–CO–). Coenzyme A also "activates" acyl groups because these thioesters release a large amount of energy when they are hydrolyzed, resulting in an energetically favorable transfer of the acyl group to a new acceptor.

not a vitamin. Lipoic acid accepts and oxidizes an intermediate from thiamine pyrophosphate, whereby lipoic acid is reduced to dihydrolipoic acid. **Arsenite** (O=As–O–), a potent poison, prevents lipoic acid from participating in this reaction. The E3 subunits contain bound flavin adenine dinucleotide (**FAD**; Fig. 22.5), which helps oxidize dihydrolipoic acid back to lipoic acid. FAD is derived from **riboflavin (vitamin B$_2$)**. Riboflavin is mainly found in milk, dairy products, meat, fish, and dark-green vegetables. Riboflavin deficiency is described in Section 5.

**FAD** (see Fig. 22.5) is typically covalently bound to an enzyme, where it often plays a role in forming C=C double bonds and disulfide bonds. Thus, FAD is also required for the activity of succinate dehydrogenase in the citric acid cycle and the electron transport chain of oxidative phosphorylation (see Chapter 23); glycerol phosphate dehydrogenase in the glycerol phosphate shuttle (see Chapter 19); acyl-CoA dehydrogenases in fatty acid β-oxidation both in mitochondria and peroxisomes (see Chapter 27); and in methylenetetrahydrofolate reductase in one-carbon metabolism (see Chapter 36).

**Flavin mononucleotide (FMN)**, a moiety of FAD, is a prosthetic group of the NADH dehydrogenase complex in the electron transport chain of oxidative phosphorylation (see Chapter 23), and of NADPH-cytochrome P450 reductase, which plays a role in steroid synthesis.

The regulation of the activity of the PDH complex is described in Section 4.

In patients who have **primary biliary cirrhosis** due to an autoimmune disease, the **E2** component of the **pyruvate dehydrogenase complex (PDC or PDC-E2)** is the dominant antigen. Primary biliary cirrhosis primarily affects middle-aged women, and the measurement of autoantibodies against the E2 component of PDC is often part of the diagnosis. In this disease, the epithelial cells that line the small bile ducts inside the liver are selectively destroyed. Eventually, this leads to fibrosis and secondary liver damage.

**α-Ketoglutarate dehydrogenase** (an enzyme of the citric acid cycle, see Section 2) and **branched-chain ketoacid dehydrogenase** (see Chapter 35) resemble the PDH complex in that they too require coenzyme A, thiamine pyrophosphate, lipoic acid, and FAD.

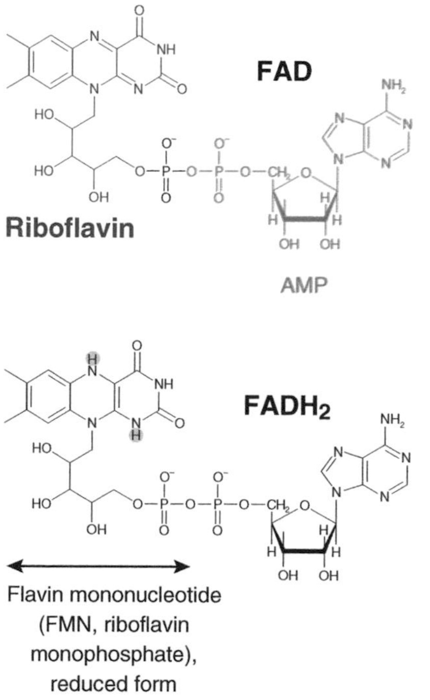

## 2. REACTIONS OF THE CITRIC ACID CYCLE

*The citric acid cycle can oxidize acetyl-CoA to CO$_2$ and thereby produce GTP, NADH, and FADH$_2$. Enzymes of the citric acid cycle use derivatives of the vitamins thiamine, niacin, riboflavin, and pantothenic acid.*

The citric acid cycle is also referred to as the **tricarboxylic acid cycle** (TCA cycle) or **Krebs cycle** (named after Dr. Hans Krebs, who realized the cyclic nature of the pathway).

The citric acid cycle takes place inside **mitochondria**.

The citric acid cycle can oxidize the acetyl group of acetyl-CoA to CO$_2$. Depending on the tissue and the feeding/fasting state, acetyl-CoA stems from pyruvate, fatty acids, ketone bodies, or ketogenic amino acids (see Chapters 19, 27, and 35). During the oxidation of the acetyl group, the citric acid cycle produces GTP, which can phosphorylate ADP to ATP. Furthermore, the citric acid cycle produces NADH and FADH$_2$, which can transfer their reducing power to the pathway of **oxidative phosphorylation** for the production of additional ATP (see Chapter 23). Fig. 22.6 shows the reactions of the citric acid cycle in detail.

Several pathways *feed* the citric acid cycle with intermediates, while others *drain* intermediates from it. This is the topic of Section 3.

Flux through the citric acid cycle depends substantially on flux through oxidative phosphorylation. This is the topic of Section 4.

The citric acid cycle requires the same vitamins as the PDH complex. NAD$^+$ and NADH derive from **niacin** (see Chapter 19). The **α-ketoglutarate dehydrogenase complex** in the citric acid cycle resembles the PDH complex and thus requires **pantothenic acid, thiamine,** and **riboflavin** as precursors of prosthetic groups (see Figs. 22.3 to 22.5). Like the α-ketoglutarate dehydrogenase complex, succinate dehydrogenase has a covalently bound prosthetic group of FAD, which is derived from riboflavin. Deficiencies of these vitamins are discussed in Section 5.

## 3. OXALOACETATE HELPS REPLENISH CITRIC ACID CYCLE INTERMEDIATES

*Intermediates of the citric acid cycle are used for gluconeogenesis and the biosynthesis of fatty acids, amino acids, and heme. To this end, carboxylation of pyruvate supplies the citric acid cycle with oxaloacetate.*

**Fig. 22.5** Structure of flavin adenine dinucleotide (FAD) and related compounds.

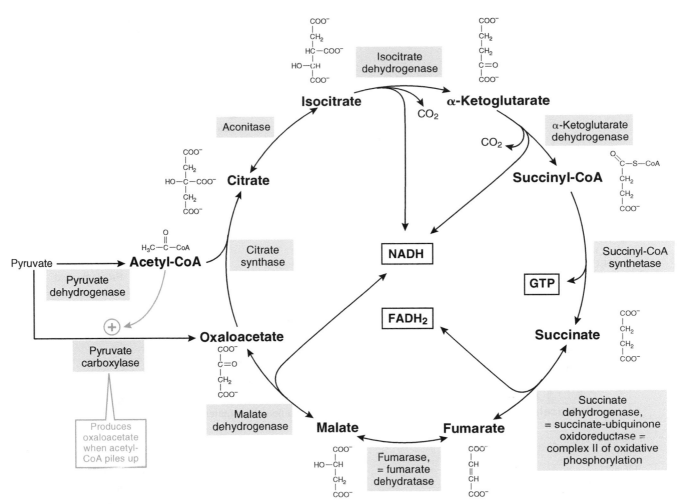

**Fig. 22.6** **Reactions of the citric acid cycle.** NADH is free to diffuse through the matrix of the mitochondria. In contrast, FADH$_2$ is covalently bound to succinate dehydrogenase.

While the full citric acid cycle is used for energy generation, parts of it also play a role in other metabolic pathways. As shown in Fig. 22.7, intermediates of the citric acid cycle serve as a starting point for the synthesis of fatty acids (see Chapter 27), amino acids (see Chapter 34), heme (see Chapter 14), or glucose (see Chapter 25). Conversely, the degradation of some amino acids yields intermediates of the citric acid cycle ($\alpha$-ketoglutarate, succinyl-CoA, fumarate, and oxaloacetate).

**Pyruvate carboxylase** converts pyruvate to **oxaloacetate** and thereby replenishes the citric acid cycle (see Fig. 22.7). Such replenishment is called **anaplerosis**. A rising concentration of **acetyl-CoA** increases the activity of pyruvate carboxylase, which then forms more oxaloacetate. Pyruvate carboxylase activity is not only important for sustained energy production by the citric acid cycle, but also for the synthesis of **cholesterol** and the elongation of **fatty acids** from exported citrate, for **gluconeogenesis** from exported oxaloacetate and malate, for cytosolic NADPH production from exported malate, and for nitrogen elimination by the **urea cycle**, which depends on the amination of oxaloacetate.

Pyruvate carboxylase requires the vitamin **biotin** as a cofactor (Fig. 22.8). Biotin is present in many different foods.

Intestinal microorganisms synthesize biotin as well, but it is unclear whether this becomes available to humans.

Biotin (Fig. 22.8) is covalently bound to a lysine residue near the active site of several different carboxylases. The reaction between biotin and the carboxylase is catalyzed by **holocarboxylase synthetase**. In addition to pyruvate carboxylase, other carboxylases that use biotin as a prosthetic group are **acetyl-CoA carboxylase** (the rate-limiting enzyme in fatty acid synthesis; see Chapter 27), **propionyl-CoA carboxylase** (involved in the degradation of branched-chain amino acids, methionine, fatty acids with an odd number of carbons, and propionic acid that bacteria in the intestine produce from undigested carbohydrate; see Chapter 36), and **3-methylcrotonyl-CoA carboxylase** (involved in the degradation of leucine; see Chapter 35).

When biotin-containing enzymes are degraded, biotin is recovered and recycled. Protein degradation yields **biocytin** (biotinyl-lysine). **Biotinidase** then cleaves biocytin into biotin and lysine; this enzyme also liberates biotin from short, biotin-containing peptides.

Biotin deficiency and its causes are described in Section 5.2.5.

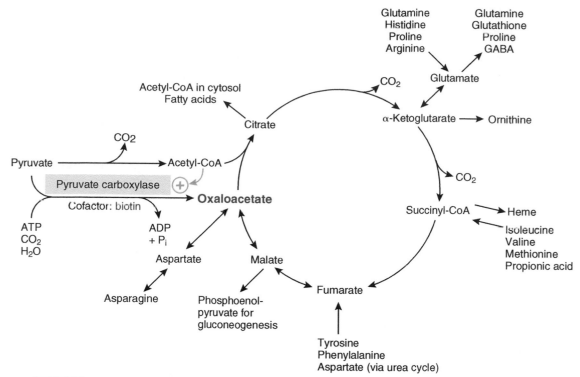

**Fig. 22.7** **Connections of citric acid cycle intermediates to metabolism, and the supply of oxaloacetate to the cycle.** GABA (γ-aminobutyric acid) is a neurotransmitter.

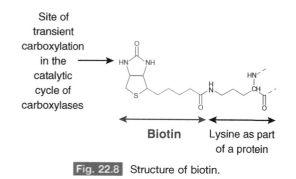

Site of transient carboxylation in the catalytic cycle of carboxylases

**Biotin**    Lysine as part of a protein

**Fig. 22.8** Structure of biotin.

## 4. REGULATION OF THE CITRIC ACID CYCLE AND THE USE OF PYRUVATE

*PDH activity determines the rate of pyruvate use for the production of acetyl-CoA. In muscle, the activity of PDH is highest during intense exercise, when acetyl-CoA is used for energy production. In the liver, the activity of PDH is highest in the fed state, when acetyl-CoA is used to produce citrate for fatty acid synthesis.*

*An elevated concentration of NADH inhibits PDH and the citric acid cycle. The concentration of NADH is highest when the rate of NADH consumption by oxidative phosphorylation is very low (i.e., when the cell uses little ATP). Hence, flux through the citric acid cycle normally depends on a cell's use of ATP. Flux through PDH depends not only on ATP consumption, but also on the consumption of intermediates of the citric acid cycle, and in some tissues on the concentrations of insulin and glucagon.*

The citric acid cycle is almost exclusively regulated on a short-term basis. The *amount* of enzymes in the citric acid cycle does not appreciably change between the fed and the fasting state.

In untrained individuals, aerobic **exercise training** increases the volume of mitochondria in skeletal muscle, thus enabling cells to produce ATP at a higher rate.

The citric acid cycle is chiefly inhibited by an increasing concentration of **NADH** (Fig. 22.10). NADH product inhibits PDH (see Fig. 22.2), as well as several enzymes of the citric acid cycle.

The citric acid cycle depends on the rate of **oxidative phosphorylation**, which in turn depends on the rate of **ATP consumption**. As shown in Section 2, the citric acid cycle produces NADH and FADH₂. As detailed in Chapter 23, oxidative phosphorylation uses the reducing power of NADH and FADH₂ to drive the phosphorylation of ADP to ATP. In cells with mitochondria, this process generates the majority of ATP. When a cell hydrolyzes ATP at a high rate and therefore produces ADP at a high rate, oxidative phosphorylation uses a large amount of NADH and FADH₂, and the citric acid cycle is very active. On the other hand, when a cell uses little ATP and therefore produces little ADP, oxidative phosphorylation also uses little NADH and FADH₂, the concentration of NADH rises, and the citric acid cycle activity declines.

**Acetyl-CoA**, the main carbon input to the citric acid cycle, can be derived from pyruvate (which in turn derives from glucose, glycogen, lactate, or alanine; see Section 1), from fatty acid β-oxidation or, in nonhepatic tissues, from the oxidation of ketone bodies (see Chapter 27). In most cells, controls are such that fatty acids and ketone bodies from the blood are preferred over pyruvate as a source of acetyl-CoA. In the fasting state, this is critical for preserving glucose because the body has large stores to produce fatty acids and ketone bodies but comparatively small stores from which it can produce glucose.

Acetyl-CoA product inhibits the PDH complex (Fig. 22.11). This prevents the conversion of pyruvate to acetyl-CoA when acetyl-CoA is abundant. It also enables cells to produce acetyl-CoA preferentially from fatty acids and ketone bodies rather than pyruvate (see Chapter 27). This effect allows pyruvate to be used for other purposes and thus helps prevent hypoglycemia in the fasting state (see Chapter 25).

Acetyl-CoA activates **pyruvate carboxylase** (see Fig. 22.9). Pyruvate carboxylase is important to the proper function of several metabolic pathways (see Section 3). The concentration of acetyl-CoA determines how much pyruvate is converted to acetyl-CoA and how much to oxaloacetate.

Two intermediates of the citric acid cycle, **citrate,** and **succinyl-CoA,** inhibit the enzymes that generate them. This inhibition prevents the buildup of high concentrations of intermediates in the citric acid cycle.

In the **liver,** acting via PDH phosphatases and a PDH kinase, **insulin, epinephrine,** and **ADP** all increase PDH activity. In the fed state, PDH tends to be high, while in the fasting state it tends to be low to preserve pyruvate for gluconeogenesis (see Chapter 25).

In contracting **skeletal muscle,** the elevated concentration of **Ca²⁺,** acting via a PDH kinase and a PDH phosphatase, leads to increased PDH activity.

# 5. PROBLEMS ASSOCIATED WITH THE CITRIC ACID CYCLE

*The citric acid cycle plays a crucial role in energy generation by mitochondria. If flux through the citric acid cycle is impaired, organs with high ATP needs (e.g., the central nervous system, the heart, and skeletal muscles) suffer damage. Clinically, the most commonly encountered diseases that have a relationship to the citric acid cycle are hypoxia, thiamine deficiency, riboflavin deficiency, niacin deficiency, paragangliomas, and pheochromocytomas.*

## 5.1. Inhibition of the Citric Acid Cycle Secondary to Impaired Oxidative Phosphorylation

An impairment of oxidative phosphorylation leads to a marked shift in energy production from the citric acid cycle plus oxidative phosphorylation toward anaerobic glycolysis. If a substantial amount of cells in the body switch to anaerobic glycolysis, production of lactic acid surpasses consumption, leading to lactic acidosis and then lactic acidemia (see Chapter 19). Inhibition of oxidative phosphorylation is seen in patients with acute or chronic **hypoxia**. Acute hypoxia may be due to stroke, heart attack, asphyxia, or drowning; chronic hypoxia may be due to cardiac, pulmonary, renal, or hemolytic disease. Oxidative phosphorylation can also be impaired by a poison, such as cyanide or uncouplers (see Chapter 23).

## 5.2. Clinically Significant Vitamin Deficiencies

### 5.2.1. Overview

Fig. 22.10 provides an overview of the vitamins that are required for reactions of the citric acid cycle, the PDH complex, and pyruvate carboxylase.

### 5.2.2. Deficiency of Thiamine (Vitamin B₁)

The most significant amounts of thiamine are found in whole grains, most vegetables, pork (not in beef, poultry, or fish), and milk. In developed nations, food supplementation is common. In North America and Europe, approximately half of the daily thiamine intake stems from the consumption of grains, and about a quarter each from the consumption of vegetables and animal products. Thiamine uptake in the small

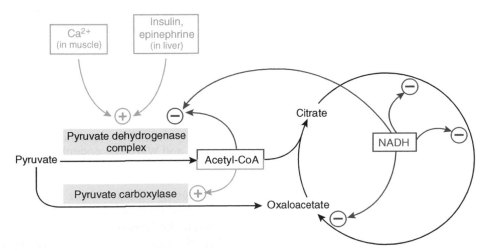

**Fig. 22.9**  **Overview of the vitamins that are cofactors of pyruvate dehydrogenase, pyruvate carboxylase, or enzymes of the citric acid cycle.**

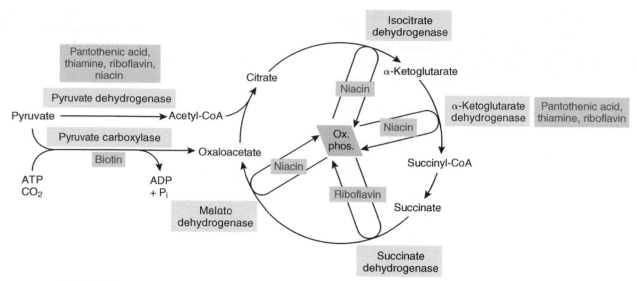

**Fig. 22.10** **Regulation of the activity of pyruvate dehydrogenase and the citric acid cycle.** When oxidative phosphorylation does not use NADH, the citric acid cycle comes to a virtual standstill. Ox. phos., oxidative phosphorylation.

intestine is reduced in the presence of **alcohol**. It is also reduced in patients of advanced **age**. Furthermore, **diuretics** increase the loss of thiamine into the urine.

In the developed world, thiamine deficiency is most commonly seen in patients who regularly abuse **alcohol**. The diet of these patients does not contain an adequate amount of thiamine, and thiamine absorption by the intestines is impaired. The treatment of these patients is outlined below.

Patients who undergo frequent **hemodialysis** and patients who have advanced **cancer** are also susceptible to thiamine deficiency.

In **refugee** populations, thiamine deficiency due to inadequate dietary intake is quite common. Affected people often consume mainly only milled white grains.

For the diagnosis of a thiamine deficiency, one commonly compares the activities of red blood cell **transketolase** (an enzyme that requires thiamine pyrophosphate; see Chapter 21) with and without extra thiamine pyrophosphate (added to a sample in the laboratory).

A chronic thiamine deficiency is usually accompanied by Wernicke cardiomyopathy, which is characterized by an enlarged heart, shortness of breath, and fatigue. In alcoholics, chronic thiamine deficiency typically also leads to **peripheral neuropathy** (see Fig. 22.11).

**Wernicke encephalopathy** (see Fig. 22.11) is typically provoked by administration of a large amount of carbohydrates to a thiamine-deficient person (i.e., a person who may already have peripheral neuropathy or Wernicke cardiomyopathy; see above). Wernicke encephalopathy is accompanied by petechial hemorrhage in the brain. If initially conscious, affected patients become agitated, confused, and ataxic. Wernicke encephalopathy is a particularly well-known complication of infusing an **alcohol**-dependent (and therefore often thiamine-deficient) patient with glucose in the hospital. About 5% of the adults in North America and Australia regularly abuse alcohol.

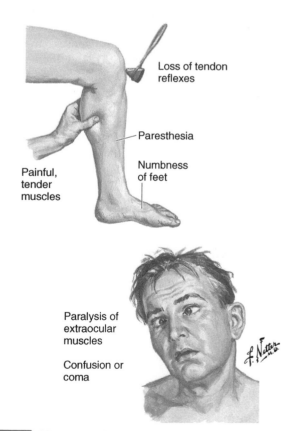

**Fig. 22.11** **Thiamine deficiency can lead to peripheral neuropathy and Wernicke encephalopathy.**

Autopsies reveal that 20% or more of these individuals have had at least one episode of Wernicke encephalopathy.

**Wernicke-Korsakoff syndrome** refers to a combination of Wernicke encephalopathy (initiated by thiamine deficiency) and **Korsakoff psychosis**. The psychosis is a result of the encephalopathy and becomes apparent while the patient recovers. Korsakoff psychosis is characterized by greatly impaired short-term memory. When patients in an **alcoholic coma** or with **alcohol withdrawal syndrome** are infused with glucose, they are routinely also given thiamine to prevent Wernicke-Korsakoff syndrome.

Emergency personnel responding to comatose patients often administer a "**coma cocktail**" that contains glucose and thiamine (as well as naloxone).

### 5.2.3. Deficiency of Riboflavin (Vitamin B₂)

A deficiency of riboflavin is also called **ariboflavinosis**.

A deficiency of riboflavin, the precursor of FMN and FAD, is endemic in many regions of the world, particularly in people who have little access to milk, dairy products, and meats, which are especially rich in riboflavin. Accordingly, vegans and vegetarians are also at greater risk of ariboflavinosis than omnivores. Poor riboflavin status is pervasive among children and the elderly even in developed nations. Riboflavin is present in many foods, with almonds, green leafy vegetables, and some legumes containing more riboflavin than other plant foods. In some countries, white flour and cereals are fortified with riboflavin.

Frank riboflavin deficiency is accompanied by lesions of the mouth, lips, skin, and genitalia (Fig. 22.12).

The preferred method of assessing riboflavin status is to compare the activity of red blood cell **glutathione reductase** before and after the addition of extra FAD. This sensitive test shows abnormal readings within only a few days of dietary deprivation.

Since the endogenous production of niacin from tryptophan requires riboflavin, riboflavin deficiency can lead to a **niacin deficiency** (see Chapter 19).

### 5.2.4. Deficiency of Niacin (Vitamin B₃, Nicotinic Acid)

A deficiency of niacin is called **pellagra** and is described in Section 1 of Chapter 20. Since niacin is a precursor for NAD⁺,

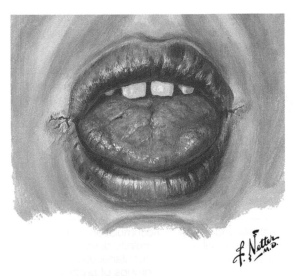

**Ariboflavinosis.**

patients with pellagra presumably have impaired flux through PDH, isocitrate dehydrogenase, and α-ketoglutarate dehydrogenase, which would curtail ATP production by the combination of citric acid cycle and oxidative phosphorylation. This may contribute to the observed diarrhea, dermatitis, and dementia.

### 5.2.5. Deficiency of Biotin

As outlined in Section 3, biotin homeostasis requires both an adequate *intake* of biotin and adequate *recycling* of protein-bound biotin; thereby recycling is quantitatively more important. A **nutritional deficiency** of biotin is unusual. Excessive consumption of **raw eggs** can cause a biotin deficiency because egg white contains the protein **avidin**. Avidin binds biotin and prevents its uptake in the intestine. Avidin is largely destroyed when eggs are cooked.

Symptoms of a pronounced biotin deficiency are most often provoked by a severe deficiency of **holocarboxylase synthetase**, the enzyme that conjugates various carboxylases with biotin, or by a deficiency of **biotinidase**, the enzyme that recycles biotin (see Section 3). A severe deficiency of holocarboxylase synthetase manifests itself during the first few days to weeks of life with tachypnea, lethargy, and signs of abnormal central nervous system function. The deficiency affects about 1 in 90,000 persons. Biotinidase deficiency affects about 1 in 60,000 persons. A complete biotinidase deficiency causes symptoms at a few weeks of age or later. Biotinidase deficiency leads to ataxia, seizures, hearing loss, delayed development, and alopecia. Increased protein degradation (e.g., during an illness) exacerbates the biotin deficiency for reasons explained below.

A severe deficiency of biotin, whether caused by excessive consumption of raw eggs, holocarboxylase synthetase deficiency, or biotinidase deficiency, causes an **organic acidemia** and **hyperammonemia**. The acidemia is characterized by elevated concentrations of lactic acid, propionic acid, and ketone bodies (i.e., acetoacetic acid and β-hydroxybutyric acid). The pathogenesis may be explained as follows. The concentration of lactic acid is elevated because the biotin-dependent pyruvate carboxylase does not produce sufficient oxaloacetate; hence, losses of citric acid cycle intermediates are not made up, and acetyl-CoA cannot adequately enter the citric acid cycle. This has two effects: (1) the concentration of acetyl-CoA becomes elevated so that acetyl-CoA inhibits the PDH complex, and (2) the production of ATP by mitochondria decreases. These effects shift ATP production to anaerobic glycolysis in the cytosol, which produces lactate at a high rate (see Chapter 19). The concentration of propionic acid is high because the metabolism of this compound requires biotin (see Chapter 36). At an elevated concentration of propionyl-CoA (the activated form of propionic acid), citrate synthase condenses some oxaloacetate with propionyl-CoA instead of acetyl-CoA; this produces methyl citrate. Methyl citrate inhibits the citric acid cycle; again, this leads to an increase in anaerobic glycolysis. The high concentration of propionic acid also causes hyperammonemia. The increased concentration of ketone bodies is in part due to a decrease in the rate of their oxidation. The combination of acidosis, decreased energy production in mitochondria, and hyperammonemia foremost impairs the function of neurons.

**Screening of newborns** often includes tests for deficiencies of holocarboxylase synthetase and biotinidase. Both deficiencies can be treated with high doses of exogenous biotin.

## 5.3. Pyruvate Carboxylase Deficiency

The pathology of pyruvate carboxylase deficiency attests to the importance of this enzyme and the citric acid cycle in several metabolic processes. Most affected patients have **lactic acidosis** because the lack of oxaloacetate prevents the use of acetyl-CoA, which in turn inhibits PDH, thereby preventing significant entry of pyruvate into mitochondria. The more severely affected patients also have fasting **ketoacidosis**, because a high concentration of acetyl-CoA from fatty acid oxidation in the liver causes overproduction of ketone bodies, whereas a high concentration of acetyl-CoA in other cells inhibits the oxidation of ketone bodies (compare to Figs. 27.14 and 27.16). Patients develop **fasting hypoglycemia** because there is not enough oxaloacetate or malate for gluconeogenesis (see Fig. 25.3). Severely affected patients have **hyperammonemia** because there is not enough oxaloacetate to accept an amino group and form aspartate for nitrogen elimination via the urea cycle (see Fig. 35.7). The low concentration of oxaloacetate also leads to depletion of α-ketoglutarate, from which glutamate and the neurotransmitter γ-aminobutyric acid (**GABA**) are made (see Fig. 35.6). The deficiency in pyru-

vate carboxylase activity also causes deficient production of **NADPH** via the sequence malate$_{mito}$ → oxaloacetate$_{cytosol}$ → pyruvate → oxaloacetate$_{mito}$ → malate$_{mito}$ (see Section 2 in Chapter 27). Without such production of NADPH in the cytosol, there is a diminished defense against **reactive oxygen species** (ROS; see Section 2.3 in Chapter 21) and a reduced elongation of **fatty acids** (see Fig. 27.6) for the production of **myelin**. The increased ROS, impaired myelin production, hyperammonemia, and deficient GABA synthesis give rise to impaired development and maintenance of the **central nervous system**.

## 5.4. Acute Poisoning With Arsenic

Acute poisoning with arsenic leads to an inhibition of the **PDH** complex, the **α-ketoglutarate dehydrogenase** complex (see Section 1), and **branched-chain ketoacid dehydrogenase** (see Chapter 35). In addition, acute poisoning leads to the inhibition and partial uncoupling of **oxidative phosphorylation**. Affected patients show an impaired function of the gastrointestinal tract, nervous system, heart, and kidneys, possibly due to impaired energy production.

## 5.5. Tumorigenic Mutations in Isocitrate Dehydrogenase, Succinate Dehydrogenase, or Fumarase

Heterozygous gain-of-function mutations in isocitrate dehydrogenases (IDH) are linked to sporadic cancers, whereas heterozygous inactivating mutations in succinate dehydrogenase (SDH) or fumarase (FH) are linked to hereditary cancer syndromes (Table 22.1). In hereditary cancer syndromes,

**Table 22.1** Mutations in Isocitrate Dehydrogenase (IDH), Succinate Dehydrogenase (SDH), or Fumarase Linked to Cancer

| Mutated Gene | Enzyme Name | Tumors That May Contain a Mutant Enzyme | Pathway of Tumorigenesis |
|---|---|---|---|
| IDH1 | IDH1 (in cytosol and peroxisomes) | Gliomas, acute myeloid leukemias, tumors that arise in the cavity or on the surface of bone, and melanomas | Formation of 2-hydroxy-glutarate, which inhibits dioxygenases |
| IDH2 | IDH2 (in mitochondria) | | |
| SDHA | SDH subunit A | Paragangliomas, pheochromocytomas, and gastrointestinal stromal tumors | Accumulation of succinate, which inhibits dioxygenases |
| SDHB | SDH subunit B | | |
| SDHC | SDH subunit C | | |
| SDHD, if inherited from the father | SDH subunit D | | |
| SDHAF2 | SDH assembly factor 2 | | |
| FH | Fumarase = fumarate hydratase (in mitochondria and the cytosol) | Hereditary leiomyomatosis and renal cell cancer, papillary renal cell cancer, Leydig cell tumors | Accumulation of fumarate, which inhibits dioxygenases; fumarate spontaneously reacts with –SH groups of proteins |

tumors arise when somatic cells acquire a second mutation that leads to a complete loss of function.

Tumorigenic mutations in IDH, SDH, or FH are similar in that mutant enzymes give rise to metabolites that competitively inhibit **dioxygenases** that use α-ketoglutarate (**2-oxoglutarate**) as one of their substrates. These dioxygenases encompass, for example, **HIF prolyl hydroxylase** and the **ten-eleven translocation** (TET) enzymes, which demethylate DNA. As explained in Chapter 16, decreased hydroxylation of hypoxia-inducible factor alpha (HIF-α) leads to increased survival of HIF-α, translocation of HIF-α into the nucleus, and increased transcription of genes, the products of which help the body alleviate hypoxia or cope with it. Many tumor cells exist in a hypoxic environment and therefore benefit from increased HIF-α–induced transcription.

Methylation of promoter regions reduces the rate of transcription of associated tumor suppressor genes and thus favors tumorigenesis. Methylation status is determined by both DNA (cytosine-5-)-methyltransferases (DNMTs) that methylate cytosines in CpG islands of DNA, and by **TET enzymes** that catalyze a multistep demethylation of 5-methyl cytosine by forming 5-hydroxymethyl cytosine, then 5-formyl cytosine, and finally 5-carboxy cytosine. The pathway for the physiologically most relevant re-formation of cytosine from one or more of these intermediates remains to be elucidated. Tumorigenic mutations in IDH, SDH, or FH lead to reduced TET enzyme activity and thus to an increased methylation of DNA near tumor suppressor genes.

Humans have three IDH isoenzymes, but to date only mutations in the genes for IDH 1 and 2 are known to give rise to the oncogenic metabolite **2-hydroxy glutarate** (see Table 22.1). IDH 3 is the main enzyme that is involved in catalyzing a reaction of the citric acid cycle. The normal product of the IDH is 2-oxo-glutarate (α-ketoglutarate). Most pathogenic mutations affect an arginine residue in the active site of the enzyme. These mutations are **acquired** (not inherited) and typically affect only one allele.

Patients who are heterozygous for a germline loss-of-function mutation in one of the five subunits of **SDH** have a high risk of losing the function of the normal allele in certain critical cells; this in turn gives rise to a **paraganglioma** or a **pheochromocytoma** (see Table 22.1). However, only a fraction of patients who have a paraganglioma or a pheochromocytoma has inherited a nonfunctional allele of an SDH subunit. In patients who are heterozygous for an SDH mutation, the loss of the normal allele in some somatic cells is an example of a **loss of heterozygosity** (see Chapters 2 and 8). Pheochromocytomas are derived from the adrenal medulla and are composed of chromaffin cells that release catecholamines (Fig. 22.13). The resulting high concentration of circulating catecholamines causes hypertension, but only about 1 in 500 patients with hypertension has a pheochromocytoma. Paragangliomas are vascular tumors in the head or neck, most frequently at the carotid bifurcation. They too may produce catecholamines, or they may simply be a painless, abnormal mass that can impair normal body function. The expression of pathogenic *SDHD* mutations is unique in that only a

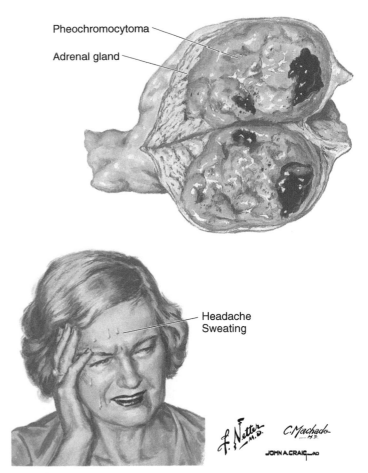

Pheochromocytoma

Adrenal gland

Headache
Sweating

**Fig. 22.13** **Pheochromocytoma.** Pheochromocytomas secrete catecholamines, which cause hypertension, headaches, sweating, and palpitations.

paternal mutation is pathogenic, due to **imprinting** of the maternal allele (imprinting is discussed in Chapter 5). Many patients who have a recognized pheochromocytoma or paraganglioma undergo genetic testing for several known heritable mutations, including mutations in SDH dehydrogenase.

Patients who are *homozygous* (or compound heterozygous) for mutations in the *SDHA* gene that result in partial SDH deficiency have **juvenile encephalomyopathy**. This is a very rare disease that appears to be due to impaired energy production in the brain and muscle.

*Heterozygous* inborn **fumarase** (FH) deficiency gives rise to **hereditary leiomyomatosis and renal cell carcinoma** (HLRCC; see Table 22.1). Fumarase is required inside *mitochondria* for the citric acid cycle and in the *cytosol* of cells that contain the urea cycle (see Chapter 35). Fumarase in the mitochondria and the cytosol is derived from the same gene. When cells lose the function of the remaining normal fumarase allele, the concentration of fumarate increases to a tumorigenic level. With dioxygenase activity inhibited by fumarate, HIF prolyl hydroxylase activity is low so that HIF stimulates the transcription of certain genes (see Fig. 16.5) and thereby promotes angiogenesis. Affected patients develop benign leiomyomas (tumors that derive from smooth muscle) in the **skin**.

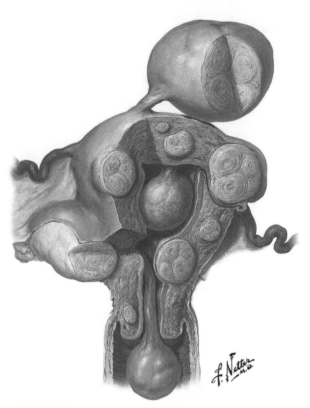

**Fig. 22.14** **Leiomyomas in the uterus (fibroids).**

Affected women also develop benign leiomyomas in the **uterus** (**fibroids**; Fig. 22.14). In addition, some male and female patients develop aggressive, metastatic renal cell cancer. In the absence of skin leiomyomas, most of the commonly occurring uterine leiomyomas and most renal cell carcinomas are not associated with mutations in fumarase.

*Homozygous* germline mutations that result in **near-complete fumarase deficiency** lead to a severe dysfunction of neurons. The dysfunction may be due to impaired energy production. Affected patients often die in early childhood.

## 5.6. Deficiency of the Pyruvate Dehydrogenase Complex

A deficiency of the PDH complex compromises ATP production, can cause **intellectual disability**, and often leads to **lactic acidosis** and **lactic acidemia**. Most deficiencies of the PDH complex result from mutations in the *PDHA1* gene on the X chromosome, the gene that encodes the $\alpha$-subunit of the E1-component. PDH deficiency is rare, and most mutations occur de novo. In patients with a *severe* deficiency, all pyruvate must be reduced to lactate, causing massive lactic acidosis at birth and death during the neonatal period. A *mild* deficiency primarily affects the function of the brain, which depends on pyruvate for energy production. Ketone bodies (see Chapter 27) can diminish the need for pyruvate; ketogenic diets therefore help some patients.

## SUMMARY

- The pyruvate dehydrogenase (PDH) complex converts pyruvate to acetyl-CoA and thereby produces NADH. Both acetyl-CoA and NADH product inhibit PDH. In the liver, insulin increases PDH activity. In skeletal and cardiac muscle, exercise (acting via $Ca^{2+}$) increases PDH activity.
- Complete oxidation of acetyl-CoA in the citric acid cycle yields $CO_2$, GTP, NADH, and $FADH_2$. NADH and $FADH_2$ transfer reducing power to the electron transport chain of oxidative phosphorylation for the production of ATP (see Chapter 23). The combination of the citric acid cycle and oxidative phosphorylation produces most of the body's ATP. In comparison, ATP production from glycolysis is small.
- The PDH complex is most active when the concentrations of acetyl-CoA and NADH inside the mitochondria are low.
- Pyruvate carboxylase converts pyruvate to oxaloacetate to help replenish citric acid cycle intermediates that are withdrawn for biosyntheses. Without oxaloacetate, acetyl-CoA cannot enter the citric acid cycle. The concentration of acetyl-CoA is the main regulator of pyruvate carboxylase activity.
- An elevated concentration of NADH leads to a decrease in flux through the citric acid cycle.
- Flux through the citric acid cycle strongly depends on flux through oxidative phosphorylation. Flux through oxidative phosphorylation in turn strongly depends on the rate of ATP hydrolysis. A low rate of flux through oxidative phosphorylation limits citric acid cycle activity mainly through an increase in the concentration of NADH.
- PDH, pyruvate carboxylase, and some enzymes of the citric acid cycle require vitamins as cofactors. Clinically, the most important vitamin deficiencies are thiamine deficiency, riboflavin deficiency, and biotin deficiency. Thiamine deficiency leads to impaired ATP generation and chiefly affects the heart and the central nervous system. Riboflavin deficiency causes lesions of the mouth, lips, skin, and genitalia. Biotin deficiency affects pyruvate carboxylase as well as carboxylases in other pathways. It primarily impairs the central nervous system.
- Certain cancers show acquired mutations in the isocitrate dehydrogenase genes *IDH1* and *IDH2* that lead to the production of 2-hydroxyglutarate, which inhibits 2-oxoglutarate–dependent dioxygenases and thereby leads to DNA hypermethylation and increased transcription of genes that are part of the hypoxia response.
- Heterozygosity for an inactivating mutation in certain subunits of succinate dehydrogenase (SDH) is associated with an increased susceptibility to the formation of pheochromocytomas or paragangliomas.
- Heterozygosity for an inactivating mutation in fumarase is associated with the formation of fibroids and an increased susceptibility to the development of renal cell cancer.
- A congenital deficiency of PDH is rare. Patients in crisis have lactic acidemia.

## FURTHER READING

- Barletta JA, Hornick JL. Succinate dehydrogenase-deficient tumors: diagnostic advances and clinical implications. *Adv Anat Pathol.* 2012;19:193-203.
- Kornberg H. Krebs and his trinity of cycles. *Nat Rev Mol Cell Biol.* 2000;1:225-228.
- Schmidt LS, Linehan WM. Hereditary leiomyomatosis and renal cell carcinoma. *Int J Nephrol Renovasc Dis.* 2014;7:253-260.
- Scourzic L, Mouly E, Bernard OA. TET proteins and the control of cytosine demethylation in cancer. *Genome Med.* 2015;7:9.

# Review Questions

1. In patients who are at risk of developing Wernicke encephalopathy, a preventive infusion of thiamine ensures adequate activity of which of the following enzymes?

   A. Citrate synthase and malate dehydrogenase
   B. Fumarase and succinate dehydrogenase
   C. α-Ketoglutarate dehydrogenase and pyruvate
   D. Pyruvate carboxylase and succinate dehydrogenase
   E. Transketolase and isocitrate dehydrogenase

2. A patient has severe hypoxia. In this situation, which of the following is the major inhibitor of the citric acid cycle?

   A. α-Ketoglutarate
   B. Acetyl-CoA
   C. ADP
   D. NADH
   E. Pyruvate

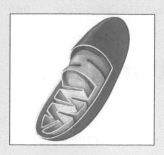

## SYNOPSIS

- Mitochondria are basically stripped-down gram-negative bacteria that specialize in energy production. Human mitochondria consist of an internal compartment (the mitochondrial matrix) that contains the enzymes of the citric acid cycle, fatty acid β-oxidation, ketone body metabolism, and parts of several biosynthetic pathways. The matrix is enclosed by the inner mitochondrial membrane, which contains the proteins for oxidative phosphorylation. The inner mitochondrial membrane is surrounded by an outer mitochondrial membrane that is permeable to small molecules. The region between the two membranes is the intermembrane space.

- Oxidative phosphorylation takes place in the mitochondria and couples the oxidation of reduced nicotinamide adenine dinucleotide (NADH) and other reduced compounds to the production of adenosine triphosphate (ATP; Fig. 23.1). As NADH is oxidized, protons ($H^+$) are pumped out of the matrix into the intermembrane space as part of a series of oxidation-reduction reactions. An ATP synthase allows protons to flow back into the mitochondrial matrix, and it uses the energy that is freed in this process to phosphorylate adenine diphosphate (ADP) to ATP.

- Mitochondria contain their own DNA. Mitochondria are inherited from only the mother. Some of the proteins needed for oxidative phosphorylation are encoded by the DNA in the mitochondria, but most are derived from the DNA in the nucleus.

- Mitochondrial diseases give rise to deficient oxidative phosphorylation and consequently affect primarily cells and tissues that require a high rate of ATP production, such as the central nervous system, the heart, and skeletal muscle. Pancreatic β-cells are also often affected, since ATP synthesis is required for glucose sensing and insulin secretion.

## LEARNING OBJECTIVES

*For mastery of this topic, you should be able to do the following:*
- Describe the function, cellular location, and tissue distribution of the electron transport chain and ATP synthase.
- Summarize how components of the electron transport chain undergo oxidation-reduction reactions and how the energy from such reactions is used to pump protons to the intermembrane space.
- Explain the coupling of electron transport and ATP synthase activity.
- Explain the role of creatine kinase, creatine, and phosphocreatine in intracellular energy transport, and list tissues in which these molecules are especially abundant.
- Differentiate the normal regulation and interplay of ATP synthase activity, flux in the electron transport chain, flux in the citric acid cycle, and flux in glycolysis.
- Assess the influence of a limiting concentration of oxygen on oxidative phosphorylation.
- Describe the effects of uncouplers and electron transport chain inhibitors on flux through the electron transport chain and on the rate of oxidative phosphorylation; predict the effects of these agents on flux in glycolysis, in the citric acid cycle, and in the conversion of pyruvate to lactate.
- Describe the role of the supplement coenzyme Q (ubiquinone) in oxidative phosphorylation and in protecting lipid integrity.
- Identify a pattern of mitochondrial inheritance.
- Explain why some mitochondrial diseases are inherited with an X-linked or autosomal recessive pattern, while others show maternal inheritance.
- Explain heteroplasmy and show how it relates to variations in onset, phenotype, and severity of mitochondrial diseases caused by mutations in mitochondrial DNA.

## 1. OXIDATIVE PHOSPHORYLATION

*Oxidative phosphorylation consists of an oxygen-requiring electron transport chain and an ATP synthase. The electron transport chain uses the reducing power (electrons and protons) of NADH and a few other reducing agents to reduce $O_2$ to $H_2O$. During these reactions, $H^+$ is pumped out of the mitochondrial matrix space into the mitochondrial intermembrane space. The ATP synthase allows $H^+$ to flow back into the matrix while using the electrochemical $H^+$ gradient to synthesize ATP from ADP and phosphate. Inhibitors of the electron transport chain and uncouplers of oxidative phosphorylation both reduce ATP production by oxidative phosphorylation.*

### 1.1. Structure and Function of Mitochondria

Mitochondria are present in most cells. Mature red blood cells do not have mitochondria. Fast white muscle cells have very few mitochondria. In contrast, organs such as the brain and heart contain many mitochondria.

Mitochondria contain an inner and an outer membrane, creating a matrix space and an intermembrane space (Fig. 23.2).

While mitochondria are often drawn in the shape of an elongated bean, they actually form a highly dynamic tubular **reticulum** inside of cells.

The matrix space contains the enzymes of the citric acid cycle (see Chapter 22); fatty acid β-oxidation, ketone body synthesis, and ketone body oxidation (see Chapter 27); parts of heme synthesis (see Chapter 14); steroid synthesis (see Chapter 31); protein metabolism (see Chapters 34 and 35); and the urea cycle (see Chapter 35). The inner mitochondrial membrane contains the components of oxidative phosphorylation discussed in this chapter. The outer membrane is permeable to small molecules.

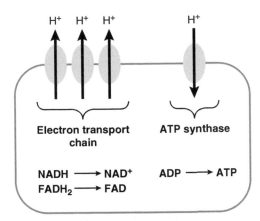

**Fig. 23.1** Formation of ATP via oxidative phosphorylation.

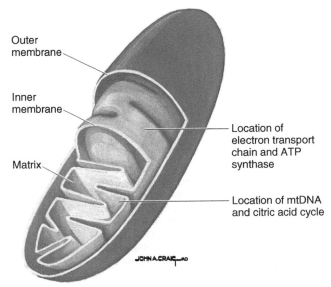

**Fig. 23.2** Structure of mitochondria.

## 1.2. Electron Transport Chain

The electron transport chain is sometimes called the **respiratory chain**.

The electron transport chain (Fig. 23.3) has a single end-point (the reduction of $O_2$ to water by complex IV), but it has multiple proteins that accept "reducing power" and thereby funnel electrons into the chain. These proteins include complex I (also called NADH dehydrogenase), electron-transferring flavoprotein dehydrogenase, mitochondrial glycerol 3-phosphate dehydrogenase (which is part of the glycerol phosphate shuttle), and complex II (also called succinate dehydrogenase, an enzyme that is part of the citric acid cycle). Complexes III and IV are part of the common and final part of the electron transport chain. Complex III is also called coenzyme Q:cytochrome c oxidoreductase, or cytochrome bc1 complex. Complex IV is also called cytochrome c oxidase.

The electron transport chain contains two electron carriers. Reduced coenzyme Q ($QH_2$, ubiquinol; see below) is a lipid that freely diffuses in the inner mitochondrial membrane. Every input of the electron transport chain gives rise to $QH_2$.

Catalyzed by complex III, $QH_2$ then donates its electrons to cytochrome c. Reduced cytochrome c is a protein that is mostly bound to the outside of the inner mitochondrial membrane. Reduced cytochrome c transports electrons from complex III to complex IV.

Only complexes I, III, and IV **pump protons** ($H^+$) out of the matrix into the intermembrane space. As described in Section 1.4, the energy of the resulting electrochemical gradient is used for the synthesis of ATP.

**Coenzyme Q** is a lipid-soluble compound (Fig. 23.4) that diffuses within the inner mitochondrial membrane. Coenzyme Q is also called **ubiquinone**. Coenzyme Q can be reduced to **coenzyme QH$_2$**, which is also called **ubiquinol**. In humans, coenzyme Q has a **polyisoprene** "tail" of 10 units, which gives rise to the designations coenzyme Q10 and CoQ10. Humans synthesize the ring structure of coenzyme Q from tyrosine and derive the polyisoprene tail from the **cholesterol synthesis** pathway (see Chapter 29). Ubiquinol is also present in other membranes and acts as an antioxidant that protects for instance unsaturated fatty acids in phospholipids (see Chapter 21).

**Supplemental coenzyme Q10** is used in the treatment of certain disorders of mitochondrial energy production and several rare forms of **heritable deficiencies of coenzyme Q10 synthesis**. CoQ10 supplementation may also have a long-term beneficial effect in **migraine** prophylaxis. In contrast, it is uncertain whether supplementary coenzyme Q10 reduces oxidative damage or is effective in the treatment of **statin-induced myopathy**.

**Cytochrome c** is a small (104-amino acid) protein in the mitochondrial intermembrane space that is normally bound electrostatically to the outside of the inner mitochondrial membrane. Cytochrome c contains a heme prosthetic group with iron that can be reduced ($Fe^{2+}$) or oxidized ($Fe^{3+}$). Cytochrome c is strongly positively charged, and this facilitates its binding to the negatively charged phospholipid **cardiolipin** in the inner mitochondrial membrane. The structure of cardiolipin is shown in Fig. 11.3.

Cytochrome c is not only part of the electron transport chain, but it is also an intracellular signal for **apoptosis**. During apoptosis, cytochrome c can pass through enlarged pores in the mitochondrial outer membrane (see Chapter 8). In the cytosol, cytochrome c binds to apoptotic protease-activating factor 1 (APAF1) and thus gives rise to an apoptosome that favors self-destruction of the cell.

The electron transport chain creates an electrochemical $H^+$ gradient (i.e., an electrical charge difference and a pH difference). When this gradient equals the chemical driving force for electron transport, electron transport slows and eventually stops (i.e., an equilibrium is reached).

## 1.3. Clinically Relevant Inhibitors of the Electron Transport Chain

During electron transport by the electron transport chain, some 1% to 4% of electrons do not stay in the chain but are instead accidentally transferred to $O_2$, giving rise to $\cdot O_2^-$ (i.e.,

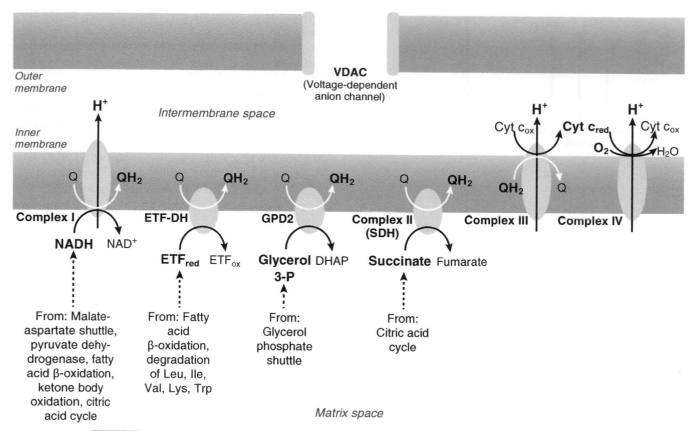

**Fig. 23.3**  **Key elements of the mitochondrial electron transport chain.** Coenzyme $QH_2$ transports hydrogen atoms inside the inner membrane. Cytochrome c transports electrons in the intermembrane space. Fatty acid β-oxidation gives rise to both NADH and reduced ETF. Reducing power from NADH that is produced in glycolysis enters the electron transport chain via the malate-aspartate shuttle or the glycerol 3-phosphate shuttle. Q, coenzyme Q (oxidized form); $QH_2$, coenzyme Q (reduced form); ETF, electron-transferring flavoprotein; ETF-DH, ETF-dehydrogenase; GPD2, mitochondrial glycerol 3-phosphate dehydrogenase; DHAP, dihydroxyacetonephosphate; SDH, succinate dehydrogenase; Cyt c, cytochrome c.

a **superoxide anion**). The superoxide anion is a reactive oxygen species that readily gives rise to a more damaging hydroxyl radical (•OH), which reacts with lipids, proteins, and DNA (see Chapter 21). The main producers of superoxide anions in the electron transport chain are complex I, semiquinol (a radical produced from ubiquinone by the addition of a single H atom), and complex III. An impairment of the electron transport chain increases the production of superoxide anions.

**Metformin** inhibits complex I, while cyanide, **carbon monoxide**, and **sodium azide** inhibit complex IV. Aggressive **oxygen therapy** is always a part of the treatment of poisoning with cyanide, carbon monoxide, or azide. Sometimes, oxygen therapy is performed in a pressure chamber at up to three times the atmospheric pressure at sea level, a treatment called **hyperbaric oxygen**.

**Metformin** is used as an antidiabetic agent. It is very effective at suppressing the excessive endogenous glucose production (i.e., chiefly glycogenolysis and gluconeogenesis in the liver) that is seen in type 2 diabetes (see Chapter 39). The mechanism of action of metformin is still debated but is thought to involve the inhibition of complex I that leads to the activation of adenosine monophosphate (AMP)-dependent protein kinase (AMPK), which then inhibits gluconeogenesis.

**Cyanide** can be produced in building fires, be a part of pesticides, or even be contained in some foods. Cyanide binds predominantly to complex IV (cytochrome c oxidase) and thus blocks the entire electron transport chain, resulting in marked lactic acidemia. Mitochondria contain thiosulfate sulfurtransferase (also called rhodanase), which detoxifies cyanide ($CN^-$) by converting it to thiocyanate ($SCN^-$), which is excreted in the urine. The half-life of cyanide in blood plasma is 20 to 60 minutes. Conversion of cyanide to thiocyanate can be enhanced with IV **sodium thiosulfate** ($S_2O_3^{2-}$), a substrate of thiosulfate sulfurtransferase. Furthermore, cyanide can be bound to cobalamin, which can be given intravenously as **hydroxocobalamin**. The resulting cyanocobalamin (the traditional form of a vitamin $B_{12}$ supplement) is not toxic. First responders often carry hydroxocobalamin. Cyanide can also be bound to **methemoglobin**. Methemoglobin is formed in the body in response to a therapeutic application of **amyl nitrite** (via inspired air) or **sodium nitrite** (intravenous; see Chapter 16). A common therapeutic goal in adults is to convert about 10% to 30% of hemoglobin to methemoglobin.

**Carbon monoxide** results from incomplete combustion in many types of fires (including cigarettes). Carbon monoxide binds to both hemoglobin and complex IV, and

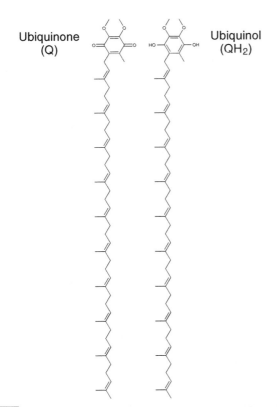

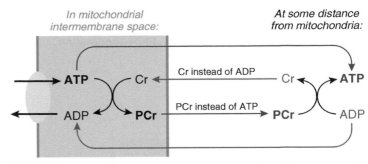

**Fig. 23.5** **Transport of energy from mitochondria to the cell periphery.** Cr, creatine; PCr, phosphocreatine.

**Fig. 23.4** **Coenzyme Q10 (ubiquinone) and its reduced form, ubiquinol.** Both molecules are dissolved in the membrane.

it impairs both oxygen delivery and oxidative phosphorylation. Oxygen therapy enhances the exchange of CO for $O_2$ on hemoglobin.

**Sodium azide** also inhibits complex IV and induces hypotension. Azide is used in explosives (including automobile airbags), as a preservative (often in laboratory settings), and sometimes as a pesticide.

**Hydrogen sulfide** gas also inhibits complex IV. Hydrogen sulfide is formed in some industrial processes and in places where manure is stored. Poisoned patients are treated with oxygen and can be given sodium nitrite, which gives rise to methemoglobin, which in turn binds sulfide. Furthermore, nitrite gives rise to NO, which can displace sulfide from complex IV.

## 1.4. ATP Synthase

An **ATP synthase** in the inner mitochondrial membrane allows $H^+$ to flow from the intermembrane space down the electrochemical gradient into the matrix; it uses the energy of this process to synthesize ATP. Interestingly, the ATP synthase consists in part of subunits that are embedded in the membrane and are essentially static, whereas other subunits form a rotating complex in which $H^+$ flux powers rotation, the mechanical energy of which causes changes in the conformation of the static complex that drives ATP synthesis.

The terms **chemiosmotic coupling** and the **Mitchell hypothesis** apply to ATP production by a combination of a

proton-pumping electron transport chain and a proton-driven ATP synthase. Peter Mitchell first proposed his theory in 1961, at a time when other investigators looked into other ways of harnessing the reducing power of NADH to produce ATP.

In healthy tissue, oxidative phosphorylation is set up such that the ATP synthase keeps the concentration of **ADP** low. The ATP synthase becomes more active whenever more ADP becomes available. When the ATP synthase makes ATP and thereby diminishes the electrochemical $H^+$ gradient, the electron transport chain becomes more active and reestablishes the gradient. Thus, the rate of ADP production determines the flux of electrons in the electron transport chain and the rate of oxygen consumption.

Although oxygen consumption is not part of the mitochondrial ATP synthase-catalyzed reaction itself, reduction of $O_2$ by the electron transport chain is the driving force for this ATP synthesis. Hence, the term *oxidative phosphorylation* is appropriate. Oxidative phosphorylation is not to be confused with substrate-level phosphorylation, which produces ATP from a high-energy phosphorylated substrate such as phosphoenolpyruvate (see Section 1 in Chapter 19).

It is estimated that feeding 1 NADH into the electron transport chain gives rise to the synthesis of about 2.5 ATP and that the oxidation of 1 $QH_2$ (ubiquinol) gives rise to about 1.5 ATP.

In most tissues, the vast majority of ATP (typically >90%) is produced by oxidative phosphorylation. In comparison, ATP production from substrate-level phosphorylation in glycolysis is small.

## 1.5. Transport of Chemical Energy in the Form of ATP and Phosphocreatine

Although ATP is made inside mitochondria, it is mostly consumed outside mitochondria and therefore must be transported across the mitochondrial membranes. The **adenine nucleotide translocator** exchanges ADP for ATP across the inner mitochondrial membrane. The outer membrane has large pores through which ADP and ATP can easily pass. A **phosphate carrier** brings phosphate into the mitochondria for ATP synthesis.

Outside the mitochondria, transport of "energy" occurs via two paths (Fig. 23.5): (1) ATP away from mitochondria versus ADP and phosphate toward mitochondria, and (2)

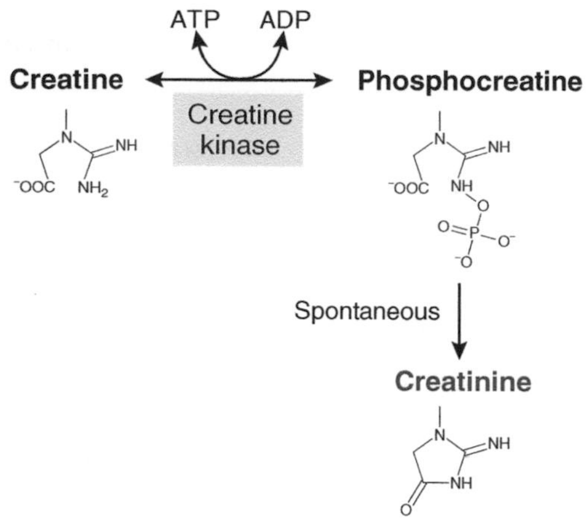

ATP      ADP

**Creatine** ⟷ **Phosphocreatine**

Creatine kinase

Spontaneous ↓

**Creatinine**

**Fig. 23.6** **Formation of creatinine.**

phosphocreatine away from mitochondria versus creatine and phosphate toward mitochondria. The structures of creatine and phosphocreatine are shown in Fig. 23.6. Like ATP, **phosphocreatine** has a high-energy phosphate bond. The concentration of ATP is in the millimolar range, but the free concentration of ADP is usually less than 0.1 mM, which severely curtails transport by diffusion. In contrast, creatine and phosphocreatine can be present in millimolar concentrations. Phosphocreatine and creatine are primarily found in muscle and in the brain, where phosphocreatine is also the primary form of energy storage.

Intake of **exogenous creatine** increases the creatine and phosphocreatine content of various tissues, including muscle. Some athletes take extra creatine to increase their muscle power. Creatine increases power output during repeated short bouts of very intense exercise. Serum **creatinine** levels can rise with creatine supplementation, which complicates the estimation of kidney function that is based on creatinine levels.

Phosphocreatine spontaneously cyclizes to form **creatinine** (see Fig. 23.6), which cannot be remade into creatine and is excreted in the urine. In most people, creatinine is made at a comparable rate; consequently, the amount of creatinine in the blood can be used as a measure of **kidney function** (with significantly decreased filtration, the measured serum concentration of creatinine becomes abnormally high). To make up for the loss of creatinine, the body synthesizes creatine (see Chapter 36).

**Creatine kinase** catalyzes the phosphorylation of creatine and the dephosphorylation of phosphocreatine (see Fig. 23.6). There are two isoenzymes: one in the intermembrane space of mitochondria and one in the cytosol. Creatine kinase is especially abundant in tissues that have a high concentration of creatine and phosphocreatine (e.g., muscle and the brain).

Measurements of creatine kinase in the serum are used to diagnose and follow various **muscle diseases**. Injury to muscle is accompanied by the release of myocyte contents into the extracellular space and blood. There is a muscle-type (M) and a brain-type (B) creatine kinase in the cytosol. Muscle contains mostly MM dimers; severe exercise or injury may lead to an increased fraction of MB dimers.

## 1.6. Uncouplers of Oxidative Phosphorylation

Uncouplers are molecules that allow protons to flow from the intermembrane space back into the matrix, bypassing the ATP synthase (i.e., they uncouple electron transport from ATP synthesis). Uncouplers impair ATP synthesis and also stimulate the electron transport chain, which attempts to reestablish a normal electrochemical $H^+$ gradient. An uncoupler thus increases oxygen consumption.

**Brown adipose tissue** contains an uncoupling protein, **UCP-1**, that, when active, allows $H^+$ to flow from the intermembrane space into the matrix space. Active UCP-1 increases thermogenesis because both the electron transport chain itself and the collapse of the electrochemical $H^+$ gradient generate heat. Brown fat cells are brown or beige because they contain many mitochondria with cytochromes. UCP-1 is activated when norepinephrine activates β-adrenergic receptors on brown fat cells. Uncoupling of the mitochondria in brown fat cells leads to increased oxidation of glucose and fatty acids to $CO_2$.

**Infants** have a significant amount of brown fat, but most adults have only relatively small remnants of it, mostly in the neck and above the clavicles. Growing evidence shows that some drugs can induce white fat cells to turn toward a brown phenotype, becoming beige or "brite" adipocytes.

In **positron emission tomography scans**, brown fat often shows up as a tissue that picks up a considerable amount of the radioactive fluorodeoxyglucose tracer. Brown fat oxidizes glucose, and tracer accumulation from labeled fluorodeoxyglucose parallels glucose use (see Section 6.3 in Chapter 19).

**2,4-Dinitrophenol** is a small-molecule uncoupler that was once tested as a weight-loss drug. It is not currently an approved drug but is available illegally. This drug is dangerous because it can severely impair ATP synthesis and also lead to severe hyperthermia due to stimulation of the respiratory chain.

## 2. INTERPLAY OF GLYCOLYSIS, CITRIC ACID CYCLE, AND OXIDATIVE PHOSPHORYLATION

*As shown above, ATP consumption gives rise to ADP, which in turn stimulates ATP synthase to convert ADP into ATP, thereby consuming a small part of the $H^+$ gradient. The electron transport chain immediately attempts to reestablish the $H^+$ electrochemical gradient by oxidizing NADH, electron-transferring flavoprotein, glycerol 3-phosphate, or succinate. Oxidation lowers the concentration of NADH, which in turn increases citric acid cycle activity.*

Flux in **glycolysis** is mainly determined by phosphofructokinase activity. As long as oxidative phosphorylation keeps the concentration of ATP high and that of ADP low, flux in glycolysis is small. However, when the concentration of ADP rises, for instance because the citric acid cycle does not get enough acetyl-CoA and thus lowers flux in the electron transport chain and in ATP synthesis, flux in glycolysis increases (Fig. 23.7).

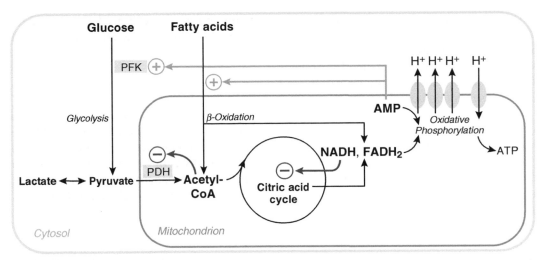

**Fig. 23.7** **Mutual dependence of glycolysis, fatty acid β-oxidation, citric acid cycle, and oxidative phosphorylation.** Fatty acid β-oxidation is also limited by the availability of NAD⁺ and FAD (not shown). PFK, phosphofructokinase.

In place of glucose, many cells can use **fatty acids** to produce reducing power for oxidative phosphorylation. In most of these cells, the concentrations of AMP, NAD⁺, and flavin adenine dinucleotide (FAD) play a role in regulating the rate of fatty acid β-oxidation (see Chapter 27).

Patients who have impaired oxidative phosphorylation produce more of their ATP via **anaerobic glycolysis**, which may lead to **lactic acidemia** (see Fig. 23.7). Oxidative phosphorylation may be impaired because of **hypoxia** or **anoxia**, or because of an inhibitor of the electron transport chain (e.g., **cyanide, carbon monoxide,** or **metformin** overdose). When flux in the electron transport chain decreases, the concentration of NADH increases, and flux in both the citric acid cycle and in pyruvate dehydrogenase decreases. The impaired electron transport chain leads to a decrease in mitochondrial ATP synthesis, which increases the concentration of free ADP and free AMP. AMP, in turn, activates phosphofructokinase and thus flux in glycolysis. Reducing power from NADH produced in glycolysis can no longer be moved into the mitochondria but must be used to reduce pyruvate to lactate. Appreciable inhibition of the body's capacity for oxidative phosphorylation leads to very marked lactic acidemia. The acidemia is the cause of death in an anoxic patient.

Although **cancer** cells usually have enough oxygen, they often produce much more pyruvate from glycolysis than they can oxidize via the citric acid cycle and oxidative phosphorylation, a paradox called the **Warburg effect**. One of the current hypotheses is that metabolic reprogramming is advantageous to cancer cells because it provides them with more precursors and NADPH for biosynthetic pathways. These precursors can be intermediates of glycolysis, intermediates of pathways that interface with glycolysis, or intermediates of the citric acid cycle. The precursors can then be used for the biosynthesis of amino acids, nucleotides, or lipids. The metabolic reprogramming is achieved by a mutation or altered expression of genes that play a role in metabolism and signaling.

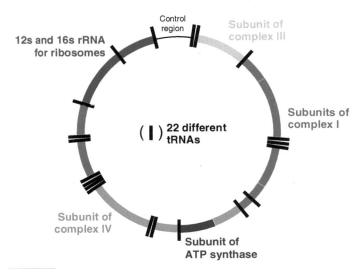

**Fig. 23.8** **Structure of human mitochondrial DNA (mtDNA).** mtDNA consists of two complementary strands. *(Modified from www.mitomap.org.)*

## 3. MITOCHONDRIAL DNA AND ITS INHERITANCE

*Mitochondrial DNA is closed, circular, and contains almost 40 genes that encode mitochondrial tRNAs, rRNAs, and 13 subunits of electron transport complexes and the mitochondrial ATP synthase. Mitochondria are passed onto offspring only via the mother. Most cells have thousands of copies of mitochondrial DNA.*

Mitochondria contain their own DNA (mtDNA), which is circular and encodes a few proteins and all of the tRNAs needed for translation (Fig. 23.8). The genetic codes for translation of mitochondrial- and nucleus-encoded RNAs differ in two codons. Most proteins in the mitochondria are encoded by genes in the nucleus, synthesized in the cytosol, and then imported into mitochondria. Similarly, most mitochondrial diseases are due to mutations in nuclear genes and therefore show Mendelian inheritance.

The mitochondrial DNA encodes two rRNAs for its ribosomes, 22 tRNAs for translation, and 13 proteins. The proteins are subunits of the ATP synthase and of complexes I, III, and IV. Other subunits of these protein complexes are encoded in nuclear DNA.

Mitochondria import RNA polymerase, transcription factors, all aminoacyl-tRNA synthetases, initiation factors, and elongation factors (see Section 2 in Chapter 6). The nucleus-encoded DNA polymerase G (or gamma) enters the mitochondria and replicates mtDNA.

Human mtDNA contains about 16,000 nucleotides. On average, unrelated humans differ by about 50 nucleotides. Hence, the mtDNA sequence can serve to identify individuals.

A typical cell contains more than 1000-fold more copies of mtDNA than nuclear DNA.

Mitochondria are **inherited** only from the **mother**. A sperm has fewer copies of mitochondrial DNA than does the egg, few of the mitochondria in sperm enter the egg, and mitochondria from the sperm are rapidly destroyed in the egg. A human egg typically contains more than 100,000 copies of mitochondrial DNA.

The term **homoplasmy** refers to a cell in which all mitochondrial DNA molecules are the same, whereas **heteroplasmy** refers to a cell that contains a mixture of mitochondrial DNA molecules.

During **cell division**, mitochondria and their DNA molecules are divided by chance. Offspring of a mother can therefore have more or less mutant mtDNA than the mother. Furthermore, some cells or tissues in a person may have more or less mutant mtDNA than others. The level of mutant mtDNA in a tissue may even change over time. Clinically, this means that offspring may have greater or lesser severity of disease than the mother. Furthermore, symptoms vary greatly among patients with the same disorder. Due to these chance events described, the terms *dominant* and *recessive* inheritance are not used for diseases attributable to mutant mtDNA.

## 4. DISEASES INVOLVING MITOCHONDRIA

*Diseases involving mitochondria are often associated with impaired energy production and affect cells and tissues that use ATP at a high rate. These diseases are acquired or inherited via DNA in the nucleus or mitochondria. Affected patients may benefit from supplements that improve the capacity for oxidative phosphorylation.*

### 4.1. Overview

Mitochondrial diseases are a group of disorders that stem largely from a loss of normal mitochondrial function, particularly oxidative phosphorylation. Major deficiencies of oxidative phosphorylation often impair the nervous system, muscle contraction, insulin secretion from pancreatic β-cells, vision, or hearing (Fig. 23.9). Mitochondria with impaired oxidative phosphorylation may induce **apoptosis** (cell death). Furthermore, such mitochondria can produce **reactive oxygen species (ROS)** at an increased rate. The nervous system is particularly sensitive to ROS because it contains an abundance of polyunsaturated fatty acids.

Syndromes of dysfunctional mitochondria are named according to clinical observations rather than cause. This explains why some of these syndromes have more than one cause.

Mitochondria turn over constantly; autophagosomes engulf mitochondria and deliver them to the lysosomes for destruction in a process called **mitophagy**. Impaired function of lysosomes or autophagy appears to impair tissue function.

**Mitochondrial disease** may arise from **mutations** in mitochondrial or nuclear DNA that affect a wide variety of mitochondrial processes; they can be **acquired** (e.g., by drug

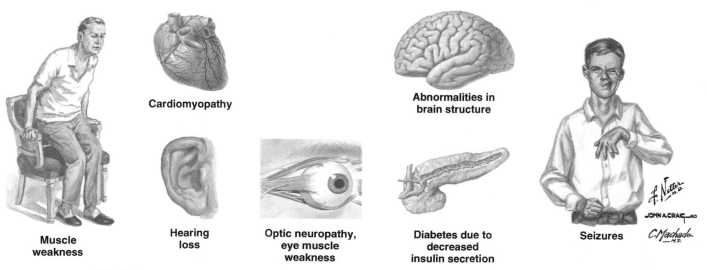

**Cardiomyopathy**

**Abnormalities in brain structure**

**Muscle weakness**

**Hearing loss**

**Optic neuropathy, eye muscle weakness**

**Diabetes due to decreased insulin secretion**

**Seizures**

**Fig. 23.9** **Manifestations of diseases involving mitochondria.** Such a disease may affect more than one organ system.

treatment), or they can be of unknown origin. Mutations in **nuclear DNA** show a mendelian pattern of inheritance, whereas mutations in **mtDNA** show a maternal pattern of inheritance. For defects in oxidative phosphorylation to become clinically manifest, there is usually a **threshold** effect (i.e., a certain minimal amount of mutant mtDNA must be present). This threshold depends on the energy needs of a tissue. Hence, the pattern of inheritance of mtDNA mutations may be difficult to interpret because patients with a mutant mtDNA load below the threshold do not exhibit the disease.

Some patients who have a mitochondrial disease benefit from supplements. Supplemental **thiamine** may increase the activity of pyruvate dehydrogenase and α-ketoglutarate dehydrogenase. **Riboflavin** gives rise to flavin mononucleotide (FMN) and FAD, which are used by enzymes that feed into the electron transport chain. Reduced **coenzyme Q10** has a role both as an antioxidant and as an electron transporter. **Ascorbate** works as an antioxidant (see Chapter 21). **Creatine** supplements can markedly increase the creatine content of muscle and brain tissue, which may improve delivery of ATP to peripheral points of cells. **Carnitine** can free up CoA when high concentrations of acyl-CoA are present due to acidemia (see Chapter 27).

## 4.2. Diseases Associated With mtDNA Mutations

Disease is generally apparent when more than about 60% of the mtDNA is mutant mtDNA, but the thresholds vary by tissue.

Mitochondrial diseases that are symptomatic in the newborn period are often accompanied by lactic acidosis, cardiomyopathy, and hyperammonemia.

The **diagnosis** of a mitochondrial disease often involves an **analysis of mtDNA**. The mtDNA can be obtained from kidney epithelial cells in the urine, white blood cells, buccal cells, or muscle cells.

When diseased mitochondria accumulate in myocytes, they give rise to so-called **ragged red fibers** in a trichrome-stained muscle biopsy.

All patients with **Kearns-Sayre syndrome** have a progressive external ophthalmoplegia, show atypical pigment degeneration of the retinae, and experience the onset of symptoms before age 20 years. Many patients have a conduction disorder of the heart or are at high risk of developing one, followed by premature death. Most of these patients have a **large deletion of mtDNA** (often ~5 kb, which is ~30% of the mtDNA) that occurs sporadically (i.e., the disease is not inherited).

The **A3243G mutation in mtDNA** gives rise to maternally inherited diabetes and deafness (**MIDD**) and sometimes mitochondrial myopathy, encephalopathy, lactic acidosis, and stroke-like episodes (**MELAS**). The A3243G mutation is in the gene that encodes one of the two mitochondrial tRNA$^{Leu}$. The mutation is found in 1 in 500 to 15,000 people, depending on the population, with many patients remaining undiagnosed. The mutation leads to diminished synthesis of all proteins of oxidative phosphorylation that are encoded by mtDNA. The milder deficiency in oxidative phosphorylation manifests

itself with MIDD in adulthood, whereas more severe deficiencies are associated with MELAS and onset during childhood or young adulthood.

**Leigh syndrome** is a progressive neurodegenerative disorder. There are many different genetic causes of Leigh syndrome. Mutations can be in the mtDNA or nuclear DNA, and they affect a gene that encodes a protein of the electron transport chain, the ATP synthase, or the pyruvate dehydrogenase complex. In many patients, the genetic cause of the disease is unknown. Disease onset is typically before age 2 years. There is a wide spectrum of disease manifestations, of which the more common are regression of development, seizures, impaired control of muscles, and lactic acidosis. The diagnosis rests in part on magnetic resonance imaging showing symmetric necrotic lesions in the brain.

## 4.3. Diseases Associated With Dysfunctional Mitochondria Due to Mutation in the Nucleus

Mutations in genes in the nucleus can affect one of the many components of the electron transport chain, ATP synthase, proteins that play a role in the transport and assembly of proteins in mitochondria, or anything else that affects the function of mitochondria.

**Huntington disease** (Fig. 23.10) is an autosomal dominantly inherited disorder that is due to an expanded trinucleotide repeat in an exon of the huntingtin gene, which leads to an aggregation of huntingtin and severe defects in the neurons of the striatum. It affects about 1 in 15,000 people. The disease often becomes evident when patients are in their 40s. Patients lose control of their movements and some

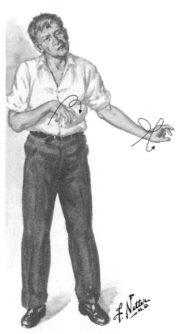

**Fig. 23.10** **Huntington disease.** Affected patients lose control over motor movements.

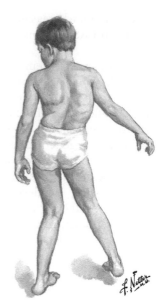

**Fig. 23.11** **Friedreich ataxia.** The disease presents with progressive ataxia, a wide gait, and scoliosis.

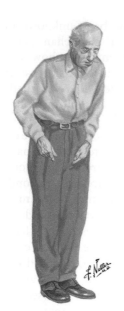

**Fig. 23.12** **Parkinson disease.** Patients have tremors and gait disturbances.

cognitive functions. Mitochondria most likely play a role in the neurodegeneration. There is a reduced capacity for oxidative phosphorylation, but the role of this deficit in the overall disease process is unclear.

**Friedreich ataxia** (Fig. 23.11) is an autosomal recessively inherited disease that is due to a trinucleotide repeat expansion in the *FXN* gene that leads to a **frataxin** deficiency in mitochondria. The prevalence is about 1 in 50,000. Frataxin likely plays a role in the insertion of iron into proteins that contain iron-sulfur clusters, such as complexes I, II, and III of the electron transport chain, and aconitase of the citric acid cycle (see Chapter 22). Frataxin deficiency also leads to iron overload of the mitochondria, which may increase oxidative stress. Friedreich ataxia is associated with the degeneration of the peripheral nervous system, central nervous system, heart, and pancreatic β-cells.

## 4.4. Idiopathic or Acquired Diseases of Mitochondria

In **Parkinson disease** (Fig. 23.12) the membrane potential of mitochondria is reduced (suggesting impaired ATP production via oxidative phosphorylation), and there is evidence that an inadequate turnover of mitochondria (mitophagy), impaired $Ca^{2+}$ homeostasis by mitochondria, an increased load of mutant mtDNA, and mitochondria-induced increased apoptosis contribute to the pathology.

**Turnover of mitochondria** can be impaired, for example, by certain lysosomal storage diseases (e.g., Gaucher disease, due to the deficient degradation of glucocerebroside to glucose and ceramide) or by mutations in proteins that regulate turnover of mitochondria (e.g., parkin or PINK1, both of which are associated with hereditary, early-onset forms of Parkinson disease).

Some **drugs** are known to impair the function of mitochondria. Mitochondria evolved from bacteria. **Aminoglycosides** (e.g., streptomycin, kanamycin, neomycin, gentamicin, tobramycin, and amikacin) inhibit the function of mitochondrial ribosomes and can impair hearing when used systemically; they are also neurotoxic and nephrotoxic. **Chloramphenicol** affects mitochondria such that hematopoiesis may be impaired. **Linezolid** decreases protein synthesis in mitochondria and may lead to lactic acidemia or even peripheral and optic neuropathy. Of the **antiretroviral drugs** that have been developed for the treatment of HIV, those with the highest affinity for DNA-polymerase gamma (the DNA polymerase for replication of mtDNA inside mitochondria) showed considerable toxicity to mitochondria, such that their use is no longer recommended.

## SUMMARY

- Oxidative phosphorylation takes place in the mitochondria and provides most of the body's ATP. The electron transport chain reduces oxygen to water and thereby pumps protons into the intermembrane space. The ATP synthase uses the proton electrochemical gradient for the synthesis of ATP.
- The electron transport chain receives input chiefly from NADH, reduced electron-transferring flavoprotein, glyceraldehyde 3-phosphate, and succinate.
- The electron transport chain consists of four multisubunit complexes (three of which pump protons), and the two electron carriers ubiquinol and reduced cytochrome c.
- An adenine nucleotide translocator transports ADP into and ATP out of mitochondria. Chiefly in muscle and the brain, creatine and phosphocreatine facilitate the transport

of chemical energy from the mitochondria to sites of consumption in the cytosol; phosphocreatine is also an energy reserve.

■ Hypoxia, uncouplers, and inhibitors of oxidative phosphorylation reduce ATP production in mitochondria, which leads to a compensatory activation of anaerobic glycolysis that may lead to lactic acidemia. Inhibitors of oxidative phosphorylation decrease oxygen consumption, and uncouplers increase it. Clinically relevant inhibitors of oxidative phosphorylation are metformin, cyanide, carbon monoxide, sodium azide, and hydrogen sulfide. The uncoupling protein UCP-1 serves the purpose of heat production in brown fat.

■ Mitochondria contain their own DNA, which encodes subunits of complexes I, II, and IV as well as the ATP synthase. In addition, mtDNA encodes the rRNAs and tRNAs needed for translation inside mitochondria. Each cell typically contains thousands of copies of mtDNA. mtDNA is passed to offspring by their mothers.

■ Impaired oxidative phosphorylation plays a role in the pathogenesis of most mitochondrial diseases. However, an impaired turnover of mitochondria, impaired control of $Ca^{2+}$ in the cytosol, acquired mutations in mtDNA, excessive apoptosis, and increased production of reactive oxygen species (ROS) often also participate.

■ Mitochondrial diseases preferentially involve tissues that have high demands for energy and depend on mitochondria for proper function. Affected patients often present with dysfunction of the nervous system, musculature, auditory perception, or pancreatic β-cells.

■ Antimicrobial drugs such as aminoglycosides, chloramphenicol, and linezolid impair the function of mitochondria and must be administered with appropriate precautions.

■ A mutation in a mitochondrial tRNA$^{Leu}$ gives rise to maternally inherited diabetes and deafness (MIDD) or mitochondrial myopathy, encephalopathy, lactic acidosis, and stroke-like episodes (MELAS). A large deletion of mtDNA gives rise to Kearns-Sayre syndrome.

■ Leigh syndrome is characterized by symmetrical necrotic lesions in the brain and has many different causes, either in nuclear or mitochondrial DNA.

■ Friedreich ataxia is due to defective iron metabolism in mitochondria caused by mutant nuclear-encoded frataxin.

■ Huntington disease is due to mutant, nuclear-encoded huntingtin, and impaired oxidative phosphorylation plays a role in the loss of motor control.

■ Parkinson disease is most often an idiopathic or acquired disease with multifaceted dysfunction of mitochondria.

## FURTHER READING

■ Borron SW, Bebarta VS. Asphyxiants. *Emerg Med Clin North Am.* 2015;33:89-115.

■ DiMauro S, Schon EA, Carelli V, Hirano M. The clinical maze of mitochondrial neurology. *Nat Rev Neurol.* 2013;9:429-444.

■ Perier C, Vila M. Mitochondrial biology and Parkinson's disease. *Cold Spring Harb Perspect Med.* 2012;4:a009332.

# Review Questions

1. A patient with carbon monoxide poisoning is best treated with which one of the following?

   A. Hydroxocobalamin
   B. $O_2$
   C. Sodium nitrite
   D. Sodium thiosulfate

2. A 5-month-old infant with a selective deficiency in one of the subunits of complex I most likely presents with which of the following?

   A. Leigh syndrome
   B. Mitochondrial myopathy, encephalopathy, lactic acidosis, and stroke-like episodes (MELAS)
   C. Maternally inherited diabetes and deafness (MIDD)

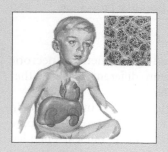

# Chapter 24

# Glycogen Metabolism and Glycogen Storage Diseases

## SYNOPSIS

- Glycogen is a branched polymer of glucose that is present in a granular form in the cytosol of virtually every cell. The largest glycogen stores are in muscle and the liver.
- Fig. 24.1 shows the basic reactions of glycogen metabolism along with connections to other metabolic pathways in the liver.
- After a meal, muscle and liver synthesize glycogen. During exercise, muscle degrades its glycogen for its own use, and the liver degrades some of its glycogen to provide muscle with glucose. During an overnight fast, the liver degrades some of its glycogen and releases glucose into the blood for the benefit of other tissues.
- Lysosomes continually degrade glycogen particles at a low rate.
- Glycogen storage diseases (glycogenoses) are quite rare; their combined incidence is about 1:20,000. Affected patients may be glucose intolerant (and thus at an increased risk of developing diabetes), have fasting hypoglycemia, develop a myopathy, or have seizures.

## LEARNING OBJECTIVES

*For mastery of this topic, you should be able to do the following:*

- Describe the reactants, products, and tissue distribution of glycogen synthesis and glycogenolysis.
- Compare and contrast how feeding, fasting, and exercise influence glycogen synthesis and glycogenolysis in the liver and skeletal muscle.
- Explain the contribution of glycogenesis and glycogenolysis to blood glucose homeostasis during the fed state, the fasting state, and exercise.
- Explain the role of muscle glycogen in exercise.
- Explain the pathogenesis of hypoglycemia in patients who have glucose 6-phosphatase deficiency.
- List the enzyme deficiencies that give rise to the most common hereditary glycogenoses and predict their effects on blood glucose concentration, the amount of tissue glycogen, and damage to tissues.
- Compare and contrast the pathogenesis and pathology of Pompe disease (lysosomal acid maltase deficiency) and Lafora disease.

## 1. SYNTHESIS OF GLYCOGEN (GLYCOGENESIS)

*A glycogen particle consists of glycogenin and a branched polymer of glucose. Under most circumstances of glycogen synthesis, an existing glycogen particle is enlarged. Less often, a new particle is started from glycogenin. Glycogen is synthesized in the liver and muscle after a carbohydrate meal and in muscle also after exercise. Glycogen synthase adds glucose from an activated form, uridine diphosphate (UDP)-glucose. Glycogen branching enzyme creates a branch from a linear glucose polymer chain.*

## 1.1. Structure and Role of Glycogen

Glycogen consists of a branched polymer of glucose that is formed on a tyrosine side chain of the **glycogenin** protein (Fig. 24.2). The glucose residues are mostly linked in $\alpha(1{\rightarrow}4)$ fashion, and occasionally in $\alpha(1{\rightarrow}6)$ fashion to create branch points. Branching increases the solubility of glycogen.

During glycogen synthesis and degradation, there are limits for particle size. The smallest particles contain about 2,000 glucosyl residues, the largest about 60,000. Small glycogen particles are also called **proglycogen**, large ones **macroglycogen**.

Glycogen particles are visible by electron microscopy after staining with a heavy metal, or by light microscopy after treatment with **periodic acid–Schiff (PAS) stain**, which generates a colored complex (Fig. 24.3). The iodine binds into the left-handed helices of glucose moieties in the linear portions of glycogen. Normal muscle glycogen particles have a diameter of up to 0.04 μm. In the liver, rosettes form that contain 20 to 40 such particles.

Muscle and liver store the largest amounts of glycogen; most other cells store only a small amount of glycogen. The liver of a typical, healthy, postprandial adult contains up to about 100 g of glycogen (i.e., about 7% of the wet weight of the liver); in the absence of exercise, the skeletal muscles contain up to about 400 g of glycogen (or about 2% of the wet weight of muscle). If a person exercises to exhaustion and then consumes a meal very rich in carbohydrates, the exercised muscles can contain as much as 5% of their wet weight as glycogen.

Glycogen synthesis and breakdown help even out the concentration of glucose in the blood in the course of a day. Glycogen in liver and muscles is synthesized chiefly during the first few hours after a meal (Fig. 24.4). In the subsequent fasting period, when glucose use exceeds glucose influx from the intestine, liver glycogen is degraded to glucose, which is released into the blood; this helps maintain a normal fasting concentration of glucose in the blood. Muscles degrade their glycogen during exercise to provide energy for contraction. Muscles do not release glucose into the blood, but the degradation of intracellular glycogen reduces the need for glucose uptake from the blood into muscle.

## 1.2. Reactions of Glycogen Synthesis

Glucose is activated to UDP-glucose, from which an additional glucose residue can be added to glycogen (Fig. 24.5). Glycogen synthesis takes place in the cytosol. Glycogen synthesis requires a modest amount of energy in the form of UTP,

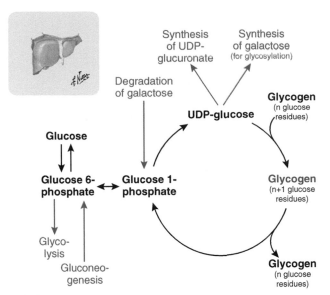

**Fig. 24.1** **Position of glycogen metabolism in overall metabolism in the liver.** UDP, uridine diphosphate.

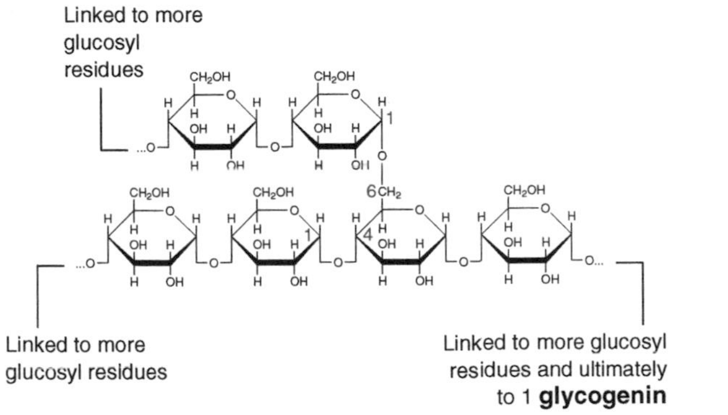

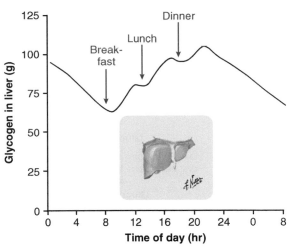

**Fig. 24.4** **Approximate daily time course of the amount of glycogen in the liver of resting volunteers.** Data are based on 13C magnetic resonance spectroscopic measurements. Volunteers consumed weight-maintaining mixed meals. (Data from Hwang J-H, Perseghin G, Rothman DL, et al. Impaired net hepatic glycogen synthesis in insulin-dependent diabetic subjects during mixed meal ingestion; a 13C nuclear magnetic resonance spectroscopy study. *J Clin Invest.* 1995;95:783-787; Taylor R, Magnusson I, Rothman DL, et al. Direct assessment of liver glycogen storage by 13C nuclear magnetic resonance spectroscopy and regulation of glucose homeostasis after a mixed meal in normal subjects. *J Clin Invest.* 1996;97:126-132; and Krssak M, Brehm A, Bernroider E, et al. Alterations in postprandial hepatic glycogen metabolism in type 2 diabetes. *Diabetes.* 2004;53:3048-3056.)

**Fig. 24.2** **Partial structure of glycogen.** Red numbers reflect the standard nomenclature for numbering carbons in sugars.

which in turn is made with the help of ATP. Significant glycogen synthesis occurs in muscle and the liver.

The **glycogen branching enzyme** (recommended name: **1,4-α-glucan branching enzyme**) introduces α(1→6) branches (Fig. 24.6). The branching enzyme cuts a stretch of linear, α(1→4)-linked terminal glucose residues and links carbon-1 of this stretch to carbon-6 of an upstream glucose residue, thus generating an α(1→6) glucosidic linkage that starts a new branch. Such branching increases the solubility of glycogen. A deficiency in branching is associated with cell damage (see Section 3.3).

In a healthy person, the center of a glycogen particle is more highly branched than the periphery, and the peripheral half of the weight of a glycogen particle consists of linear branches.

### 1.3. Regulation of Glycogen Synthesis

**Skeletal muscle** synthesizes glycogen in response to depleted glycogen stores; this synthesis is strongly enhanced by insulin. Antecedent exercise and an elevated concentration of insulin each increase both the number of **glucose transporters** in the plasma membrane and the activity of **glycogen synthase** in the cytosol (see Fig. 24.5). As a result of these control mechanisms, postexercise glycogen synthesis proceeds at a relatively low rate in the fasting state, and at a markedly higher rate after a carbohydrate-containing meal. During extended exercise, an elevated concentration of epinephrine prevents glycogen synthesis.

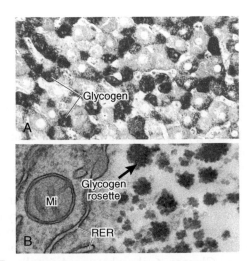

**Fig. 24.3** **Glycogen in the liver.** (A) Light microscope image of PAS (periodic acid–Schiff)-stained tissue. (B) Transmission electron micrograph. Mi, mitochondrion; RER, rough endoplasmic reticulum.

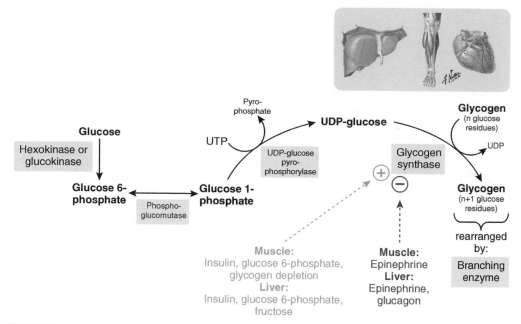

**Fig. 24.5** **Glycogen synthesis.** For details of the branching enzyme, see Fig. 24.6. UDP, uridine diphosphate; UTP, uridine triphosphate.

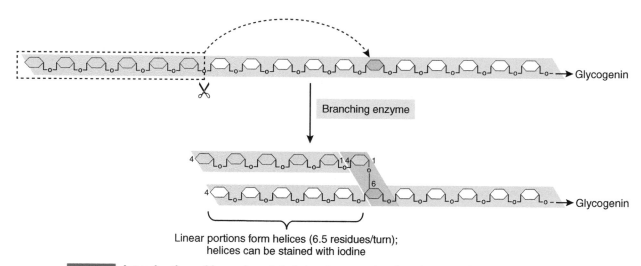

Linear portions form helices (6.5 residues/turn);
helices can be stained with iodine

**Fig. 24.6** **Introduction of branch points into glycogen by the glycogen branching enzyme.**

The higher the carbohydrate content of the diet, the higher the muscle glycogen stores. In the short term, a **diet** with greater than 90% of calories from carbohydrate can lead to three- to fourfold greater muscle glycogen stores than a diet of less than 10% carbohydrate. In the long term, differences between low- and high-carbohydrate diets are smaller.

Athletes can maximize their endurance by maximizing their muscle glycogen stores. To this end, they can deplete muscles of glycogen through intense exercise, followed by 2 to 3 days of rest during which they consume a high-carbohydrate diet. Such a regimen leads to approximately double the normal glycogen stores, a phenomenon called **supercompensation**. To make glycogen stores peak near the start of a competition,

athletes often consume a high-carbohydrate meal a few hours before exercise starts.

In the **heart**, glycogen depletion due to an acute increase in workload or due to ischemia subsequently stimulates glycogen synthesis. Filled glycogen stores have a favorable effect on maximal power output and hypoxia tolerance.

In the **liver** (see Fig. 24.5), glucose, fructose, and insulin are the main stimuli for glycogen synthesis. Dietary fructose, glucose, and insulin receptor signaling activate glucokinase, which leads to an increased concentration of glucose 6-phosphate. Glucose 6-phosphate and insulin signaling enhance glycogen synthase activity, which is the main determinant of the rate of glycogen synthesis.

## 2. DEGRADATION OF GLYCOGEN (GLYCOGENOLYSIS)

*Glycogen phosphorylase degrades the linear portions of glycogen to glucose 1-phosphate, which is in equilibrium with glucose 6-phosphate. Glycogen phosphorylase ends its activity a few residues before a branch point. The glycogen debranching enzyme then moves the remaining short, linear chain of glucosyl residues to the end of another linear chain and produces glucose from the glucosyl residue at the branch point. In the liver, glucose 6-phosphatase dephosphorylates glucose 6-phosphate to glucose for export into the blood. Muscle does not have glucose 6-phosphatase and does not export glucose.*

*As part of the turnover of cell components, lysosomes occasionally engulf glycogen particles. Inside lysosomes, acid α-glucosidase degrades glycogen particles to glucose.*

### 2.1. Degradation of Glycogen to Glucose 6-Phosphate and Glucose

Glycogen degradation takes place in muscle during exercise and in the liver during the first day of fasting.

**Glycogen phosphorylase** catalyzes the phosphorolysis of glycogen to form glucose 1-phosphate, which is then isomerized to glucose 6-phosphate (Fig. 24.7). Glycogen phosphorylase activity is rate limiting. The isomerization of glucose 6-phosphate and glucose 1-phosphate (a reversible reaction) is part of both glycogen synthesis and glycogen degradation (as well as the degradation of galactose; see Chapter 20).

The degradation of glycogen near α(1→6) branch points requires glycogen debranching enzyme activity. Once a linear branch of glycogen is only four glucosyl residues long, glycogen phosphorylase can no longer shorten it. Glycogen that has all of its linear branches shortened maximally by glycogen phosphorylase is called a **limit dextrin**. The **debranching enzyme** (Fig. 24.8) cleaves the remaining stretch of three linearly linked glucosyl residues (i.e., a maltotriose unit) and transfers it to the C-4 end of another linear portion of glycogen. Next, the debranching enzyme produces glucose from the remaining glucosyl residue that forms the branch point. The degradation of glycogen by the combined actions of glycogen phosphorylase and debranching enzyme thus yields mostly glucose 1-phosphate and some glucose.

A glucose 6-phosphatase in the endoplasmic reticulum hydrolyzes glucose 6-phosphate to produce glucose (Fig. 24.9). The hydrolysis requires three different activities: (1) a **glucose 6-phosphate/phosphate antiporter** (encoded by the *SLC37A4* gene) in the membrane of the endoplasmic reticulum, (2) **glucose 6-phosphatase** activity that hydrolyzes glucose 6-phosphate to glucose + phosphate, and (3) a **glucose transporter** that releases glucose from the endoplasmic reticulum into the cytosol.

Glucose 6-phosphatase activity is somewhat increased by glucagon and epinephrine, whereas insulin decreases it.

Major hydrolysis of glucose 6-phosphate to glucose is seen in the liver (for glycogenolysis and gluconeogenesis) and the kidneys (for gluconeogenesis; see Chapter 25).

### 2.2. Regulation of Glycogenolysis

Glycogenolysis is mostly regulated by intracellular signals in muscle and extracellular signals in the liver.

In muscle, the three main types of **muscle fibers** (Table 24.1) differ in their metabolism. Most muscles contain several types of fibers, whereby the proportions depend on the function of the muscle (see Section 5.5 in Chapter 19). Exercise typically involves the use of several muscles, which together derive energy from intracellular glycogen and triglycerides, as well as from blood-derived glucose and fatty acids.

**Blood flow** to muscle becomes maximal only several minutes after the start of exercise; in the meantime, muscle glycogen provides the necessary extra fuel for adenosine triphosphate (ATP) generation, in part via anaerobic

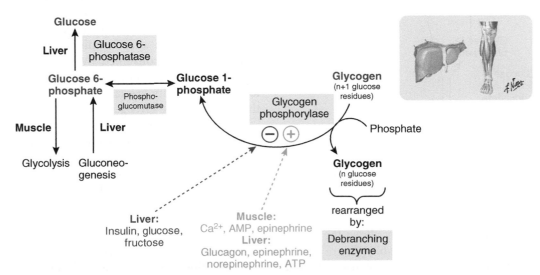

**Fig. 24.7 Degradation of glycogen (glycogenolysis).** For details of the debranching enzyme, see Fig. 24.8. AMP, adenosine monophosphate; ATP, adenosine triphosphate.

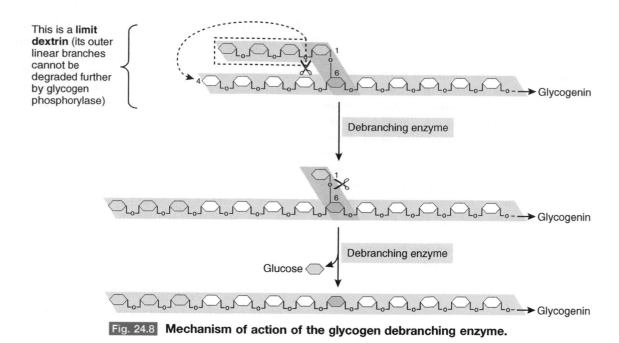

This is a **limit dextrin** (its outer linear branches cannot be degraded further by glycogen phosphorylase)

Debranching enzyme

Glycogenin

Debranching enzyme

Glucose

Debranching enzyme

Glycogenin

**Fig. 24.8** Mechanism of action of the glycogen debranching enzyme.

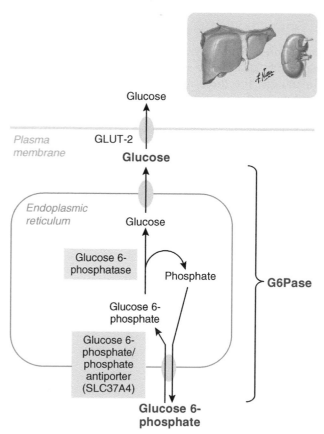

Glucose

Plasma membrane     GLUT-2

**Glucose**

Endoplasmic reticulum     Glucose

Glucose 6-phosphatase

Phosphate

**G6Pase**

Glucose 6-phosphate

Glucose 6-phosphate/phosphate antiporter (SLC37A4)

**Glucose 6-phosphate**

**Fig. 24.9** **Production of glucose by glucose 6-phosphatase.** Glucose 6-phosphatase also plays a role in gluconeogenesis (see Chapter 25).

increased hydrolysis of circulating very-low-density lipoprotein (VLDL) and intermediate-density lipoprotein (IDL) particles by muscle lipoprotein lipase, and from the increased hydrolysis of triglycerides inside the adipose tissue (see Chapter 28).

Persistent, intense exercise requires that some of the energy be produced from the degradation of muscle glycogen. Without glycogen degradation in muscles, a person's power output is limited to about half the output at the person's maximal oxidative capacity. This is partly explained by the fact that a given amount of oxygen produces more ATP from glucose than from fatty acids.

With increasing **intensity** of exercise, muscles degrade glycogen at a faster rate. With exercise at less than 25% of a person's maximal aerobic capacity, glycogen use is small and ceases after about 30 minutes. Glycolysis then mainly degrades glucose that is taken up from the blood. In contrast, with exercise at ~80% of a person's maximal aerobic capacity, glycogen degradation after 30 minutes still accounts for about half the calories consumed by muscle. When most of the muscle glycogen is consumed, muscle **fatigue** sets in. Therefore, high-intensity exercise endurance critically depends on the size of muscle glycogen stores.

Skeletal muscles do not have glucose 6-phosphatase and therefore cannot convert glycogen-derived glucose 6-phosphate to glucose. Although glycogen debranching enzyme produces glucose from the (1→6)-branch points, the concentration of glucose in the cytosol of exercising muscle is still lower than in the extracellular space; hence, this glycogen-derived glucose does not leave the muscle (it enters glycolysis).

Within contracting muscle, an increase in the cytosolic concentration of **Ca²⁺** activates glycogenolysis (see Fig. 24.7). The Ca²⁺ stems from the endoplasmic reticulum in response to neural input.

glycolysis. Increased blood flow eventually allows the muscle to use more oxygen and glucose from the blood.

With increasing **duration** of moderate-intensity exercise, muscles shift some of their energy production from carbohydrate to **fatty acid oxidation**. These fatty acids derive from

**Table 24.1  Muscle Fiber Types**

| Fiber Type | Composition and Metabolism | Fiber Speed | Onset of Fatigue | Example |
|---|---|---|---|---|
| 1 | Rich in mitochondria; oxidize carbohydrates, fatty acids, ketone bodies to $CO_2$ | Slow twitch | Last | Soleus |
| 2a | Combination of metabolism of type 1 and type 2x fibers | Intermediate twitch | Intermediate | |
| 2x | Few mitochondria; mostly glycolysis | Fast twitch | First | Gastrocnemius |

In contracting muscle, an increase in the concentration of adenosine monophosphate (**AMP**) activates both glycogen phosphorylase and glucose transport (see Fig. 24.7). Since contraction uses ATP, the concentrations of ADP and AMP in the cytosol are higher during exercise than at rest. ADP and AMP are in equilibrium via the reaction 2 ADP $\leftrightarrow$ AMP + ATP (see Section 1 in Chapter 38). Incorporation of GLUT-4 transporters into the plasma membrane permits increased uptake of glucose from the blood.

During exercise, nerves stimulate the adrenal medulla to release **epinephrine**; epinephrine activates β-adrenergic receptors that in turn lead to increased glycogen phosphorylase activity and decreased glycogen synthase activity (see Figs. 24.5 and 24.7). Within 15 minutes of intense exercise, the concentration of epinephrine in the serum increases by a factor of ~10 (see Fig. 26.8).

Skeletal muscle expresses virtually no **glucagon receptors**; therefore, glucagon has no appreciable effect on muscle glycogen metabolism.

In the **heart**, ischemia or an acute increase in workload both stimulate glycogen degradation. At a low workload, the heart mostly uses fatty acids for energy generation, but as the workload increases, the heart uses progressively more glucose and glycogen because ATP generation from glucose requires less oxygen than ATP generation from fatty acids. During ischemia, the heart degrades glucose 6-phosphate from glycogen mostly to lactate.

In the **liver**, as postprandial carbohydrate influx from the intestine fades, liver glycogen increasingly serves as a source of glucose to maintain a physiological concentration of glucose in the blood. After a 15-hour fast, liver glycogenolysis typically accounts for about one-third of the body's glucose production (the other two-thirds stem from gluconeogenesis; see Chapter 25).

**Glucagon, epinephrine, norepinephrine**, and extracellular **ATP** stimulate liver glycogenolysis, while **insulin** inhibits it (see Figs. 24.7). A pharmacological dose of glucagon can immediately activate liver glycogenolysis. **Diabetic** patients take advantage of this effect to counter insulin-induced hypoglycemia. A glucagon injection can also be used to test whether a patient's liver can degrade glycogen to glucose. Epinephrine and norepinephrine are released from the adrenal glands during exercise or hypoglycemia. Like glucagon, epinephrine is effective even in the presence of a significant concentration of insulin (epinephrine is not routinely used to counter hypo-

glycemia because it also affects pulse rate and blood pressure). During **exercise**, norepinephrine and ATP are released from splanchnic nerve endings into the extracellular space.

**Glucose** and **fructose** both inhibit glycogenolysis (see Fig. 24.7). Glucose inhibits glycogen phosphorylase partly through direct allosteric inhibition and partly by creating a glucose-glycogen phosphorylase complex that is more readily inactivated through phosphorylation by protein phosphatase 1. The fructose effect is partly due to direct inhibition of glycogen phosphorylase by fructose 1-phosphate, but a further understanding is currently lacking.

Some glycogen particles are engulfed by **lysosomes** and then degraded by **acid α-glucosidase** (also called **acid maltase**), which hydrolyzes both α(1→4) and α(1→6) glucosidic linkages, thereby exclusively producing glucose. This process is presumably part of the normal turnover of all components of a cell; it does not contribute significantly to glucose production when glycogenolysis is activated. Lysosomes have a low pH (about 5). The word "acid" in acid maltase refers to the lysosomal enzyme having optimum activity at a lower pH than does maltase on the brush border of small intestinal enterocytes (see Chapter 18); in fact, the two enzymes are encoded by different genes.

## 3. DISORDERS OF GLYCOGEN METABOLISM

*Diabetes is associated with reduced glycogen synthesis and degradation. Glycogen storage diseases are rare; glucose 6-phosphatase deficiency, debranching enzyme deficiency, and lysosomal α-glucosidase deficiency are the most common of these disorders. Disorders that affect the liver result in hepatomegaly and fasting hypoglycemia; disorders that affect muscle cause weakness and cardiomyopathy.*

### 3.1. Diabetes and Glycogen Metabolism

After a meal, patients with insulin-resistant **type 2 diabetes**, as well as those with **type 1 diabetes** who inject too little insulin, generally form less liver and muscle glycogen than healthy patients. Similarly, in the fasting state, patients with type 1 or type 2 diabetes degrade glycogen at an abnormally low rate.

Patients who are heterozygous for a mutant liver **glucokinase** with physiologically insufficient activity typically have

**maturity-onset diabetes of the young subtype 2 (MODY-2)** and form less glycogen in the liver (see Chapter 39). Although this is the most common form of MODY, fewer than 1% of patients with diabetes have MODY-2. In accordance with the notion that glucokinase activity in the liver is a key regulator of glycogen synthesis, patients with MODY-2 store glycogen in the liver at a reduced rate. Muscle glycogen synthesis in patients with MODY-2 is not appreciably affected because muscle normally does not express glucokinase.

## 3.2. Fructose and Glycogen Metabolism

Patients with **hereditary fructose intolerance** (see Chapter 20) who are given fructose after an overnight fast have a reduced rate of glycogenolysis and become markedly hypoglycemic. The hypoglycemia is in part due to diminished glycogenolysis, which is in turn due to the inhibition of glycogen phosphorylase by a persistently high concentration of fructose 1-phosphate. Since most phosphate is trapped in fructose 1-phosphate, the intracellular concentration of phosphate is low, which further lowers the activity of glycogen phosphorylase.

Patients with **fructose 1,6-bisphosphatase deficiency** also become hypoglycemic when given fructose after an overnight fast because they have a reduced rate of glycogenolysis and gluconeogenesis. In the fasting state, these patients perform little or no gluconeogenesis (see Chapter 25) and thus depend largely on glycogenolysis for glucose production. Glycogen phosphorylase is inhibited to a dangerous degree by a combination of an abnormally low concentration of free phosphate, a nearly normal concentration of fructose 1-phosphate, and elevated concentrations of fructose 1,6-bisphosphate and glycerol 3-phosphate (both of which are intermediates of gluconeogenesis; see Chapter 25).

## 3.3. Glycogenoses

In Europe, the combined incidence of all **glycogen storage disorders** (also called **glycogenoses**) is about $1:20,000$. Almost all of these disorders are inherited in an autosomal recessive fashion, and the carrier frequency is therefore about 1%. Among patients with glycogen storage diseases, the following enzyme deficiencies make up about 90% of all patients in roughly comparable fractions: glucose 6-phosphatase deficiency, lysosomal acid α-glucosidase deficiency, debranching enzyme deficiency, and liver glycogen phosphorylase or phosphorylase kinase deficiency (Fig. 24.10, shown in red).

**Type I** glycogen storage disease (synonyms: **von Gierke disease, glucose 6-phosphatase deficiency**) has an incidence of about 1 in 100,000. In the fasting state, patients with glucose 6-phosphatase deficiency still release an appreciable amount of glucose into the blood, in part from yet unknown sources. Nonetheless, starting at a few months of age, affected patients become severely hypoglycemic in the postabsorptive phase because their liver and kidneys cannot release sufficient glucose (from glycogenolysis or gluconeogenesis) into the blood. Hypoglycemia is particularly dangerous to the brain. During the day, small frequent meals help patients avoid hypoglycemia. At night, patients receive a constant infusion of glucose via a nasogastric tube, or they drink uncooked cornstarch in water every few hours (uncooked cornstarch is slowly hydrolyzed to glucose; see Chapter 18). The liver has excessive glycogen stores because the elevated concentration of glucose 6-phosphate stimulates glycogen synthesis (Fig. 24.5). Fasting may be accompanied by lactic acidosis because gluconeogenesis is blocked (see Section 4.1.5 in Chapter 25). Similarly, the blockage in gluconeogenesis can generate ATP-consuming futile cycles that lead to hyperuricemia and an increased risk of gout (see Section 4.1 in Chapter 38). Severe

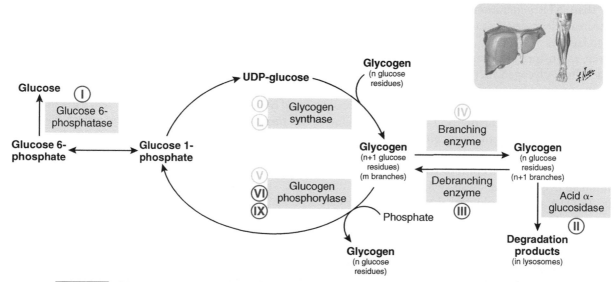

**Fig. 24.10** **Glycogen storage diseases.** Disease types are shown as Roman numerals inside circles, next to the deficient enzyme; L designates Lafora disease. The enzyme deficiencies shown in red together account for about 90% of all cases. Some of the more rare diseases are shown in orange. Types 0, I, VI, and IX affect only the liver; type V affects only muscle. UDP, uridine diphosphate.

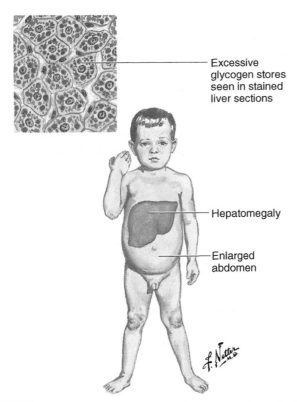

Excessive glycogen stores seen in stained liver sections

Hepatomegaly

Enlarged abdomen

**Fig. 24.11** **Glucose 6-phosphatase deficiency (type I glycogen storage disease, von Gierke disease).** Glycogen is stained with carminic acid, yielding a bright red product.

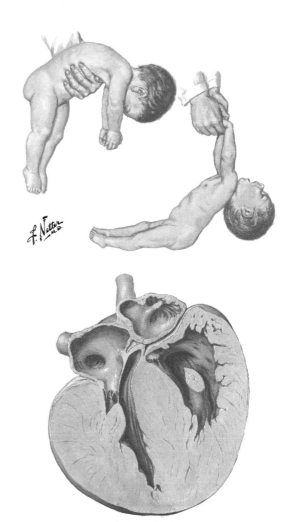

**Fig. 24.12** **Type II glycogen storage disease (Pompe disease, acid α-glucosidase deficiency, acid maltase deficiency).** In classic, infantile Pompe disease, the accumulation of glycogen particles in the lysosomes leads to profound generalized myopathy and cardiomyopathy.

hyperlipidemia and hepatomegaly (Fig. 24.11) are discussed in Section 4.1.5 of Chapter 25.

**Type II** glycogen storage disease (synonyms: deficiency of lysosomal **α-glucosidase**, deficiency of lysosomal **acid maltase**, **Pompe disease**) has an incidence of about 1 in 40,000. In the infantile-onset form, the heart, liver, and muscles are enlarged (Fig. 24.12) and contain excessive amounts of glycogen in the lysosomes (visible with periodic acid staining; see also Fig. 24.3). Due to generalized muscle weakness, babies are "floppy" and, if not treated, die by age 2 years from cardiorespiratory insufficiency. Glucose metabolism is normal. Creatine kinase activity in the serum is increased due to the loss from damaged muscle. In patients with late onset (≥1 year of age), the heart is less severely affected, but respiratory weakness still leads to premature death. Treatment with alglucosidase alfa, a recombinant glucosidase (administered intravenously), dramatically alters the course of the disease. The enzyme replacement therapy greatly reduces damage to the heart, but the skeletal muscle is less responsive to treatment. A high-protein diet is used to favor maintenance of muscle mass.

**Type III** glycogen storage disease (synonyms: **debranching enzyme deficiency, Cori disease, Forbes disease, limit dextrinosis**) is the most common glycogen storage disease that affects both the liver and muscle (skeletal and cardiac). Hepatomegaly is common among children but not adults. Starting in childhood, patients have difficulty exercising, but muscle loss and cardiomyopathy often set in only during the 30s or

40s. Fasting hypoglycemia is more moderate than in a glucose 6-phosphatase deficiency because the outer linear branches of glycogen can still be degraded. Compared with a healthy individual, gluconeogenesis (see Chapter 25), lipolysis (see Chapter 28), and ketogenesis (see Chapter 27) are activated abnormally early. Glycogen particles are unusually large because branch points can be created but not degraded. Liver cirrhosis is occasionally seen in adults. Damage to the liver, muscle, and heart is often blamed on the long, poorly water-soluble, linear outer branches of glycogen, because such damage, although more severe, is also seen in the more rare branching enzyme deficiency (i.e., type IV glycogen storage disease, which is not discussed here). Oral glucose tolerance is mildly abnormal because glycogen particles rapidly reach a finite size, to which UDP-glucose can no longer be added. Treatment is largely geared toward avoiding hypoglycemia, which is accomplished with frequent meals containing slowly absorbed carbohydrates, and often also with nocturnal infusions or feedings containing carbohydrates (as in type I glycogen storage disease). In addition, patients are given a diet high in protein

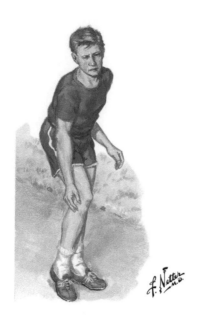

**Fig. 24.13** Muscle glycogen phosphorylase deficiency (McArdle disease, type V glycogen storage disease) causes fatigue and cramping several minutes after the start of exercise.

(to minimize muscle protein loss; see also Chapter 35) and low in saturated fatty acids and cholesterol (to lessen the frequently accompanying hypercholesterolemia).

**Type V** glycogenosis (synonyms: **McArdle** disease, deficiency of **muscle glycogen phosphorylase**) is very rare; it is mentioned here because it illustrates the importance of muscle glycogen in powering muscle contraction. Affected patients (Fig. 24.13) have muscle cramps when they exercise (e.g., sprinting, heavy lifting, walking uphill), often more so during the early phase of exercise, when muscle glycogen is a particularly important contributor of fuel for energy production (see Section 2.2). If vigorous exercise is maintained, rhabdomyolysis sets in with the loss of myoglobin into the blood and from there into the urine (giving urine a burgundy color).

**Type VI** and **type IX** glycogen storage diseases are due to deficiencies of liver glycogen phosphorylase and its activating enzyme, phosphorylase kinase, respectively. Affected patients usually have hepatomegaly, yet hypoglycemia is mild. Patients avoid episodes of hypoglycemia with small, frequent meals.

**Lafora disease** (also called **Lafora progressive myoclonus epilepsy**) is often lumped together with the glycogen storage diseases. Lafora disease is due to homozygosity or compound heterozygosity for mutant **laforin** or **malin**. Laforin is a glycogen phosphatase that removes excess phosphate groups from glycogen. Although the origin of phosphate groups on glycogen is not fully understood, recent studies have shown that glycogen synthase can erroneously and very rarely incorporate phosphate groups into glycogen. Malin is an E3-ubiquitin ligase that plays a role in the degradation of laforin. Loss-of-function mutations in laforin or malin lead to accumulation of aberrant glycogen that precipitates in the cytosol of cells, forming Lafora bodies. Such Lafora bodies accumulate in the brain, liver, heart, muscle, and skin. The

Lafora bodies contain excessive amounts of unbranched (therefore poorly soluble) and hyperphosphorylated glycogen, and they can be visualized by periodic acid staining (see Section 1.1). The brain is affected foremost, possibly due to a noxious effect of unbranched glycogen. Symptoms typically set in suddenly with apparently healthy teenagers; this is usually followed by myoclonic epilepsy, dementia, and death within about 10 years. Lafora disease is found especially frequently around the Mediterranean, in the Middle East, and in Southeast Asia.

## SUMMARY

- Glycogen is a polymer of up to about 60,000 glucose residues that are formed on a side chain of the protein glycogenin. The most appreciable glycogen stores are found in the liver and skeletal muscle.
- The liver synthesizes glycogen after a meal, typically from dietary glucose. Liver glycogen synthesis is largely controlled by the activities of glucokinase and glycogen synthase. Glucokinase is activated by dietary fructose and by insulin. Glycogen synthase is activated by insulin but can be inhibited completely by epinephrine and glucagon.
- The liver degrades glycogen to glucose during the early phases of a fast and also during exercise. The liver releases glucose into the blood; this helps maintain normoglycemia, in the fasting state for the benefit of red blood cells and the brain, and during exercise also for the benefit of the skeletal muscles. Glycogen phosphorylase is the chief controller of glycogen degradation. An increased concentration of glucagon and epinephrine in the blood and increased release of norepinephrine and ATP from the vagus nerve in the liver all lead to an activation of glycogen phosphorylase.
- Skeletal muscles degrade their glycogen during exercise. Glucose 6-phosphate obtained in the degradation of glycogen is particularly important during the first few minutes of exercise when blood flow and glucose uptake are not yet maximal. With increasing duration of mild exercise, skeletal muscles derive more of their energy from glucose and free fatty acids (both taken up from the blood). Once muscle glycogen stores have reached a very small size, fatigue sets in.
- The skeletal muscles synthesize glycogen mainly after a meal from glucose that they take up from the blood. Prior exercise and depletion of glycogen stores render skeletal muscle cells especially sensitive to insulin.

## FURTHER READING

- Ørtenblad N, Westerblad H, Nielsen J. Muscle glycogen stores and fatigue. *J Physiol.* 2013;591:4405-4413.
- Sanders L. The girl with unexplained hair loss. *N Y Times Mag.* 2011 (a case of juvenile-onset Pompe disease).
- Zois CE, Favaro E, Harris AL. Glycogen metabolism in cancer. *Biochem Pharmacol.* 2014;92:3-11.

# Review Questions

1. In skeletal muscle, glycogenolysis is stimulated by an elevated concentration of which one of the following?

   A. AMP
   B. Glucagon
   C. Glucose 6-phosphate
   D. Insulin

2. A 10-year-old boy has signs of a muscle disorder. His lung function and his muscle strength are also decreased. He has difficulty getting up and walking. A muscle biopsy shows that the glycogen is of normal structure, and the size of the glycogen particles is within the normal range. In an oral glucose tolerance test, the patient's 0-, 1-, and 2-hour blood glucose values were all within the range of values seen in 10 healthy volunteers. This patient could have a deficiency of which one of the following enzymes in his muscles?

   A. Debranching enzyme
   B. Glycogen branching enzyme
   C. Glycogen synthase
   D. Lysosomal acid α-glucosidase

3. A 5-month-old boy is found to have hepatomegaly, fasting hypoglycemia, and high levels of free fatty acids in his blood. His liver glycogen content was found to be high, but the glycogen had a normal structure. After an overnight fast, there was no detectable increase in the serum glucose concentration after an oral administration of galactose (which gives rise to glucose 6-phosphate). The disease is most likely the result of a deficiency of which one of the following enzymes?

   A. Glucokinase
   B. Glucose 6-phosphatase
   C. Glycogen debranching enzyme
   D. Glycogen synthase

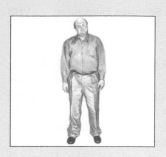

## Chapter 25

# Gluconeogenesis and Fasting Hypoglycemia

## SYNOPSIS

■ Gluconeogenesis is a process by which lactate, many amino acids (chiefly alanine and glutamine), and glycerol give rise to glucose. Gluconeogenesis takes place in the liver and the kidneys. Gluconeogenesis benefits glucose-dependent tissues, such as the brain, red blood cells, and exercising muscle.

■ Gluconeogenesis proceeds via the reversible reactions of glycolysis and via unique, irreversible reactions that bypass the irreversible reactions of glycolysis.

■ Gluconeogenesis depends on the breakdown of body protein (mostly muscle protein) or, in persons who eat a high-protein, low-carbohydrate diet, on the breakdown of dietary protein. Gluconeogenesis also depends on an adequate supply of adenosine triphosphate (ATP), which stems from the β-oxidation of fatty acids.

■ Gluconeogenesis is activated by glucagon, epinephrine, and cortisol; it is inhibited by insulin. As a result, gluconeogenesis is most strongly suppressed after a meal, and it is near-maximally active after a 2-day fast, as well as during prolonged, intense exercise.

■ Gluconeogenesis is excessive in patients who secrete too little insulin or who secrete too much cortisol, thyroid hormone, epinephrine, norepinephrine, or glucagon.

■ Gluconeogenesis can be inadequate in patients who are intoxicated with alcohol, who are hyperinsulinemic, who release too little cortisol, or who have an inherited metabolic defect in the gluconeogenic pathway.

## LEARNING OBJECTIVES

*For mastery of this topic, you should be able to do the following:*
■ Describe the reactants, products, and tissue distribution of gluconeogenesis.
■ Describe the roles of protein degradation and fatty acid oxidation vis-à-vis gluconeogenesis.
■ Compare and contrast glycolysis and gluconeogenesis with regard to reactants, products, pathways, and regulation.
■ Explain the contribution of gluconeogenesis to blood glucose homeostasis.
■ Explain the pathogenesis of lactic acidosis and hyperalaninemia in patients who have a deficiency of one of the enzymes of gluconeogenesis.
■ Explain the pathologic alterations of gluconeogenesis in patients who have diabetes, Cushing syndrome, a pheochromocytoma, a glucagonoma, Addison disease, severe liver dysfunction, or a glucose 6-phosphatase deficiency.
■ Describe the effect of metformin on gluconeogenesis.
■ Discuss abnormalities of gluconeogenesis in newborns.

## 1. PATHWAY OF GLUCONEOGENESIS

*Gluconeogenesis is a process in which lactate, glycerol, or amino acids are turned into glucose. The energy for this process is derived chiefly from the oxidation of fatty acids. As part of gluconeogenesis, pyruvate is carboxylated inside mitochondria to oxaloacetate, which in turn is converted to phosphoenolpyruvate in the cytoplasm. From phosphoenolpyruvate, glucose is synthesized via the reversible reactions of glycolysis and the irreversible reactions that are unique to gluconeogenesis. The liver and the kidneys are the two main organs that are known to carry out gluconeogenesis. There is some evidence that the intestine also performs gluconeogenesis.*

In the transition from the fed to the fasting state, the body reduces its **glucose consumption**. After a meal, many organs consume glucose at a high rate. Muscle and liver store some glucose as glycogen, and the liver converts a small amount of glucose into fatty acids. In the presence of a high concentration of insulin, the body can use more than 100 μmol glucose/kg/min (i.e., ~1.3 g/min for a 70-kg person). In contrast, in the fasting state, the body uses only ~10 μmol glucose/kg/min because many organs produce ATP through the oxidation of fatty acids and ketone bodies rather than glucose.

Some cells, such as neurons in the brain, red blood cells, cells in the medulla of the kidney, and cells in the dermis of the skin, need glucose even in the fasting state. This glucose derives from **glycogenolysis** in the liver and from **gluconeogenesis** in the liver and in the kidney cortex (the kidney cortex does not store a significant amount of glycogen).

During an extended fast, gluconeogenesis accounts for almost all of the endogenous glucose production. Fig. 25.1A shows the time course of glucose production by glycogenolysis and gluconeogenesis during a 2-day fast. In the evening of day 1, volunteers consumed a standardized meal followed by an overnight fast. In the morning of day 2, measurements were started and continued until almost noon on day 3. By that point, glycogenolysis produced virtually no glucose, and gluconeogenesis accounted for almost all the endogenous glucose production.

After a fast, the intake of food leads to a decrease in glucose production from glycogenolysis and gluconeogenesis. Fig. 25.1B shows the time course of an experiment with healthy, adult volunteers who were treated similarly to those described above. After fasting, the volunteers were given 75 g of glucose in water by mouth (similar to a standard oral glucose tolerance test; see Chapter 39). After 3 hours, about half of the glucose had been transported from the intestine into the blood. Over the same period, glucose production from glycogenolysis and

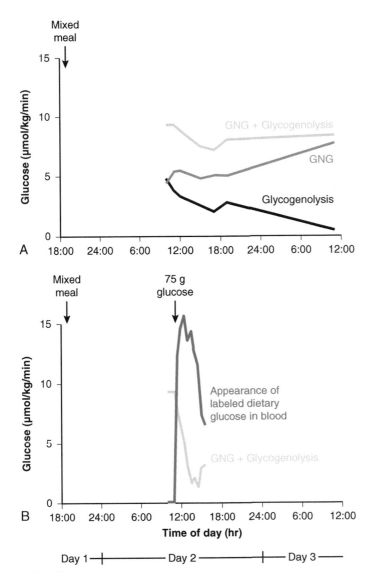

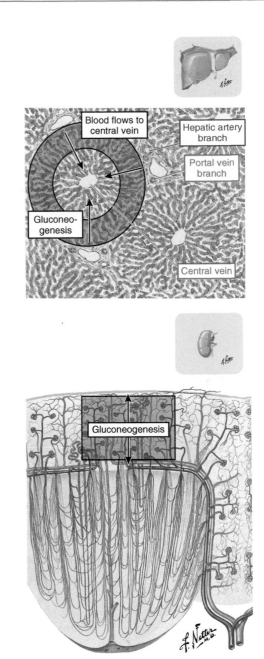

**Fig. 25.1** **Effect of fasting and feeding on endogenous glucose production.** (A) Endogenous glucose production from glycogenolysis and gluconeogenesis (GNG), as measured with various tracer methods. (B) Appearance of dietary glucose and suppression of endogenous glucose production. (Based on data of Bisschop PH, Pereira Arias AM, et al. The effects of carbohydrate variation in isocaloric diets on glycogenolysis and gluconeogenesis in healthy men. *J Clin Endocrin Metabol.* 2000;85:1963-1967; Kunert O, Stingl H, Rosian E, et al. Measurement of fractional whole-body gluconeogenesis in humans from blood samples using 2H nuclear magnetic resonance spectroscopy. *Diabetes.* 2003;52:2475-2482; Boden G, Chen X, Capulong E, Mozzoli M. Effects of free fatty acids on gluconeogenesis and autoregulation of glucose production in type 2 diabetes. *Diabetes.* 2001;50:810-816; Wajngot A, Chandramouli V, Schumann WC, et al. Quantitative contributions of gluconeogenesis to glucose production during fasting in type 2 diabetes mellitus. *Metabolism.* 2001;50:47-52; Katz J, Tayek JA. Gluconeogenesis and the Cori cycle in 12-, 20-, and 40-h-fasted humans. *Am J Physiol.* 1998;275: E537-E542; and Meyer C, Woerle HJ, Dostou JM, et al. Abnormal renal, hepatic, and muscle glucose metabolism following glucose ingestion in type 2 diabetes. *Am J Physiol.* 2004;287:E1049-E1056.

**Fig. 25.2** **Gluconeogenesis takes place in the liver and the kidneys.** *Top,* Hematoxylin and eosin-stained thin section of the liver. Each lobule consists of plates of cells that resemble a stack of pancakes. Blood flows from the periphery to the center of the stack. Gluconeogenesis takes place in the well-oxygenated peripheral portion of the lobules indicated by the red ring, and glycolysis predominates in the central portion of the lobule. *Bottom,* Structure of a pyramid and the associated cortex in the kidney. Gluconeogenesis takes place in the well-oxygenated cortex indicated by the red rectangle.

gluconeogenesis declined to about one-fourth of its initial value. Most of this decrease is due to a decreased rate of glycogenolysis.

Gluconeogenesis takes place in the well-oxygenated **periportal cells** of the **liver** and the **cortical cells** of the **kidneys**

(Fig. 25.2). The liver and the kidneys are heterogeneous in that some cells produce glucose, while others consume it. Periportal cells of the liver and cortical cells of the kidneys both have sufficient oxygen to oxidize fatty acids to produce ATP for gluconeogenesis. In contrast, perivenous cells of the liver and cells in the medulla of the kidneys operate at lower concentrations of oxygen, depend at least partially on anaerobic glycolysis for ATP production, and cannot carry out gluconeogenesis.

The **small intestine** expresses all enzymes of gluconeogenesis; however, little is known about the small intestine's contribution to gluconeogenesis under physiological conditions.

The **reactions of gluconeogenesis** start with lactate, alanine, various other amino acids, or glycerol (Fig. 25.3). Several steps in gluconeogenesis require energy in the form of guanosine triphosphate (GTP) or ATP.

The physiologically **irreversible reactions** of gluconeogenesis (see Fig. 25.3) differ from those of glycolysis, whereas the reversible reactions are the same as for glycolysis (see Fig. 19.2) and they are also catalyzed by the same enzymes. The

physiologically irreversible reactions of glycolysis are not used for gluconeogenesis. The physiologically irreversible reactions of gluconeogenesis are pyruvate → phosphoenolpyruvate (in several steps, two of which are irreversible), fructose 1,6-bisphosphate → fructose 6-phosphate, and glucose 6-phosphate → glucose.

**Pyruvate** is converted to **phosphoenolpyruvate** in several enzyme-catalyzed steps that take place in the mitochondria and the cytosol (see Fig. 25.3). Pyruvate enters the mitochondria, where **pyruvate carboxylase** carboxylates it to oxaloacetate. This is the same reaction that also supplies the citric acid

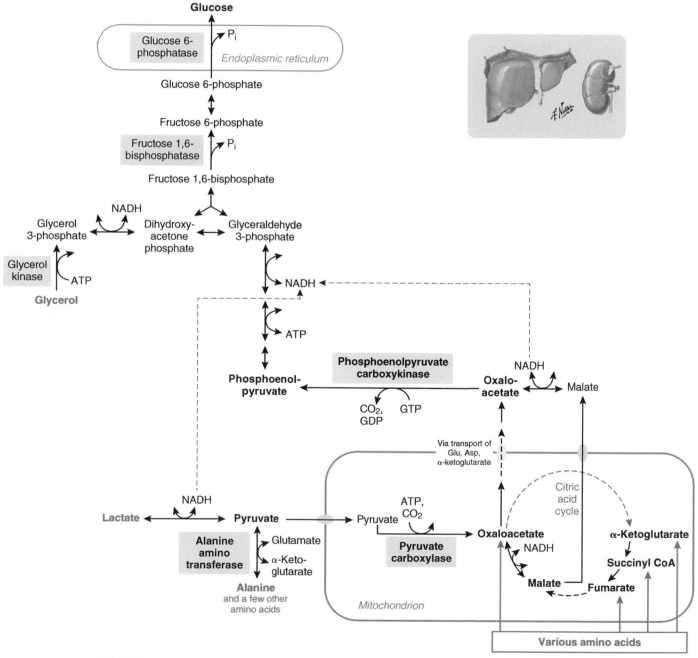

**Fig. 25.3  Pathway of gluconeogenesis.** The direction of pathway flow is from the bottom to the top. Compounds with carbon skeletons that give rise to glucose are shown in blue. Further details about the amino acids that give rise to pyruvate or feed into the citric acid cycle are shown in Fig. 25.5.

cycle with oxaloacetate (see Section 3 in Chapter 22). A high concentration of acetyl-coenzyme A (CoA) stimulates pyruvate carboxylase. Mitochondria do not have a transporter for oxaloacetate. Hence, oxaloacetate is converted to either aspartate or malate, which can be exported into the cytosol. The choice of export system depends on the need for NADH in the cytosol. In the cytosol, both aspartate and malate give rise to oxaloacetate. Oxaloacetate is then converted to phosphoenolpyruvate by **phosphoenolpyruvate carboxykinase** (**PEPCK**).

## 2. SUBSTRATE AND ENERGY SOURCES FOR GLUCONEOGENESIS

*The substrates of gluconeogenesis are, in decreasing order of quantity used, lactate, alanine, glutamine, glycerol, and other glucogenic amino acids. Lactate stems from red blood cells, the skin, the intestine, and exercising muscle. Alanine, glutamine, and other glucogenic amino acids are derived from skeletal muscle protein or the diet. Glycerol results from the hydrolysis of adipose tissue triglycerides, which also yields fatty acids. Energy for gluconeogenesis stems from the β-oxidation of fatty acids inside the mitochondria.*

### 2.1. Lactate

In the course of a day, a sedentary adult produces about 115 g of lactate. The major producers of lactate are, in decreasing order, red blood cells, skin, brain, skeletal muscle type 2X fibers, kidney medulla, and the intestine. The liver, kidney cortex, and skeletal muscle type 1 fibers oxidize most of the lactate (lactate → pyruvate → acetyl-CoA → $CO_2$). The liver uses about 20% of the daily lactate production for the synthesis of glucose via gluconeogenesis.

The term **Cori cycle** refers to the cycling of carbon skeletons between glucose and lactate via glycolysis and gluconeogenesis (Fig. 25.4).

The fate of lactate depends on the hormonal state of the body. Shortly after a meal, most of the lactate is oxidized in the citric acid cycle. Conversely, during a long-term fast or strenuous exercise most of the lactate that reaches the liver is converted to glucose via gluconeogenesis.

### 2.2. Amino Acids

**Glucogenic amino acids** are amino acids from which net glucose synthesis is possible via gluconeogenesis (see also Chapter 35). These amino acids are shown in Fig. 25.5. All of these amino acids can eventually give rise to oxaloacetate, from which phosphoenolpyruvate is made (see Fig. 25.3). It is not possible to net produce oxaloacetate from acetyl-CoA.

Amino acids that are used for gluconeogenesis can stem from the diet but, in the long run, they are derived from the degradation of skeletal muscle protein. Cortisol stimulates proteolysis in muscle, while **insulin** inhibits it (see Chapter 35). Cortisol also stimulates the transcription and translation of transaminases that transfer amino groups from amino acids

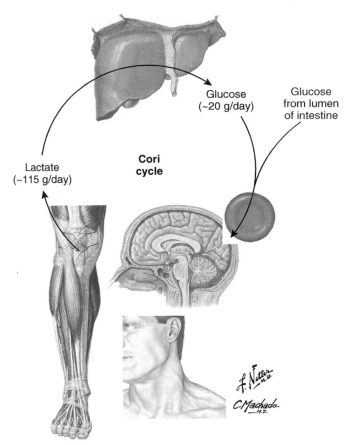

**Fig. 25.4** **The Cori cycle.**

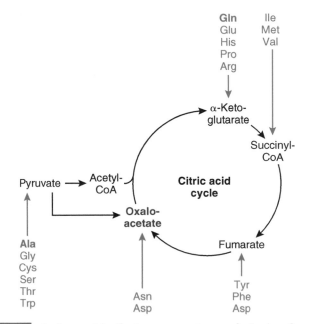

**Fig. 25.5** **Amino acids that can serve as substrates for gluconeogenesis.** Among the 20 genetically encoded amino acids, only leucine and lysine cannot serve as substrates for gluconeogenesis. Quantitatively the most important glucogenic amino acids are alanine and glutamine. (Aspartate is listed twice because it can give rise to either oxaloacetate or fumarate.)

to pyruvate and glutamate. Muscle exports mostly **alanine** and **glutamine** (Fig. 25.6; see also Fig. 35.3 and Section 2 in Chapter 35).

The term **glucose-alanine cycle** refers to the pathway in which muscle exports alanine and the liver takes up alanine and converts it to glucose; the liver then releases glucose into the blood, and muscle takes up a portion of this glucose from the blood (Fig. 25.6).

**Glutamine** can also give rise to glucose. In the fasting state, glutamine in the blood stems mainly from muscle (see Fig. 25.6). The small intestine converts some of this glutamine to alanine. The liver uses this alanine to synthesize glucose via gluconeogenesis. The kidneys also take up glutamine, but they convert it to α-ketoglutarate and then, via a portion of the citric acid cycle, to oxaloacetate (see Fig. 25.3), which is used for the synthesis of glucose via gluconeogenesis. Both the liver and the kidneys release glucose from gluconeogenesis into the blood.

## 2.3. Glycerol

Glycerol stems from the hydrolysis of triglycerides (see Section 5 in Chapter 28). The liver converts glycerol to dihydroxyacetone phosphate, which is an intermediate of gluconeogenesis (see Fig. 25.3). Glycerol is a precursor of quantitatively minor importance. Thus, after a 16-hour fast, only ~10% of the glucose produced by gluconeogenesis stems from glycerol.

## 2.4. Fatty Acids as a Source of ATP

The oxidation of **fatty acids** provides ATP but not carbon skeletons for gluconeogenesis. Glucose can be converted into

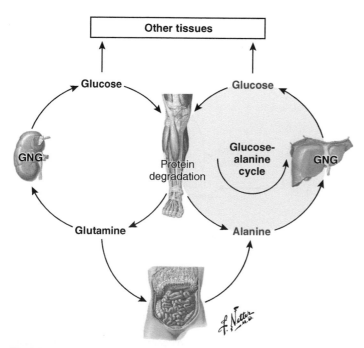

Fig. 25.6 **Major interorgan flux of amino acids when gluconeogenesis (GNG) is active.**

fatty acids (see Section 2 in Chapter 27), but **fatty acids cannot be converted into glucose.** There are two reasons for this: (1) acetyl-CoA cannot be converted to pyruvate (this reaction is physiologically irreversible and proceeds only from pyruvate to acetyl-CoA), and (2) net production of a citric acid cycle intermediate from acetyl-CoA alone is impossible (oxaloacetate is required to feed acetyl-CoA into the citric acid cycle, and acetyl-CoA is not entirely lost before oxaloacetate is reformed).

## 3. REGULATION OF GLUCONEOGENESIS

*The rate of gluconeogenesis is lowest after a high-carbohydrate meal and highest during prolonged strenuous exercise and prolonged fasting. Flux through gluconeogenesis changes largely as a result of long-term controls, which include an effect of hormones on the production of transaminases, PEPCK, and glucose 6-phosphatase. Normally, PEPCK activity exerts the strongest control over the rate of gluconeogenesis. Short-term controls have modest effects and include an effect of insulin, glucagon, and epinephrine on the activity of fructose 1,6-bisphosphatase, as well as an allosteric effect of acetyl-CoA on pyruvate carboxylase.*

Gluconeogenesis must be regulated to avoid excessive substrate cycling with glycolysis, quickly correct hypoglycemia and support ongoing strenuous exercise, avoid the excessive consumption of amino acids from body protein, and accommodate the input of different substrates. As a consequence, the regulation of gluconeogenesis is complex; Fig. 25.7 shows a simplified version of it. The regulated enzymes are pyruvate carboxylase, PEPCK, fructose 1,6-bisphosphatase (FBPase), and glucose 6-phosphatase (G6Pase), all of which catalyze physiologically irreversible reactions.

The long-term rate of gluconeogenesis is regulated chiefly via changes in the rate of transcription of transaminases, PEPCK, and G6Pase. It takes about 30 minutes from the time transcription starts to the time these enzymes are synthesized de novo and thus become active. The half-lives of these enzymes are on a scale of hours. Changes in the amount of PEPCK exert the main control over the rate of gluconeogenesis. Transaminase activity is important for the export of amino acids (mostly alanine and glutamine) from muscle and the import of amino acids into the liver, the kidney cortex, and the intestine (see Fig. 25.6).

Short-term, gluconeogenesis is regulated via phosphorylation/dephosphorylation and allosteric regulators of enzymes. FBPase is largely controlled by this mechanism (see Fig. 25.7).

During the transitions between feeding and fasting, glycolysis and gluconeogenesis are both appreciably active in the liver. This state permits the fine and rapid control of glucose production, but it wastes ATP due to metabolite cycling between glycolysis and gluconeogenesis.

**Glucagon, epinephrine, cortisol,** and **thyroid hormone** activate gluconeogenesis (see Fig. 25.7). In contrast, **insulin** and adenine monophosphate (**AMP**) or **AMP-dependent protein kinase** (**AMPK**) inhibit gluconeogenesis.

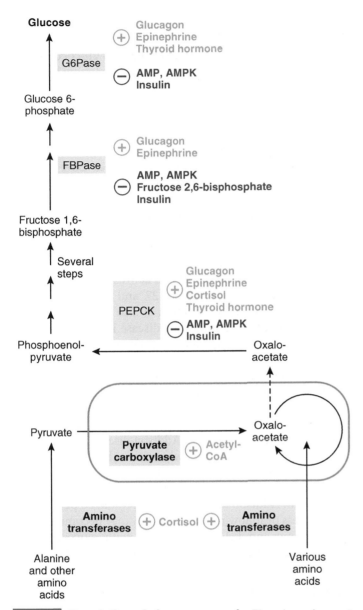

**Regulation of gluconeogenesis.** Phosphoenolpyruvate carboxykinase (PEPCK) has the greatest control strength over the rate of gluconeogenesis. AMPK, adenine monophosphate (AMP)-activated protein kinase; CoA, coenzyme A; FBPase, fructose 1,6-bisphosphatase; G6Pase, glucose 6-phosphatase.

Details about the regulation of gluconeogenesis by hormones are as follows. Pancreatic α-cells secrete **glucagon** in response to *hypo*glycemia (see Chapter 26). Glucagon stimulates gluconeogenesis by binding to glucagon receptors. The medulla of the adrenal glands secretes **epinephrine** in response to hypoglycemia or exercise (see Chapter 26). Epinephrine stimulates gluconeogenesis via β-adrenergic receptors. The cortex of the adrenal glands secretes **cortisol** in a diurnal pattern; the concentration of cortisol in the blood is lowest in the early evening and highest in the early morning (see Chapter 31). Fasting enhances cortisol release most pronouncedly in the afternoon and during the night. The

concentration of cortisol also increases with intense exercise. Cortisol activates glucocorticoid receptors, which in turn increase transcription of genes that are associated with a promoter that contains a glucocorticoid response element. Cortisol notably leads to increased synthesis of transaminases. **Triiodothyronine** (T3, the active metabolite of thyroid hormone) activates thyroid hormone receptors in the nucleus, which in turn increases the transcription of genes that are associated with a thyroid hormone response element–containing promoter. The concentration of T3 gradually decreases with long-term fasting. Pancreatic β-cells secrete **insulin** in response to *hyper*glycemia (see Chapter 26), and insulin binds to insulin receptors, which lead to a decreased rate of gluconeogenesis.

Gluconeogenesis is never completely suppressed, but it is least active 1 to 2 hours after a high-carbohydrate **meal** and most active 2 to 3 days into a prolonged **fast**. Gluconeogenesis is also very active during prolonged strenuous **exercise**. For instance, after an overnight fast, 1 hour of strenuous exercise approximately doubles the rate of gluconeogenesis.

Persons who previously exclusively consumed a **very-low-carbohydrate diet** (e.g., an **Atkins**-type diet) show a somewhat increased rate of gluconeogenesis after an overnight fast. This reflects a partial compensation of a decreased rate of glycogenolysis.

An increased concentration of epinephrine, in conjunction with a decreased concentration of insulin, not only promotes gluconeogenesis but also stimulates **lipolysis** of triglycerides in the adipose tissue (see Chapter 27). As a result, the adipose tissue releases **fatty acids** and **glycerol** into the blood. Mitochondrial oxidation of fatty acids provides **ATP** for gluconeogenesis, and it also raises the concentration of **acetyl-CoA**, which in turn activates pyruvate carboxylase (see Fig. 25.7). When periportal hepatocytes or cells in the kidney cortex cannot produce enough ATP, they do not participate in gluconeogenesis. In the liver, the concentration of acetyl-CoA is highest during a long-term fast, when the rate of fatty acid β-oxidation is high and the need for acetyl-CoA oxidation in the citric acid cycle is limited (see Chapter 27).

The **liver autoregulates** the balance between hepatic glycogenolysis and gluconeogenesis. Thus, in a healthy person, an increase in the concentration of fatty acids or of precursors for gluconeogenesis (lactate, amino acids, or glycerol) in the blood leads to an increase in the rate of gluconeogenesis and a concomitant decrease in the rate of glycogenolysis. These changes cannot be explained by altered concentrations of hormones alone. The mechanism by which the liver autoregulates its glucose production is unknown.

While the rate of gluconeogenesis is high in the long-term fasting state, the rate of **glycolysis** is low (see Sections 3 and 5 in Chapter 19). In the fasting state, **glucokinase** in the liver is inactive because it is inhibited by its regulatory protein GKRP and is sequestered in the nucleus (see Section 5.6 in Chapter 19). **Phosphofructokinase 1** (PFK 1) has low activity due to a lack of its powerful allosteric activator, fructose 2,6-bisphosphate. **Pyruvate kinase** has low activity because of glucagon-induced phosphorylation.

# 4. DISEASES ASSOCIATED WITH AN ABNORMAL RATE OF GLUCONEOGENESIS

*Gluconeogenesis is impaired and can be a cause of hypoglycemia in patients with insufficient cortisol. Gluconeogenesis is also impaired in patients who have impaired ATP production from fatty acids (e.g., alcohol-intoxicated patients, patients who have deficient fatty acid β-oxidation), and in patients who have a hereditary deficiency of an enzyme of gluconeogenesis. Deficiencies in enzymes of gluconeogenesis between pyruvate and glucose lead to life-threatening lactic acidosis and hypoglycemia in the fasting state. On the other hand, gluconeogenesis is inappropriately elevated and a cause of hyperglycemia in patients with insufficient insulin secretion (diabetes), excessive thyroid hormone (hyperthyroidism), excessive cortisol (Cushing syndrome), or excessive glucagon (glucagonoma).*

## 4.1. Diseases Associated With Inadequate Gluconeogenesis

### 4.1.1. General Comments

Inadequate gluconeogenesis during a fast leads to **hypoglycemia**, which is particularly damaging to the brain.

Knowledge of the regulation of gluconeogenesis (see Fig. 25.7) suggests that an excessive concentration of insulin or abnormally low concentrations of cortisol, thyroid hormone, epinephrine, or glucagon can lead to an abnormally low rate of gluconeogenesis. In addition, impaired gluconeogenesis can also be the result of liver dysfunction or impaired enzyme activity. Diseases that lead to such impairment of gluconeogenesis are described in detail below.

Inadequate gluconeogenesis causes hypoglycemia as soon as glycogenolysis can no longer provide glucose at an adequate rate. Patients with chronically impaired gluconeogenesis need to consume carbohydrates with adequate frequency. **Low-carbohydrate meals**, **dieting**, and extended periods of **fasting** may be life threatening. Intense, prolonged **exercise** likewise requires that these patients frequently take in extra carbohydrates. **Newborns** and **children** are at a greater risk of hypoglycemia than adults due to the large size of their brain relative to the size of their liver and kidneys.

### 4.1.2. Hyperinsulinemia

Because insulin stimulates glucose use and exerts a dominant inhibitory effect over glycogenolysis and gluconeogenesis, an excessive concentration of insulin can lead to hypoglycemia. The concentration of insulin is excessive in patients with **diabetes** who inject too much insulin (causing an **insulin reaction**; see Chapter 39), in **newborns** of mothers who had **chronic gestational hyperglycemia** (see Chapter 39), in patients who have an **insulinoma** (a tumor of the pancreas that secretes insulin; see Section 6.1.1 in Chapter 26), and in patients who have persistent hyperinsulinemia due to a **β-cell defect** (see Section 6.1.3 in Chapter 26).

### 4.1.3. Hypocortisolism

Patients who take a large dose of **exogenous glucocorticoids** should **taper** them off gradually to avoid developing hypocortisolism. The exogenous glucocorticoids suppress the secretion of adrenocorticotrophic hormone (ACTH) from the pituitary gland, which normally stimulates cortisol release from the adrenal glands (see Fig. 31.12). ACTH secretion adjusts over a period of days.

Toddlers and young children sometimes have delayed development of **cortisol** production. Cortisol is needed to stimulate muscle protein breakdown and induce the transcription of transaminases in muscle and the liver, which convert pyruvate to alanine and vice versa (see Section 2.3 and Chapter 35). With a prolonged fast (e.g., ≥15 hours), these children experience life-threatening hypoglycemia. At the same time, they also show hypoalaninemia and ketosis (a consequence of increased lipolysis; see Chapters 27 and 28). This delayed maturation of cortisol production is also known as **ketotic hypoglycemia of childhood**. The disease is usually apparent at 2 to 5 years of age and remits spontaneously by 10 years of age.

Patients who have **Addison disease** chronically produce insufficient quantities of **glucocorticoids**, of which cortisol is the major one (see Fig. 31.20 and Section 4.2 in Chapter 31). In Europe, about 1 in 10,000 persons has a diagnosis of Addison disease. Patients with Addison disease lose the function of their adrenal cortex slowly, so that the disease is often discovered only during a crisis. If there is also a mineralocorticoid deficiency, there is a decrease in blood pressure. If patients with Addison disease fast for a prolonged period (e.g., due to illness or following surgery), they may become severely hypoglycemic and ketotic. Treatment with glucocorticoids and mineralocorticoids is essential for these patients.

### 4.1.4. Liver Disease

Severe dysfunction of the liver leads to hypoglycemia. This can happen in patients with toxic **hepatitis**, fulminant viral hepatitis, or **sepsis**.

### 4.1.5. Impaired Production of ATP and Intermediates of Gluconeogenesis (Impaired Oxidation of Fatty Acids, Alcohol Intoxication, and Enzyme Deficiencies)

Patients who have impaired fatty acid β-oxidation (e.g., **medium-chain acyl-CoA dehydrogenase [MCAD]** deficiency; see Section 7.1 in Chapter 27) develop hypoglycemia in the fasting state due to excessive use of glucose and insufficient flux in gluconeogenesis. Gluconeogenesis is impaired because β-oxidation does not permit adequate ATP production, and because the concentration of acetyl-CoA is too low to inhibit pyruvate dehydrogenase and activate pyruvate carboxylase.

Consumption of **excess alcohol** leads to a decrease in the rate of gluconeogenesis (see Section 3.1 in Chapter 30). The rate of gluconeogenesis is low because the concentration of pyruvate is low and that of AMP is high. Early on, due to the autoregulation of glucose production by the liver, endogenous glucose production is maintained through an increase in the rate of glycogenolysis. In a later phase, glycogen stores are depleted and hypoglycemia sets in, particularly in patients who consume large quantities of alcohol without any food.

Newborns, especially **preterm infants**, frequently have hypoglycemia during the first day or so of life. Several factors appear to be the cause. One is the delayed expression of enzymes of gluconeogenesis, including glucose 6-phosphatase (which is also needed for glucose release from glycogenolysis).

During a fast, patients who have an inherited deficiency of an **enzyme** that catalyzes one of the irreversible steps in gluconeogenesis develop **hyperalaninemia** and **lactic acidosis**. The hyperalaninemia is due to decreased use of alanine in gluconeogenesis and increased production of alanine in muscle (secondary to a low concentration of insulin because of hypoglycemia). The lactic acidosis also has two causes: the decreased use of lactate in gluconeogenesis and the increased formation from glycolysis (activated by elevated concentrations of intermediates and by AMP from ATP-consuming cycles between gluconeogenesis and glycolysis). Reduced secretion of insulin and increased secretion of epinephrine also lead to increased lipolysis and hence increased ketone body production (see Chapter 27). The high concentrations in the blood of lactic acid, acetoacetic acid, and β-hydroxybutyric acid in turn impair the renal excretion of uric acid (see Section 2.3 in Chapter 38). Hence, **hyperuricemia** often accompanies hereditary deficiencies of enzymes of gluconeogenesis.

Hereditary **glucose 6-phosphatase deficiency** (**von Gierke disease, glycogen storage disease type I**) affects glucose production from both glycogenolysis (see Section 3.3 in Chapter 24) and gluconeogenesis. In the fasting state, the disease is accompanied by severe lactic acidosis (see above). A glucose 6-phosphatase deficiency leads to increased concentrations of all metabolites between phosphoenolpyruvate and FBPase (see Fig. 25.7). In turn, this leads to a high concentration of glycerol 3-phosphate. The severe fasting hypoglycemia leads to increased release of fatty acids into the blood (see Section 5 in Chapter 28) and hence an increased concentration of fatty acids inside hepatocytes. The combination of increased intracellular concentrations of glycerol 3-phosphate and fatty acids favors the excessive formation of triglycerides in the fasting state, causing **hypertriglyceridemia** and hepatomegaly.

Hereditary **FBPase deficiency** presents much like a glucose 6-phosphatase deficiency, except that affected patients develop hypoglycemia more slowly. The disease is rare, and the mortality rate is high early in life. As survivors age, the weight ratio of glucose producing organs/glucose-consuming organs becomes more favorable, and episodes of hypoglycemia are milder and occur less frequently. For glucose homeostasis, children with FBPase deficiency depend on glycogenolysis to an unusually high degree. Because the metabolism of dietary fructose normally leads to an inhibition of glycogenolysis, patients with hereditary FBPase deficiency should refrain from consuming fructose, sucrose, or sorbitol (see Section 3.3 in Chapter 20).

## 4.2. Diseases Associated With Excessive Gluconeogenesis

### 4.2.1. General Comments

Excessive gluconeogenesis causes **hyperglycemia**, which can lead to diabetes and its concomitant long-term complications (see Chapter 39).

As can be expected from knowledge of the regulation of gluconeogenesis (see Fig. 25.7), excessive gluconeogenesis is seen in patients who secrete too little insulin or do not respond well to circulating insulin and in patients who have excessive concentrations in the blood of cortisol, thyroid hormone, epinephrine, or glucagon. These diseases are described below.

### 4.2.2. Insulin Deficiency With Diabetes

Patients who have **diabetes** (see Chapter 39) and who are insulin deficient have an excess rate of gluconeogenesis. This applies to patients with type 1 diabetes who inject too little insulin, particularly when they are ill or stressed (when extra epinephrine, glucagon, and cortisol are released). It also applies to patients with type 2 diabetes who are insulin resistant and show absolute or relative insulin deficiency. Both an inordinately low concentration of insulin and an inadequate response of cells to circulating insulin (i.e., insulin resistance) cause excessive glucose production via gluconeogenesis (see Fig. 25.7).

To normalize the rate of glucose production from gluconeogenesis with drugs, patients with type 1 diabetes can be treated with an adequate amount of exogenous insulin; patients with type 2 diabetes can be treated with exogenous insulin, drugs that boost insulin secretion, drugs that increase insulin sensitivity, or, as is currently most common, with the hypoglycemic agent **metformin**. Metformin leads to an activation of AMPK, thereby inhibiting gluconeogenesis at the level of PEPCK, FBPase, and G6Pase (see Fig. 25.7).

In patients who have type 2 diabetes and who develop the acute **hyperosmolar hyperglycemic state** (see Chapter 39), gluconeogenesis plays a special role in causing severe hyperglycemia and dehydration. Over the course of a few days, a persistently low concentration of insulin leads to an abnormally increased rate of gluconeogenesis, decreased glucose use, and a mildly increased rate of lipolysis (not enough to cause pronounced ketoacidosis). The concentration of glucose in the blood reaches such a high concentration that a massive loss of glucose and water in the urine ensues, which eventually causes life-threatening dehydration and hyperosmolarity.

### 4.2.3. Cushing Syndrome

Patients who have **Cushing syndrome** secrete an excessive amount of **cortisol** (see Fig. 31.16) and therefore have an increased rate of gluconeogenesis. The abnormally high concentration of cortisol stimulates the breakdown of muscle protein to amino acids. The increased availability of amino acids leads to an increased rate of gluconeogenesis. Due to autoregulation by the liver, this in turn decreases the rate of glycogenolysis. The abnormally high concentration of cortisol also leads to a poor response to insulin (i.e., insulin resistance); the mechanism of this alteration remains unknown. Hence, patients with untreated Cushing syndrome tend to be glucose intolerant and develop diabetes.

Patients who receive long-term treatment with high doses of a **glucocorticoid**, such as dexamethasone or prednisone, show symptoms similar to patients with Cushing disease. Thus, they show excessive degradation of muscle protein with concomitant muscle weakness, they become insulin resistant, and tend to have hyperglycemia and diabetes.

### 4.2.4. Hyperthyroidism

Patients who have pronounced **hyperthyroidism** (e.g., in thyrotoxicosis or thyroid storm; Fig. 25.8) are hyperglycemic. These patients have elevated concentrations of cortisol and epinephrine in the blood, which stimulate glycogenolysis and gluconeogenesis. Furthermore, thyroid hormone makes the liver more sensitive to epinephrine. Epinephrine inhibits insulin secretion. As a result, endogenous glucose production is increased, whereas glucose use is decreased.

### 4.2.5. Pheochromocytoma

Patients who have a **pheochromocytoma** (see Fig. 22.13), an uncommon chromaffin cell tumor that secretes epinephrine and norepinephrine, can have life-threatening episodes of hypertension and heart disease. Elevated concentrations in the blood of epinephrine and norepinephrine may also cause chronic hyperglycemia (in the liver, norepinephrine binds to the same receptor as epinephrine, though with lower affinity). Pheochromocytomas occur at various sites in the body.

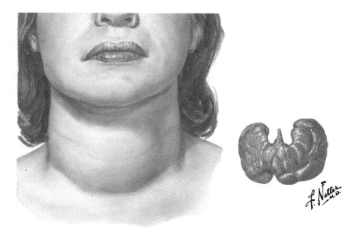

**Fig. 25.8** **Pronounced hyperthyroidism is typically associated with an increased rate of gluconeogenesis that leads to hyperglycemia.**

### 4.2.6. Glucagonoma

Patients who have a **glucagonoma**, a rare tumor of the pancreatic islets that produces predominantly glucagon, have an excessive rate of gluconeogenesis and readily develop diabetes. These patients come to medical attention due to diabetes or a migratory skin rash. The rash appears to be due to **hypoaminoacidemia**. The concentration of glucagon is usually elevated approximately 20-fold. Glucagon primarily stimulates gluconeogenesis (and glycogenolysis) in the liver and, at a high concentration, lipolysis in adipose tissue. Muscle does not have many glucagon receptors. Patients with a glucagonoma have mild hyperglycemia that is caused by a combination of increased gluconeogenesis, as well as increased lipolysis and decreased tissue glucose use (largely due to the glucose-sparing effect of the increased concentration of circulating fatty acids that accompany the increase in lipolysis). The hyperglycemia necessitates increased insulin secretion and, within months, is accompanied by β-cell failure and diabetes. The hypoaminoacidemia appears to be due to persistent, increased use of amino acids for gluconeogenesis and the concomitant loss of muscle protein (patients lose both lean body mass and fat). The loss of muscle protein is probably a consequence of hypoaminoacidemia.

## SUMMARY

- Gluconeogenesis produces glucose from lactate, glycerol, alanine, glutamine, and other glucogenic amino acids.
- Gluconeogenesis takes place in the periportal cells of the liver and the cortex of the kidneys.
- Gluconeogenesis requires ATP, which is normally derived from the β-oxidation of fatty acids.
- Insulin and cortisol control the degradation of muscle protein into amino acids. Cortisol controls the synthesis of transaminases, which transfer amino groups from various amino acids onto pyruvate or glutamate so that muscle chiefly exports alanine and glutamine.
- The hormones insulin, glucagon, epinephrine, cortisol, and thyroid hormone control the synthesis of phosphoenolpyruvate carboxykinase (PEPCK) and glucose 6-phosphatase, which catalyze irreversible steps in gluconeogenesis. In an instant, insulin and glucagon control the activity of FBPase. PEPCK activity is the most important determinant of the rate of gluconeogenesis.
- Gluconeogenesis is impaired in patients who have hyperinsulinemia, hypocortisolism, severe liver dysfunction, a deficiency of an enzyme of gluconeogenesis, deficient fatty acid β-oxidation, or alcohol intoxication along with low carbohydrate intake. In the fasting state, an inadequate rate of gluconeogenesis leads to hypoglycemia. Patients with a deficiency of an enzyme of gluconeogenesis also develop lactic acidosis during fasting.
- Gluconeogenesis is inappropriately high and hence a cause of hyperglycemia in patients who have poorly controlled diabetes, have a high concentration of circulating

cortisol (i.e., patients with Cushing disease or those who are treated with high doses of glucocorticoids), or have pronounced hyperthyroidism, a pheochromocytoma, or a glucagonoma.

### FURTHER READING

■ Jitrapakdee S. Transcription factors and coactivators controlling nutrient and hormonal regulation of hepatic gluconeogenesis. *Int J Biochem Cell Biol.* 2012;44:33-45.

■ Mitrakou A. Kidney: its impact on glucose homeostasis and hormonal regulation. *Diabetes Res Clin Pract.* 2011;93(suppl 1):S66-S72.

# Review Questions

1. An abnormally high rate of gluconeogenesis is observed in patients with which one of the following abnormalities?

   A. Acute alcohol intoxication
   B. Addison disease
   C. Fulminant viral hepatitis
   D. Glucagonoma
   E. Insulin reaction and type 1 diabetes

2. In the fasting state, infants who have a glucose 6-phosphatase deficiency develop which one of the following?

   A. Hyperglycemia
   B. Hyperinsulinemia
   C. Hypoalaninemia
   D. Lactic acidosis

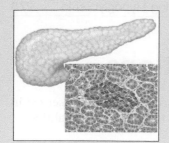

# Chapter 26

# Insulin and Counterregulatory Hormones

## SYNOPSIS

- The body uses insulin, glucagon, epinephrine, and cortisol to control the flow, storage, and use of fuels. Cells in the *pancreas* secrete insulin and glucagon, depending on the concentration of glucose and other fuels. Cells in the intestine secrete incretins, which modify insulin and glucagon secretion. Cells in the brain secrete hormones that regulate the secretion of epinephrine and cortisol from the adrenal glands.

- Glucagon, epinephrine, norepinephrine, and cortisol are "counterregulatory hormones" because they increase the concentration of glucose in the blood in contrast to insulin, which lowers it.

- The pancreas contains islets, which are small nests of cells that secrete insulin, glucagon, and other hormones into the bloodstream. Islet β-cells secrete insulin in response to an elevated concentration of glucose, and this secretion is enhanced by amino acids, fatty acids, and ketone bodies. Epinephrine inhibits insulin secretion. Islet α-cells secrete glucagon in response to amino acids or epinephrine, and hypoglycemia enhances this effect.

- Inherited and acquired defects of β-cell fuel sensing can lead to life-threatening hypoglycemia, neonatal diabetes, maturity-onset diabetes of the young (MODY), or other forms of diabetes.

- In response to food, the intestine secretes incretins, which enhance glucose-induced insulin secretion. Patients who receive glucose as part of parenteral nutrition may need to be given exogenous insulin, in part because the bypassed intestine does not secrete incretins.

- Insulin can *stimulate* glucose uptake, glucose use, glycogen synthesis, fatty acid synthesis, triglyceride deposition, protein synthesis, and cell growth. Insulin can *inhibit* glycogenolysis, lipolysis, and gluconeogenesis.

- Tissues of patients who are pregnant or obese or who have polycystic ovary syndrome show a diminished response to insulin.

- Glucagon favors the release of glucose from the liver. The liver makes glucose via glycogenolysis or gluconeogenesis.

- Insulin-secreting tumors are uncommon and cause hypoglycemia. Glucagon-secreting tumors are very rare and lead to hypoaminoacidemia and hyperglycemia.

## LEARNING OBJECTIVES

*For mastery of this topic, you should be able to do the following:*

- Explain how glucagon, glucagon-like peptide 1 (GLP-1), and insulin are synthesized, processed, and stored.
- Compare and contrast how glucose, amino acids, ketone bodies, epinephrine, and GLP-1 affect glucagon and insulin secretion, relating hormone secretion to food intake, exercise, and fasting.
- Describe the basic mechanism by which sulfonylurea and glinide hypoglycemic drugs work, noting their most common side effect.
- Explain why C-peptide is a useful measure of endogenous insulin secretion.

- Outline the molecular events that are set in motion after insulin, glucagon, epinephrine, and cortisol bind to their respective receptors.
- Explain the mechanism of action and pharmacologic use of GLP-1 receptor agonists.
- Explain the mechanism of action and pharmacologic use of dipeptidylpeptidase-4 inhibitors.
- Describe the effect of polycystic ovary syndrome on insulin signaling.
- Characterize the clinical presentation of patients who have an asymptomatic insulinoma; do the same for glucagonoma.
- Describe abnormalities of β-cell proteins that cause hypoglycemia; do the same for hyperglycemia.
- Describe the effects of adrenal insufficiency, a pheochromocytoma, or Cushing syndrome on plasma glucose.

## 1. STRUCTURE OF THE HUMAN PANCREAS

*The pancreas contains islets of Langerhans. These islets contain α-cells that store glucagon and β-cells that store insulin inside secretory vesicles.*

The human pancreas consists of an **exocrine** and an **endocrine** portion. The *exocrine* cells make up about 99% of the volume of the pancreas and secrete *digestive enzymes* via the pancreatic duct into the lumen of the intestine. These digestive enzymes are composed of amylase, lipases, nucleases, and proteases or precursors of proteases (see Chapters 18, 28, and 34). The *endocrine* cells of the pancreas account for about 1% of the volume of the pancreas and secrete *hormones* into the bloodstream; these hormones control fuel metabolism and growth.

The endocrine cells occur in nests of cells called **islets of Langerhans** (Fig. 26.1). Each such islet contains **β-cells** (previously called B-cells, but not to be confused with B-lymphocytes) that secrete insulin and some amylin, **δ-cells** (previously called D-cells) that secrete somatostatin, and either **α-cells** (previously called A-cells) that secrete glucagon, or **PP-cells** (F-cells) that secrete pancreatic polypeptide (PP). Some islets contain both α- and PP-cells. The average human islet contains about 2,000 cells, but individual islets may contain a half a dozen cells to tens of thousands of cells. The entire pancreas contains roughly 1 million islets.

## 2. SYNTHESIS OF GLUCAGON, GLUCAGON-LIKE PEPTIDES, INSULIN, EPINEPHRINE, AND CORTISOL

*In α-cells, the proteolytic processing of preproglucagon gives rise to glucagon; in intestinal L-cells, it gives rise*

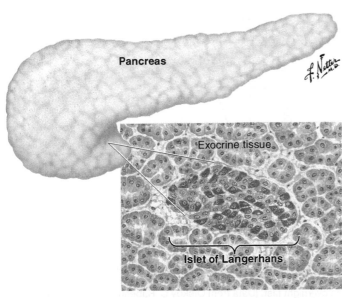

Fig. 26.1 Structure of the human pancreas and an islet of Langerhans.

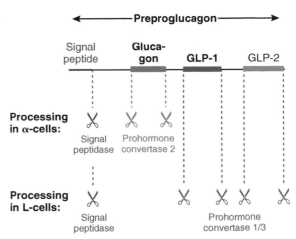

| Cell type | Fraction of islet volume | Hormone content |
|-----------|--------------------------|-----------------|
| α-cells | ~20% | Glucagon |
| β-cells | ~65% | Insulin, C-peptide, amylin |
| δ-cells | ~10% | Somatostatin |
| PP-cells | ~5% | Pancreatic polypeptide |

**Fig. 26.1** **Structure of the human pancreas and an islet of Langerhans.** In this islet, the β-cells appear deep purple from an aldehyde fuchsin stain.

*to glucagon-like peptides 1 and 2. Proteolytic processing of preproinsulin gives rise to insulin, which consists of disulfide-linked A- and B-chains, as well as C-peptide. In the adrenal glands, epinephrine is synthesized from tyrosine, and cortisol is made from cholesterol.*

## 2.1. Synthesis of Glucagon and Glucagon-Like Peptides

The glucagon gene encodes **glucagon, glucagon-like peptide 1 (GLP-1)**, and **glucagon-like peptide 2 (GLP-2)**. GLP-1 and GLP-2 have appreciable amino acid sequence homology to glucagon, but they activate different receptors and have different effects. Glucagon and the GLPs evolved via DNA sequence duplication.

Glucagon and the glucagon-like peptides are synthesized from **preproglucagon**. The **"pre" sequence,** or **signal sequence,** of preproglucagon ensures the insertion of the nascent peptide into the endoplasmic reticulum (see Chapter 7). After cleavage of the "pre" sequence, **proglucagon** (containing the sequences for glucagon, GLP-1, and GLP-2) is sorted through the Golgi apparatus and ends up in **secretory vesicles** (also called **secretory** *granules*). Several different tissues produce proglucagon.

Inside secretory vesicles, proglucagon is proteolyzed to tissue-specific products (Fig. 26.2). α-Cells in the pancreas contain prohormone convertase 2 (PC2) and process proglucagon into **glucagon. L-cells** in the small and large intestine

**Fig. 26.2** **Tissue-specific processing of proglucagon.** GLP, glucagon-like peptide.

instead contain prohormone convertase 1/3 (PC1/3, meaning PC1 is identical with PC3) and process proglucagon into GLP-1 and GLP-2.

## 2.2. Synthesis of Insulin and Amylin

Insulin consists of two peptides, the **A-chain,** and the **B-chain,** that derive from a single precursor, **preproinsulin** (Fig. 26.3), which derives from the insulin gene. The insulin gene is almost exclusively transcribed in pancreatic β-cells. Translation of insulin mRNA gives rise to preproinsulin. The "pre" sequence ensures the insertion of the nascent peptide into the endoplasmic reticulum and is cleaved (see also Chapter 7). The remaining peptide, **proinsulin,** contains the A- and B-chains, as well as a connecting peptide, called **C-peptide.** The A- and B-chains contain cysteine residues that form disulfide bridges. These bridges form properly in high yield only from folded proinsulin but not from isolated A- and B-chains. Proinsulin is transported through the Golgi apparatus and ends up in secretory vesicles.

The secretory granules inside β-cells contain the **prohormone convertases PC1/3 and PC2,** which hydrolyze proinsulin into an A-chain, a B-chain, and C-peptide. The A- and B-chains remain disulfide-linked and together are called **insulin.** Insulin binds **zinc** (see Fig. 26.3) and crystallizes inside the granules. **C-peptide** remains soluble and is secreted together with insulin.

In patients who have diabetes and inject pharmaceutical-grade insulin, measurement of the concentration of **C-peptide in blood** plasma provides information about the patient's insulin secretion. Although commercially available insulins are generated from proinsulins, they do not contain the C-peptide.

β-Cells are packed with about a week's supply of insulin-containing secretory vesicles. When a patient's pancreas cannot adequately control the concentration of glucose in the blood, it is almost never due to a lack of insulin inside β-cells; rather, it is due to a problem with the number of β-cells (e.g., type 1 diabetes) or the response of β-cells to physiological stimuli (e.g., MODY and type 2 diabetes; see Chapter 39).

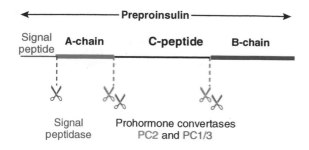

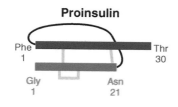

**2 Zn: 6 Insulin crystal**

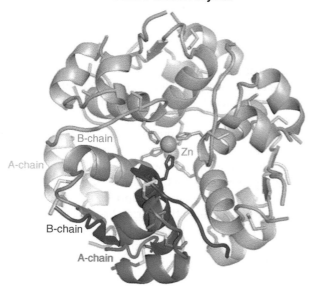

**Fig. 26.3** **Synthesis of insulin in pancreatic β-cells.** Yellow lines indicate disulfide bonds. (Based on Protein Data Bank [www.rcsb.org] file 1MSO from Smith, GD, Pangborn WA, Blessing RH. The structure of T6 human insulin at 1.0 A resolution. *Acta Crystallogr D Biol Crystallogr.* 2003;59:474-482.)

Besides insulin, pancreatic β-cells also synthesize a small amount of **amylin**. Amylin is also called **islet amyloid polypeptide (IAPP)**. Amylin is a small peptide that derives from preproamylin. On a molar basis, the β-cell secretory granules contain up to 100 times more insulin than amylin. The pancreatic β-cells are the primary but not the exclusive producer of amylin. Because the secretory granules of pancreatic β-cells contain both insulin and amylin, these two hormones are also secreted at the same time.

Amylin is found as part of extracellular **amyloid** deposits (see Chapter 9) in the islets of patients who secrete a large amount of insulin, commonly because of insulin resistance or an insulinoma (see Section 6 below).

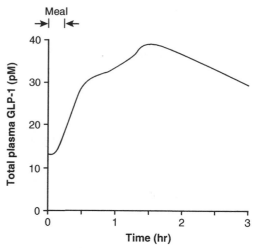

**Fig. 26.4** **Effect of a mixed meal on plasma glucagon-like peptide 1 (GLP-1).** Volunteers consumed a 450-kcal breakfast after an overnight fast. (Data from Orskov C, Rabenhøj L, Wettergren A, Kofod H, Holst JJ. Tissue and plasma concentrations of amidated and glycine-extended glucagon-like peptide I in humans. *Diabetes.* 1994;43:535-9; and Højberg PV, Vilsbøll T, Zander M, et al. Four weeks of near-normalization of blood glucose has no effect on postprandial GLP-1 and GIP secretion, but augments pancreatic B-cell responsiveness to a meal in patients with type 2 diabetes. *Diabet Med.* 2008;25:1268-1275.)

## 2.3. Synthesis of Epinephrine and Cortisol in the Adrenal Glands

The adrenal glands sit on top of the kidneys (see Fig. 31.12 and 31.15) and contain a medulla (inner region) that synthesizes norepinephrine and epinephrine from tyrosine (see Section 4.2 in Chapter 35), and a cortex (outer region) that synthesizes cortisol from cholesterol (see Section 3 in Chapter 31). Norepinephrine and epinephrine are both **catecholamines** (dopamine is another catecholamine). The adrenal glands store catecholamines inside secretory vesicles. Cortisol is membrane permeable and therefore cannot be stored in secretory granules. Instead, it is synthesized as needed.

## 3. SECRETION OF GLUCAGON, GLUCAGON-LIKE PEPTIDES, INSULIN, EPINEPHRINE, AND CORTISOL

*α- and β-cells in the islets of the pancreas secrete glucagon and insulin, respectively, in response to nutrients, incretins, and epinephrine, depending on the prevailing concentration of glucose. L-cells in the intestine secrete GLP-1 in response to nutrients in the diet. The hypothalamus and anterior pituitary gland control the secretion of epinephrine and cortisol.*

### 3.1. Secretion of Glucagon-Like Peptide 1

L-cells in the distal ileum and colon secrete GLP-1 in response to fats and sugars, whereas amino acids have little effect. Fig. 26.4 shows the effect of a mixed meal on the concentration of GLP-1 in plasma.

## 3.2. Secretion of Glucagon

**Amino acids** are the principal fuel stimulus of glucagon secretion from α-cells. α-Cells appear to recognize amino acids much like β-cells do (see Fig. 26.7). **Glucose** decreases amino acid–induced glucagon secretion (the mechanism for this is still debated). Physiologically, the concentration of glucose is a major regulator of glucagon secretion. For instance, at the 1-hour time point of a 75-g **oral glucose tolerance test** given to fasting volunteers, the concentration of glucagon in peripheral blood reached a low of about 60% of the pretest concentration.

Acting through the β2-adrenergic receptors, **epinephrine** and **norepinephrine** stimulate glucagon secretion from α-cells. This occurs through the production of cyclic adenosine monophosphate (cAMP), activation of protein kinase A (PKA), and subsequent potentiation of exocytosis.

Glucagon from pancreatic islets enters the hepatic portal vein; the liver therefore experiences the highest concentration of glucagon. Under physiological conditions, changes in the concentration of glucagon in the peripheral circulation are small.

Fig. 26.5 shows the concentration of glucagon in the peripheral blood in response to a mixed meal. The time course of the glucagon concentration is determined by a combination of decreased glucagon secretion due to meal-induced hyperglycemia and increased glucagon secretion due to the presence of amino acids. The data make it apparent that glucagon secretion is ongoing, and that metabolism is regulated by small changes in glucagon concentration rather than an absence or presence of this hormone.

## 3.3. Secretion of Insulin

### 3.3.1. Stimulatory Effect of Glucose

The principal stimulus for insulin secretion is an elevated concentration of glucose in the blood. Fig. 26.6 shows the relationship between the steady-state concentrations of glucose and insulin in blood plasma in overnight-fasted volunteers.

Inside β-cells, **glucokinase** serves as a glucose sensor (Fig. 26.7). GLUT-2 glucose transporters equilibrate glucose between blood plasma and the cytoplasm of β-cells. Glucokinase shows a small degree of cooperativity toward glucose, and it is half-maximally active at about the same concentration of glucose that half-maximally stimulates insulin secretion (i.e., ~10 mM or ~180 mg glucose/dL). Mutations that increase the affinity of glucokinase for glucose cause hypoglycemia (see Section 6.1), whereas mutations that decrease the affinity for glucose cause diabetes (MODY-2; see Section 6.2 and Chapter 39). Unlike hepatocytes, β-cells do not express the glucokinase regulatory protein (GKRP; see Chapter 19).

Pancreatic β-cells contain adenosine triphosphate (**ATP**)-sensitive K+-channels ($K_{ATP}$-channels) that regulate insulin secretion (see Fig. 26.7). The pore of these channels oscillates between open and closed states. These channels conduct more K+ when the concentration of ATP is relatively low and the

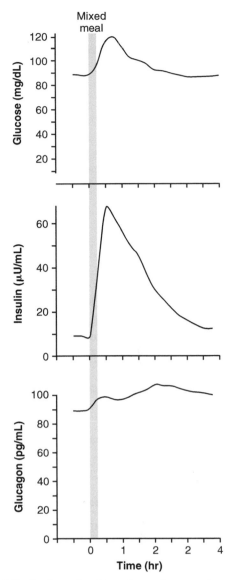

**Fig. 26.5** **Effect of a mixed meal on plasma glucose, insulin, and glucagon concentrations.** Lean volunteers aged ~27 years were given a mixed meal of 400-500 kcal, of which approximately 50% was from carbohydrates and 17% from protein. (Data from Gerich JE, Lorenzi M, Karam JH, Schneider V, Forsham PH. Abnormal pancreatic glucagon secretion and postprandial hyperglycemia in diabetes mellitus. *JAMA.* 1975;234:159-165; and Cooperberg BA, Cryer PE. β-Cell-mediated signaling predominates over direct α-cell signaling in the regulation of glucagon secretion in humans. *Diabetes Care.* 2009;32:2275-2280.)

concentration of adenosine diphosphate (ADP) is relatively high. At a very low concentration of glucose, the concentration of ADP inside β-cells is relatively high and that of ATP slightly low. Under these conditions, $K_{ATP}$ channels pass enough K+ that they can polarize β-cells to about −70 mV; such polarized cells do not secrete insulin. In contrast, at a high concentration of glucose, the concentration of ADP is low and that of ATP is normal. The $K_{ATP}$ channels are therefore almost always closed now in place of K+ flowing through $K_{ATP}$-channels, yet uncharacterized currents play a greater role in determining the membrane potential, and these currents depolarize the plasma membrane. Once the membrane potential reaches about −40 mV, voltage-sensitive $Ca^{2+}$ channels open and allow **$Ca^{2+}$** to flow from the extracellular space into the cytoplasm. There, the elevated concentration of $Ca^{2+}$ activates **exocytosis**, which moves insulin-containing granules to the plasma membrane.

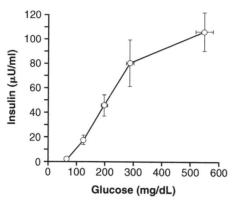

**Fig. 26.6** **Relationship between the steady-state concentrations of glucose and insulin in blood plasma.** Volunteers were infused with glucose at various rates to near steady state. Blood samples were drawn and the concentrations of glucose and insulin determined. (Modified from Cerasi E, Luft R, Efendic S. Decreased sensitivity of the pancreatic beta cells to glucose in prediabetic and diabetic subjects; a glucose dose-response study. *Diabetes.* 1972;21:224-234.)

$K_{ATP}$ channels are inhibited pharmacologically by the **sulfonylurea** and the **glinide anti-diabetes drugs** that are sometimes used to treat patients with type 2 diabetes (see Chapter 39). Each β-cell $K_{ATP}$ channel consists of Kir6.2 peptides that form a K+-selective pore, and sulfonylurea-receptor 1 (SUR1) peptides that regulate the opening and closing of the K+ pore. The sulfonylureas and the glinides bind to the SUR1 peptides of the $K_{ATP}$ channels. These drugs boost insulin secretion by reducing the probability that $K_{ATP}$ channels are open (hyperglycemia normally has this same effect). Obviously, a dangerous side effect of these drugs is excessive insulin secretion that leads to severe **hypoglycemia**.

**Diazoxide**, a potassium channel–opening drug, also binds to the SUR1 peptides of $K_{ATP}$ channels in β-cells, but it *increases* the probability that the $K_{ATP}$ channels are open. Consequently, diazoxide *inhibits* insulin secretion. Diazoxide is used in the rare patient who has persistent hypoglycemia from secretion of excessive amounts of insulin, most commonly as a result of heritable faulty sensing of amino acids (see Section 6.1).

During hormone secretion, secretory vesicles dock to the plasma membrane and empty their contents. Docking is aided by a protein on the vesicle surface and two proteins on the cytosolic plasma membrane surface that contain one or two **SNARE sequences**, which form a coiled coil structure (see Fig. 9.7).

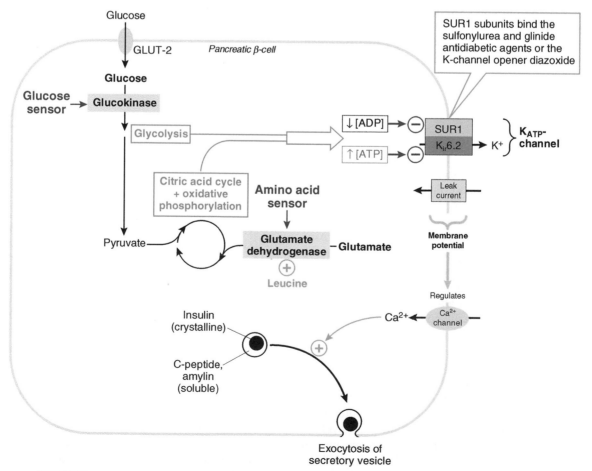

**Fig. 26.7** **Regulation of the membrane potential of pancreatic β-cells by adenosine triphosphate (ATP)-sensitive K+-channels ($K_{ATP}$ channels).**

### 3.3.2. Amplification of Glucose-Induced Insulin Secretion

Incretins, amino acids, fatty acids, and ketone bodies can amplify glucose-induced insulin secretion, but by themselves, they cannot induce sustained insulin secretion.

The incretins **GLP-1** and **GIP** (gastric inhibitory peptide, glucose-dependent insulinotropic peptide) boost glucose-induced insulin secretion. Incretins are defined as hormones that are secreted from the intestine and regulate insulin secretion. GLP-1 and GIP are secreted when the gastrointestinal tract contains nutrients. GIP is secreted from **K-cells** in the duodenum and upper jejunum. GLP-1 is secreted mainly from L-cells in the ileum. GLP-1 and GIP increase insulin secretion only when the concentration of glucose is above ~90 mg/dL (~5 mM).

If a patient receives an intravenous infusion of glucose, incretins are not secreted. As a result, the same dose of glucose given intravenously results in lower insulin secretion than the same dose given orally.

In **parenteral nutrition,** insulin is sometimes infused together with glucose to increase glucose utilization and diminish hyperglycemia.

Some patients who have type 2 diabetes are treated with **GLP-1 receptor agonists.** These agonists are peptides and must be injected.

In the bloodstream, GLP-1 and GIP are rapidly degraded by dipeptidylpeptidase-4 (DPP-4). **DPP-4 inhibitors,** known as *gliptins,* are used to treat type 2 diabetes (see Chapter 39).

Among amino acids, the combination of **leucine** and **glutamine** is particularly effective at potentiating glucose-induced insulin secretion. Leucine is an essential amino acid. Its concentration in the blood rises significantly after a protein meal; this increase may serve as a signal of protein intake. (In the fasting state, muscle cells degrade protein and release amino acids into the blood, but they largely transaminate leucine and release only its corresponding ketoacid, α-ketoisocaproic acid.) Glutamine is the most abundant amino acid in the blood. Inside β-cells, glutamine is deaminated into glutamate. In the mitochondria, glutamate dehydrogenase, allosterically activated by leucine, converts glutamate to α-ketoglutarate, which is part of the citric acid cycle (see Fig. 26.7 and Fig. 22.7). In pancreatic β-cells, glutamate dehydrogenase is a sensor of amino acids; excessive activity of this enzyme leads to excessive insulin secretion and concomitant severe hypoglycemia (see Section 6.1.3). Besides insulin secretion, leucine and glutamine regulate other processes as well as insulin secretion. Thus, leucine also stimulates protein synthesis in skeletal muscle (see Chapter 34). Similarly, glutamine affects gene expression, protein synthesis, metabolism, and cell survival in many tissues of the body.

Besides leucine and glutamine, **arginine** and **lysine** also stimulate insulin secretion. The most commonly invoked explanation for the effects of these positively charged amino acids on insulin secretion is that their uptake depolarizes the β-cell plasma membrane and thus stimulates insulin secretion.

As evident from the above discussion, an elevated concentration of amino acids stimulates both insulin and glucagon secretion. As will become evident below, insulin stimulates not only the use of amino acids for protein synthesis, but also the removal of glucose from the blood; glucagon counteracts this last effect by favoring glucose production. The net result is the removal of amino acids and maintenance of normoglycemia.

**Fatty acids** and **ketone bodies** each have only a mild stimulatory effect on insulin secretion, but this effect is crucial in attenuating adipose tissue lipolysis in the fasting state to prevent ketoacidosis (see Chapter 27).

### 3.3.3. Inhibition of Insulin Secretion by Catecholamines

Epinephrine and norepinephrine potently inhibit insulin secretion, regardless of the β-cell stimulus. Epinephrine and norepinephrine both work through $\alpha_2$-adrenergic receptors. Pancreatic β-cells are exposed to increased concentrations of epinephrine and norepinephrine during exercise, hypoglycemia, trauma, or stress.

Fig. 26.5 shows the concentrations of glucose and insulin in healthy volunteers in response to a mixed meal. Glucose in the meal is the principal stimulus for insulin secretion, and both incretins and amino acids enhance glucose-induced insulin secretion. Fatty acids and ketone bodies significantly stimulate insulin secretion only in the fasting state. Fig. 39.6 shows 1-day profiles of the concentrations of glucose and insulin in volunteers who consumed three mixed meals.

### 3.4. Secretion of Epinephrine and Norepinephrine

During exercise or hypoglycemia, nerves from the sympathetic division of the autonomic nervous system stimulate chromaffin cells in the medulla of the adrenal glands to secrete epinephrine and norepinephrine.

Fig. 26.8 shows the effects of short duration, high-intensity **exercise** on the plasma concentrations of glucose, insulin, glucagon, and epinephrine. During intense exercise, the concentration of glucose rises somewhat, but an increased concentration of epinephrine ensures that insulin secretion decreases. The concentration of glucose in the blood reflects the balance of glucose production and consumption by muscles. Glucose enters the blood from the intestine after a meal; otherwise, the liver produces glucose from glycogenolysis, and both the liver and the kidneys produce glucose from gluconeogenesis. During the recovery phase, glucose production initially far surpasses glucose consumption, thus increasing the concentration of glucose in the blood. In response to the elevated concentration of glucose and no longer inhibited by a high concentration of epinephrine, insulin is secreted. Insulin then attenuates glucose production.

For type 1 diabetic patients who no longer secrete insulin, it is challenging to manage blood glucose during and after exercise, which they must do by adjusting carbohydrate intake and the size of the subcutaneous insulin depot.

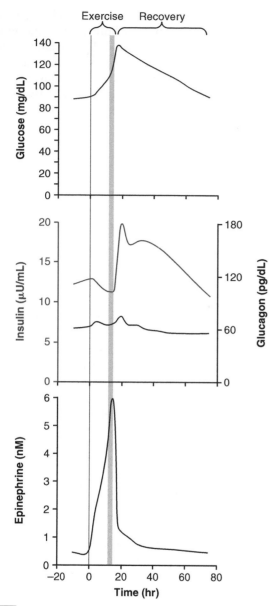

**Fig. 26.8** **Glucose, insulin, glucagon, and epinephrine in volunteers who exercised to exhaustion.** Exhaustion occurred after 12-16 minutes of exercise (range indicated by gray bar). (Modified from Sigal RJ, Fisher SJ, Manzon A, et al. Glucoregulation during and after intense exercise: effects of alpha-adrenergic blockade. *Metabolism.* 2000;49:386-394.)

## 3.5. Secretion of Cortisol

The hypothalamus and the pituitary gland regulate the secretion of cortisol form the adrenal glands (see Chapter 31). The hypothalamus secretes corticotropin-releasing hormone (CRH), which stimulates the pituitary gland to secrete adrenocorticotropic hormone (ACTH). ACTH stimulates the synthesis and secretion of cortisol.

Cortisol is secreted in a diurnal pattern (see Fig. 31.13). With a normal sleep cycle, the lowest concentration of cortisol is observed around the time of sleep onset, and the highest shortly after awakening in the morning. In addition, long-term stress increases cortisol secretion (short-term stress increases the secretion of epinephrine and norepinephrine).

## 4. EFFECTS OF INSULIN AND COUNTERREGULATORY HORMONES ON TISSUES

*Insulin lowers the concentration of glucose in the blood by affecting multiple metabolic pathways that consume glucose. The binding of insulin to insulin receptors activates intracellular signaling pathways that dephosphorylate certain enzymes of metabolism and alter the rate of transcription of certain genes. Glucagon increases the concentration of glucose in the blood by stimulating glycogenolysis and gluconeogenesis in the liver. Activated glucagon receptors signal through G-proteins that lead to altered rates of transcription of certain genes and phosphorylation of certain enzymes for metabolism. Epinephrine and norepinephrine signal through G protein–coupled receptors, and cortisol exerts its effects through receptors that are transcription factors.*

### 4.1. Biological Effects of Glucagon-Like Peptides

**GLP-1** potentiates glucose-induced insulin secretion, stimulates the growth of pancreatic β-cells, slows gastric emptying, decreases food intake, and favors glycogen synthesis in the liver rather than in muscle.

GLP-1 exerts its biological effects via a G protein–coupled **GLP-1 receptor** (see Chapter 33). In pancreatic β-cells, binding of GLP-1 to the GLP-1 receptor leads to an increased concentration of **cAMP** and activation of **protein kinase A (PKA)**, which enhances glucose-induced insulin secretion.

**DPP-4** cleaves two amino acids from GLP-1 and thus renders it inactive. DPP-4 is present as a soluble protein in blood and as an integral membrane protein on the surface of many cells. **DPP-4 inhibitors** are used in the treatment of type 2 diabetes (see Chapter 39).

**GLP-2** stimulates the growth of intestinal cells and is useful in the treatment of patients who have short bowel syndrome.

### 4.2. Biological Effects of Glucagon

Glucagon receptors are G protein–coupled receptors that signal via **cAMP** (similar to GLP-1 receptors; Fig. 26.9; see also Chapter 33). cAMP activates **PKA**, which phosphorylates various enzymes of metabolism, thereby either increasing or decreasing their activity. In addition, cAMP binds to **cAMP-response element-binding (CREB) protein**, which in turn binds to the promoter of certain genes and thereby alters the rate at which they are transcribed.

In the liver, glucagon stimulates **glycogenolysis** and **gluconeogenesis** while inhibiting **glycolysis** (see Chapters 24 and 25).

Glucagon and **GLP-1** receptors are each highly selective for glucagon and GLP-1, respectively, but they are not completely specific for either peptide due to peptide homology.

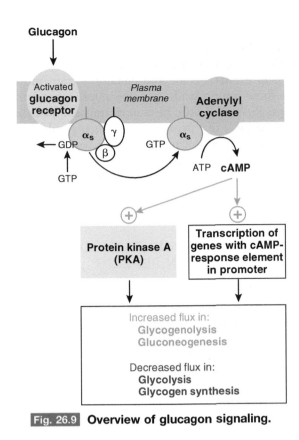

**Fig. 26.9** Overview of glucagon signaling.

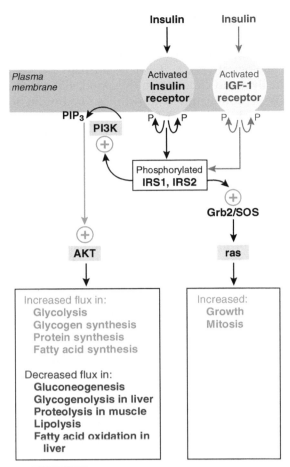

**Fig. 26.10** Biological effects of insulin.

Glucagon is the most important hormone in the body's defense against hypoglycemia; epinephrine is the second most important such hormone. The hormones glucagon, epinephrine, norepinephrine, and cortisol are called **counterregulatory hormones**.

**Radiologists** often use glucagon injected intravenously to relax and dilate the small intestine and reduce bowel motion.

**Type 1 diabetic** patients sometimes use glucagon to counteract **hypoglycemia**. Regardless of the concentration of insulin in the blood, glucagon stimulates glycogenolysis in the liver, which leads to an increase in blood glucose.

Once released into the blood, glucagon has a half-life of about 6 minutes. Glucagon is degraded by the liver, the kidneys, and enzymes in the blood vessels (mostly by DPP-4, the same enzyme that also degrades GLP-1).

## 4.3. Biological Effects of Insulin

Almost all cells have insulin receptors because insulin is a regulator of metabolism as well as cell proliferation. However, the number of insulin receptors varies among tissues.

With its diverse effects on almost all tissues, insulin takes a prominent position in hormone signaling. Insulin is a **growth factor** (see Chapter 8), promotes protein synthesis (see Chapters 7 and 34), and regulates metabolism. Fig. 26.10 lists the major effects of insulin on metabolism. Further details on these metabolic pathways are given in separate chapters. The balance of metabolic and mitogenic effects of analogs of human insulin is of concern in the treatment of diabetes (see Chapter 39).

The insulin receptor is a tetramer of two α- and two β-subunits. Proteolytic processing of the insulin receptor precursor gives rise to one α- and one β-subunit. The α- and β-subunits aggregate to form active insulin receptors that span the plasma membrane.

When the insulin receptor binds insulin, it has tyrosine kinase activity, it phosphorylates itself, and it also phosphorylates **insulin receptor substrate** (**IRS**) proteins. Then, phosphorylated IRS acts as a signal and activates enzymes in two pathways: phosphatidylinositol 3-kinase (PI3K) and Grb2-SOS (a complex with guanine nucleotide exchange factor activity). PI3K phosphorylates the phospholipid phosphatidylinositol 4,5-bisphosphate (PIP2) to produce PIP3, which attracts protein kinase B (AKT, PKB) to the membrane and activates it. AKT, in turn, affects the activity of various enzymes of metabolism. Grb2-SOS activates Ras in the ERK1/2 pathway, which alters the rate of transcription of certain genes.

Although not shown in Fig. 26.10, each signaling branch is also subject to stimulation and inhibition by other signaling pathways. Furthermore, each cell type has a tailored network of signaling pathways, thanks to the cell-specific expression of signaling proteins.

In response to a rising concentration of insulin, enzymes that play a role in fuel metabolism are usually **dephosphorylated**. In contrast, an increase in the concentration of glucagon or epinephrine often leads to the *phosphorylation* of enzymes of metabolism (see below).

Insulin and **insulin-like growth factor 1** (IGF-1) can have similar biological effects. IGF-1 is normally derived mainly from the liver and circulates in the blood, along with insulin. IGF-1 is predominantly a growth factor. Insulin receptors prefer to bind insulin over IGF-1, and the reverse is true for IGF-1 receptors. Insulin and IGF-1 receptors signal in a similar, though not identical, fashion. Furthermore, cells can form heterodimeric insulin/IGF-1 receptors. For this reason, patients who have a tumor that secretes IGF-1 may have hypoglycemia. Furthermore, synthetic analogs of insulin used in the treatment of diabetes may be more mitogenic (and thus possibly tumorigenic) than normal insulin.

Signaling by insulin receptors is modulated by internalization and by the phosphorylation state of several residues. Occupation of the insulin receptor by insulin leads to the **internalization** of the receptor. Internalized receptors can either be returned to the plasma membrane or be degraded. **Phosphotyrosine phosphatases** dephosphorylate tyrosine-phosphorylated insulin receptors and thus render them inactive. Various **protein kinases** phosphorylate the insulin receptor on certain *serine* residues and thus render it less active.

In the blood, insulin has a half-life of about 4 minutes. After endocytosis of an insulin receptor-insulin complex, insulin is mostly degraded intracellularly by insulin-degrading enzyme and other enzymes. By the time blood from the hepatic portal vein reaches the hepatic vein, the liver has extracted approximately half of the insulin. The other half is removed principally by the kidneys and further passages through the liver.

## 4.4. Biological Effects of Epinephrine and Norepinephrine

Epinephrine and norepinephrine bind to α- and β-adrenergic G protein–coupled receptors, and these receptors and their subtypes couple to different α-subunits of heterotrimeric G proteins (see Chapter 33). $\alpha_2$-Adrenergic receptors inhibit insulin secretion from β-cells by activating $G_i$ and $G_0$ proteins. β-Adrenergic receptors enhance glycogenolysis and gluconeogenesis in the liver, lipolysis in adipose tissue, and glucagon secretion from α-cells.

Cells, particularly in the liver, take up circulating catecholamines and then inactivate them by methylating norepinephrine to **normetanephrine** and epinephrine to **metanephrine**; some of these metabolites end up in the urine. Measurement of normetanephrine or metanephrine in urine and/or blood plasma is part of the diagnosis of **pheochromocytoma** (a tumor that secretes mostly epinephrine and a lesser amount of norepinephrine; see Fig. 22.13).

## 4.5. Biological Effects of Cortisol

Cortisol crosses membranes and binds to the glucocorticoid receptor in the cytosol, which then moves into the nucleus, binds to a glucocorticoid response element, and thus stimulates transcription (see Chapters 6 and 31).

Cortisol enhances the transcription of transaminases, which help export alanine and glutamine from muscle and import these amino acids into the intestine and the liver (see Figs. 35.4 and 35.10). In muscle, transaminases facilitate the amination of pyruvate (producing alanine) and α-ketoglutarate (producing glutamate, which gives rise to glutamine). In the intestine and liver, transaminases facilitate the reverse processes. Transfer of amino acids from muscle to the liver is essential for gluconeogenesis (see Chapter 25).

## 5. PHYSIOLOGICAL AND PATHOLOGICAL CHANGES IN INSULIN SENSING

*Insulin resistance is a state of diminished cellular responses to circulating insulin. Because pancreatic β-cells attempt to maintain the concentration of glucose in the blood at a normal concentration, β-cells in an insulin-resistant person must secrete more insulin. Insulin resistance is seen in normal pregnancy, in obese persons, and in those who have polycystic ovary syndrome.*

### 5.1. General Commen+ts About Insulin Resistance

The term **insulin resistance** refers to a state of poor response to insulin. The terms insulin *resistance* and insulin *insensitivity* mean the same, whereas the term insulin *sensitivity* means the opposite of insulin resistance. In clinical practice, insulin resistance refers to the effect of insulin on glucose transport; other effects of insulin on a patient's cells are currently measured only rarely. Compared with a patient with a normal response to insulin, an insulin-resistant patient needs a higher concentration of insulin to move a given amount of glucose out of the blood. The insulin resistance may be due to a problem with insulin receptors or with the insulin receptor–activated signaling pathway.

Insulin resistance can be organ specific or affect multiple organs. In humans, there is evidence that common forms of "whole body" insulin resistance are associated with insulin resistance of at least the liver, muscles, and adipose tissue.

**Puberty** is associated with mild insulin resistance. Insulin resistance is most pronounced around Tanner stage III. Girls are more insulin resistant than boys.

**Pregnancy** is associated with marked insulin resistance. Pregnant women in their third trimester secrete about eight times more insulin than nonpregnant women, although the mass of pancreatic β-cells increases by only about 25% with pregnancy. If the pancreas does not provide the required extra insulin, **gestational diabetes** ensues (see Chapter 39).

Pharmacological doses of **corticosteroids** induce insulin resistance. Patients who take corticosteroids for years are at an increased risk of developing diabetes.

In developed countries, **obesity** is the most common cause of insulin resistance (see Chapter 39). The cause of this association is still debated. It may be that triglyceride-laden adipocytes have altered secretion of hormones and fatty acids. Furthermore, triglyceride accumulation inside muscle and the liver may impair signaling from activated insulin receptors.

Severe insulin resistance is often accompanied by **acanthosis nigricans** (thickening and darkening of the skin, most often in the axillae and the skin folds of the neck and groin Fig. 26.11); **ovarian dysfunction, hyperandrogenism**, and **hirsutism** (male-pattern hair growth; Fig. 26.12); and **lipoatrophy.**

**Exercise** depletes the glycogen stores of skeletal muscle; as a consequence, after a meal, more glucose can be deposited as glycogen in exercised than in unexercised muscle. Persons who exercise regularly are less likely to be insulin resistant than **sedentary** persons. Most insulin-resistant persons can increase their insulin sensitivity with exercise.

In medical practice, insulin sensitivity, if quantified, can be estimated in one of the following ways.

1. In patients who have **type 2 diabetes** and treat their disease with insulin, the **daily dose** of insulin required for blood glucose control gives the treating physician an idea of the patient's insulin sensitivity. A lean adult without β-cells requires about 30 units of insulin per day.
2. Glucose and insulin can be measured in plasma after an overnight fast, and an insulin sensitivity index can then be calculated.
3. Glucose and insulin in plasma can be measured before and during an oral glucose tolerance test, and the data can be used to calculate another insulin sensitivity index.
4. Rarely, an **insulin tolerance test** is applied, which consists of measuring the degree of hypoglycemia after an injection of insulin. At first, a fasting patient is injected with only a small amount of insulin (often ~0.1 U/kg body weight). If hypoglycemia does not occur, the patient is injected with increasingly higher amounts of insulin. Insulin-resistant patients need an abnormally large amount of insulin to cause hypoglycemia. Unfortunately, there are no generally accepted ranges that define normal insulin sensitivity.

Only a minority of patients with **hereditary severe insulin resistance** have mutant insulin receptors. Instead, they are likely to have mutations in other proteins that are involved in insulin signaling.

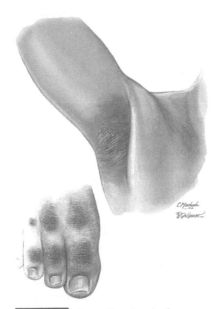

**Fig. 26.11**  **Acanthosis nigricans.**

## 5.2. Polycystic Ovary Syndrome

Polycystic ovary syndrome (PCOS) affects about 5% to 10% of women during their reproductive years. In women who do not take birth control pills, a polycystic ovary is defined as an ovary that has a volume greater than 10 mL and/or contains 12 or more follicles 2 to 9 mm in diameter (see Further Reading for a reference to the currently used 2003 Rotterdam criteria). The ovarian dysfunction is commonly associated with an abnormally high concentration of androgens in the blood (see Chapter 31). PCOS may be accompanied by irregular menses, infertility, obesity, and hirsutism (i.e., male-pattern hair growth; see Fig. 26.12). About 40% of patients with PCOS have impaired glucose tolerance or diabetes.

PCOS most likely represents a family of diseases of yet unknown cause. The syndrome shows multigenic inheritance with a strong environmental component.

Among patients with PCOS, **insulin resistance** is common, even though this is not part of the diagnosis. If insulin resistance is assessed, the measurements usually refer only to the relationship between insulin and glucose metabolism, whereby metabolism in skeletal muscle contributes the most. How these measurements relate to the insulin sensitivity of the androgen-producing theca cells in the ovaries is uncertain.

Enlarged, polycystic ovary

Hirsutism

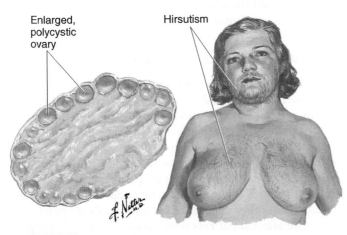

**Fig. 26.12**  **Patient with polycystic ovary syndrome.**

In overweight or obese patients with PCOS, an increase in insulin sensitivity can be achieved with weight loss and exercise. This is accompanied by increased fertility. Oral contraceptives with progestin and estrogen can be used to treat the hyperandrogenism and hirsutism.

# 6. PATHOLOGY OF THE SECRETION OF INSULIN AND COUNTERREGULATORY HORMONES

*Insulin-secreting tumors occasionally develop in middle-aged patients and cause hypoglycemia. Multiple endocrine neoplasia (MEN-1) is a syndrome of tumor formation in two or more endocrine organs. Mutations in one of several proteins that are involved in β-cell development or insulin secretion can give rise to either insufficient or excessive insulin secretion (i.e., to hypoglycemia or hyperglycemia). Adrenal insufficiency can give rise to hypoglycemia, and an excess of epinephrine or cortisol can cause hyperglycemia.*

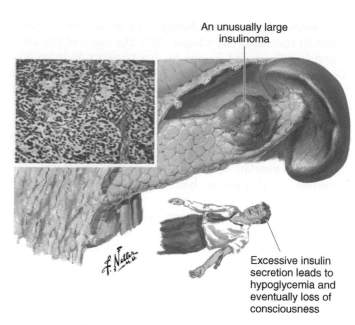

An unusually large insulinoma

Excessive insulin secretion leads to hypoglycemia and eventually loss of consciousness

**Fig. 26.13**  **Patient with an insulinoma.**

## 6.1. Disorders Associated With Hypoglycemia

When determining the cause of hypoglycemia, physicians sometimes first distinguish between ketotic and nonketotic hypoglycemia.

In **ketotic hypoglycemia**, the concentration of insulin must be low because it is a prerequisite for a high rate of lipolysis that, in turn, gives rise to the conversion of fatty acids to ketone bodies (see Chapter 27). Hence, in ketotic hypoglycemia the problem is usually with glucose production, (i.e., in glycogenolysis and/or gluconeogenesis; see Chapters 24 and 25).

In **nonketotic** or **hypoketotic hypoglycemia**, there is usually a problem with excessive insulin (which inhibits lipolysis and glucose production) or a problem with the oxidation of fatty acids (see Chapter 27).

### 6.1.1. Insulinoma

Many pancreatic endocrine tumors secrete a variety of hormones, but the secretion of one hormone usually far outpaces that of all others.

Insulinomas cause hypoglycemia. Excessive secretion of insulin from an insulinoma is usually due to an abnormal regulation of insulin secretion by glucose. The response of the nervous system to hypoglycemia causes patients to be hungry, sweaty, and anxious and have a tremor. Food intake temporarily alleviates the hypoglycemia; many patients who have an insulinoma therefore become overweight or obese. Marked hypoglycemia impairs primarily the central nervous system and can manifest itself in confusion, unusual behavior, visual disturbances, and eventually seizures and loss of consciousness.

Despite the hypoglycemia, patients with an insulinoma do *not* show ketosis. The high concentration of insulin inhibits lipolysis (see Chapter 28). When the concentration of free fatty acids in the blood is low, the liver does not produce ketone bodies.

Insulinomas are commonly diagnosed based on symptoms of hypoglycemia in the fasting state that are accompanied by measurable hypoglycemia and excessive concentrations of both insulin and C-peptide in the blood whereby infusion of glucose or glucagon provides rapid relief of symptoms. Diagnosis of an insulinoma also requires ruling out the surreptitious administration of an anti-diabetes drug, such as a sulfonylurea.

Surgical removal of the insulinoma usually cures the hypoglycemia. About 90% of all insulinomas are benign. About 95% of insulinomas are sporadic, and about 5% are associated with MEN-1 (see below). Perhaps 1 in 4,000 persons develops an insulinoma during his or her lifetime. The median age at diagnosis is about 50 years. The median diameter of insulinomas is only about 1.3 cm, and they are therefore often difficult to locate (Fig. 26.13). Patients who cannot undergo surgery can be treated with **diazoxide** (a K⁺ channel opener and activator of $K_{ATP}$ channels; see Fig. 26.7).

### 6.1.2. Multiple Endocrine Neoplasia

**MEN-1,** also called **Wermer syndrome,** affects at least 1 in 30,000 persons. Affected patients most often inherit one nonfunctional copy of the tumor suppressor and transcription factor menin. The physiological role of menin is only poorly understood. In persons with MEN-1, the function of the normal menin allele is lost sporadically in endocrine glands, particularly the parathyroid glands, pancreatic islets, and anterior pituitary. Neoplasms may then develop by additional mutations in other genes (see Chapter 8). By 40 years of age, almost all affected patients develop symptomatic hyperplasias and adenomas. Patients often have multiple adenomas, which complicate surgical excision. Pancreatic islet adenomas secrete multiple hormones and cause hypoglycemia only if they secrete sufficient insulin. Islet adenomas are often malignant and deadly. However, of all patients who have an insulinoma, only a minority have MEN-1.

### 6.1.3. Congenital Hyperinsulinism

Known heritable abnormalities of β-cell proteins are very rare, but they tell us a lot about the mechanisms that control insulin secretion. Four such abnormalities cause excessive insulin secretion and thus pose a risk of deadly hypoglycemia: mutations that affect $K_{ATP}$ channels, glucokinase, glutamate dehydrogenase, or a monocarboxylate transporter.

Patients with insufficiently active $K_{ATP}$ channels due to autosomal recessive mutations in the Kir6.2 or SUR1 subunits cannot adequately suppress insulin secretion during hypoglycemia. This disease is present in utero and causes macrosomia by excessive insulin stimulation of fatty acid synthesis and triglyceride deposition in the adipose tissue. Shortly after birth, affected infants become severely hypoglycemic. The hypoglycemia must be counteracted with infusions of glucose. Insulin secretion can be inhibited by a calcium channel inhibitor, epinephrine, or a somatostatin analog. The excessive concentration of circulating insulin can be partially balanced with an infusion of glucagon or epinephrine. In most patients, the $K_{ATP}$ channel opener diazoxide is ineffective. Many affected patients require partial pancreatectomy to control blood glucose, but this means that they may later develop diabetes. For reasons that are not understood, the hyperinsulinemia abates with age.

Patients who are heterozygous for a mutant **glucokinase** that is overly sensitive to glucose secrete insulin even during hypoglycemia. This disease is usually evident in the newborn period. Many affected patients can be successfully treated with diazoxide, which opens $K_{ATP}$ channels in pancreatic endocrine cells (see Fig. 26.7).

Patients with overly active, mutant **glutamate dehydrogenase** may secrete an excessive amount of insulin in response to elevated concentrations of leucine and glutamine in the blood. The disease is inherited in autosomal dominant fashion. Hypoglycemia most commonly sets in after a high-protein, low-carbohydrate meal, but it also occurs during an extended period of fasting. Some patients show hypoglycemia already in the newborn period, whereas others receive a diagnosis only as adults. Patients with mutant glutamate dehydrogenase also can be treated with diazoxide (an opener of $K_{ATP}$ channels). These patients should avoid long fasts or high-protein, low-carbohydrate meals.

Some patients have **exercise-induced hypoglycemia** due to inappropriate expression of the **monocarboxylate transporter 1**, which moves lactate and pyruvate across the β-cell plasma membrane. The mutation is in the promoter region of the *SLC16A1* gene, which encodes the monocarboxylate transporter. As a result, the β-cells secrete insulin when the concentration of pyruvate or lactate in the blood is increased (e.g., due to exercise). Within 30 minutes of a short bout of anaerobic exercise, affected patients become hypoglycemic. The disorder is inherited in a dominant fashion.

### 6.1.4. Adrenal Insufficiency

Patients who have adrenal insufficiency, especially children, often develop hypoglycemia in the fasting state.

## 6.2. Disorders Associated With Hyperglycemia

### 6.2.1. Diabetes Due to Heritable β-Cell Abnormalities

As described in Section 5, insulin resistance requires a compensatory increase in insulin secretion. It is unclear how insulin resistance eventually leads to β-cell failure. This section describes causes of abnormal insulin secretion that originate in the *β-cell*.

Infants who are diagnosed with diabetes during the first 6 months of life are said to have **neonatal diabetes**, which is usually due to heritable abnormalities in β-cell proteins. Table 44-1 in Chapter 39 provides more details.

In Europe, roughly half of the infants diagnosed with neonatal diabetes are heterozygous for mutations that lead to overactive $K_{ATP}$ **channels**. When $K_{ATP}$ channels are overly active, they keep the β-cells overly polarized, and the β-cells therefore do not secrete enough insulin (see Fig. 26.7). The patients can be treated with insulin, but many achieve better control of blood glucose if they are given a relatively high dose of a sulfonylurea drug.

Heritable mutations in genes that code for yet other proteins that are important for β-cell development, insulin synthesis, or insulin secretion cause **MODY**. This form of diabetes is due to heritable mutations in proteins of the liver and/or β-cells that are essential to glucose homeostasis. MODY resembles type 2 diabetes, which is typically seen in older (i.e., mature) patients, but MODY can present at any age (including newborns). There is some overlap in the genes that are mutated in neonatal diabetes and MODY. Patients with MODY make up a few percent of all patients with diabetes, at most. Section 6 in Chapter 39 provides further details about the most common subtypes of MODY. The phenotypes of these mutations confirm and shape our concepts of the mechanism of pancreatic hormone secretion.

### 6.2.2. Hyperglycemia Due to Glucagonoma

Glucagonomas are rare, usually malignant, and often recognized only after metastases have formed. The very high concentration of glucagon excessively stimulates gluconeogenesis and to some extent, lipolysis. The elevated rate of lipolysis leads to a high concentration of free fatty acids in the blood. The excessive rate of gluconeogenesis leads to hyperglycemia and hypoaminoacidemia. The hypoaminoacidemia decreases the synthesis of new protein in muscle. Patients with a glucagonoma typically lose weight due to a diminishing mass of both adipose tissue and skeletal muscle. The low concentration of amino acids in the blood often gives rise to a **migratory**

**skin rash**, which frequently brings patients to medical attention. Other patients first come to medical attention because of type 2 diabetes. Diabetes is thought to be due to β-cell failure after chronic stimulation of β-cells by hyperglycemia.

### 6.2.3. Hyperglycemia Due to Pheochromocytoma or Cushing Syndrome

Due to the overproduction of epinephrine and norepinephrine, some patients with a **pheochromocytoma** (see Fig. 22.13) also have hyperglycemia (but hypertension is the main presenting symptom).

Hyperglycemia is quite common in patients with **Cushing syndrome** (i.e., hypercortisolism; see Chapter 31). Cortisol favors funneling amino acids into gluconeogenesis, thus increasing glucose production. In addition, cortisol induces insulin resistance, which is initially overcome by increased insulin secretion but eventually leads to impaired glucose-induced insulin secretion.

## SUMMARY

- Endocrine cells, organized into islets, make up about 1% of the pancreas. They produce insulin, amylin, and glucagon as well as other peptide hormones and store them in secretory vesicles. These peptides are derived from larger precursors (preprohormones) by proteolysis. Signal peptide peptidase in the endoplasmic reticulum cleaves the signal sequence, whereas prohormone convertases PC1/3 and PC2 in secretory vesicles cleave prohormones.
- Glucose (≥5 mM, or 90 mg/dL) by itself stimulates insulin secretion. Amino acids, fatty acids, and ketone bodies all potentiate glucose-induced insulin secretion. The gastrointestinal tract secretes the incretins glucagon-like peptide 1 (GLP-1) and gastric inhibitory peptide (GIP), which also amplify glucose-induced insulin secretion. Epinephrine inhibits insulin secretion.
- Pancreatic β-cells use glucokinase as a glucose sensor. They also use glutamate dehydrogenase as a leucine- and glutamine-dependent sensor of amino acids. ATP-sensitive $K^+$ channels ($K_{ATP}$ channels) sense cytosolic ADP and ATP. When active, $K_{ATP}$ channels polarize the plasma membrane and prevent insulin secretion. When inactive, $K_{ATP}$ channels permit membrane depolarization, which is followed by calcium influx and the exocytosis of secretory granules. Certain anti-diabetes drugs (e.g., sulfonylureas, repaglinide, and nateglinide) decrease the opening frequency of $K_{ATP}$ channels and thus boost insulin secretion.
- Amino acids, epinephrine, and hypoglycemia-sensing neuronal pathways stimulate glucagon secretion. In contrast, glucose inhibits glucagon secretion.
- Insulin binds to a receptor in the plasma membrane of a cell. All cells have insulin receptors, although at different densities. The cytoplasmic portion of the insulin receptor has tyrosine kinase activity that phosphorylates insulin receptor substrate (IRS). Grb2-SOS and phosphatidylinositol 3-kinase (PI3K) bind to phosphorylated IRS and thereby become active themselves. Signaling from Grb2-SOS stimulates cell growth and facilitates cell survival. Signaling from PI3K via AKT eventually leads to *de*phosphorylation of enzymes of metabolism. Some enzymes are activated by dephosphorylation, and others are inactivated. In muscle and adipose tissue, PI3K-derived signals also lead to the insertion of insulin-sensitive glucose transporters (GLUT-4) into the plasma membrane.

- The liver is physiologically the most important target of glucagon. Muscle cells have only an insignificant number of glucagon receptors. Glucagon binds to a G-protein–coupled receptor in the plasma membrane that leads to signaling via cAMP, protein kinase A (PKA), and cAMP-response element-binding (CREB) protein. Activation of glucagon receptors leads to the phosphorylation of target enzymes of metabolism and to increased transcription of genes that are linked to a promoter that has a cAMP-response element.

- Patients who are insulin resistant require a higher concentration of insulin to control the concentration of glucose in the blood than patients who have a normal response to insulin. Puberty is associated with mild insulin resistance. Pregnancy and obesity cause moderate insulin resistance. Polycystic ovary syndrome (PCOS) is usually associated with insulin resistance.

- Patients with insulinomas have episodes of nonketotic hypoglycemia. Patients with inactivating mutations in $K_{ATP}$ channels, or with activating mutations in glucokinase or glutamate dehydrogenase, may have congenital persistent or episodic nonketotic hypoglycemia. Activating mutations in $K_{ATP}$ channels and inactivating mutations in glucokinase, as well as mutations in other factors that impair β-cell development, insulin synthesis, or insulin secretion may cause hyperglycemia and thus diabetes.

- Patients with glucagonoma are hyperglycemic and hypoaminoacidemic. They also frequently have a migratory skin rash and diabetes.

## FURTHER READING

- Bliss M. *The Discovery of Insulin*. Chicago: University of Chicago Press; 1982. This is a comprehensive, very well-written account.
- Raju TNK. A mysterious something: the discovery of insulin and the 1923 Nobel prize for Frederick G. Banting (1891-1941) and John J.R. Macleod (1876-1935). *Acta Paediatr*. 2006;95:1155-1156. This is a review of the history of the discovery of insulin.
- Shah P, Demirbilek H, Hussain K. Persistent hyperinsulinaemic hypoglycaemia in infancy. *Semin Pediatr Surg*. 2014;23:76-82.
- Thakker RV. Multiple endocrine neoplasia type 1 (MEN1) and type 4 (MEN4). *Mol Cell Endocrinol*. 2014;386:2-15.

- The Rotterdam ESHRE/ASRM-sponsored PCOS consensus workshop group. Revised 2003 consensus on diagnostic criteria and long-term health risks related to polycystic ovary syndrome (PCOS). *Hum Reprod.* 2004;19: 41-47.
- Trikudanathan S. Polycystic ovarian syndrome. *Med Clin North Am* 2015;99:221-235.

# Review Questions

1. Under physiological circumstances, which of the following increase both insulin and glucagon secretion?

   **A.** Amino acids
   **B.** Epinephrine
   **C.** Fatty acids
   **D.** GLP-1
   **E.** Glucose

2. A 28-year-old woman has hyperglycemia (160 mg/dL, or 8.9 mM). Immune assays show that the patient has extreme hyperinsulinemia. When injected with a dose of a recombinant human insulin analog that induces mild hypoglycemia in insulin-sensitive persons, this patient develops a similar mild hypoglycemia. This patient most likely has an inborn abnormality of which of the following?

   **A.** Glucose transporter
   **B.** Grb2/SOS
   **C.** Insulin
   **D.** Insulin receptor
   **E.** Phosphatidylinositol 3-kinase

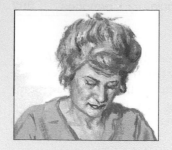

# Chapter 27 Fatty Acids, Ketone Bodies, and Ketoacidosis

## SYNOPSIS

■ Fatty acid synthesis occurs mostly in the liver after a carbohydrate-rich meal, stimulated by insulin. The lactating mammary glands also synthesize fatty acids.

■ Fatty acids are synthesized in two-carbon steps. To this end, glucose gives rise to malonyl-CoA in the cytosol (Fig. 27.1). Condensation of several malonyl-CoA yields long-chain fatty acids of about 16 carbons. These fatty acids, along with dietary fatty acids, are stored as triglycerides in adipose tissue.

■ Many cells can elongate long-chain fatty acids and introduce double bonds in the cis configuration in certain places.

■ Particularly in the fasting state and during prolonged exercise, but to a small degree also on an ongoing basis, the adipose tissue hydrolyzes triglycerides and releases fatty acids into the blood (see Fig. 27.1). Many different tissues oxidize these fatty acids to acetyl-CoA in their mitochondria. The liver also converts acetyl-CoA to ketone bodies that the brain and muscle oxidize to acetyl-CoA. Fatty acids and ketone bodies are the principal fuel for energy production during prolonged starvation; this helps the body conserve glucose for cells that depend on it, such as erythrocytes and the central nervous system.

■ Patients who have a disorder of fatty acid oxidation may develop hypoglycemia when fasting and show dysfunction of the heart and skeletal muscle.

■ Fatty acids with double bonds in the trans configuration are found in foods that are derived from ruminants or contain chemically partially hydrogenated oils.

## LEARNING OBJECTIVES

*For mastery of this topic, you should be able to do the following:*

■ Interpret common chemical notations pertaining to fatty acids, such as 18:2, $\Delta^9$, ω-3, and n-6.

■ List common sources of cis and trans unsaturated fatty acids.

■ Describe the overall purpose of fatty acid synthesis as well as its reactants and products, cellular location, tissue distribution, and regulation.

■ Describe the elongation and desaturation of fatty acids as well as their reactants and products, cellular location, and tissue distribution.

■ Define the term "essential fatty acids," list two classes of essential fatty acids, and provide an example of a fatty acid in each class.

■ Describe the overall purpose of fatty acid β-oxidation as well as its reactants and products, cellular location, tissue distribution, and regulation.

■ Describe the overall purpose of ketone body synthesis and ketone body oxidation as well as their reactants and products, cellular location, tissue distribution, and regulation.

■ Explain the terms ketosis, ketoacidosis, ketonemia, and ketonuria. Compare and contrast the metabolic basis of ketosis and ketoacidosis.

■ Describe the blood glucose concentration and the rate of endogenous glucose production in the fed and fasting state of a patient who has a deficient rate of fatty acid β-oxidation.

■ Describe the β-oxidation of very-long-chain fatty acids in peroxisomes and compare it with β-oxidation of long-chain fatty acids inside mitochondria.

■ Name the cause of X-linked adrenoleukodystrophy and the cause of Zellweger syndrome.

■ Describe the link between oxidative phosphorylation and fatty acid β-oxidation, and predict the change in the rate of β-oxidation when a tissue becomes hypoxic.

## 1. USE AND NOMENCLATURE OF FATTY ACIDS

*Fatty acids consist of a hydrophilic –COOH group and a hydrophobic tail that may contain one or more double bonds, mostly in the cis configuration. Partial chemical hydrogenation of oils generates some trans fatty acids. Fatty acids are needed for the synthesis of eicosanoids, phospholipids, and triglycerides.*

Table 27.1 lists physiologically important fatty acids along with their structure, use, and properties.

The body uses fatty acids to **anchor** certain proteins in the membrane and to form **phospholipids** for membranes, **eicosanoids** and **docosanoids** for signaling, or **triglycerides** as an energy store. Fig. 27.2 shows the structures of these compounds. Most of the fat we eat is in the form of triglycerides.

**Short-chain** fatty acids contain 5 or fewer carbons, **medium-chain** contain ~6 to 12 carbons, **long-chain** contain ~14 to 20 carbons, and **very-long-chain** fatty acids contain 22 or more carbons.

Fatty acids are **detergents** and can therefore be detrimental to cell function. Hence, fatty acids are mostly bound to **albumin** in the blood and **fatty acid binding proteins** inside cells (see Figs. 9.6 and 9.8).

Fatty acids without double bonds are called **saturated**, those with one double bond are called **monounsaturated** (**MUFA**), and those with two or more double bonds are called **polyunsaturated** (**PUFA**).

The location of **double bonds** in fatty acids can be described according to the classical chemical method for acids or a special **omega** terminology. A notation of 18:1 indicates that a fatty acid has 18 carbons and one double bond. The location of the double bond is often indicated by a notation such as $\Delta^9$, which indicates that the double bond is between carbons 9 and 10, with carbon 1 being the carbon of the carboxyl (–COOH) end of the fatty acid. In contrast, the C at the end of the hydrophobic tail of a fatty acid is called ω-1, omega-1, or n-1. For a discussion of fatty acid metabolism, the omega numbering

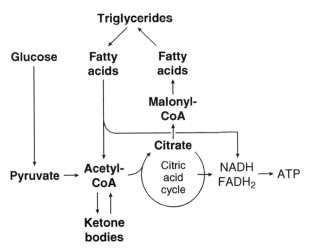

**Fig. 27.1** Overview of the synthesis, storage, mobilization, and oxidation of fatty acids.

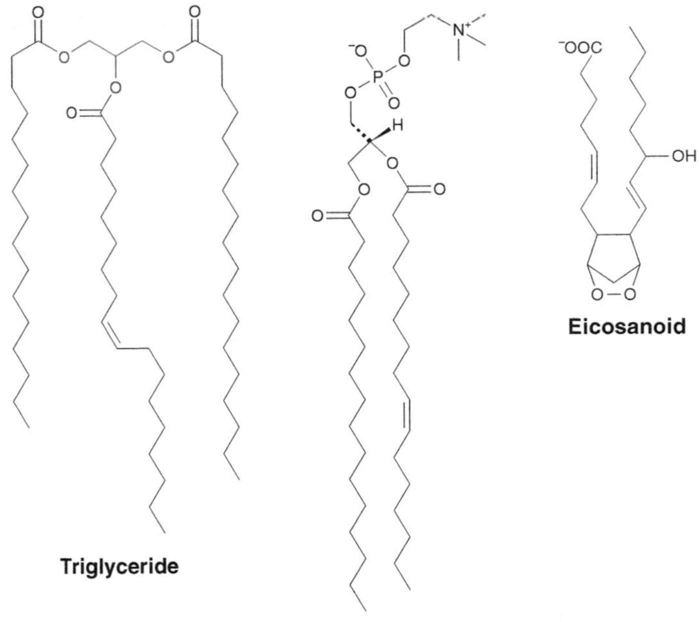

Eicosanoid

Triglyceride

Phospholipid

**Fig. 27.2** Structures of physiologically important lipids derived from fatty acids.

## Table 27.1 Physiologically Important Fatty Acids

| Structure | Fatty Acid | Number of Carbons | Number of Double Bonds | Comments |
|---|---|---|---|---|
| 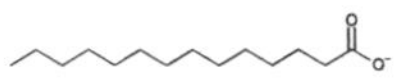 | Myristic acid | 14 | 0 | Membrane anchor for some proteins |
| 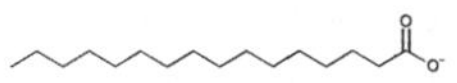 | Palmitic acid | 16 | 0 | Saturated, abundant in triglycerides, a membrane anchor for some proteins |
| 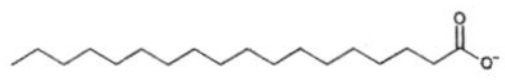 | Stearic acid | 18 | 0 | Saturated, abundant in triglycerides |
| 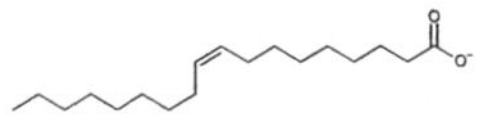 | Oleic acid | 18 | 1 | Monounsaturated, abundant in triglycerides, the main fatty acid in olive oil |
| 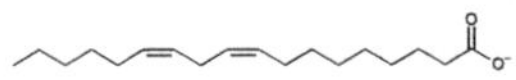 | Linoleic acid | 18 | 2 | Polyunsaturated, ω-6 |
| 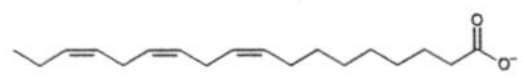 | α-Linolenic acid | 18 | 3 | Polyunsaturated, ω-3 |
| 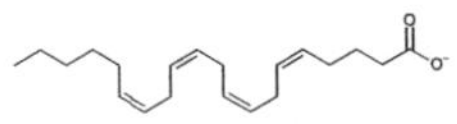 | Arachidonic acid | 20 | 4 | Polyunsaturated, ω-6, a precursor for ω-6 eicosanoids |
| 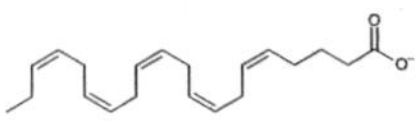 | Eicosapentaenoic acid | 20 | 5 | Often abbreviated as EPA, used as ω-3 fatty acid supplement, precursor for ω-3 eicosanoids |
| 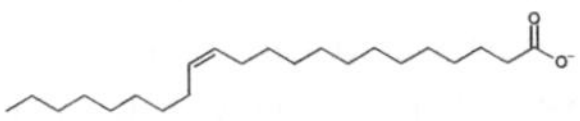 | Erucic acid | 22 | 1 | Triglycerides containing oleic and erucic acid make up "Lorenzo's oil" |
| 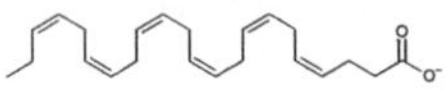 | Docosahexaenoic acid | 22 | 6 | Often abbreviated as DHA, used as ω-3 fatty acid supplement, precursor for ω-3 eicosanoids |

**Table 27.2   Fatty Acid Composition of Some Foods**

| Food | Saturated | Monounsaturated | Polyunsaturated | Trans |
|------|-----------|-----------------|-----------------|-------|
| Canola oil | 7% | 63% | 28% | 0% |
| Margarine | 19% | 48% | 30% | 18% |
| Butter | 63% | 26% | 4% | 4% |
| Cheddar cheese | 57% | 25% | 4% | 3% |
| Milk, 2% fat | 63% | 28% | 4% | 4% |
| Eggs | 33% | 38% | 20% | 0% |
| Potato chips | 10% | 56% | 24% | 0% |

Values are derived from the United States Department of Agriculture National Nutrient Database for Standard Reference Release 27.

is more convenient than the standard chemical numbering because of the way cells elongate fatty acids and introduce double bonds (see Section 3 and Figs. 27.6 and 27.7).

Double bonds in naturally occurring fatty acids are typically in the **cis** configuration, which places a kink in the hydrophobic chain (see Table 27.1 and Figs. 27.2, 27.7, and 27.8). As a result, triglycerides or phospholipids that contain cis unsaturated fatty acids have lower **melting points** than those that contain only saturated fatty acids. Trans fatty acids (see below) have physical properties that are similar to those of saturated fatty acids.

Chemically **partially hydrogenated fats** (e.g., margarine) and unsaturated fats that are heated to high temperatures (e.g., during frying) contain a mixture of cis and **trans** double bonds. The body metabolizes fatty acids with either cis or trans double bonds, but cis and trans fatty acids can affect the membrane structure, signaling pathways, and lipoprotein metabolism differently. The degree of fatty acid saturation affects the shelf life and physical characteristics of fat-containing foods. Chemical **hydrogenation** of unsaturated fatty acids reduces the number of double bonds. Fully hydrogenated fatty acids are saturated and have no double bonds. Partially hydrogenated fatty acids contain some double bonds in the trans configuration due to a side reaction that occurs during hydrogenation. In place of using partially hydrogenated oils, manufacturers can obtain desired physical properties of fats by blending fully hydrogenated and natural unsaturated oils; the resulting mixture is free of trans fatty acids. Alternatively, manufacturers can use enzymes to switch fatty acids with cis double bonds among triglycerides from a liquid oil and a solid fat; this process is called **interesterification**.

Table 27.2 lists the fatty acid composition of some foods.

## 2. FATTY ACID SYNTHESIS

*After a carbohydrate-rich meal, the liver synthesizes fatty acids from excess glucose. Glycolysis gives rise to acetyl-coenzyme A (CoA), which is converted to citrate inside mitochondria. Citrate is exported into the cytosol, where it gives rise to malonyl-CoA. Fatty acid synthase uses malonyl-CoA to generate fatty acids. This process requires NADPH, which derives from the pentose phosphate shunt and malic enzyme. Fatty acid synthesis is controlled largely by insulin, which favors glycolysis and synthesis of malonyl-CoA. Besides the liver, the lactating mammary glands can also synthesize fatty acids.*

In humans, nearly all fatty acid synthesis takes place in the **liver** and the **lactating mammary glands**. The adipose tissue carries out only a minor amount of fatty acid synthesis, but it imports fatty acids and stores them as triglycerides (see Chapter 28). A part of the **epidermis** also seems to be able to synthesize fatty acids for local use. Little is known about the regulation of fatty acid synthesis in human mammary glands and epidermis. For this reason, the following discussion is focused on the liver.

The liver synthesizes fatty acids in the fed state by using glycolysis, the oxidative branch of the pentose phosphate pathway, and a part of the citric acid cycle. These pathways provide acetyl-CoA, malonyl-CoA, and NADPH for fatty acid synthesis. Here, fatty acid synthesis is presented in two steps: first, the synthesis of malonyl-CoA, and second, the synthesis of fatty acids by fatty acid synthase.

In the liver, stimulated by **insulin**, excess dietary glucose gives rise to **malonyl-CoA** (Fig. 27.3). Insulin stimulates the formation of fructose 2,6-bisphosphate, which in turn activates phosphofructokinase 1 (see Chapter 19). This enables the liver to increase glycolysis beyond the rate that would be required for adenosine triphosphate (ATP) production alone. Pyruvate from glycolysis enters mitochondria. About half of this pyruvate is converted to acetyl-CoA and the other half to oxaloacetate; together, acetyl-CoA and oxaloacetate form **citrate**. Citrate is exported into the cytosol, where it gives rise to **acetyl-CoA**. This production of acetyl-CoA is also useful for the synthesis of cholesterol (see Chapter 29). Stimulated by insulin, **acetyl-CoA carboxylase (ACC)** converts

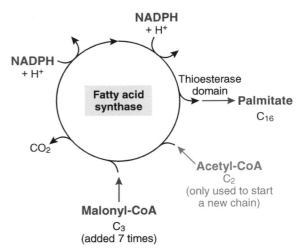

**Fig. 27.4 Synthesis of fatty acids from malonyl-coenzyme A (CoA).** Synthesis of palmitate requires acetyl-CoA plus seven cycles of malonyl-CoA addition.

**Pantothenic acid**
(vitamin B$_5$)

**Phosphopantetheine**

Attaches to fatty acid synthase

Attaches to fatty acid

**Fig. 27.5 Role of pantothenic acid in fatty acid synthesis.**

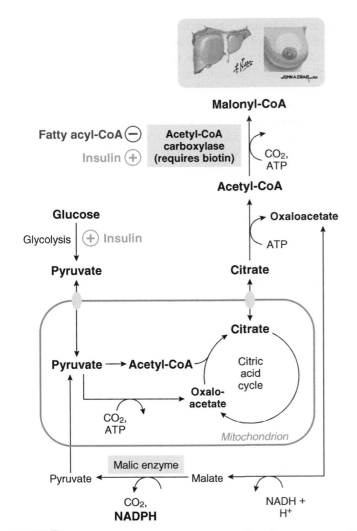

**Fig. 27.3 conversion of glucose to malonyl-coenzyme A (CoA) as part of fatty acid synthesis.** Oxaloacetate in the cytosol can be moved back into mitochondria after conversion to pyruvate with the production of NADPH. Alternatively, malate can enter mitochondria via the malate-aspartate shuttle (not shown).

acetyl-CoA to malonyl-CoA. Like other carboxylases, ACC requires the vitamin **biotin**. ACC activity is the main determinant of the rate of fatty acid synthesis. In the fasting state, lack of stimulation by insulin and inhibition by cytosolic fatty acyl-CoA attenuate ACC activity.

**Fatty acid synthase** in the cytosol produces fatty acids by the sequential addition of two-carbon units (Fig. 27.4). Fatty acid synthase is a single protein that contains multiple enzymatic activities. Synthesis starts with acetyl-CoA (two carbons), to which malonyl-CoA is added (three carbons). Decarboxylation, hydration, and reduction with NADPH yields a four-carbon fatty acid that remains bound to fatty acid synthase. Malonyl-CoA is added in further such steps. Thereby, the concentration of malonyl-CoA limits the rate of fatty acid synthesis. An arm-like domain of the synthase, called **acyl-carrier protein** (ACP), contains a **phosphopantetheine** prosthetic group (Fig. 27.5) that binds the first acetyl group and then presents the growing fatty acid chain to the different enzyme domains of the fatty acid synthase. This arrangement is thought to greatly enhance the catalytic efficiency of the enzyme. Phosphopantetheine is derived from the vitamin **pantothenic acid**. Pantothenic acid is also part of CoA (see Fig. 22.3). A thioesterase activity of the fatty acid synthase cleaves the bond between the ACP and the fatty acid when the growing fatty acid chain is about 16 carbons long.

**NADPH** for fatty acid synthesis stems from the oxidative branch of the **pentose phosphate pathway** (see Fig. 21.3) and from **malate dehydrogenase (decarboxylating)**, which is often called **malic enzyme** (see Fig. 27.3). Malic enzyme is located in the cytoplasm.

Tracer-based measurements in nonlactating humans have so far shown only a **small rate** of fatty acid de novo synthesis. This small rate was highest when volunteers consumed a diet that provided more than 80% of calories from carbohydrates.

Many **tumor** cells express markedly more fatty acid synthase than their normal counterparts. Efforts are underway to test whether inhibition of fatty acid synthase should be part of the treatment of neoplasms.

## 3. FATTY ACID ACTIVATION, ELONGATION, AND DESATURATION

*For metabolism, fatty acids must be activated with CoA to form fatty acyl-CoA. Fatty acyl-CoA can be elongated, and double bonds can be inserted between carbons that are 5, 6, or 9 carbons from the COOH end. Essential fatty acids cannot be synthesized by humans because of the position of their double bonds. Humans need these essential fatty acids for the synthesis of eicosanoids and docosanoids, which participate in short-distance signaling (see Chapter 32).*

Metabolic reactions involving fatty acids require that the fatty acids be converted to **fatty acyl-CoAs**. This is necessary for elongation, desaturation, β-oxidation (see Section 4 below), and the synthesis of triglycerides (see Chapter 28), phospholipids, and glycolipids. The formation of acyl-CoA is catalyzed by acyl-CoA synthetase and requires ATP (Fig. 27.6).

There are multiple acyl-CoA synthase isozymes that differ in subcellular location and specificity for the fatty acid chain length. An isozyme on the cytosolic surface of the endoplasmic reticulum facilitates fatty acid elongation and desaturation. Other isozymes of acyl-CoA synthetase are involved in fatty acid oxidation (see below) and are located on the mitochondrial outer membrane, as well as on the inside of the inner mitochondrial membrane.

Most cells can modify fatty acids by elongation, desaturation, or a combination of elongation and desaturation in any order. Both newly synthesized fatty acids and fatty acids acquired from the diet can be modified after activation with fatty acyl-CoA.

**Elongation** of existing fatty acids occurs by the sequential addition of two carbon units that are derived from malonyl-CoA (see Fig. 27.6) and is catalyzed by elongases on the cytosolic face of the endoplasmic reticulum. Humans have seven elongase isozymes. The structure of these enzymes likely resembles that of fatty acid synthase. Most tissues elongate fatty acids to 18 to 24 carbons, mainly for use in phospholipids and glycolipids. The skin, brain, retina, and sperm synthesize small amounts of fatty acids with up to 40 carbons; the function of these lipids is largely a mystery.

**Desaturation** can occur at carbons 5, 6, or 9 from the carboxyl end of fatty acids (see Fig. 27.7). Most double bonds are introduced into C-9 of palmitate (16:0) or stearate (18:0), thus giving rise to palmitoleate (16:1, $\Delta^9$) and oleate (18:1, $\Delta^9$), respectively. In the entire body, about 25% of the fatty acids are palmitate (16:0) and about 50% are oleate (18:1). Like fatty acid elongases, fatty acid desaturases are bound to the cytosolic face of the endoplasmic reticulum.

Since fatty acid synthase produces mostly 16-carbon saturated fatty acids, and because desaturases cannot insert double bonds beyond carbon 9, humans cannot synthesize long-chain unsaturated fatty acids with a double bond near the omega end. These fatty acids are therefore essential and must be taken up from the diet. **Linoleic acid** (18:2, $\Delta^{9,12}$) and **α-linolenic acid** (18:3, $\Delta^{9,12,15}$) are both **essential fatty acids**. Linoleic acid is an **ω-6 fatty acid**, and α-linolenic acid is an **ω-3 fatty acid** (see Fig. 27.8). Although α-linolenic acid has a double bond at position ω-6, it is never called a ω-6 fatty acid. In other words, only the double bond closest to the ω-end is considered when classifying essential fatty acids into ω-3 and ω-6.

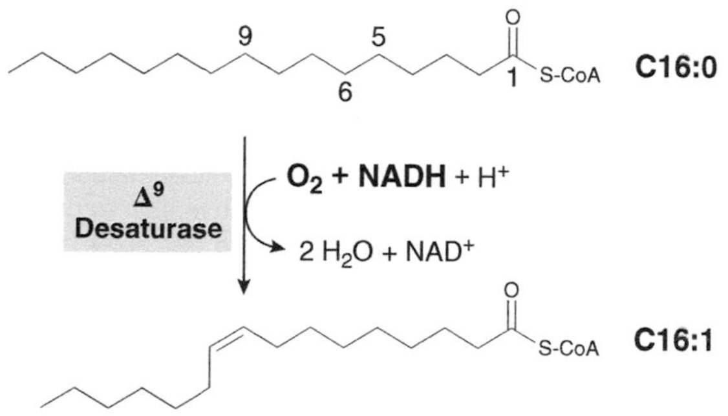

**Fig. 27.7** Desaturation of fatty acids.

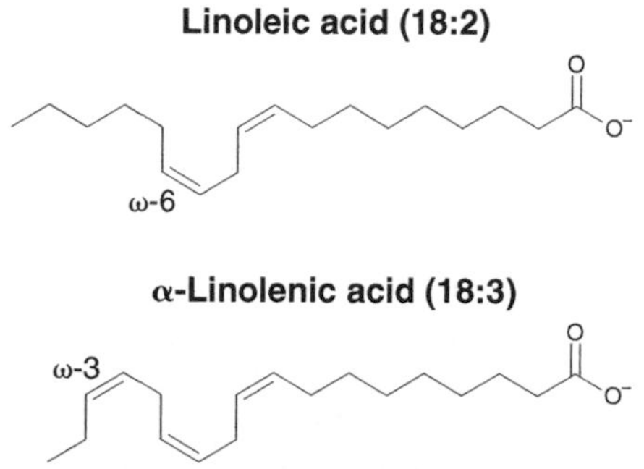

**Fig. 27.8** **Essential fatty acids linoleic and α-linolenic acid.** While this figure shows the fatty acids in extended conformations, polyunsaturated fatty acids that are part of phospholipids in membranes also assume looped conformations. The transitions between these conformations occurs rapidly.

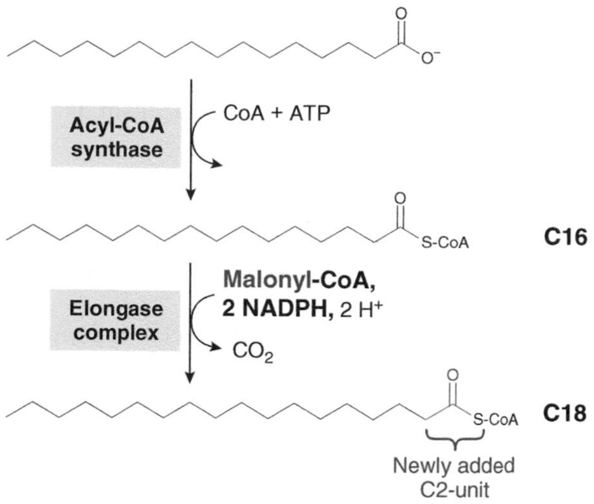

**Fig. 27.6** Activation and elongation of fatty acids.

Bacteria, algae, and plants make some ω-3 fatty acids and lots of ω-6 fatty acids, and we acquire these essential fatty acids either directly from food or indirectly via the food chain. **Table 32.1** shows the ω-3 and ω-6 fatty acid content of various foods, and **Section 1** in Chapter 32 discusses the recommended intake of these fatty acids.

Essential fatty acids can be desaturated and elongated like nonessential fatty acids. In this fashion, linoleic acid gives rise to **arachidonic acid** (20:4, still an ω-6 fatty acid; see structure in Table 27.1). Similarly, α-linolenic acid gives rise to **eicosapentaenoic acid** (**EPA**; 20:5) and **docosahexaenoic acid** (**DHA**; 22:6, still an ω-3 fatty acid). Since elongation occurs at the carboxyl-end, an ω-3 fatty acid always remains an ω-3 fatty acid, and an ω-6 fatty acid always remains an ω-6 fatty acid. The same is true for desaturation because human desaturases cannot introduce double bonds beyond carbon 9. Metabolites of ω-3 and ω-6 fatty acids act as lipid messengers or as short-lived local hormones (see Chapter 32).

Some use the term essential fatty acid only for linoleic and linolenic acid; others use it more broadly for all ω-3 and ω-6 fatty acids in the body.

## 4. FATTY ACID OXIDATION

*To enter the mitochondria, long-chain fatty acids must be converted from acyl-CoA to acyl-carnitine, a process that is inhibited by malonyl-CoA. As a result, the liver moves fatty acids into mitochondria only when the concentration of insulin is low, and muscle does it only when the concentration of adenosine monophosphate (AMP) is elevated. Mitochondria oxidize fatty acids to produce acetyl-CoA, reduced flavin adenine dinucleotide (FADH₂), and NADH. FADH₂ and NADH enter oxidative phosphorylation. Acetyl-CoA enters the citric acid cycle. The liver can also convert acetyl-CoA to ketone bodies (see Section 5 below).*

In the fasting state, the adipose tissue hydrolyzes stored triglycerides and releases the fatty acids (also called **free fatty acid**s [**FFAs**] or **nonesterified fatty acids** [**NEFAs**]) into the blood, where they bind to **albumin** (see Chapter 28). These fatty acids can be oxidized by a variety of cells.

The blood contains triglyceride-rich lipoprotein particles that can also give rise to fatty acids for use as fuel. Triglycerides are mostly contained in chylomicrons and very-low-density lipoprotein particles (see Chapter 28). These triglycerides can be hydrolyzed by lipoprotein lipase, which is tethered to the wall of capillaries in the adipose tissue and muscle and by hepatic lipase in the capillaries of the liver. Most of the resulting fatty acids enter the tissues in which they are hydrolyzed, but perhaps ~20% enter the general circulation. The rate of hydrolysis of triglycerides in lipoprotein particles changes markedly with feeding and fasting, as does the use of the resulting fatty acids. Details are provided in Chapter 28.

Fatty acid oxidation occurs primarily in muscle and liver cells, which extract the fatty acids from the blood. Fatty acid oxidation in the **liver** is maximal during a prolonged fast; in **muscle**, it is maximal during endurance exercise.

Fatty acid transporters enhance the transport of fatty acids across plasma membranes, and some of the transporters likely play a role in forming fatty acyl-CoA. As with glucose transporters (see Chapter 18), some fatty acid transporters are always inserted into the plasma membrane, and others are inserted only on demand (e.g., in the heart, when AMP-dependent protein kinase [AMPK] is active). Fatty acids that contain eight or fewer carbons can efficiently cross membranes without the need for a transporter.

Inside cells, the concentration of **malonyl-CoA** controls the uptake of fatty acids into mitochondria (Fig. 27.9). Fatty acids are transported through the cytosol bound to fatty acid–binding proteins. At the cytosolic face of the mitochondrial outer membrane, an acyl-CoA synthetase activates fatty acids to fatty acyl-CoAs. Fatty acyl-CoAs pass freely through pores in the *mitochondrial outer* membrane, but they do not cross the *inner* mitochondrial membrane. For fatty acids to cross the inner membrane, **carnitine palmitoyltransferase I (CPT-I)** must convert fatty acyl-CoAs to fatty acyl carnitines. After transport into the mitochondrial matrix, fatty acyl carnitines are converted back into fatty acyl-CoAs. Malonyl-CoA inhibits CPT-I and thus prevents the oxidation of fatty acids. As shown in Section 2, malonyl-CoA is also a substrate of fatty

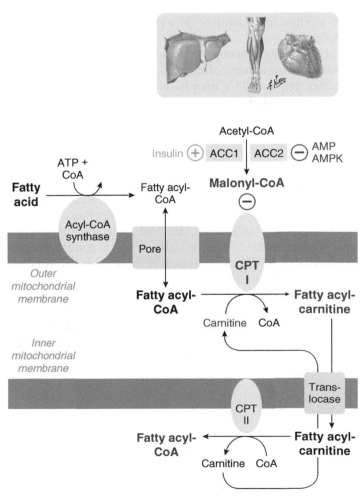

**Fig. 27.9** Malonyl-coenzyme A (CoA) regulates the transport of fatty acids across the inner mitochondrial membrane.

acid synthase and via its concentration determines the activity of fatty acid synthase.

In the liver, the concentration of malonyl-CoA depends on **insulin**, while in other cells, it depends on the cell's **energy state** (see Fig. 27.9). In the liver, insulin stimulates the formation of malonyl-CoA via **acetyl-CoA carboxylase 1 (ACC1)**. Hence, insulin inhibits the uptake of fatty acids into mitochondria and thus prevents the oxidation of fatty acids. In the fed state, newly synthesized fatty acids can therefore not enter mitochondria. In all other cells that synthesize malonyl-CoA, there is no significant de novo fatty acid synthesis, and malonyl-CoA is simply a regulator of fatty acid transport into mitochondria. In these cells, **acetyl-CoA carboxylase 2 (ACC2)** produces malonyl-CoA depending on the energy state of the cell, as reflected in the concentration of **AMP** and the activity of **AMPK**. Muscle also has an AMPK-activated malonyl-CoA decarboxylase that destroys malonyl-CoA.

**Carnitine** (Figs. 27.9 and 27.10) stems from the degradation of proteins that contain trimethylated lysine residues. These proteins are found both in the human body and in dietary meats. Vegans consume virtually no carnitine in their diet. Under normal circumstances, humans can synthesize enough carnitine and also recover enough of it from the glomerular filtrate in the kidneys; carnitine is therefore not a vitamin. Carnitine is available commercially as a supplement.

In medicine, carnitine supplementation is occasionally used in the treatment of diseases in which excess acyl-CoA depletes free CoA in a harmful way (see Section 7.1). Carnitine then leads to the formation of acyl-carnitines with a concomitant increase in available free CoA.

The **β-oxidation** of fatty acyl-CoA involves the sequential removal of two-carbon units, yielding acetyl-CoA, NADH, and FADH$_2$ (Fig. 27.11). NADH and FADH$_2$ both enter oxidative phosphorylation (see Fig. 23.3 and Section 1 in Chapter 23) and thus provide about one-third of the ATP that can be derived from the complete oxidation of fatty acids to CO$_2$. Acetyl-CoA can enter the citric acid cycle and thereby give rise to yet more NADH and FADH$_2$, as well as some guanosine triphosphate (GTP). β-Oxidation of fatty acids can occur in all cells that have mitochondria.

There are four isozymes of acyl-CoA dehydrogenase (see Fig. 27.11) that differ with respect to the range of acyl chain lengths they recognize: **very-long-chain acyl-CoA dehydrogenase (VLCAD)**, **long-chain acyl-CoA dehydrogenase (LCAD)**, **medium-chain acyl-CoA dehydrogenase (MCAD)**,

and **short-chain acyl-CoA dehydrogenase (SCAD)**. Deficiencies of these enzymes are described in Section 7.

**Fibrates** are a class of drugs that increase the rate of fatty acid β-oxidation and are used to lower the concentration of triglycerides in the blood. Fibrates act on the transcription factor **PPARα (peroxisome proliferator-activated receptor α)**, which stimulates the proliferation of peroxisomes and transcription of genes that encode proteins that play a role in fatty acid oxidation, such as CPT-I (see Fig. 27.9).

When a cell is **hypoxic**, it has a decreased capacity to oxidize fatty acids and glucose and must resort to anaerobic glycolysis (see Chapter 19). During hypoxia, the concentrations of NADH and FADH$_2$ increase, and those of NAD$^+$ and FAD decrease, which reduces the rate of fatty acid β-oxidation.

The β-oxidation of **unsaturated fatty acids** proceeds similar to that of saturated fatty acids, except that NADH is needed to reduce the double bond in additional, enzyme-catalyzed steps.

The β-oxidation of fatty acids with an **odd number of carbons** also proceeds similar to that of saturated fatty acids, but it yields a final propionyl-CoA (three carbons), which is then converted to succinyl-CoA (see Fig. 36.12). Odd-chain fatty acid metabolism produces only a minor amount of propionyl-CoA; a much greater amount is produced from the metabolism of isoleucine, valine, and methionine.

**Very-long-chain fatty acids** of 22 or more carbons are oxidized to medium-chain fatty acids in **peroxisomes** and then transferred to mitochondria (Fig. 27.12). Very-long-chain fatty acids are present primarily in neural tissue. These fatty acids enter peroxisomes, are activated, and get shortened to medium-chain acyl-CoA, thereby giving rise to acetyl-CoA and NADH. In a poorly understood manner, the

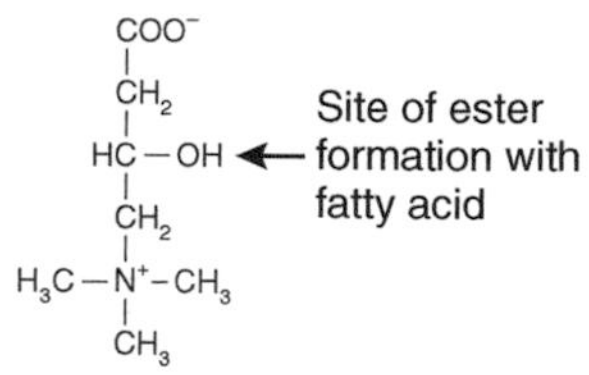

COO$^-$
|
CH$_2$
|
HC — OH ◄— Site of ester formation with fatty acid
|
CH$_2$
|
H$_3$C — N$^+$ — CH$_3$
|
CH$_3$

**Fig. 27.10** **Carnitine.**

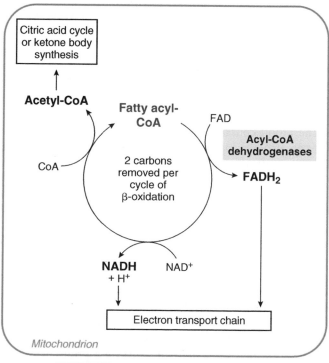

**Fig. 27.11** **β-Oxidation of fatty acids.**

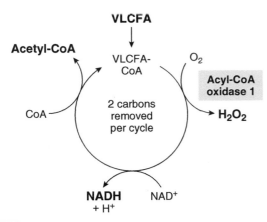

**Fig. 27.12** β-Oxidation of very-long-chain fatty acids (VLCFA) in peroxisomes. β-Oxidation of VLCFA only proceeds to a medium-chain length.

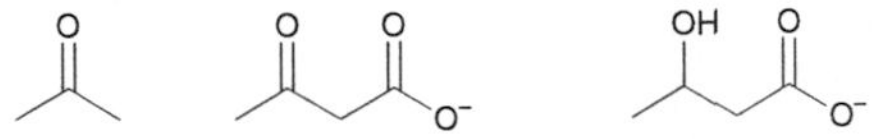

**Acetone    Acetoacetate    β-Hydroxybutyrate**

**Fig. 27.13**    Ketone bodies.

medium-chain fatty acids get transferred to mitochondria for β-oxidation as described above. The reducing power of NADH is also transferred from the peroxisomes to the mitochondria (the exact mechanism is not well understood).

# 5. SYNTHESIS AND DEGRADATION OF KETONE BODIES

*Mitochondria in the liver synthesize the ketone bodies aceto-acetate and β-hydroxybutyrate when the concentration of fatty acids in the blood is elevated. During starvation, ketone bodies are an important source of energy for several extrahepatic tissues, especially the brain, thereby reducing the body's need for glucose. Dipstick tests can provide an indication of the concentration of acetoacetate. More refined laboratory tests report the concentration of β-hydroxybutyrate.*

## 5.1. Ketone Body Synthesis (Ketogenesis)

The term ketone bodies encompasses the compounds **β-hydroxybutyrate** (also known as **3-hydroxybutyrate**), **ace-toacetate**, and **acetone** (Fig. 27.13). The acetone is produced nonenzymatically from acetoacetate through the loss of $CO_2$. Acetone is not used by the body. The liver is the only organ that produces an appreciable amount of ketone bodies.

During starvation, liver mitochondria convert some of the acetoacetyl-CoA and acetyl-CoA from the β-oxidation of fatty acids to ketone bodies (Fig. 27.14). In the liver, fatty acid oxidation occurs at a relatively rapid pace. After a 1- to 2-day fast, β-oxidation alone can supply most of the $FADH_2$ and NADH that oxidative phosphorylation needs. As a result, NADH is present at a relatively high concentration and inhibits the citric acid cycle (see Chapter 22). Then, acetyl-CoA from

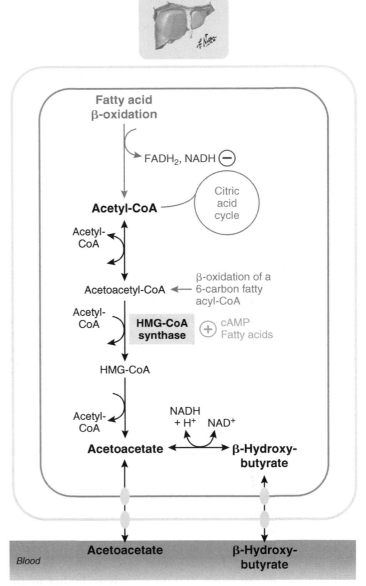

**Fig. 27.14    Synthesis of ketone bodies.** HMG-CoA, hydroxymethylglutaryl-CoA.

β-oxidation does not enter the citric acid cycle and instead gives rise to ketone bodies.

In liver mitochondria, two acetyl-CoA give rise to acetoacetyl-CoA, and the addition of a third acetyl-CoA yields HMG-CoA (3-hydroxy-3-methylglutaryl-CoA; see Fig. 27.14). Hydrolysis of HMG-CoA then returns an acetyl-CoA and gives rise to acetoacetate. NADH is used to reduce acetoacetate to β-hydroxybutyrate, such that the ratio β-hydroxybutyrate/acetoacetate reflects the $NADH/NAD^+$ ratio inside mitochondria.

There are two distinct pools of **HMG-CoA** in liver cells: a pool in mitochondria that leads to ketone body synthesis and a pool in the **cytosol** that leads to **cholesterol** synthesis (see Chapter 29).

The concentration of **acetyl-CoA** in liver mitochondria is the main controller of ketone body synthesis. The

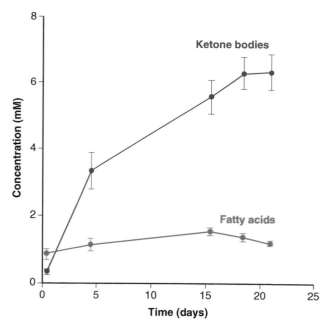

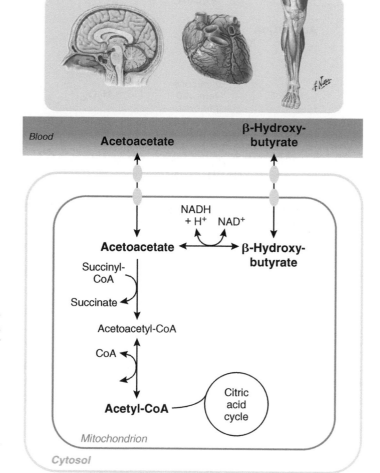

**Fig. 27.16** **Oxidation of ketone bodies.**

concentration of acetyl-CoA in the liver is considerably
higher in the fasting state than in the fed state. In addition, an
elevated concentration of **fatty acids** or **cyclic adenosine
monophosphate (cAMP)** increases the transcription of
HMG-CoA synthase, the rate-limiting enzyme of ketone
body synthesis.

In persons who consume a typical Western diet (roughly
30% of calories from fat, 15% from protein, and 55% from
carbohydrates), the concentration of ketone bodies in the
plasma substantially increases only with a fast of more than 1
day (Fig. 27.15).

## 5.2. Oxidation of Ketone Bodies by Extra-Hepatic Tissues

The brain, heart, muscle, and kidneys are particularly active
in using ketone body oxidation (also called ketolysis) for ATP
production. Degradation of ketone bodies generates acetyl-
CoA, which enters the citric acid cycle, and NADH, which
delivers reducing power to oxidative phosphorylation (Fig.
27.16). The rate of ketone body oxidation is roughly proportional to the ketone body concentration in the blood (see Fig.
27.15). The liver does not use the ketone bodies that it synthesizes because it does not possess the enzyme that transfers
CoA from succinyl-CoA to acetoacetate.

**Glucose** cannot be generated from ketone bodies. Ketone
body metabolism leads solely to the production of acetyl-
CoA, and the carbon skeleton of acetyl-CoA cannot give rise
to the carbon skeleton of glucose (see Chapter 25).

## 5.3. Laboratory Tests for Ketone Bodies

Tests for ketone bodies measure the concentration of either
acetoacetate or β-hydroxybutyrate. Most tests based on nitro-
prusside (sodium nitroferricyanide) are predominantly sensitive to acetoacetate. **Dipsticks** and **tablets** based on this test
are widely available for detecting acetoacetate in the urine,
based on the production of a dark-red color. **Clinical laboratories** measure β-hydroxybutyrate and acetoacetate separately.
There are also **test strips** for β-hydroxybutyrate that use a
small amount of capillary blood and are analyzed in a hand-
held meter.

The concentration ratio **β-hydroxybutyrate/acetoacetate**
in the blood is proportional to the concentration ratio NADH/
NAD$^+$ in mitochondria. During a normal fast in a healthy
person, there is approximately three times more β-
hydroxybutyrate than acetoacetate. Conditions that lead to
ketoacidosis, particularly alcoholic ketoacidosis, typically lead
to an increase in the NADH/NAD$^+$ ratio, and β-hydroxybutyrate
then makes up an even greater fraction of ketone bodies.
Hence, a test that measures only the acetoacetate has to be
interpreted with caution.

## 5.4. Ketosis, Ketonemia, and Ketonuria

**Ketosis** is a state of increased production of ketone bodies; this can be normal or abnormal.

In persons who consume a typical, weight-maintaining Western diet (more than about 50% of calories from carbohydrates), ketosis occurs physiologically only with prolonged **fasting** (see Fig. 27.15). Persons who consume a diet that contains little carbohydrate (e.g., an **Atkins**-type diet), particularly if it is associated with weight loss, have ongoing ketosis.

If ketosis is stable for a prolonged period, the control of lipolysis by **insulin** is usually intact.

Ketosis occurs abnormally rapidly in patients who have deficient **glycogenolysis** or **gluconeogenesis** while fasting.

**Ketonemia** is a readily detectable concentration of ketone bodies in the blood; this can be normal or abnormal.

**Ketonuria** is a readily detectable concentration of ketone bodies in the urine; this too can be normal or abnormal. Ketonuria occurs during ketosis when the rate of filtration of ketone bodies in the kidneys exceeds the rate of recovery of ketone bodies from the filtrate. Ketone bodies in the urine increase the loss of $Na^+$, $K^+$, and water in the urine.

**Ketoacidosis** is discussed in Section 7.3.

## 6. OVERVIEW OF FUEL USE BY TISSUES

Fuel use by most tissues is highly complex, depending on cell type, energy output, time, circulating hormones (especially insulin), and concentrations of circulating glucose, fatty acids, and ketone bodies. Hence, the following descriptions are simplified.

The **heart** has a relatively high need for ATP production. Between rest and exercise, this need varies about fivefold. In the heart of a resting person, typically about 60% of the ATP is produced from the β-oxidation of fatty acids, 20% from the oxidation of lactate, and 20% from the oxidation of glucose. After a meal, when the concentration of insulin is high, the heart increases its oxidation of glucose. Oxidation of ketone bodies depends on availability. Compared with other tissues, the heart has a higher rate of ketone body oxidation per gram of tissue. Oxidation of ketone bodies reduces the oxidation of fatty acids and glucose by the heart. As the heart enters high contractile activity, it makes more ATP from the oxidation of glucose than from fatty acids, because oxygen becomes limiting and ATP production from glucose requires less oxygen than ATP production from fatty acids.

**Skeletal muscles** during rest and sustained aerobic exercise use mostly fatty acids for ATP production. In contrast, the early phase of exercise is fueled mostly by the metabolism of blood glucose and muscle glycogen. Later, some of the blood glucose derives from liver glycogen and from gluconeogenesis in both the liver and kidneys.

The **brain** uses a substantial amount of energy, accounting for approximately 20% of total body oxygen use of a person who is at rest. ATP use by neurons is roughly comparable to ATP use by intensely exercising muscle. The brain contains neurons and glial cells, which support the neurons. There is some evidence that glial cells convert glucose to lactate and transfer the lactate to neurons, which oxidize lactate via acetyl-CoA in the citric acid cycle. Contrary to earlier beliefs, fatty acids readily cross the blood brain barrier. Most of the brain β-oxidation of fatty acids takes place in astrocytes, a type of glial cell that is abundant. Still, compared to the heart, the rate of fatty acid β-oxidation is low, and it is not a major source of energy for the brain. This seems to be due to low CPT-I activity (therefore a low rate of fatty acid uptake into mitochondria) and a very low activity of one of the enzymes of fatty acid oxidation. Both glial cells and neurons can oxidize ketone bodies, which can meet up to about 75% of the caloric needs of the brain; glucose must provide most of the balance of calories.

The **liver** mainly oxidizes glucose, lactate, and fatty acids; it cannot oxidize ketone bodies. Glucose oxidation is highest in the postprandial period, and fatty acid β-oxidation is highest during a prolonged fast. In the fasting state, ATP from fatty acid β-oxidation is needed to power gluconeogenesis.

**Brown fat** oxidizes both glucose and fatty acids. These adipocytes are brown because they contain a significant amount of mitochondria. Brown fat stores triglycerides. When the body temperature needs to increase, mitochondria in brown fat are partially uncoupled to generate heat in place of ATP (see Chapter 23).

## 7. METABOLIC DISTURBANCES OF FATTY ACID AND KETONE BODY METABOLISM

*A severe deficiency of any one of the enzymes of fatty acid or ketone body oxidation can produce a metabolic disorder. Of these disorders, the most common are carnitine deficiency and MCAD deficiency. X-linked adrenoleukodystrophy results from an inability to import very-long-chain fatty acids into peroxisomes for oxidation. The buildup of very-long-chain fatty acids then affects myelination, leading to neurological symptoms. In patients who have ketoacidosis, ketone body production significantly exceeds ketone body use. This life-threatening condition most commonly occurs in patients who have type 1 diabetes.*

### 7.1. Hypoketotic Hypoglycemia and Disorders of Fatty Acid Oxidation

When trying to determine the cause of hypoglycemia, physicians often first distinguish **ketotic hypoglycemia** from **hypoketotic** (or **nonketotic**) **hypoglycemia**. Patients who have ketotic hypoglycemia can evidently perform lipolysis and produce ketone bodies, which rules out excess insulin as a cause of the hypoglycemia. Patients with ketotic hypoglycemia may have a problem with glucose production. In contrast, patients who have hypoketotic hypoglycemia may have an excessive concentration of circulating insulin or a defect in lipolysis, fatty acid β-oxidation, ketone body synthesis, or ketone body oxidation. An excess of insulin is most common (see Sections 4.3, 5.3, and 7 in Chapter 39), and a defect in β-oxidation is the second most common.

Most patients who have impaired fatty acid β-oxidation develop **rhabdomyolysis** after sustained exercise. Those with more severe disease may also have hypoketotic hypoglycemia in childhood, along with liver dysfunction; those with the most severe disease may have **cardiomyopathy** at birth and die at a young age.

Patients who cannot gain much energy from fatty acid oxidation have a compensatory increase in **glucose oxidation** and impaired **gluconeogenesis**. The impairment of gluconeogenesis is due to a combination of inadequate ATP synthesis and an unusually low concentration of acetyl-CoA, which thus fails to activate pyruvate carboxylase (see Fig. 25.3). Affected patients should therefore avoid long fasts because they lead to severe nonketotic or hypoketotic hypoglycemia.

An **acquired carnitine deficiency** may develop in patients who receive an inadequate amount of carnitine in parenteral nutrition (particularly in newborns) and in patients who lose acyl-carnitines in their urine due to a disorder of fatty β-oxidation (see below).

The following disorders of fatty acid β-oxidation are inherited in an autosomal recessive fashion (i.e., patients are homozygous or compound heterozygous for pathogenic mutant alleles).

**Primary carnitine deficiency** is caused by mutant alleles of the *SLC22A5* gene, which encodes the organic cation transporter 2 (OCTN2). OCTN2 transports carnitine from the extracellular space into the cytosol. The prevalence is about 1 in 50,000 worldwide but about 1 in 300 on the Faroe Islands. Affected patients are treated with supplementary carnitine, which is then transported into cells by other organic cation transporters, although less efficiently.

**Mitochondrial trifunctional protein deficiency** is due to homozygosity or compound heterozygosity for mutant alleles of the *HADHA* or *HADHB* gene and impairs the oxidation of long-chain fatty acids. The *HADHA* and *HADHB* genes encode the α- and β-subunit, respectively, of the mitochondrial trifunctional protein.

**Multiple acyl-CoA dehydrogenase deficiencies (MADD)** is caused by a deficiency of electron transport flavoprotein (ETF) dehydrogenase, the subunits of which are encoded by the genes *ETFA*, *ETFB*, and *ETFDH*.

**Very-long-chain acyl-CoA dehydrogenase deficiency (VLCADD)** is due to mutant ACADVL alleles. About 1 in 50,000 people have this deficiency. In newborn screening (of blood) with tandem mass spectroscopy, it is detectable based on the amount of C14:1 acyl-carnitines.

**Medium-chain acyl-CoA dehydrogenase deficiency (MCADD)** is due to mutant ACADM alleles and has a prevalence of about 1 in 15,000, but some of these patients are asymptomatic. Fever often leads to metabolic decompensation, in part because the mutant enzyme shows an excessive loss of activity with increased temperature. Patients with MCADD should avoid prolonged fasting. When they are sick, they should be hospitalized and infused with glucose. In

newborn screening, the acyl-carnitine ratios C8/C10 and C8/C2 are the most reliable markers. Patients are supplemented with carnitine to normalize the concentration of free carnitine.

**Short-chain acyl-CoA dehydrogenase deficiency (SCADD)** is due to mutant ACADS alleles. The enzyme dehydrogenates butyryl-CoA (C4), and SCADD leads to an accumulation of butyric acid and butyryl-carnitine. Among newborns, the prevalence is about 1 in 45,000.

## 7.2. Diseases of Very-Long-Chain Fatty Acid Oxidation in Peroxisomes

**Zellweger syndrome** is due to a **deficiency in peroxisome biogenesis**. This deficiency causes several problems, including defective oxidation of very-long-chain fatty acids. Most affected infants die by age 6 months. The prevalence is about 1 in 50,000 births.

**X-linked adrenoleukodystrophy** is due to defective transport of very-long-chain fatty acids into peroxisomes. The defective transporter is called adrenoleukodystrophy protein (ALDP), which is encoded by the *ABCD1* gene. The disease affects at least about 1 in 20,000 males and about 1 in 14,000 females, whereby females have a milder form of the disease. Very-long-chain fatty acids accumulate primarily in the central nervous system and the adrenal cortex. The disorder leads to impaired function of the adrenal cortex (which produces cortisol and the blood pressure–regulating steroid aldosterone) and to demyelination of the nervous system. Affected patients show an elevated concentration of very-long-chain fatty acids in the blood. Diagnosis is typically based on symptoms and measurements of the concentration of C22:0, C24:0, and C26:0 fatty acids in plasma.

In males, the onset of symptoms of X-linked adrenoleukodystrophy varies greatly; the most severe form shows an onset at about 7 years of age, while a milder adult form shows onset around 30 years of age. About half of all heterozygous females develop some neurologic symptoms, usually during adult life.

There is currently no highly effective treatment for adrenoleukodystrophy. Some patients might delay the onset of symptoms with the consumption of **Lorenzo's oil**, a mixture of four parts triglyceride that is made from oleic acid and one part of triglyceride that is made from erucic acid (22:1, $\Delta^{13}$).

## 7.3. Ketoacidosis

**Ketoacidosis** is a ketosis that is associated with ketone body production well in excess of ketone body use so that the blood is depleted of **bicarbonate** and has an abnormally low **pH**.

Acetoacetic acid and β-hydroxybutyric acid both have pK values below five. Hence, in blood, they are mostly deprotonated. When acetoacetic acid and β-hydroxybutyric acid are transported from the liver into the blood, they release their protons ($H^+$) into the blood. The protons are buffered by bicarbonate ($HCO_3^-$), generating $H_2CO_3$, which is in equilibrium with $CO_2$. $CO_2$ can be lost via the lungs. When peripheral tissues take up ketone bodies from the blood, they take up acetoacetic acid and β-hydroxybutyric acid. Hence, the combination of secretion and uptake of acetoacetic acid and β-hydroxybutyric acid does not affect the pH of the blood. However, when the kidneys fail to recover filtered acetoacetate and β-hydroxybutyrate, blood pH is not restored. It is estimated that the liver can produce ketone bodies at about five times the rate at which the kidneys can excrete protons. For this reason, if ketone bodies are not oxidized, bicarbonate in the blood can be used up within as little as 3 hours.

Patients who have ketoacidosis have such a high concentration of circulating acetoacetate that they produce a noticeable amount of **acetone** through the spontaneous decarboxylation of acetoacetate. When a patient's breath smells of acetone (the traditional nail-polish remover), the patient's blood likely contains a high concentration of ketone bodies.

Ketoacidosis is always abnormal and may be life-threatening. In practice, a finding of ketoacidosis most often implies that the feedback inhibition of lipolysis by insulin does not work (i.e., there is **runaway lipolysis**; see Chapter 28).

Patients with **type 1 diabetes** have virtually no functioning β-cells and develop ketoacidosis when they do not get any (or only a grossly inadequate amount) exogenous insulin. The lack of insulin leads to runaway lipolysis, which is then followed by ketone body synthesis far in excess of ketone body consumption (see also Section 2.1 in Chapter 39). Patients with type 1 diabetes and ketoacidosis also have pronounced hyperglycemia; this combination of metabolic abnormalities is called **diabetic ketoacidosis**. The high concentration of glucose diminishes the rate of ketone body oxidation. In contrast, patients with **type 2 diabetes** have β-cells with impaired (not abolished) insulin secretion; these patients typically secrete enough insulin to attenuate lipolysis. Hence, type 2 diabetic patients only very rarely develop ketoacidosis (see Chapter 39).

A diagnosis of **diabetic ketoacidosis** typically involves finding the following abnormal **laboratory data**: blood glucose greater than 200 mg/dL (>11 mM), blood pH less than 7.3 or bicarbonate less than 15 mEq/L, ketonemia (generally ≥3 mM β-hydroxybutyrate), and ketonuria (generally +2 or greater on urine dipstick). The β-hydroxybutyrate/acetoacetate ratio is often approximately 3 (i.e., normal).

The typical patient who has **alcoholic ketoacidosis** is a regular abuser of alcohol, is malnourished, and has gone through an episode of alcohol binge drinking that ended in vomiting, followed by 2 to 3 days of fasting and low or no fluid intake. The patient is often alert and lucid. The concentration of glucose may be low, normal, or high (though not nearly as high as in diabetic ketoacidosis). In patients with alcoholic ketoacidosis, the concentration ratio β-hydroxybutyrate/acetoacetate is approximately 7 (i.e., two to three times higher than in diabetic ketoacidosis, because alcohol metabolism generates a high NADH:NAD⁺ ratio). Nitroprusside-based ketone body screening therefore must be interpreted with caution, and a laboratory determination of β-hydroxybutyrate is needed for an accurate assessment of ketoacidosis. The concentration of lactate is usually elevated, as well as the lactate/pyruvate ratio (see Chapters 25 and 30). In emergency

departments, alcoholic ketoacidosis is much less commonly seen than acute alcohol intoxication.

## SUMMARY

- A fatty acid designation of $18:3, \Delta^{9,12,15}$ indicates a fatty acid with 18 carbons and three double bonds, which start at positions 9, 12, and 15 from the carboxyl end and extend to carbons 10, 13, and 16, respectively. In an alternative nomenclature, these double bonds are at positions ω-9, ω-6, and ω-3 (or n in place of ω), and the fatty acid is therefore classified as a ω-3 fatty acid (but not as a ω-6 fatty acid).

- Humans make only cis unsaturated fatty acids. Trans unsaturated fatty acids are found in chemically partially hydrogenated fats and in foods made from ruminant meat or milk.

- After a carbohydrate-rich meal, stimulated by insulin, the liver uses excess glucose to synthesize saturated 16-carbon fatty acids. In the grand scheme of fuel metabolism, the rate of fatty acid de novo synthesis in the liver appears to be very small. The production of malonyl-CoA by acetyl-CoA carboxylase (ACC) is the rate-limiting step. The adipose tissue synthesizes a much smaller amount of fatty acids than the liver. However, the mammary glands synthesize an appreciable amount of fatty acids during lactation. Fatty acid synthesis requires NADPH, which derives from the oxidative branch of the pentose phosphate pathway, and from the malic enzyme, which uses malate that is exported from mitochondria.

- Most cells can elongate fatty acids to about 24 carbons and can introduce double bonds at positions 5, 6, or 9. Skin, brain, and retina can produce fatty acids as long as 40 carbons. Fatty acids with double bonds that humans cannot make are essential fatty acids of the ω-3 or ω-6 type. Essential fatty acids, such as linoleic or α-linolenic acid, can be elongated and further desaturated. Thus, linoleic acid is converted to arachidonic acid, whereas α-linolenic acid gives rise to eicosapentaenoic acid (EPA) and docosahexaenoic acid (DHA).

- Significant fatty acid β-oxidation for the production of ATP takes place in most tissues, but not in the brain. Fatty acid β-oxidation yields NADH, FADH₂, and acetyl-CoA. At the cellular level, the rate of fatty acid β-oxidation is controlled mostly by malonyl-CoA, which inhibits carnitinepolmitoyl transferase I (CPT-I) activity, a key determinant of fatty acid transport into mitochondria. In the liver, insulin-induced synthesis of malonyl-CoA ensures that fatty acids are oxidized only in the fasting state but not in the fed state. In other cells, the energy state regulates the concentration of malonyl-CoA such that energy depletion favors the transport and oxidation of fatty acids.

- The term *ketone bodies* lumps together acetoacetate, β-hydroxybutyrate, and acetone; acetone is the product of a spontaneous decay reaction. The liver makes a significant amount of ketone bodies when the concentration of circulating fatty acids is high, such as after a 2-day or longer fast.

The brain uses ketone bodies in place of glucose; this significantly reduces the body's need for gluconeogenesis during a prolonged fast.

- Ketoacidosis occurs when ketone body production significantly exceeds ketone body use such that the concentration of bicarbonate and the pH of the blood become abnormally low. Ketoacidosis is seen in patients who have type 1 diabetes and a grossly inadequate amount of insulin. On occasion it is also seen in alcohol-addicted patients who are fasting.
- The milder disorders of impaired fatty acid oxidation manifest with rhabdomyolysis, the moderately severe ones also with hypoketotic hypoglycemia, and the most severe ones also with cardiomyopathy and early death. Newborn screening for inherited disorders of fatty acid oxidation is based on absolute concentrations and/or concentration ratios of fatty acyl-carnitines.
- Very long-chain fatty acids accumulate in patients who cannot degrade these fatty acids in peroxisomes, such as patients who have Zellweger syndrome or X-linked adrenoleukodystrophy.

## FURTHER READING

- Kersten S. Integrated physiology and systems biology of PPARα. *Mol Metab.* 2014;3:354-371.
- Kihara A. Very long-chain fatty acids: elongation, physiology and related disorders. *J Biochem.* 2012;152:387-395.
- *Lorenzo's Oil* is a 1992 film dramatization of Lorenzo Odone's parents' quest for a treatment of his X-linked adrenoleukodystrophy. This is a wonderful example of patient activism.

# Review Questions

1. After a high-carbohydrate meal, a patient's liver synthesizes palmitate de novo. Which of the following is the main factor that prevents the β-oxidation of newly synthesized palmitate in liver mitochondria?

   A. A high concentration of malonyl-CoA inhibits the activity of CPT-I.
   B. The arm of the ACP is too short to allow fatty acids access to enzymes of fatty acid β-oxidation.
   C. The high concentration of insulin prevents the insertion of a fatty acid transporter into the inner mitochondrial membrane.
   D. The liver does not express an enzyme that uses succinyl-CoA to activate fatty acids.

2. A blood sample from a patient shows a bicarbonate concentration of 7 mEq/L (normal, 22-28 mEq/L) and a concentration of β-hydroxybutyrate of 18 mM (normal, < 0.5 mM). This patient has which of the following?

   A. Ketoacidosis, ketonemia, and ketonuria
   B. Ketoacidosis without ketonuria
   C. Ketonemia and ketosis without acidosis
   D. Ketonuria and ketosis without acidosis

3. After an accident, a 45-year-old patient was hospitalized and underwent surgery. Subsequently, the patient felt too ill to consume any food or calorie-containing beverages. Two days after admission, which one of the following scenarios best describes some of the pathways that are active in this patient's liver? (0 = no or very little activity, + = active)

| Option | Fatty Acid Synthesis | Ketone Body Synthesis | Ketone Body Oxidation |
|--------|----------------------|-----------------------|-----------------------|
| A. | 0 | 0 | + |
| B. | 0 | + | 0 |
| C. | 0 | + | + |
| D. | + | 0 | + |
| E. | + | + | 0 |

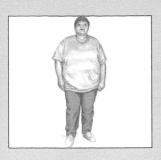

# Chapter 28

# Triglycerides and Hypertriglyceridemia

## SYNOPSIS

■ A triglyceride, also known as triacylglycerol, consists of glycerol that is esterified with three fatty acids.

■ Triglycerides are a major part of our diet and a major source of energy. They are stored in adipose tissue. They serve as a fuel during fasting and prolonged exercise.

■ Triglycerides are too hydrophobic to cross cell membranes. Moving triglycerides across cell membranes can be accomplished in two ways: (1) hydrolysis, transport of components, and re-esterification; and (2) secretion inside a lipoprotein particle into the extracellular space.

■ Dietary triglycerides are digested in the intestinal lumen, resynthesized in intestinal epithelial cells, and then released into the lymph in the form of chylomicrons.

■ The liver synthesizes some fatty acids from excess dietary carbohydrate and esterifies these fatty acids with glycerol to form triglycerides. The liver also receives a substantial amount of fatty acids from the blood. The liver esterifies some of these fatty acids into triglycerides. The liver packages triglycerides into very-low-density lipoproteins, which it releases into the blood.

■ Inside adipocytes, triglycerides are stored as lipid droplets. During times of fasting, these triglycerides are hydrolyzed, and the resulting fatty acids and glycerol are released into the blood.

■ Triglycerides make up about 40% to 50% of the calories in breast milk. The mammary glands synthesize triglycerides from fatty acids that are derived from the diet, from de novo synthesis in the liver and the mammary glands, and from hydrolysis of triglycerides in the adipose tissue.

■ The absorption of lipid-soluble vitamins follows much of the same mechanism as the absorption of triglycerides.

■ An abnormally high concentration of triglycerides is common. It is a risk factor for arteriosclerotic vascular disease. Lifestyle modification is a cornerstone of treatment.

## LEARNING OBJECTIVES

*For mastery of this topic, you should be able to do the following:*
■ Describe the hydrolysis of triglycerides in the intestine and the absorption of the resulting products.
■ Describe the mechanism of action and use of the drug orlistat.
■ Describe the purpose of triglyceride synthesis as well as its reactants and products, cellular location, tissue distribution, and regulation.
■ Compare and contrast the lipoproteins that transport triglycerides between tissues.
■ Describe the overall purpose of lipolysis as well as its reactants and products, cellular location, tissue distribution, and regulation. Describe the transport of fatty acids in the blood.
■ Distinguish the effects of feeding, fasting, and exercise on triglyceride metabolism.
■ Describe how triglycerides are formed and delivered to milk in the lactating mammary gland.

■ List risk factors for hypertriglyceridemia, fatty liver, and hypertriglyceridemia-induced pancreatitis.
■ Identify the vitamin deficiencies that may develop in a patient who has fat malabsorption. Describe the resulting symptoms.

## 1. STRUCTURE AND ROLE OF TRIGLYCERIDES

*Triglycerides are esters of glycerol with fatty acids. Triglycerides in the diet are a major part of our intake of calories. Triglycerides in the adipose tissue are an energy store that is mostly used in prolonged exercise and during a long-term calorie deficit.*

A **triglyceride** (**triacylglycerol**) consists of a glycerol with each of the three of its hydroxyl groups covalently linked to a fatty acid via an ester bond (Fig. 28.1). Each hydroxyl group of glycerol can carry a different fatty acid.

The most common fatty acids in triglycerides in adipose tissue are usually palmitic acid (C16:0) and oleic acid (C18:1). The fractions of the diverse fatty acids depend on dietary intake. The nomenclature of fatty acids is explained in Section 1 of Chapter 27, and Table 27.1 cites names and corresponding chemical structures.

Triglycerides move across cell membranes either inside lipoprotein particles or as products of triglyceride hydrolysis. Triglycerides are highly hydrophobic and essentially insoluble in water, where they aggregate and form lipid droplets. There is no transporter for single triglyceride molecules. Hepatocytes and epithelial cells of the intestine can secrete lipoprotein particles that contain a core lipid droplet with triglycerides. Otherwise, the translocation of triglycerides is accomplished by hydrolysis to fatty acids and monoglycerides or glycerol, transport of fatty acids (and monoglycerides in the intestine), and the re-esterification of fatty acids into triglycerides inside cells.

Triglycerides are the major storage form of fatty acids. By **weight**, triglycerides yield about six times more adenosine triphosphate (ATP) than glycogen.

Triglycerides are largely ingested with the **diet**, and a small amount is also **synthesized** in the liver from excess dietary carbohydrate (Fig. 28.2). After a meal, triglycerides are largely stored in the adipose tissue.

During protracted exercise or a fast, the adipose tissue hydrolyzes triglycerides to glycerol and fatty acids, which are released into the blood (Fig. 28.3). Fatty acid β-oxidation is a major source of energy for cells that contain mitochondria (see Chapter 27), except the brain. The liver can convert fatty acids to ketone bodies. The brain and other organs can use ketone bodies as a source of energy.

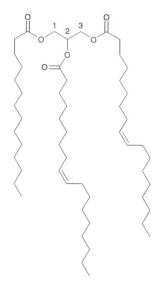

**Fig. 28.1** **Structure of a triglyceride.** Red, glycerol; black, fatty acids.

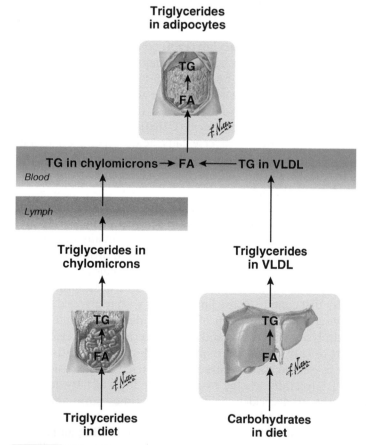

**Fig. 28.2** **Overview of the formation of triglyceride (TG) deposits in the adipose tissue.** FA. Fatty acids; VLDL, very-low-density lipoprotein.

## 2. DIGESTION OF TRIGLYCERIDES AND ABSORPTION OF FATTY ACIDS AND MONOGLYCERIDES

*In the digestive tract, catalyzed largely by enzymes from the pancreas, triglycerides are hydrolyzed into fatty acids and*

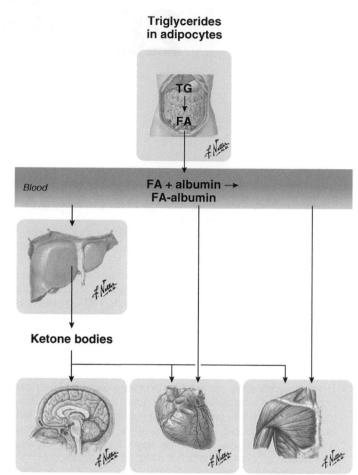

**Fig. 28.3** **Overview of lipolysis and the use of fatty acids.** FA, fatty acids; TG, triglycerides.

*monoglycerides. Similarly, the hydrolysis of phospholipids and cholesteryl esters gives rise to fatty acids. Bile, released from the gallbladder, facilitates the hydrolysis and absorption of dietary lipids.*

### 2.1. Partial Digestion of Triglycerides in the Stomach

The human diet contains a sizable fraction of water-insoluble molecules. The term **lipid** refers to the collection of these water-insoluble compounds, which include phospholipids, cholesterol, cholesteryl esters, glycolipids, and fat-soluble vitamins. About 90% of the lipids in the diet are triglycerides.

Digestion of triglycerides begins with the action of lingual and gastric **lipases**. Lipases are enzymes that hydrolyze the ester bonds between fatty acids and an alcohol, such as glycerol or cholesterol. Lingual and gastric lipases originate from the lingual glands of the mouth and the chief cells of the stomach, respectively. These lipases generate diglycerides and fatty acids, and they account for about 20% of triglyceride hydrolysis in the digestive tract. The fatty acids act as detergents, which help to break up lipid globules into smaller particles that are more readily digested by pancreatic enzymes.

## 2.2. Digestion of Triglycerides in the Intestine

The bulk of lipid digestion occurs in the intestine. When lipids and proteins reach the intestine, they stimulate endocrine cells in the lower duodenum and in the jejunum to release the peptide hormone cholecystokinin (CCK) into the blood. CCK stimulates the **pancreas** to secrete digestive enzymes. CCK also causes the **gallbladder** to contract, which propels bile into the duodenum. **Bile** contains mixed micelles composed of bile salts, phospholipids, and cholesterol (see Section 4.1 in Chapter 29).

In the intestine, **pancreatic lipase** hydrolyzes fatty acids from positions 1 and 3 of the triglycerides (Fig. 28.4). Pancreatic lipase requires the protein **colipase,** which is also secreted by the pancreas. Colipase anchors lipase to the surfaces of lipid particles that are emulsified by bile salts. Pancreatic lipase yields **fatty acids** and **monoglycerides**, which enter mixed micelles that also contain bile salts, cholesterol, phospholipids, and the lipid-soluble vitamins A, D, E, and K.

The weight-loss drug **orlistat** inhibits pancreatic lipase when it reaches the intestine. At the recommended doses, orlistat prevents about a third of the dietary triglycerides from being digested.

In the intestine, **phospholipase A₂** and **lysophospholipase** hydrolyze dietary **glycerophospholipids**, producing fatty acids and glycerophosphodiesters with a phospholipid head group (e.g., glycerophosphocholine; see Figs. 11.1 and 11.2). Lysophospholipids are phospholipids that have lost one of their constituent fatty acids due to phospholipase A1 or A2 activity. The pancreas secretes both prophospholipase A₂ and lysophospholipase. In the intestinal lumen, trypsin cleaves prophospholipase A₂, to produce active phospholipase A₂.

**Carboxyl ester lipase** hydrolyzes fatty acids from a wide variety of fatty acid–containing lipids, including **cholesteryl esters** (see Section 1 in Chapter 29). Cholesteryl esters make up about 10% of the total dietary cholesterol.

**Bile salt–stimulated lipase** is a component of breast milk. In breastfed infants, it supplements the action of pancreatic enzymes. Since the activity of this enzyme depends on the presence of bile salts, it does not digest the triglycerides in milk until they reach the intestine. Infants receive about 50% of their calories from triglycerides.

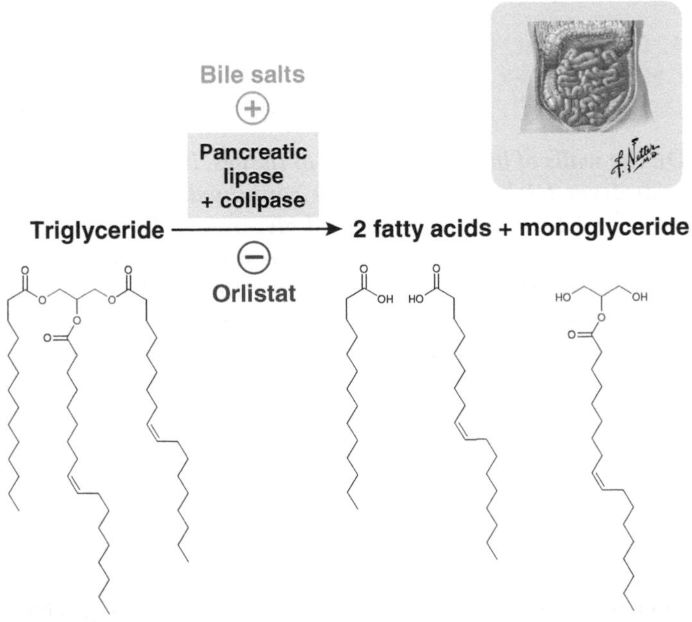

## 2.3. Absorption of Fatty Acids and Monoglycerides

The jejunum absorbs nearly all of the fatty acids and monoglycerides from mixed micelles via facilitated and passive diffusion across the plasma membrane of the epithelial cells. Fatty acids and likely also monoglycerides are substrates of **fatty acid transporters**. Cholesterol enters intestinal epithelial cells with the help of the Niemann-Pick C1–like (NPC1L1) carrier-mediated sterol transporter (see Fig. 29.1). The bile salts are absorbed in the ileum and return to the liver via the enterohepatic circulation (see Fig. 29.10).

Inside the epithelial cells of the intestine, fatty acids bind to **fatty acid binding proteins**. This increases the effective solubility of fatty acids and protects the cell from the detergent effects of the fatty acids.

## 3. PRODUCTION AND EXPORT OF TRIGLYCERIDES FROM THE INTESTINE, LIVER, AND MAMMARY GLANDS

*Intestinal epithelial cells resynthesize triglycerides and release them into the lymphatic system inside chylomicrons. The liver and the mammary glands produce triglycerides primarily from fatty acids in the blood. The liver exports its triglycerides inside very-low-density lipoproteins (VLDLs). The mammary glands export triglycerides into breast milk in the form of fat globules that are surrounded by a membrane.*

## 3.1. Triglycerides Made in the Intestine

Intestinal epithelial cells resynthesize triglycerides from absorbed fatty acids and monoglycerides (Fig. 28.5; see also Fig. 28.2).

On the cytosolic surface of the endoplasmic reticulum, an acyl-coenzyme A (acyl-CoA) synthetase conjugates fatty acids with CoA to form acyl-CoAs, a process that is often called

Bile salts
⊕

Pancreatic lipase + colipase

Triglyceride ⟶ 2 fatty acids + monoglyceride

⊖
Orlistat

**Fig. 28.4** **Digestion of triglycerides in the lumen of the intestine.**

| Mono-glyceride | + | 2 Fatty acyl-CoA | ⟶ | Tri-glyceride | Epithelial cells of the intestine |
|---|---|---|---|---|---|
| Glycerol 3-phosphate | + | 3 Fatty acyl-CoA | ⟶ | Tri-glyceride | Liver, adipose tissue |

**Fig. 28.5** **Synthesis of triglycerides.**

**fatty acid activation** (Fig. 27.6). Such activation of fatty acids is ubiquitous. It also happens in the endoplasmic reticulum (ER) in preparation for fatty acid elongation and desaturation, and on mitochondria for β-oxidation (see Fig. 27.9).

Intestinal epithelial cells use two pathways for the synthesis of triglycerides: they mostly produce them from monoglycerides and to a lesser extent from glycerol 3-phosphate (see Fig. 28.5). To this end, a monoglyceride is esterified with two fatty acyl-CoA, and glycerol 3-phosphate is esterified with three fatty acyl-CoA.

Intestinal epithelial cells use the **microsomal triglyceride transfer protein** (MTP) to assemble chylomicrons from **apolipoprotein B-48**, triglycerides, phospholipids, cholesterol, and cholesteryl esters. The chylomicrons are exported into the lymphatic system and from there reach the subclavian vein via the thoracic duct.

Apolipoprotein B-48 is encoded by the *APOB* gene and contains only 48% of the full-length amino acid sequence, due to **mRNA editing**. Apolipoprotein B-100 contains the full amino acid sequence and is synthesized from unedited mRNA. The editing involves the deamination of a specific C in the mRNA to a U, which creates an in-frame stop codon. Compared with apolipoprotein B-100, apolipoprotein B-48 is missing the protein domain that can bind to the LDL-receptor.

In the blood, chylomicrons gain **apolipoprotein C-II**, a small protein that is necessary for lipoprotein lipase activity, and **apolipoprotein E**, which is necessary for the uptake of chylomicron remnants by the liver. Apolipoprotein C-II is mostly made in the liver and intestine. Chylomicrons gain apolipoprotein C-II primarily from high-density lipoprotein (HDL). Apolipoprotein E in the blood mainly stems from the liver, and chylomicrons acquire it from HDL too.

**Fatty acids** of eight or fewer carbons pass through the intestinal epithelial cells and enter the portal vein directly (not via chylomicrons).

## 3.2. Triglycerides Made in the Liver

The liver produces triglycerides from glycerol 3-phosphate and fatty acids that it acquired from the blood or (to a lesser extent) synthesized de novo from excess glucose (see Chapter 27 and Figs. 27.3, 28.2, and 28.5).

For triglyceride synthesis, fatty acids are activated by a conversion to acyl-CoAs (see Fig. 27.6).

The liver produces triglycerides mainly through the esterification of glycerol 3-phosphate with three fatty acyl-CoAs (see Fig. 28.5). Glycerol 3-phosphate is formed from dihydroxyacetone phosphate, an intermediate of glycolysis and gluconeogenesis, or from glycerol, a degradation product of triglyceride hydrolysis in the blood (see Section 4) and inside adipocytes (see Section 5.1).

Hepatocytes export triglycerides into the blood inside **VLDL** that contain **apolipoprotein B-100**. Similar to the intestine (see Section 3.1), the MTP is needed for the assembly of a VLDL. VLDL contains a monolayer membrane that consists of phospholipids and cholesterol. Apolipoprotein B-100

covers a sizable part of the surface of a mature VLDL. The interior of VLDL contains triglycerides and cholesteryl esters in a ratio of approximately 5:1.

Lipoprotein particles in the blood are named based on their properties in **density** gradient centrifugation. Particles with the highest ratio of protein to lipid are the densest and those with the lowest ratio have the lowest density. Accordingly, HDL (see Section 3.2 in Chapter 29) are the most dense, followed by low-density lipoproteins (LDL; see Section 4.1), intermediate-density lipoproteins (IDL; see Section 4.1), VLDL, and chylomicrons.

In the blood, VLDL acquires **apolipoprotein C-II** and **apolipoprotein E** from HDL. A similar process takes place with chylomicrons (see Section 3.1).

## 3.3. Triglycerides Made in the Lactating Mammary Glands

Human breast milk contains about 4% (weight/volume) triglycerides, which make up about half of the calories in milk. These triglycerides are produced by the alveolar cells of the lactating mammary gland via the same glycerol 3-phosphate pathway as in the liver (see Section 3.2 and Fig. 28.5). As triglycerides are synthesized in secretory cells, they coalesce into lipid droplets in the cytosol that move to the apical plasma membrane. There, the droplets are enveloped by the cell membrane to form membrane-bound milk fat globules, which are then secreted.

The lactating mammary glands obtain the fatty acids for triglyceride production from albumin-bound fatty acids in the blood, from chylomicrons and VLDL, and from de novo synthesis. The rate of fatty acid de novo synthesis (from glucose) is highest after a high-carbohydrate meal and lowest during fasting in women who habitually consume a high-fat diet.

## 4. REMOVAL OF TRIGLYCERIDES FROM CHYLOMICRONS AND VLDL, AND DEPOSITION OF TRIGLYCERIDES INSIDE ADIPOCYTES

*On the walls of blood capillaries of tissues, lipoprotein lipase hydrolyzes triglycerides that are contained inside chylomicrons or VLDL to fatty acids and glycerol. In the capillaries of the liver, hepatic lipase catalyzes a similar reaction. Most of the fatty acids enter the cells near the capillaries where they were produced, but a fraction is swept away in the blood for uptake by other tissues. In the fed state, the adipose tissue esterifies fatty acids to triglycerides, which it stores.*

## 4.1. Removal of Triglycerides From Chylomicrons and VLDL

The capillaries of many tissues contain membrane-anchored **lipoprotein lipase** that hydrolyzes triglycerides inside **chylomicrons** and **VLDL** to fatty acids and glycerol (Fig. 28.6). Lipoprotein lipase is found primarily in the capillaries of the adipose tissue, muscle, and lactating mammary glands. The

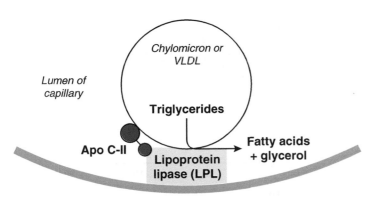

**Fig. 28.6** **Removal of triglycerides from chylomicrons and VLDL.** Apo C-II, apolipoprotein C-II.

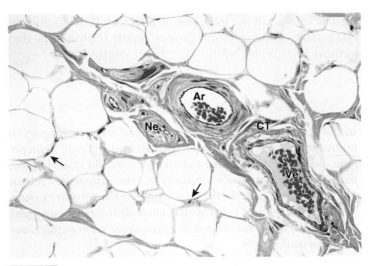

**Fig. 28.7** **Structure of white adipose tissue.** Masson trichrome stain. Arrows point to capillaries. Ar, arteriole; CT, connective tissue; Ne, nerve fascicle; Ve, venule.

lipase is synthesized inside adipocytes and myocytes and then migrates through endothelial cells that form the wall of blood capillaries. In the lumen of the capillaries, the glycosylphosphatidylinositol-anchored HDL-binding protein (GPIHBP1) positions lipoprotein lipase in the plasma membrane of endothelial cells.

In adipose tissue (but not in muscle), insulin stimulates lipoprotein lipase synthesis and thereby increases the delivery of fatty acids for triglyceride storage in the fed state. In muscle, a variety of factors, including increased activity of AMP-dependent protein kinase (AMPK) lead to increased lipoprotein lipase activity in the lumen of the capillaries.

For activity, lipoprotein lipase requires **apolipoprotein C-II** on the surface of a lipoprotein particle. The resulting fatty acids mostly enter nearby cells and to a small degree remain in the blood, bound to serum albumin. **Glycerol** that is produced remains in the blood and is then taken up by the liver and converted to dihydroxyacetone phosphate for entry into glycolysis or gluconeogenesis.

Through the removal of triglycerides by lipoprotein lipase, chylomicrons become **chylomicron remnants**, and VLDL become **IDL**, also known as VLDL remnants. As a result of the loss of triglycerides from VLDL, IDL contain about the same weight of triglycerides as of cholesterol and cholesteryl esters.

Chylomicron remnants (but not chylomicrons) are small enough to enter the space of Disse in the liver, where **hepatic lipase** removes more triglycerides. Hepatic lipase is made in hepatocytes, exported, and then bound to heparan sulfate on the cell surface. **Apolipoprotein E** on **chylomicron remnants** binds to the **LDL receptor-related protein 1 (LRP1)** on hepatocytes and the remnants enter via endocytosis. Lysosomes then degrade the chylomicron remnants.

As a rule, blood normally contains virtually no chylomicrons after a 12-hour fast. The presence of a significant amount of chylomicrons indicates a problem with the metabolism of lipoprotein particles.

The liver takes up about half of the IDL, and it uses hepatic lipase (see above) to deplete the other half of the IDL of triglycerides, thereby generating **LDL**. The uptake of IDL into the liver occurs via the binding of apolipoprotein E on the surface of IDL to the LDL receptor on the surface of

hepatocytes. LDL contain cholesterol and cholesteryl esters, but they are virtually free of triglycerides.

The liver and peripheral cells take up LDL via **LDL receptors**, when they need more **cholesterol** (see Fig. 29.3 and Section 3.1 in Chapter 29).

## 4.2. Deposition of Triglycerides Inside Adipocytes

Adipose tissue stores triglycerides that the body can use as an energy source during periods of fasting (Fig. 28.7). In the fed state, adipocytes take up fatty acids and glucose from the blood (Fig. 28.2). They convert glucose to glycerol 3-phosphate via glycolysis. Then, they esterify glycerol 3-phosphate with fatty acids to produce triglycerides (see Fig. 28.5). The triglycerides are stored in a lipid droplet that is coated by a phospholipid monolayer membrane that contains **perilipin** proteins. Perilipins control the entry of triglycerides and cholesteryl esters into the lipid droplet; they also control the exit of lipids from the droplet.

Adipocytes can import glucose only when the concentration of insulin is elevated and insulin stimulates the insertion of GLUT-4 glucose transporters into the plasma membrane. In the fasting state, adipocytes cannot produce triglycerides because they do not contain glucose to produce glycerol 3-phosphate.

Quite surprisingly, when body weight is stable, the half-life of triglycerides in adipose tissue is typically greater than 6 months.

Most triglycerides are normally stored in the adipose tissue. A much smaller amount can also be stored inside muscle.

Once the triglyceride deposits in the adipose tissue are very appreciable, there is a spillover effect so that triglycerides are increasingly deposited in other tissues. These deposits are often referred to as **ectopic fat**. They occur in skeletal and cardiac muscle, in the liver, and in pancreas. If the liver or the epithelium of the intestine cannot export triglycerides, they become likewise fat laden.

## 5. HYDROLYSIS OF STORED TRIGLYCERIDES

*In the fasting state and during prolonged exercise, adipocytes hydrolyze triglycerides into fatty acids and glycerol. Epinephrine, norepinephrine, and natriuretic peptides stimulate this process, whereas insulin inhibits it. The adipocytes release fatty acids and glycerol into the blood for use by other tissues, chiefly the liver and muscle. Muscle hydrolyzes its own small triglyceride stores to compensate for a short-term gap between demand and supply.*

### 5.1. Lipolysis

During prolonged **fasting** and persistent **exercise**, adipocytes hydrolyze stored triglycerides and release glycerol and fatty acids into the blood (Fig. 28.8; see also Fig. 28.9). The rate-limiting step is catalyzed by **adipose triglyceride lipase** (**ATGL**), which hydrolyzes the fatty acid from the C1 position of the glycerol moiety of the triglyceride. Subsequently, **hormone-sensitive lipase** (**HSL**) and **monoglyceride lipase** hydrolyze the remaining esters. Adipocytes then release fatty acids and glycerol into the blood.

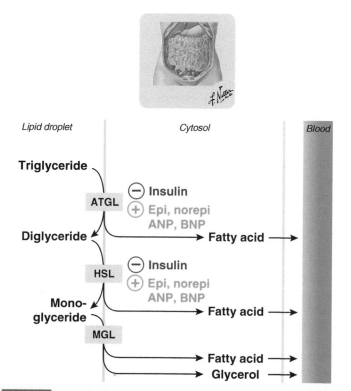

**Fig. 28.8** **Lipolysis.** ANP, atrial natriuretic peptide; ATGL, adipose triglyceride lipase; BNP, B-type natriuretic peptide; epi, epinephrine; HSL, hormone-sensitive lipase; MGL, monoglyceride lipase; norepi, norepinephrine.

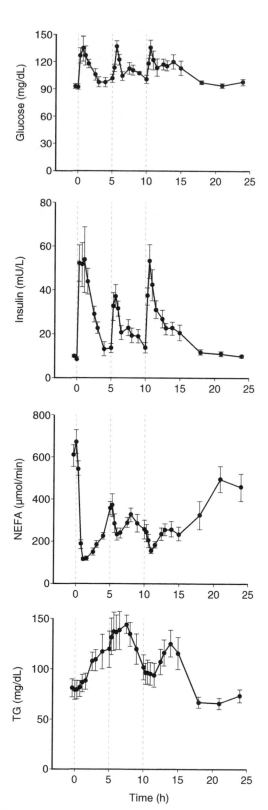

**Fig. 28.9** **Glucose, insulin, fatty acids, and triglycerides in the femoral artery in the course of a day.** Mean ± standard deviation of eight lean men who fasted overnight and then consumed three weight-maintaining meals of equal caloric value. NEFA, nonesterified fatty acid; TG, triglyceride. (From Ruge T, Hodson L, Cheeseman J, al. Fasted to fed trafficking of fatty acids in human adipose tissue reveals a novel regulatory step for enhanced fat storage. *J Clin Endocrinol Metab.* 2009;94:1781-1788.)

Epinephrine, norepinephrine, atrial natriuretic peptide (ANP), and B-type natriuretic peptide (BNP) stimulate ATGL and HSL (see Fig. 28.8). Epinephrine and norepinephrine are secreted in response to hypoglycemia or exercise and act via β-adrenergic receptors, which lead to an increase in the concentration of cAMP, and an increase in protein kinase A (PKA) activity. ANP and BNP are secreted in response to an increased output of the heart (e.g., during exercise). They work via natriuretic peptide receptors that lead to an increase in the concentration of cGMP, and protein kinase G (PKG) activity. Increases in PKA and PKG activity lead to the activation of ATGL and HSL.

Insulin inhibits lipolysis by inhibiting ATGL and HSL activity. Insulin signaling acutely leads to the activation of a phosphodiesterase that degrades cAMP and thus antagonizes signaling from epinephrine and norepinephrine (see above). By stimulating the synthesis of an inhibitory protein, insulin also has a separate, long-term dampening effect on ATGL activity.

There is appreciable debate about whether glucagon stimulates lipolysis in a physiologically relevant fashion.

Lipolysis is regulated in such a way that the heart "always" gets access to fatty acids from the adipose tissue. To this end, the effects of ANP and BNP override the effects of insulin.

Insulin and epinephrine compete for the regulation of lipolysis during fasting and exercise: epinephrine increases the rate of lipolysis, and insulin decreases it (this is akin to the regulation of gluconeogenesis by competition between glucagon and insulin).

A patient who has hypoglycemia due to hyperinsulinemia generally cannot activate lipolysis or ketogenesis and therefore has nonketotic or hypoketotic hypoglycemia (see Section 6.1 in Chapter 26). This applies to the patient who has an insulinoma and to the patient who has diabetes and injected too much insulin or took too much of a drug (e.g., a sulfonylurea) that stimulates insulin secretion independently of plasma glucose.

In the blood, fatty acids bind to albumin. Albumin is secreted by the liver and binds to various hydrophobic molecules, such as bilirubin, bile salts, and fatty acids.

The liver, heart, and skeletal muscle extract fatty acids from blood for fatty acid β-oxidation (see Chapter 27).

### 5.2. Hydrolysis of Triglycerides in Muscles

Both skeletal and heart muscle contain triglycerides. These stores complement glycogen as a short-term fuel. Muscle triglycerides turn over quickly compared with adipose tissue triglycerides, and they provide muscle with an assured supply of fatty acids even when plasma free fatty acid concentrations are low, such as during the postprandial period.

Muscle contains ATGL and HSL, which are activated by an elevated concentration of $Ca^{2+}$ in the cytosol and by an increased concentration of epinephrine in the circulation. Muscle does not release fatty acids from triglyceride hydrolysis into the blood.

### 5.3. Daily Course of Triglycerides and Fatty Acids in the Blood

As is evident from the data shown in Fig. 28.9, the concentration of fatty acids in blood plasma (bound to albumin) increases with fasting and decreases after a mixed meal; conversely, the concentration in plasma of triglycerides increases after a meal and then stabilizes during an overnight fast.

During a fast, the concentration of insulin is relatively low, which permits epinephrine- and norepinephrine-stimulated lipolysis to proceed at a low rate. After a meal, the concentration of insulin is high, and insulin leads to inhibition of ATGL and HSL so that the rate of lipolysis is now very small and leads to a decrease in the concentration of free fatty acids in plasma.

After a mixed meal, triglycerides derived from the diet enter the blood circulation inside chylomicrons. Chylomicrons have a very short half-life, but the intestine produces them for several hours after a meal. There is appreciable spilling of fatty acids from lipoprotein lipase into the blood, likely about 20%. The liver secretes VLDL on an ongoing basis. The triglycerides in these VLDL largely stem from fatty acids in the blood and to a lesser extent from de novo synthesis, from endocytosed IDL, and from the action of hepatic lipase. The total concentration of triglycerides in the plasma is largely the sum of all triglycerides in chylomicrons, VLDL, and IDL.

## 6. LABORATORY DETERMINATIONS

*The most frequently performed measurement is the concentration of all triglycerides in plasma after an overnight fast.*

Total triglycerides encompass the triglycerides inside all lipoprotein particles (i.e., chylomicrons, chylomicron remnants, VLDL, IDL, LDL, and HDL). After an overnight fast, there are normally virtually no chylomicrons or chylomicron remnants.

The normal range for total triglycerides is less than 150 mg/dL (<1.7 mM). The determination of total triglycerides is part of the measurements made for a lipid panel (or lipid profile); in that panel, it is part of estimating LDL cholesterol via the Friedewald equation (see Section 3.4 in Chapter 29).

Obesity and insulin resistance are often associated with an increased concentration of total plasma triglycerides.

## 7. ABSORPTION, TRANSPORT, AND STORAGE OF THE FAT-SOLUBLE VITAMINS A, D, E, AND K

*Absorption of the fat-soluble vitamins A, D, E, and K occurs in the small intestine, and chylomicrons transport these vitamins to the liver. The liver releases vitamin A as retinol, which binds to the retinol-binding protein in the blood. The liver hydroxylates vitamin D to 25-hydroxyvitamin D3. Both vitamin D and 25-hydroxyvitamin D₃ circulate in the*

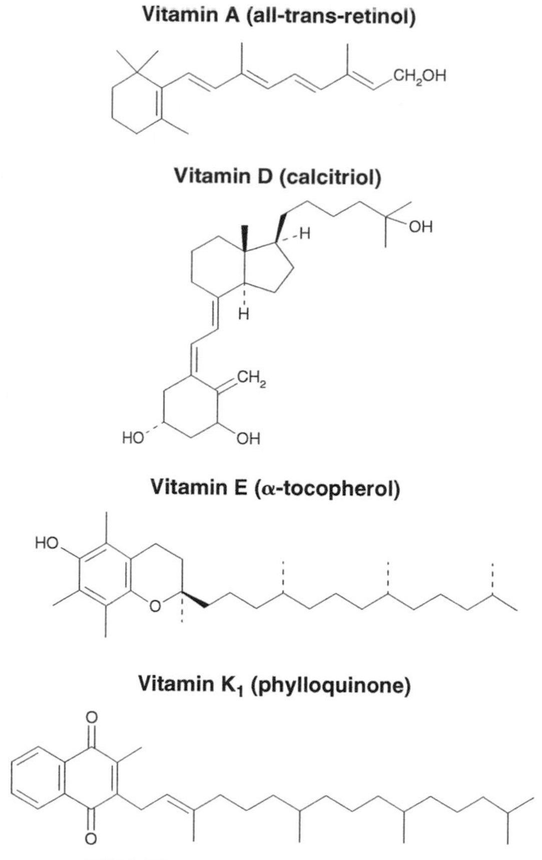

**Vitamin A (all-trans-retinol)**

**Vitamin D (calcitriol)**

**Vitamin E (α-tocopherol)**

**Vitamin K₁ (phylloquinone)**

**Fig. 28.10** Fat-soluble vitamins.

*bloodstream, bound to vitamin D–binding protein. The liver incorporates vitamins E and K into nascent VLDL and then secretes these into the bloodstream.*

The **fat-soluble vitamins** encompass **vitamins A, D, E, and K** (Fig. 28.10).

In the intestine, the fat-soluble vitamins enter the **mixed micelles** that also contain fatty acids, monoglycerides, and cholesterol. From there, they are absorbed either by diffusion through the plasma membrane of epithelial cells of the intestine or via specific transporters in those membranes.

Inside epithelial cells of the intestine, fat-soluble vitamins are packaged into **chylomicrons**, which are secreted into the lymph and eventually reach the bloodstream.

The term **retinoids** includes a number of different compounds, including **retinol (vitamin A), retinyl esters, retinal,** and **retinoic acid**. Some carotenoids, such as **β-carotene**, can give rise to retinoic acid, retinol, and retinal. Retinoids are stored principally as retinyl esters inside hepatic stellate cells.

The recommended daily allowance of vitamin A for nonlactating adults is 700 to 900 μg retinol activity equivalents (RAE), and the tolerable upper intake is 3,000 μg RAE. A large intake of carotenoids does not lead to vitamin A toxicity.

In the blood, retinoids are present in various forms, such as retinol bound to retinol-binding protein, retinoic acid bound to albumin, and retinyl esters inside lipoprotein particles. Lipoprotein lipase can hydrolyze retinyl esters in lipoproteins.

A derivative of **vitamin A, 11-cis-retinal,** is the chromophore in retinal rods and cones that change conformation upon excitation with light. The rods are needed for **vision** at night and the cones for color vision.

Night blindness is an early sign of **vitamin A deficiency**. In developing countries, hundreds of thousands of children each year become blind due to vitamin A deficiency.

**All-trans-retinoic acid** binds to **retinoic acid receptors (RAR)**, a type of nuclear hormone receptor. **9-Cis-retinoic acid** (also called **alitretinoin**) binds to **retinoid X receptors (RXR)**, which are transcription factors that form heterodimers with other nuclear hormone receptors, such as LXR (liver X receptor), FXR (farnesoid X receptor), and RAR.

Retinoic acid is required for proper development in utero. Both a deficiency and an excess of vitamin A can lead to birth defects.

The drug **13-cis-retinoic acid** (**isotretinoin**) is very effective for the treatment of acne (it seems to reduce the size of sebaceous glands and also the flow of sebum from these glands).

**Vitamin D** plays a role in the homeostasis of **calcium** and **phosphate**.

The endogenous, ultraviolet-light–dependent synthesis of **vitamin D₃** (**cholecalciferol, calciol**) is presented in Section 6 in Chapter 31.

Vitamin D from the diet stems mostly from fortified foods (e.g., milk). Oily fish (e.g., salmon) are also a good source of vitamin D. People who are exposed to little sunlight need more vitamin D in their diet.

Vitamin D₃ is hydroxylated to **25-hydroxyvitamin D₃** (**25-hydroxycholecalciferol, calcidiol**), which is stored in the blood, bound to vitamin D–binding protein (see Section 5 in Chapter 31).

**Vitamin E** is a lipid-soluble **antioxidant** that protects polyunsaturated fatty acids (see Figs. 21.6 and 21.7). The most abundant form of vitamin E is α-**tocopherol**.

For nonlactating persons aged 14 years and older, the recommended dietary allowance is 15 mg α-tocopherol per day, equivalent to about 22 IU of the natural stereoisomer of α-tocopherol or 33 IU of the synthetic racemic mixture of stereoisomers of α-tocopherol.

Good **sources** of vitamin E are sunflower oil, safflower oil, almonds, and hazelnuts.

After absorption in the intestine, vitamin E is incorporated into chylomicrons and reaches the liver via chylomicron remnants (some of it also reaches the adipose tissue when chylomicrons are depleted of triglycerides). In the liver, α-tocopherol transfer protein (TTP) transfers vitamin E (α-tocopherol) into VLDL particles, which are then secreted into the blood. Some vitamin E is again transferred into adipose tissue. Adipose tissue serves as the major site of vitamin E storage. Vitamin E that remains in LDL particles enters a variety of tissues via LDL receptor-mediated uptake of LDL particles. Some vitamin E reaches the cells via HDL and the scavenger receptor class B type I (SR-B1).

In patients with severe fat malabsorption without vitamin supplementation, a **vitamin E deficiency** develops and appears to be responsible for neurologic degeneration. **Myelin** contains many polyunsaturated fatty acids, which may form lipid peroxyl radicals; vitamin E is a lipid-soluble free radical scavenger that reacts with lipid peroxyl radicals. If there is a deficiency of vitamin E, lipid peroxyl radicals ultimately lead to the cross-linking of proteins and/or lipids (see Chapter 21).

Mutations in TTP also cause a deficiency in vitamin E.

In children who have a defective uptake in vitamin E, symptoms may develop as early as the second year of life. In contrast, in adults who have acquired fat malabsorption, it may take decades for symptoms of vitamin E deficiency to show. Concerned clinicians can request the measurement of vitamin E ($\alpha$-tocopherol) in serum.

**Vitamin K** is required for the carboxylation of certain clotting factors, regulation of bone growth and remodeling, and prevention of blood vessel calcification.

Humans get most of their vitamin K as **vitamin K$_1$ (phylloquinone)** from green vegetables and a lesser amount of **vitamin K$_2$ (menaquinone)** from cheese. Vitamins K$_1$ and K$_2$ differ in their hydrophobic side chain. The isoprene chain of menaquinone can have various lengths; the most common menaquinones found in the diet and supplements are designated as MK-4 and MK-7, indicating an isoprene chain of four and seven residues, respectively.

The intestine exports vitamin K in chylomicrons, and the liver takes up the chylomicron remnants. The liver then exports vitamin K inside VLDL, and peripheral cells gain vitamin K by taking up LDL via the LDL receptor.

In the liver, **peptidyl $\gamma$-glutamate carboxylase** uses vitamin K to attach carboxyl groups to certain Glu residues on specific proteins, turning them into $\gamma$-carboxyglutamate (Gla) residues. In this process, vitamin K becomes vitamin K epoxide. The enzyme vitamin K epoxide reductase (VKOR) converts vitamin K epoxide back to vitamin K.

Several **coagulation factors** are synthesized in the liver and require $Ca^{2+}$ to be active. $Ca^{2+}$ binds to Gla residues in these factors.

Patients who have a **deficiency of vitamin K** attach a reduced number of Gla residues on certain coagulation factors, thereby causing the blood to clot abnormally slowly.

# 8. DISORDERS OF TRIGLYCERIDE METABOLISM

*Hypertriglyceridemia is common and caused by a combination of genetic predisposition and lifestyle. Even moderate hypertriglyceridemia is a risk factor for arteriosclerotic vascular disease. A very high concentration of plasma triglycerides can cause pancreatitis. Lifestyle modification plays a key role in the treatment of hypertriglyceridemia. Fatty liver is due to an accumulation of triglycerides. Fat malabsorption may lead to a deficiency of vitamins A, D, E, or K.*

## 8.1. Hypertriglyceridemia

Patients with hypertriglyceridemia may have a normal or elevated LDL cholesterol. This section covers only hypertri-

glyceridemia in the absence of an elevated LDL cholesterol. A combination of hypertriglyceridemia and hypercholesterolemia is described in Section 6 of Chapter 29.

**Hypertriglyceridemia** is defined as total plasma triglycerides in the fasting state in excess of 150 mg/dL (1.7 mM). Severe hypertriglyceridemia is sometimes defined as greater than 1,000 mg/dL (>11 mM), and very severe hypertriglyceridemia as greater than 2,000 mg/dL (>23 mM). The hypertriglyceridemia is due to an abnormally high quantity of chylomicrons, VLDL, or both. In patients with hypertriglyceridemia, VLDL is formed at an excessive rate, or chylomicrons and VLDL are removed at an abnormally low rate. In the United States, about one-third of the adult population has hypertriglyceridemia, and approximately 0.2% has severe or very severe hypertriglyceridemia.

Due to the activity of the **CETP** (cholesterylester transfer protein) enzyme, hypertriglyceridemia leads to **low plasma HDL cholesterol** (see Fig. 29.7).

Hypertriglyceridemia increases a person's risk for **cardiovascular disease**, but the nature of the pathogenic lipoprotein is unclear.

The major risk of very severe hypertriglyceridemia is **pancreatitis**. Patients who have very severe hypertriglyceridemia may also have eruptive and tuberous **xanthomas** (see Fig. 29.14).

In most patients who have hypertriglyceridemia, the abnormality is due to a combination of **insulin resistance** (as in all **obese** and most type 2 **diabetic** patients), **hypothyroidism**, excessive **alcohol** intake, certain **medications**, **pregnancy**, and **genetic predisposition**.

The genetic predisposition is due to a large number of **risk alleles**, most of which alter the risk by a factor of two or less per allele. The most readily understandable pathogenic variants encode dysfunctional lipoprotein lipase, apolipoprotein C-II, or apolipoprotein E. Patients who have hypertriglyceridemia seem to be those who have a relatively high genetic risk in conjunction with obesity, diabetes, alcohol addiction, or hypothyroidism. Patients who have very severe hypertriglyceridemia seem to be those who have a similarly high number of common risk alleles but also have one or more alleles that are especially pathogenic.

**Pregnancy** is normally accompanied by about a three-fold increase in plasma triglycerides (to ~200 mg/dL or ~2.3 mM). Patients who already have a significant genetic predisposition may develop severe hypertriglyceridemia, mostly in the third trimester, although they had normal plasma triglycerides before pregnancy.

Since there is a strong environmental influence on plasma triglycerides, lifestyle modification is the cornerstone of treatment and can often lower triglycerides halfway toward the normal range; drug treatment is then used in an attempt to normalize plasma triglycerides. Lifestyle modification includes weight loss, exercise, a diet low in saturated fatty acids, and cessation of excessive consumption of alcohol. In patients who have **diabetes** and are in poor control of their blood glucose, better control with exogenous **insulin** is instituted. **Hypothyroidism** is corrected with levothyroxine. After reviewing the effect of these interventions, the need for further treatment is assessed. A **statin** in a high dose reduces VLDL production. A supplement of **fish oil**, which is rich in ω-3 **fatty acids**, increases lipoprotein lipase activity. **Fibrate** drugs activate **PPAR-α** transcription factors that lead to both increased lipoprotein lipase activity and an increased rate of fatty acid β-oxidation. **Nicotinic acid** (**niacin**) in large doses works in part by activating niacin receptor 1 (GPR109A), a G protein–coupled receptor that inhibits lipolysis (the release of fatty acids from adipose tissue).

**Pancreatitis** due to severe hypertriglyceridemia is initially treated in part with cessation of **food** intake. This reduces the production of chylomicrons (from dietary triglycerides) and VLDL (from dietary triglycerides and de novo synthesis from carbohydrate). Lowering of plasma triglycerides to less than 500 mg/dL (<5.6 mM) virtually eliminates a person's risk of a repeat episode of hypertriglyceridemia-induced pancreatitis.

## 8.2. Fatty Liver

While a normal liver contains up to 5% w/w fat (mostly triglycerides), an abnormal liver with a high fat content may contain about 20% fat. An abnormal accumulation of fat is called **steatosis** (Fig. 28.11). An amount of fat greater than about 5% is diagnostic for steatosis of the liver. Worldwide, about 20% of adults have steatosis of the liver, which is typically recognized at the age of 40 to 60 years.

Steatosis, a term that refers to the abnormal accumulation of fat in the liver, is subdivided into **alcoholic fatty liver disease** and **nonalcoholic fatty liver disease** (**NAFLD**). Alcoholic liver disease is common among persons who regularly abuse alcohol (see Chapter 30). The majority of persons who

are **obese** have NAFLD. Dyslipidemia and diabetes are additional risk factors for NAFLD.

NAFLD is typically detected based on abnormal laboratory values, and less commonly with imaging of the abdomen. A diagnosis of NAFLD requires abnormal liver function laboratory values, steatosis on imaging or biopsy histology, and exclusion of excessive alcohol consumption.

Patients who have NAFLD are at increased risk of developing fibrosis of the liver (**cirrhosis**) and liver **cancer**.

The treatment of NAFLD focuses on weight loss. Affected patients should also avoid excessive alcohol consumption. Patients who have alcoholic fatty liver are advised to abstain from drinking alcohol.

## 8.3. Fat Malabsorption

Malabsorption of fat is frequently seen and may be due to **inflammatory bowel disease** (a group of autoimmune disorders that includes **celiac disease**), **pancreatic insufficiency**, **short bowel syndrome**, bacterial **infection, bariatric surgery**, deficient delivery of **bile**, or an inherited deficiency in chylomicron production (see Section 8.4).

Fat malabsorption causes **steatorrhea,** an abnormally high fat content of the feces. Unabsorbed lipids are excreted in the feces.

Fat malabsorption can lead to a deficiency of lipid-soluble vitamins (A, D, E, and K) and essential fatty acids. This in turn can lead to night blindness and demyelination (see also Section 8.4).

## 8.4. Abetalipoproteinemia and Hypobetalipoproteinemia

Abetalipoproteinemia signifies an absence of lipoprotein particles that carry apolipoprotein B-48 or B-100 (i.e., chylomicrons, VLDL, IDL, and LDL). In contrast, HDL is present. Hypobetalipoproteinemia is between normal and abetalipoproteinemia. When the concentration of apoB-containing lipoprotein particles is very low, red blood cells become acanthocytic (i.e., they have spicules; Fig. 28.12). Such acanthocytosis is pathognomonic.

The term abetalipoproteinemia is typically used for the disorder that is inherited in an autosomal recessive fashion and caused by a deficiency of **MTP**. More than 30 pathogenic variants of the *MTTP* gene have been described.

The term familial hypobetalipoproteinemia is typically used for the disorder that is frequently caused by a loss of functional **apolipoprotein B**. More than 60 pathogenic truncation mutations in the *APOB* gene have been identified. Clinically, there is no difference between *MTTP* and *APOB* mutations.

Both abetalipoproteinemia and hypobetalipoproteinemia can lead to a tremendous accumulation of triglycerides in the epithelial cells of the intestine and hepatocytes, which is then usually accompanied by steatorrhea.

Without treatment, severe fat malabsorption due to abetalipoproteinemia or hypobetalipoproteinemia leads to night

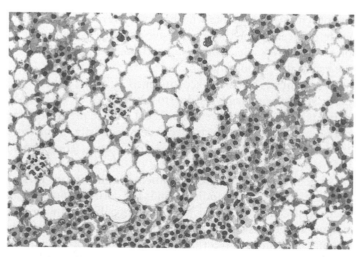

**Fig. 28.11**   **Fatty liver.** During preparation of this stained thin section, lipid droplets were washed away, leaving behind empty spaces.

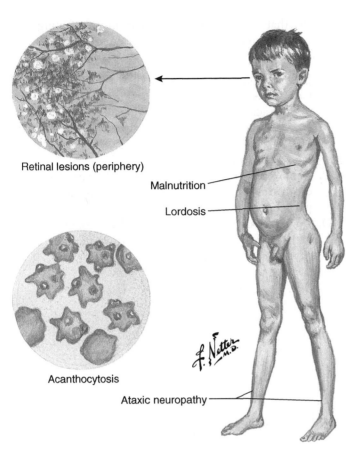

Retinal lesions (periphery)

Malnutrition

Lordosis

Acanthocytosis

Ataxic neuropathy

**Fig. 28.12** **Untreated abetalipoproteinemia.**

blindness due to **vitamin A deficiency** and severe degeneration of myelin in the nervous system due to **vitamin E deficiency** (see Fig. 28.12). Evaluation for a deficiency of fat-soluble vitamins is therefore part of standard care.

## SUMMARY

- Triglycerides comprise about 90% of the dietary lipids. Chiefly in the lumen of the intestine, triglycerides are hydrolyzed to monoglycerides and fatty acids. Hydrolysis of phospholipids and cholesteryl esters also yields fatty acids. Bile salts emulsify lipids during digestion and form mixed micelles that contain fat-soluble vitamins and the products of lipid digestion.
- Epithelial cells of the intestine take up monoglycerides and fatty acids, from which they re-form triglycerides. They package triglycerides into chylomicrons and export these into the lymphatic system, from where they reach the blood.
- The liver produces triglycerides from fatty acids in the circulation and from de novo fatty acid synthesis. The liver packages triglycerides into very-low-density lipoprotein (VLDL) and releases these into the blood.

- Lipoprotein lipase bound to the capillary walls of adipose tissue, muscle, and the lactating breast hydrolyzes triglycerides in circulating chylomicrons and VLDL, producing fatty acids and glycerol.
- Hepatic lipase removes triglycerides from intermediate-density lipoprotein (IDL) and high-density lipoprotein (HDL).
- Adipocytes take up fatty acids produced by lipoprotein lipase and use them to synthesize triglycerides for storage in membrane-delimited lipid droplets, access to which is controlled by perilipins. Adipocytes depend on a supply of glucose to generate glycerol 3-phosphate for the synthesis of triglycerides. Insulin increases the supply of fatty acids and glucose by stimulating, respectively, lipoprotein lipase synthesis and the incorporation of insulin-sensitive GLUT-4 glucose transporters into the plasma membrane.
- During fasting, inside adipocytes, the low concentration of insulin permits increased activity of adipose-triglyceride lipase (ATGL) and hormone-sensitive lipase (HSL), which together limit the rate of triglyceride hydrolysis. The resulting fatty acids and glycerol are both released into the blood. In the blood, the fatty acids bind to albumin.
- During lactation, the breast takes up fatty acids from the blood, either from hydrolysis of chylomicrons and VLDL or as fatty acids released by the adipose tissue.
- The fat-soluble vitamins A, D, E, and K are absorbed via the same routes as the triglycerides. Patients who have fat malabsorption may need to be supplemented with one or more of these vitamins. Deficiency of vitamin A causes night blindness and blindness, while a deficiency of vitamin E leads to demyelination.
- Hypertriglyceridemia is common and ascribed to a combination of genetic factors and insulin resistance, hypothyroidism, alcohol abuse, pregnancy, or certain medications. Hypertriglyceridemia is treated with lifestyle modification and drugs.
- Fatty liver is due to an excess of triglycerides in the liver. Affected patients are at increased risk for fibrosis and liver cancer.
- Patients who have abetalipoproteinemia or hypobetalipoproteinemia have mutations in the genes that encode the microsomal triglyceride transfer protein (MTP) and apolipoprotein B, respectively.

## FURTHER READING

- Lewis GF, Xiao C, Hegele RA. Hypertriglyceridemia in the genomic era: a new paradigm. *Endocr Rev*. 2015;36: 131-147.
- Nielsen TS, Jessen N, Jørgensen JO, Møller N, Lund S. Dissecting adipose tissue lipolysis: molecular regulation and implications for metabolic disease. *J Mol Endocrinol*. 2014;52:R199-R222.

# Review Questions

1. A 70-year-old patient who could not eat received an infusion of a large amount of glucose. The patient was also given insulin to control the concentration of glucose in the blood. As a result of this procedure, the patient's plasma triglycerides rose to an abnormally high level. Most of these triglycerides must have been inside which one of the following lipoprotein particles?

   A. Chylomicron remnants
   B. Chylomicrons
   C. IDL
   D. LDL
   E. VLDL

2. VLDL that circulate in the blood in the fasting state are derived mostly from which one of the following processes?

   A. β-Oxidation of fatty acids in the liver, yielding acetyl-CoA, the excess of which is used for de novo synthesis of fatty acids, followed by esterification.
   B. Hydrolysis of adipose tissue triglycerides, the transport of fatty acids to the liver, and re-esterification of excess fatty acids to triglycerides.
   C. Removal of triglycerides from LDL particles in the capillaries of the adipose tissue to produce VLDL particles.
   D. Uptake of chylomicrons into the liver, followed by the export of triglycerides that were contained in the chylomicrons.

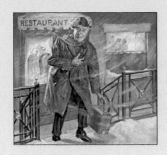

# Chapter 29

# Cholesterol Metabolism and Hypercholesterolemia

## SYNOPSIS

- Cholesterol is an essential component of plasma membranes, and it is the precursor for bile salts, vitamin D, and steroid hormones.
- Nearly all human cells can synthesize cholesterol, but the majority of cholesterol is synthesized in steroid-producing cells and in the liver for the benefit of other cells. Cholesterol is transported through the blood as part of all lipoprotein particles. The liver plays a central role in regulating the body's cholesterol metabolism.
- Dietary cholesterol is found only in foods derived from animals.
- As detailed in Chapter 28, the intestine incorporates cholesterol and cholesteryl esters into chylomicrons, and after the loss of associated triglycerides, the cholesterol-rich chylomicron remnants enter the liver. The liver exports cholesterol and cholesteryl esters in very-low-density lipoproteins (VLDL), which deliver triglycerides to adipose tissue and muscle. The VLDL then become low-density lipoproteins (LDL), which are taken up by the liver and by extrahepatic tissues.
- High-density lipoproteins (HDL) transport cholesterol from the periphery to the liver.
- Bile salts are required for the digestion of lipids. They are produced from cholesterol in the liver, secreted into the duodenum as a component of bile, and reabsorbed by the ileum.
- An abnormally high concentration of cholesterol or a low concentration of bile salts in bile leads to crystallization of cholesterol and the formation of gallstones.
- An elevated concentration of LDL cholesterol in the blood is a risk factor for atherosclerotic cardiovascular disease. Drugs that lower LDL cholesterol inhibit the de novo synthesis of cholesterol, increase the number of LDL receptors, reduce the absorption of cholesterol, or increase the elimination of bile salts in the feces.
- An elevated concentration of triglycerides in plasma leads to a low concentration of HDL cholesterol in plasma, which is a secondary risk factor for atherosclerotic cardiovascular disease.

## LEARNING OBJECTIVES

*For mastery of this topic, you should be able to do the following:*
- List the functions of cholesterol in the body.
- Describe the absorption of cholesterol in the intestine and the effect of dietary cholesterol on plasma LDL cholesterol. Describe cholesterol-rich and cholesterol-free foods. List foods and drugs that can reduce LDL cholesterol by reducing cholesterol absorption.
- Characterize the circulating lipoprotein particles that contain cholesterol and cholesteryl esters, and explain their role in cholesterol transport.
- Explain the regulation of the intracellular cholesterol concentration in the liver, steroid-producing cells, and peripheral cells.
- Explain the synthesis, storage, use, and reuse of bile salts, as well as the link between bile salt synthesis and cholesterol

metabolism. List drugs that exploit this link to lower LDL cholesterol.
- Describe abnormalities of bile metabolism, including the formation of cholesterol gallstones.
- Describe the association between the concentration of cholesterol in different types of lipoprotein particles and the incidence of atherosclerotic cardiovascular disease. List drugs that can reduce the likelihood that a patient develops this disease.

## 1. ABSORPTION OF CHOLESTEROL

*Cholesterol is required for the proper function of membranes and the synthesis of bile salts, vitamin D, and steroids. Cholesterol is derived in part from animal products in the diet and de novo synthesis (mostly in steroid-producing cells and in the liver). The liver and steroid-producing cells store cholesterol as cholesteryl esters in lipid droplets. The liver is the main regulator of the body's cholesterol metabolism.*

Cholesterol is a sterol that is present in many **membranes** (see Chapter 11), and that is the starting point for the synthesis of **steroids** (see Chapter 31). The structure of cholesterol is shown in Figs. 11.4 and 29.2.

The liver secretes cholesterol (along with bile salts) into the bile from where it reaches the duodenum, and the jejunum absorbs a portion of both secreted cholesterol and the cholesterol that is in the diet.

Only animal products contain cholesterol; plants contain many different sterols (**phytosterols**; Table 29.1), but not cholesterol. Plant sterols can interfere with cholesterol absorption, and they thus lower plasma LDL cholesterol (see Section 5.4).

In the lumen of the intestine, dietary cholesteryl esters are hydrolyzed, and cholesterol, along with other sterols, enters mixed micelles that contain bile salts, fatty acids, and monoglycerides (see Chapter 28).

Epithelial cells of the jejunum take up sterols from the lumen of the intestine rather indiscriminately via binding to **NPC1L1** (Niemann-Pick C1-like protein 1), followed by endocytosis (Fig. 29.1); then, epithelial cells expel most sterols but not cholesterol.

Approximately 0.1% of people are heterozygous for a **loss-of-function** mutation of the **NPC1L1** transporter, which is crucial to the absorption of cholesterol in the intestine. Such persons have an about 10 mg/dL lower concentration of LDL cholesterol.

In epithelial cells of the intestine, **acyl-CoA:cholesterol O-acyltransferase** (**ACAT**, also called sterol O-acyltransferase) converts some of the absorbed cholesterol into **cholesteryl**

## Table 29.1 Phytosterol Content of Selected Foods

| Food | Phytosterols (g/100 g) |
|------|------------------------|
| Sesame oil | 0.8 |
| Corn oil | 0.7 |
| Olive oil | 0.2 |
| Peanuts | 0.4 |
| Almonds | 0.3 |
| Take Control spread | 11.8 |
| Benecol spread | 6.1 |

Data from Linus Pauling Institute, Oregon State University. Avaialble at http://lpi.oregonstate.edu/mic/dietary-factors/phytochemicals/phytosterols#food-sources.

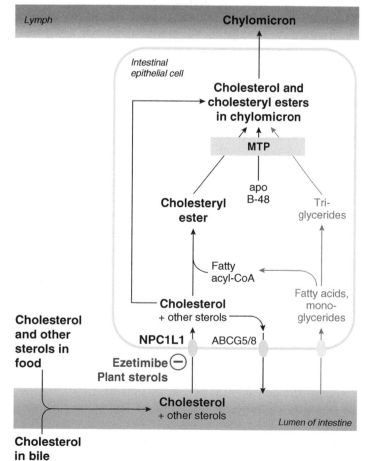

**Fig. 29.1** **Absorption of cholesterol and export into the blood.** Plant sterols compete with cholesterol for uptake via NPC1L1. MTP, microsomal triglyceride transfer protein.

esters (Fig. 29.2). Cholesteryl esters are considerably more hydrophobic than cholesterol, and cholesteryl esters therefore cannot be incorporated into membranes or transported through them. Hepatocytes and steroid-producing cells store cholesterol as cholesteryl esters inside lipid droplets in the cytosol, whereas most other cells contain virtually no cholesteryl esters.

Epithelial cells in the intestine export cholesterol and cholesteryl esters in **chylomicrons** (see Fig. 29.1). As outlined in Chapter 28, chylomicrons also contain triglycerides that are derived from fat in the diet. Chylomicrons contain **apolipoprotein B-48**, and they are assembled with the help of the **microsomal triglyceride transfer protein** (MTP). Weightwise, chylomicrons contain about twice as much cholesteryl esters as free cholesterol. The intestine releases chylomicrons into the lymph. Chylomicrons then reach the subclavian vein (and thus the bloodstream) via the thoracic duct. In the circulation, chylomicrons acquire **apolipoprotein C-II** and **apolipoprotein E** from HDL. The apolipoproteins C-II and E are essential for the removal of triglycerides (see Chapter 28) and chylomicron remnants (see below), respectively.

As **lipoprotein lipase** in the capillaries of the adipose tissue and muscle removes triglycerides, chylomicrons become cholesterol-rich **chylomicron remnants**, which are taken up by the liver. Thus, cholesterol from the diet first ends up in the liver. Similarly, some of the cholesterol that the liver secretes into bile (see above) and that is absorbed by the intestine ends up back in the liver. On hepatocytes, the **LDL receptor-related**

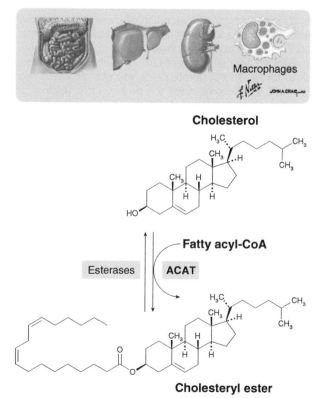

**Fig. 29.2** **Esterification of cholesterol inside cells.** ACAT, acyl-coenzyme A cholesterol acyltransferase.

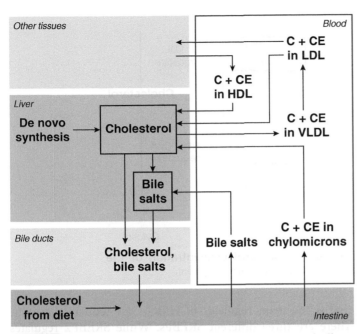

**Fig. 29.3** **Central role of the liver in cholesterol metabolism.** C, cholesterol; CE, cholesteryl esters.

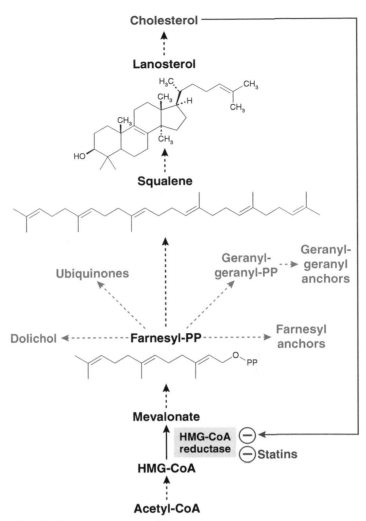

**Fig. 29.4** **Synthesis of isoprenes and cholesterol from acetyl-coenzyme A (acyl-CoA).**

protein 1 (**LRP1**) binds to **apolipoprotein E** on chylomicron remnants and then initiates endocytosis of the receptor-chylomicron remnant complex. Subsequently, lysosomes degrade chylomicron remnants.

The liver plays a central role in cholesterol metabolism in that it receives dietary cholesterol, synthesizes additional cholesterol for itself and other tissues as needed, exports cholesterol and cholesteryl esters in VLDL, and secretes both cholesterol and cholesterol-derived bile salts into the bile (Fig. 29.3). A person consuming a typical Western diet takes up about one-third of the daily needed cholesterol and de novo synthesizes the remaining two-thirds.

The autosomal recessively inherited disorder **abeta-lipoproteinemia** is characterized by an absence of lipoprotein particles that carry apoprotein B-48 or B-100 (i.e., chylomicrons, VLDL, IDL, and LDL). The disease is due to a deficiency of MTP (see Fig. 29.1). Since essentially only HDL are present, these patients have a very low plasma total cholesterol. The disease is described in greater detail in Chapter 28.

**Familial hypobetalipoproteinemia** is caused by heterozygosity of truncated apolipoprotein B. Patients develop a fatty liver due to reduced export of triglycerides.

## 2. DE NOVO SYNTHESIS OF CHOLESTEROL

*Cholesterol is synthesized in the cytosol from HMG-CoA that in turn is derived from acetyl-CoA. HMG-CoA reductase catalyzes the rate-limiting step of the pathway and is the primary point of regulation. The pathway is regulated such that cholesterol synthesis occurs in response to a lower-than-normal concentration of cholesterol in the endoplasmic reticulum (ER). An intermediate of the pathway, farnesyl*

*pyrophosphate, gives rise to several important compounds that are required for protein glycosylation, adenosine triphosphate (ATP) production, and anchoring of proteins in membranes.*

### 2.1. Pathway for the Biosynthesis of Cholesterol

Although every cell that contains mitochondria can make cholesterol, physiologically, cholesterol is predominantly synthesized in **steroid-producing cells** and the **liver** for the benefit of other cells. Every day, we synthesize 1.0 to 1.5 g of cholesterol, adjusting to dietary intake. Humans do not need cholesterol in the **diet**.

The de novo synthesis of cholesterol starts with acetyl-CoA, occurs in the cytosol, and is controlled by the activity of **HMG-CoA reductase** (Fig. 29.4), which yields **mevalonic acid**. The acetyl-CoA for cholesterol synthesis is derived from citrate exported from the mitochondria, as explained in Chapter 27 (the liver also uses this acetyl-CoA for de novo fatty acid synthesis). Chemically, the synthesis of HMG-CoA in the cytosol is similar to the synthesis of HMG-CoA in

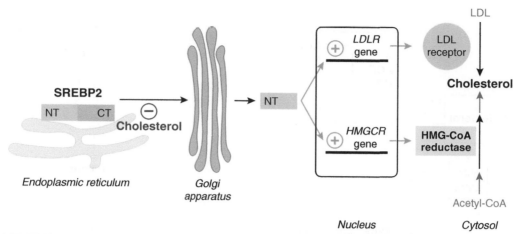

**Fig. 29.5** **Regulation of cholesterol synthesis by the cholesterol concentration of the endoplasmic reticulum membrane.** CT, C-terminal segment; NT, N-terminal segment.

mitochondria as part of the synthesis of ketone bodies, but these processes are catalyzed by isoenzymes.

Mevalonic acid gives rise to the isoprene **squalene**, which "folds up" and through a series of intramolecular reactions gives rise to **lanosterol**; lanosterol, in turn, is converted to cholesterol in many reactions (see Fig. 29.4).

Mevalonic acid gives rise not only to cholesterol, but also to **terpenes** (**isoprenoids**, sometimes also called **isoprenes**) such as farnesyl pyrophosphate, dolichol, ubiquinones, and geranylgeranyl pyrophosphate (see Fig. 29.4). **Farnesyl pyrophosphate** and **geranylgeranyl pyrophosphate** can be conjugated with proteins and then serve as lipid anchors (see Chapter 11). **Dolichyl pyrophosphate** is required for the dolichol pathway of N-linked posttranslational protein glycosylation (see Chapter 7). **Ubiquinones** can be reduced to ubiquinols, which can donate their electrons to the electron transport chain as part of oxidative phosphorylation (see Chapter 23).

Most of the cholesterol in a typical cell is in the plasma membrane; this cholesterol is in equilibrium with the cholesterol in the ER and the Golgi apparatus. Intracellular transport is facilitated by the ATP-driven **ATP-binding cassette transporter A1** (**ABCA1**), which is a floppase (see Chapter 11).

The **statin** drugs inhibit HMG-CoA reductase and thus inhibit the synthesis of terpenes and cholesterol (see Fig. 29.4). Statins are used to lower LDL cholesterol (see Section 5.4). Some of the beneficial effects as well as side effects of statins may be related to altered terpene metabolism.

Among antifungal agents, **fluconazole** is used in the treatment of **candidiasis** and inhibits the conversion of lanosterol to ergosterol in *Candida* without significantly affecting human cholesterol synthesis. In cell membranes of fungi and protozoa, ergosterol has similar essential functions as cholesterol does in mammals.

## 2.2. Regulation of Cholesterol Synthesis

Cholesterol synthesis is mainly controlled by the activity of **HMG-CoA reductase**, and **sterol regulatory element–binding protein 2** (**SREBP2**). SREBP2 is a cholesterol sensor

that is the main regulator of HMG-CoA reductase activity. There are three different SREBPs. While SREBP2 regulates cholesterol synthesis, SREBP1c regulates fatty acid synthesis, and SREBP1a regulates both cholesterol and fatty acid synthesis.

SREBP2 is an integral membrane protein of the ER that senses the concentration of cholesterol in the ER membrane (Fig. 29.5). The concentration of cholesterol in the ER membrane is rather low, but it is nonetheless reflective of the concentration of cholesterol in the plasma membrane. When the concentration of cholesterol in the ER is abnormally low, SREBP2-containing vesicles form and move to the Golgi apparatus. There, proteases cleave SREBP2. The N-terminal segment of SREBP2 then moves into the nucleus and enhances the transcription of several genes, including the genes for HMG-CoA reductase and LDL receptors. When the concentration of cholesterol is high, there is no such stimulation of transcription by an SREBP2 fragment.

**SREBP1c** is also in the ER, but it is set loose when the concentration of **insulin** is elevated. A fragment of SREBP1c activates transcription of genes that give rise to proteins that favor **fatty acid synthesis**.

**SREBP1a** is expressed in growing normal and tumor cells, and it can activate both cholesterol and fatty acid de novo synthesis.

## 3. TRANSPORT OF CHOLESTEROL VIA THE BLOOD

*The liver exports cholesterol and cholesteryl esters in VLDL. Lipases remove triglycerides, thereby converting VLDL to intermediate-density lipoprotein (IDL) and LDL. LDL contain much more cholesterol than triglycerides. When the liver and peripheral cells need more cholesterol, they endocytose the cholesterol-rich LDL. Peripheral cells export cholesterol by adding it to circulating HDL. This cholesterol is delivered mainly to the liver. As part of a "lipid panel," the concentration of total cholesterol and HDL cholesterol is often determined in plasma from fasting patients.*

## 3.1. Transport of Cholesterol From the Liver to Peripheral Cells

The chylomicron-based transport of cholesterol from the intestine to the liver is discussed in Section 1.

The liver exports cholesterol and cholesteryl esters as part of **VLDL**, which contains **apolipoprotein B-100**. VLDL also exports triglycerides from the liver (see Chapter 28). Cholesterol is mainly in the monolayer membrane that delimits VLDL, and cholesteryl esters are in the liquid core of the lipoprotein particle. On a molar basis, a VLDL particle contains about three times more cholesteryl esters than cholesterol.

**Lipoprotein lipase** in the lumen of the capillaries of the adipose tissue and muscle depletes VLDL of about 80% of its triglycerides, leaving behind all the cholesterol and cholesteryl esters and thus giving rise to **IDL**. The liver expresses **hepatic lipase**, which on one hand depletes IDL of triglycerides and on the other facilitates the receptor-mediated uptake of IDL and LDL into the liver. By weight, VLDL have about a 5:1 ratio of triglyceride/cholesterol, whereas IDL have a ratio of about 1:1 and LDL about 1:10.

Depending on their need for cholesterol, hepatocytes and peripheral cells display **LDL receptors** on their surface, which they use to bind and endocytose LDL via **apolipoprotein B-100**. Cells express LDL receptors based on the concentration of cholesterol that the **SREBP2** senses in the ER membrane. After endocytosis, lysosomal acid lipase hydrolyzes triglycerides and cholesteryl esters in lysosomes. LDL receptors can be recycled to the plasma membrane surface. The liver takes up approximately 70% of all LDL.

The liver secretes the enzyme **PCSK9** into the blood, from where the enzyme reaches LDL receptors, prevents their recycling to the plasma membrane surface, and favors their degradation in lysosomes. This pathway is an integral part of the cholesterol-dependent regulation of the number of LDL receptors.

About 3% of Caucasians are heterozygous for a **loss-of-function mutation** in the *PCSK9* gene and therefore have better survival of LDL receptors and about a 15% reduction in LDL cholesterol. About 2% of African-Americans are heterozygous for two other such mutations that result in an ~30% reduction in LDL cholesterol.

**Gain-of-function** mutations in *PCSK9* are uncommon and lead to hypercholesterolemia (see Section 5.2).

## 3.2. Export of Cholesterol From Peripheral Cells (Reverse Cholesterol Transport)

Transport of cholesterol from the liver to peripheral tissues is often called cholesterol transport; the transport of cholesterol from the peripheral tissues to the liver and steroid-producing tissues is called **reverse cholesterol transport**. Reverse transport is performed by **HDL**.

HDL form chiefly in the liver and intestine by loading phosphatidylcholine, cholesterol, and cholesteryl esters onto **apolipoprotein A-I** (Fig. 29.6). The liver and intestine synthesize apolipoprotein A-I, the chief protein of HDL. These organs use the ABCA1 transporter to enrich discoidal HDL with phosphatidylcholine and cholesterol out of the plasma membrane, thereby generating **preβ-HDL**.

In the blood, **lecithin-cholesterol acyltransferase (LCAT)** binds to preβ-HDL and then uses a fatty acid from the phospholipid lecithin (i.e., phosphatidylcholine; made available once again by an ABCA1 transporter) of a peripheral cell to esterify cholesterol to cholesteryl esters, which are stored inside HDL. This lipidation gives rise to mature HDL particles,

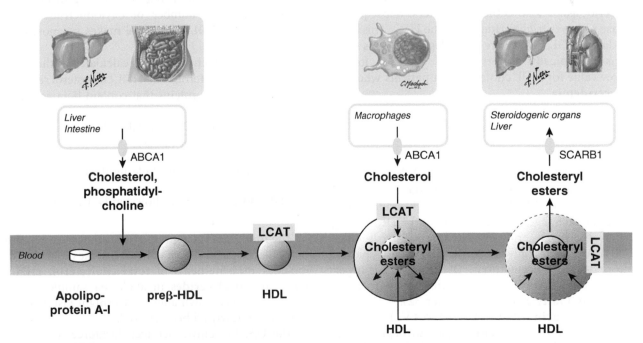

**Fig. 29.6** **Biology of high-density lipoprotein (HDL).** ABCA1, ATP-binding cassette transporter A1; LCAT, lecithin-cholesterol acyltransferase; SCARB1, scavenger receptor class B member type 1.

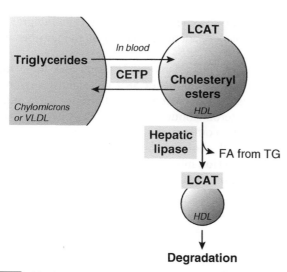

**Cholesteryl ester transfer protein (CETP)-mediated exchange of lipids between high-density lipoproteins (HDL) and chylomicrons or very-low-density lipoproteins (VLDL) leads to low HDL cholesterol.** FA, fatty acids; LCAT, lecithin-cholesterol acyltransferase; TG, triglycerides.

known as α-HDL, which have a much longer half-life than the smaller preβ-HDL. By weight, circulating HDL particles contain about twice as much protein as cholesterol.

HDL offload some of their cholesteryl esters in the liver and in steroidogenic organs, where **scavenger receptor class B member type 1 (SCARB1, SRB1, SRBI)** equilibrate cholesteryl esters in HDL with cellular cholesteryl esters (see Fig. 29.6). The resulting HDL recirculate and can transport more cholesteryl esters. However, the smaller the HDL, the shorter their lifetime in the circulation.

Catalyzed by the **cholesteryl ester transfer protein (CETP)**, VLDL exchange lipids with HDL (Fig. 29.7). HDL thus gain triglycerides and lose cholesteryl esters. Subsequently, hepatic lipase removes triglycerides from the HDL. This leaves poorly lipidated HDL, which are then degraded. This series of reactions is clinically important and accounts for the observed low value for HDL cholesterol in patients who have **hypertriglyceridemia.**

### 3.3. Treatment of a Low Concentration of HDL Cholesterol

Most patients who have HDL cholesterol levels below 20 mg/dL (0.5 mM) have severe **hypertriglyceridemia.** The low HDL is a consequence of **CETP**-catalyzed triglyceride versus cholesteryl ester exchange between VLDL and HDL (see Fig. 29.7). When the triglyceride-enriched, cholesteryl ester–depleted HDL lose their triglyceride, they are poorly lipidated and therefore degraded prematurely. The treatment of hypertriglyceridemia often involves a **statin**, a **fibric acid** drug, and supplementary **ω-3 fatty acids** (see Chapter 32).

**Nicotinic acid (niacin, vitamin B$_3$)** reduces VLDL production and increases HDL cholesterol in part through reduced CETP-mediated lipid exchange between HDL and VLDL, which allows HDL to remain in the circulation longer. Nico-

tinic acid often has side effects, such as flushing, that prevent patients from taking this drug. Nonsteroidal antiinflammatory drugs (NSAIDs) may reduce the flushing.

In previously sedentary adults, the addition of regular **exercise** increases the plasma HDL cholesterol by a modest ~2 mg/dL (~0.05 mM).

Patients who have HDL cholesterol levels lower than 20 mg/dL (0.5 mM) *without* marked hypertriglyceridemia may have a **deficiency** of functional **apolipoprotein A-I, ABCA1,** or **LCAT.**

About 1 in 400 people are **heterozygous** for an **ABCA1 deficiency.** These individuals have only about two-thirds to one-half of the normal HDL cholesterol, yet they do not have a markedly increased risk of ischemic heart disease.

### 3.4. Laboratory Measurements of Cholesterol-Containing Lipoproteins

Clinical laboratories routinely measure **total cholesterol, HDL cholesterol,** and **triglycerides** in plasma samples.

**LDL cholesterol** is usually calculated from measurements of total cholesterol, HDL cholesterol, and total triglycerides, using the plasma from **fasting** patients. The calculation is based on the **Friedewald equation** (all concentrations in **mg/dL**):

$$\text{LDL cholesterol} = \text{total cholesterol} - \text{HDL cholesterol} - (\text{total triglycerides}/5)$$

The equation thus uses an approximation of the triglyceride versus cholesterol content of VLDL, IDL, and LDL. If all concentrations are calculated in units of **mM**, the triglyceride-based correction uses a factor of 0.45 (instead of 0.2 for mg/dL). The Friedewald equation is inaccurate when the concentration of triglycerides is high (>~400 mg/dL) or when there is an appreciable number of chylomicrons. In a fasting plasma sample, LDL cholesterol makes up most of the total cholesterol.

The **non-HDL cholesterol** is calculated as the total cholesterol – HDL cholesterol. Non-HDL cholesterol represents cholesterol in the lipoproteins that contain beta-apolipoproteins (i.e., B-48 or B-100).

Occasionally, the **Castelli risk indices** are used for predicting the risk of vascular disease:

$$\text{Total cholesterol/HDL cholesterol} = \text{Castelli risk index 1}$$

$$\text{LDL cholesterol/HDL cholesterol} = \text{Castelli risk index 2}$$

The **lipid panel** is a group of tests that are often ordered to help assess a patient's risk of heart disease or stroke. The panel includes measurements of **total cholesterol, HDL cholesterol,** and **triglycerides** in a plasma sample. The patient's blood sample is drawn after an overnight fast when chylomicrons have nearly all been cleared.

The U.S. Preventive Services Taskforce recommends that the following persons be screened for lipid disorders: (1) men aged 35 years and older and (2) men aged 20 to 35 years and women aged 20 years or older who are at an increased risk for coronary heart disease.

The National Cholesterol Education Program's Adult Treatment Panel III (ATP III) recommends that all persons aged 20 years and older have a fasting lipid panel performed every 5 years. More frequent screenings are recommended if the total cholesterol is 200 mg/dL or higher, if the HDL is less than 40 mg/dL, or if the person has risk factors such as cigarette smoking, age older than 45 years for men, age older than 55 years for women, blood pressure higher than 140/90 mm Hg, blood pressure–lowering medication use, or a family history of premature heart disease.

## 4. BILE METABOLISM

*Bile salts are synthesized by the liver and secreted, together with cholesterol and phospholipids, into the bile ducts to form bile. Bile is stored in the gallbladder and then secreted into the duodenum in response to dietary protein and fat. Bile salts solubilize lipids in the intestinal lumen and thus enhance their digestion. Bile salts also form mixed micelles with lipids and thus facilitate their absorption. Insufficient production of bile acids causes lipid malabsorption. Most of the secreted bile salts are reabsorbed by the ileum and returned to the liver. If the liver produces an insufficient amount of bile salts or secretes too much cholesterol, cholesterol gallstones may form in the gallbladder or bile ducts.*

### 4.1. Production of Bile and Recirculation of Bile Salts and Cholesterol

Bile is made in the liver, secreted into bile canaliculi, stored in the gallbladder, and dispensed into the duodenum via the common bile duct (Fig. 29.8). Bile contains micelles of **bile salts**, **cholesterol**, and the phospholipid **phosphatidylcholine** (also called lecithin). Bile salts are detergents that emulsify triglycerides and cholesteryl esters. Bile salts also form mixed micelles with cholesterol, fatty acids, and monoglycerides (see Chapter 28).

The only means of removing cholesterol from the body is via the secretion of cholesterol into bile and conversion of cholesterol into bile acids, followed by the secretion into bile. There is no pathway for the degradation of cholesterol into small molecules.

The liver hydroxylates cholesterol to produce the **bile acids chenodeoxycholic acid** and **cholic acid** (Fig. 29.9); these bile acids are then conjugated with the amino acids **glycine** or **taurine** to yield **primary bile salts**. The rate-limiting enzyme for bile acid production is cholesterol 7α-hydroxylase (CYP7A1, a cytochrome P450 enzyme). Cholic acid has one more hydroxyl group than chenodeoxycholic acid and is therefore more soluble in water. Conjugation of bile acids with glycine or taurine further increases the solubility in water. Bile salts are amphipathic; they have both a hydrophobic and a hydrophilic surface. The amount of bile salts in the bile is an important determinant of the amount of water in bile and thus

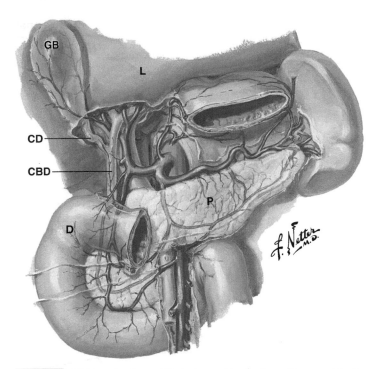

**Fig. 29.8** **Biliary system.** Bile is formed in the liver (L), stored in the gallbladder (GB), and secreted into the duodenum (D). CD, cystic duct; CBD, common bile duct; P, pancreas.

the flow of bile out of the liver. The gallbladder then concentrates bile by removing water from it. In the fasting state, most bile salts are stored in the **gallbladder**.

The composition of the micelles in bile is determined by the relative rates of export of bile salts, cholesterol, and phospholipids, each of which has its own export system from the liver (Fig. 29.10). The rate of bile salt export is determined by the activity of the bile salt export pump (**BSEP**, **ABCB11**), which increases in response to elevated concentrations of bile salts inside the cell. Cholesterol is exported from the liver via an ATP-driven transporter (a heterodimer of the ATP binding cassette proteins G5 and G8; **ABCG5/G8**). The phospholipid **phosphatidylcholine** in bile is derived from the cell membrane. The floppase **MDR3** (also called **ABCB4**) moves phosphatidylcholine from the inside of the membrane to the outside.

In response to the influx of chyme that contains protein and fat, I-cells in the duodenum secrete the peptide hormone **cholecystokinin (CCK)**, which causes the gallbladder to contract and dispense bile into the common bile duct from where it reaches the intestine. CCK also stimulates the secretion of enzymes from the pancreas.

In the lumen of the ileum and colon, **bacteria** can remove the 7α-hydroxyl group from primary bile salts to yield **secondary bile salts** (see Fig. 29.9); bacteria can also deconjugate bile salts to yield bile acids. Both of these modifications decrease the solubility of bile acids and bile salts in the gut.

The distal ileum reabsorbs over 95% of primary and secondary bile salts via a Na⁺-driven transporter (ASBT, SLC10A2) and releases the bile salts via the Ostα-Ostβ organic solute transporter into the blood so that they can move back to the

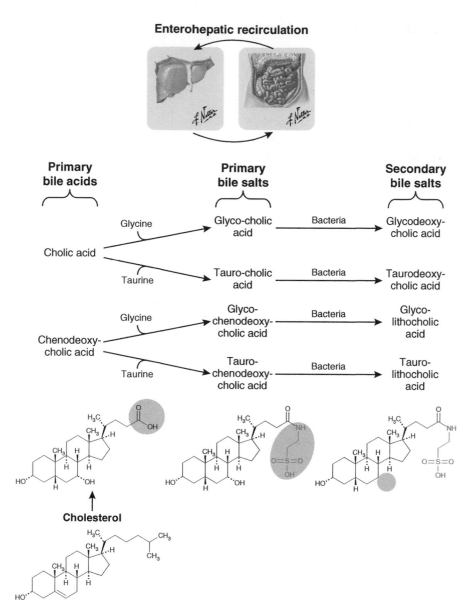

**Fig. 29.9** Production of bile acids and bile salts.

liver and be resecreted into bile (see Fig. 29.10). In the blood, bile salts bind to albumin. On average, a bile salt makes approximately eight passes per day through this **enterohepatic circulation**. The total bile salt pool is about 3 g, and the daily loss into the feces is about 0.5 g.

The conversion of cholesterol to bile salts and the transport of bile salts are in part controlled at the level of transcription by liver X receptors and farnesoid X receptors, each of which forms heterodimers with retinoic acid receptors and function as follows.

Heterodimeric **liver X receptors/retinoic acid receptors (LXR/RXRs)** are activated by **oxysterols** (e.g., 27-hydroxycholesterol) and retinoic acid, which cause them to increase the transcription of certain genes so that more cholesterol is exported in the form of bile salts. Fig. 6.5 illustrates the binding of LXR/RXR to DNA. In the absence of an activator, LXR/RXR heterodimers bind to LXR-response elements on DNA and inhibit transcription. Oxysterols that activate LXR/RXRs are intermediates in the conversion of cholesterol to steroids or bile acids. Compared with binding of a single ligand, binding of both an oxysterol and retinoic acid markedly enhances LXR/RXR activity. Some of the genes that have LXR-response elements encode proteins that play a role in cholesterol metabolism, such as *CETP* (exchanges cholesterol between VLDL and HDL; see Section 3.2), *CYP7A1* (the rate-limiting enzyme in bile acid synthesis), *ABCA1* (exports cholesterol to HDL; see Section 3.2), *ABCG1* (exports cholesterol from macrophages and the liver to circulating lipoproteins), and *ABCG8* (exports cholesterol from the liver into bile; see Fig. 29.10). Activated LXR/RXRs also affect the transcription of some genes that are not associated with an LXR response element.

Heterodimeric **farnesoid X receptors/retinoic acid receptors (FXR/RXRs)** are activated by **bile acids** and then increase

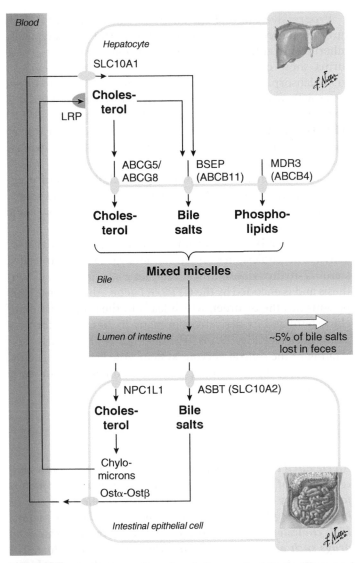

**Fig. 29.10** Enterohepatic circulation of bile salts and cholesterol.

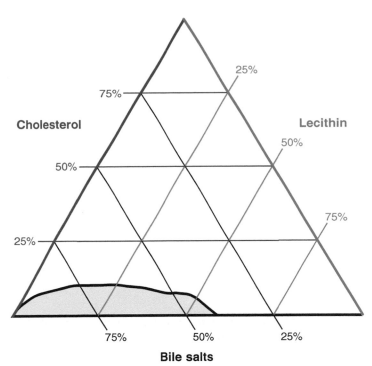

**Fig. 29.11** **Phase diagram for a model system of cholesterol in micelles in bile.** The green area represents the combinations of solutes that give rise to a single phase of micelles. The composition of bile of healthy persons is typically well within the green area, while that of persons with cholesterol gallstones is close to the border of this area or clearly outside of it. The fractions refer to the total moles of solute in a solution that is 90% water and 10% solute (cholesterol + lecithin + bile salts). (Modified from Admirand WH, Small DM. The physicochemical basis of cholesterol gallstone formation in man. *J Clin Invest.* 1968;47:1043-1052.)

the transcription of genes that have a promoter with an FXR-response element. The products of these genes protect hepatocytes and intestinal epithelial cells from the effects of a high concentration of bile acids. In the liver, bile acid–activated FXR/RXRs inhibit bile salt uptake and synthesis and favor bile salt secretion. In intestinal epithelial cells, bile acid–activated FXR/RXRs likewise inhibit bile salt uptake and stimulate bile salt efflux.

## 4.2. Diseases of Bile Metabolism

For bile to be free of crystals and stones, cholesterol must constitute less than 10% of the total moles of cholesterol, bile salts, and lecithin; furthermore, bile salts must be greater than 40% and lecithin less than 60% of this total (Fig. 29.11). On a molar basis, normal bile contains approximately 6% cholesterol, 74% bile salts, and 20% lecithin.

**Gallstones** can form when there is an excessive rate of cholesterol secretion or a decreased rate of bile salt secretion.

Gallstones are more likely to form when bile gets highly concentrated in the gallbladder, when the gallbladder empties at a low rate, or when the bile system has low motility.

The presence of gallstones (Fig. 29.12) in the gallbladder (**cholelithiasis**) or bile duct (**choledocholithiasis**) is quite common and usually does not cause symptoms. However, gallstones that block the cystic duct (which connects the gallbladder to the common bile duct) or the common bile duct (see Fig. 29.8) can cause pain. Pain is especially common after a fatty meal because the fat in the duodenum elicits the secretion of the hormone **CCK**, which stimulates the contraction of the gallbladder. Gallstones can lead to cholecystitis (inflammation of the gallbladder), cholangitis (inflammation of the bile duct), jaundice (due to impaired bilirubin excretion), and pancreatitis (due to blockage of the flow of enzymes from the pancreatic duct into the common bile duct).

About 80% of gallstones are due to the precipitation of cholesterol crystals, which appear **yellow**. Precipitates of calcium **bilirubinate** (see Chapter 14), which form **black** stones and are common in persons with a hemolytic disorder, account for the other 20%.

A decrease in bile salt secretion may occur if there is decreased reabsorption of bile salts from the intestine, as is observed in patients with diseases that affect the ileum, or

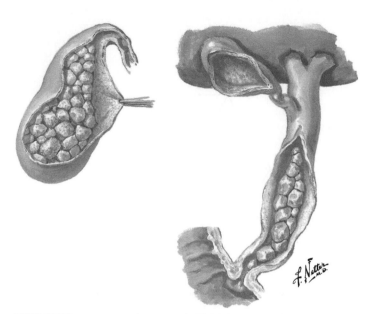

**Fig. 29.12** **Multiple cholesterol gallstones in the gallbladder and the common bile duct.**

if there is decreased synthesis of bile salts due to liver dysfunction.

An increase in cholesterol secretion may occur in patients who take one of the **fibrate** drugs (e.g., gemfibrozil or fenofibrate) to lower triglycerides in the blood. Fibrates stimulate the transcription factor PPARα (see Chapter 28), which increases the expression of the ABCG5/G8 proteins, which export cholesterol into the bile (see Fig. 29.10). This increases the risk of gallstone formation.

Noninvasive images of gallstones are usually obtained with **ultrasound**. In plain radiographs, cholesterol stones do not show sufficient contrast because they do not contain heavy elements.

Surgery is currently the preferred treatment of gallstones because drug treatment is mostly unsatisfactory. Over time, the drugs ursodeoxycholic acid and ezetimibe have favorable effects in some patients. **Ursodeoxycholic acid** (**ursodiol**) differs from chenodeoxycholic acid in the orientation of the –OH group at C7. The effect of ursodeoxycholic acid is difficult to understand because it has many diverse effects on cholesterol and bile salt metabolism. **Ezetimibe** inhibits the uptake of cholesterol in the intestine and, as a result, tends to reduce cholesterol secretion from the liver into bile.

Cholestasis (an abnormally low flow of bile from the gallbladder to the duodenum) is often accompanied by **pruritus** (itching), although the pathogenesis of this is not clear. **Bile acid sequestrants** such as cholestyramine and colestipol, which in part reduce the enterohepatic recirculation of bile acids, are a standard treatment for pruritus.

**Cholestasis** can be induced by an **intrahepatic** problem with bile formation or by **extrahepatic** obstruction. An intrahepatic problem may be due to autoimmune disease, induced by drugs (sometimes dependent on a patient's genetic makeup), or caused by a congenital deficiency in bile formation. An extrahepatic obstruction may be due to gallstones or a tumor.

**Progressive familial intrahepatic cholestasis (PFIC2)** is rare and caused by deficient bile salt export. PFIC is typically inherited in autosomal recessive fashion. The most severe forms show onset in the first year of life, and they lead to malabsorption of fat and fat-soluble vitamins, followed by growth restriction and severe liver disease. Affected patients have defects in the **bile salt export pump (BSEP) ABCB11**, in the flippase **ATP8B1,** which seems to impair ABCB11 activity, or in the floppase **ABCB4** that exports phosphatidylcholine.

Some women who have **intrahepatic cholestasis of pregnancy** are heterozygotes for a mutation in the *ABCB4* gene.

Treatment of cholestasis may include oral ursodeoxycholic acid, diversion of bile, and liver transplantation.

**Cerebrotendinous xanthomatosis** is caused by deficient activity in cholestanetriol 26-monooxygenase (also called sterol 27-hydroxylase), which catalyzes a step in bile acid synthesis and is encoded by the *CYP27A1* gene. About 1 in 25,000 persons has the disorder, which leads to the accumulation of cholesterol and its derivatives in many tissues, often forming xanthomas (see Fig. 29.14). The disorder is particularly devastating to the central nervous system. Ataxia and intellectual decline typically become apparent in adolescence or early adulthood.

## 5. HYPERCHOLESTEROLEMIA

*An elevated concentration of LDL cholesterol and a low concentration of HDL cholesterol in the plasma are risk factors for coronary artery disease (CAD). LDL cholesterol can be high due to genetic factors, diet, obesity, and other factors. LDL cholesterol can be lowered through diet, exercise, and drugs such as statins, ezetimibe, and PCSK9 inhibitors. The concentration of HDL cholesterol is most often low due to hypertriglyceridemia.*

### 5.1. Blood Cholesterol Concentration and the Risk of Coronary Artery Disease

**Newborns** have plasma **LDL cholesterol** of about 60 mg/dL. The mean serum LDL cholesterol of **adults** is strongly influenced by diet, being on the order of 95 mg/dL in Japanese fishermen who consume a low-fat diet, and about 180 mg/dL in foresters in Finland who consume a fat-rich diet.

In population studies, there is a very strong correlation between plasma **LDL cholesterol** and the incidence of CAD. The lower the LDL cholesterol, the lower the risk for CAD.

A high concentration of LDL cholesterol is associated with **atherosclerosis** (Fig. 29.13). Plaques are present already in young adults, although they do not yet give rise to clinical symptoms. It is thought that **oxidized LDL** (i.e., LDL with damage to protein and lipids from reactive oxygen species) can enter the walls of arteries and eventually be endocytosed by **macrophages** via the scavenger receptor A (SR-A). These macrophages thus become **foam cells** that secrete cytokines

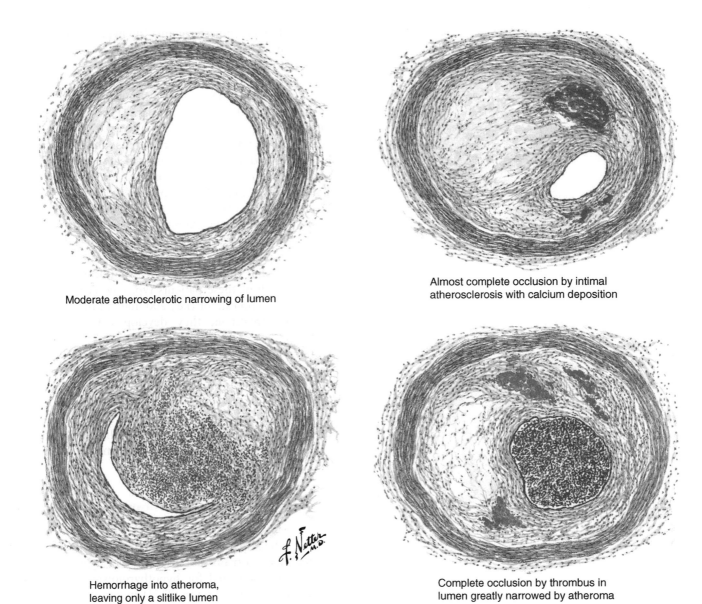

Moderate atherosclerotic narrowing of lumen

Almost complete occlusion by intimal
atherosclerosis with calcium deposition

Hemorrhage into atheroma,
leaving only a slitlike lumen

Complete occlusion by thrombus in
lumen greatly narrowed by atheroma

**Fig. 29.13** **Progressive narrowing and occlusion of the coronary artery by atherosclerotic plaque and thrombus.**

and start an inflammatory reaction. In response, smooth muscle cells proliferate, and plaques grow over time. At some point they rupture and, together with a newly forming blood **clot**, obstruct blood flow.

In industrialized countries, about 25% of all deaths are attributable to atherosclerotic plaques, which mainly cause **heart attacks**.

Besides high LDL cholesterol, low **HDL cholesterol** is also positively associated with the incidence of cardiovascular disease. The cause of this association remains to be elucidated. It is puzzling that patients who have monogenic disorders that lead to extremely low HDL cholesterol have no clear-cut increase in CAD risk. This is true for apolipoprotein A-I mutations, Tangier disease due to ABCA1 mutations (ABCA1 exports cholesterol from cells; see Fig. 29.6), and a deficiency of LCAT.

Other risk factors for heart attacks are **smoking, hypertension**, and **diabetes**.

## 5.2. Familial Hypercholesterolemia

Mutations in the genes for the LDL receptor, apolipoprotein B-100, and PCSK9 are currently known to cause congenital hypercholesterolemia. The prevalence is on the order of ~1 in 400. In adulthood, affected persons have elevated LDL cholesterol (>220 mg/dL [>5.7 mM]) and total cholesterol (>300 mg/dL [>7.8 mM]) but a normal plasma concentration of total triglycerides. Without treatment, these persons develop premature **atherosclerosis** (see Fig. 29.13) and often also xanthomas.

**Xanthomas** (Fig. 29.14) contain cholesterol-laden foam cells, and their location depends on the cause of dyslipidemia.

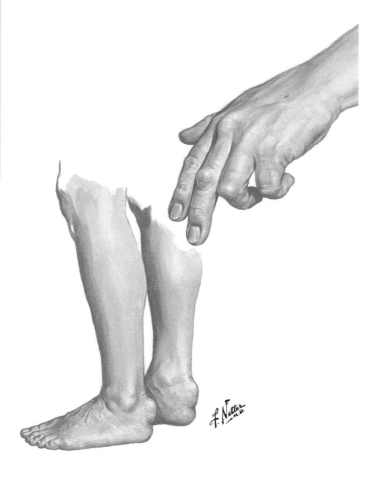

Patients with hypercholesterolemia (no hypertriglyceridemia) have tendon xanthomas, most often on the hands and feet. Patients with combined hypercholesterolemia and hypertriglyceridemia have tuberous xanthomas, which form over joints. Xanthelasmas form under the skin, typically of the eyelid, and mostly occur in patients with high LDL cholesterol.

Most patients who have **heterozygous familial hypercholesterolemia** and a known disease-causing mutation have a mutant allele for the **LDL receptor**. About 5% of these patients have a mutant **apolipoprotein B**, and approximately 2% have an overly active **PCSK9** enzyme. Sometimes, the term heterozygous familial hypercholesterolemia is applied to only those who have a mutant LDL receptor, and carriers of a pathogenic apolipoprotein B mutation are said to have **familial ligand-defective apolipoprotein B-100 (apoB-100)**. All of these patients typically have about twice the usual LDL cholesterol (i.e., 200-400 mg/dL [5-10 mM]), and without treatment they develop CAD before their late 50s.

**Homozygous familial hypercholesterolemia** has a prevalence of only ~1 in 1 million. Most often, patients with this disorder have two alleles for a defective LDL receptor. Their LDL cholesterol is approximately tenfold the usual concentration. Without treatment, these patients have heart attacks in their teens and twenties. Less often, patients are homozygous for loss-of-function mutations in apo B-100.

## 5.3. Other Causes of Hypercholesterolemia

Besides a deficient LDL receptor, uptake of LDL particles into the liver can be impaired by **hypothyroidism** or a diet high in **saturated fats** and **trans fats**. Patients with hypercholesterolemia are often screened for hypothyroidism by measuring thyroid-stimulating hormone (TSH) in serum. The effect of saturated and trans fats on LDL cholesterol depends on **genetic predisposition**.

## 5.4. Lowering the Concentration of LDL Cholesterol

Atherosclerosis is a process that takes years to develop, and it is not readily reversible. Although plaques occasionally do recede with a dramatic lowering of LDL cholesterol, epidemiologic studies show that repair is typically not sufficient to lower a patient's CAD risk to that of a person with a similarly low LDL cholesterol for decades.

Modification of food intake often lowers plasma LDL cholesterol remarkably. Patients can try the following:

- A **low-calorie diet** to achieve **weight loss** (if overweight or obese)
- A **moderate-fat diet** with some unsaturated fatty acids, especially monounsaturated fats, but low in saturated and trans fats
- A **cholesterol-free diet**, such as a **vegan diet**

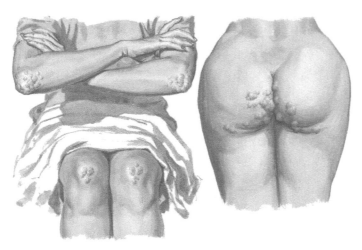

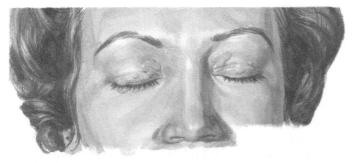

**Fig. 29.14** **Xanthomas caused by dyslipidemia.** Tendon xanthomas (hands and feet), plain and tuberous xanthomas, xanthelasmas of eyelids.

- **Plant sterols (phytosterols)**, which compete with cholesterol for uptake into intestinal epithelial cells via the NPC1L1 (see Fig. 29.1)
- **Fiber**, which binds bile acids and thus prevents their recirculation to the liver

**Exercise** helps patients lose weight and it also independently leads to a lowering of non-HDL cholesterol by approximately 4%.

**Drug treatment** guidelines for hypercholesterolemia and the prevention of **atherosclerotic cardiovascular disease (ASCVD)** vary by country and ethnic population. Agreement exists mostly on treating patients who have clinically evident ASCVD, diabetes, or familial hypercholesterolemia. Various calculators are used to estimate the 10-year **risk** of ASCVD. These estimators often use gender, age, total cholesterol, HDL cholesterol, systolic blood pressure, diabetes, and smoking history as risk factors. Patients with about a 10% 10-year risk of ASCVD are often advised to take a statin.

**Statins** (e.g., **rosuvastatin, atorvastatin, simvastatin, lovastatin, pravastatin**, and **fluvastatin**) inhibit **HMG-CoA reductase** (see Fig. 29.4), which leads to a decreased concentration of cholesterol in the ER membranes. This stimulates SREBP2-mediated transcription of various genes, including the **LDL-receptor** gene. Increased expression of LDL receptors leads to a decreased number of LDL in the blood, thus lowering LDL cholesterol. While SREBP2 also enhances synthesis of HMG-CoA reductase in the cholesterol biosynthesis pathway, this effect is very modest due to inhibition of HMG-CoA reductase by the statin. Over a 5-year period, lowering of LDL cholesterol by 40 mg/dL with statin therapy reduces the number of major vascular events by about 20%.

**Ezetimibe** inhibits the **NPC1L1** transporter in intestinal epithelial cells and therefore inhibits the absorption of cholesterol (see Fig. 29.1). Some of this cholesterol is dietary, and some stems from the enterohepatic cholesterol recirculation. For this reason, ezetimibe lowers LDL cholesterol even in persons who adhere to a cholesterol-free vegan diet.

**Bile acid sequestrants** such as **cholestyramine, colestipol**, and **colesevelam** bind bile salts in the intestine and prevent their reabsorption. Because of the lowered amount of reabsorption, bile salt synthesis from cholesterol increases. As more cholesterol is used for bile acid synthesis, the concentration of intracellular cholesterol drops, SREBP2 becomes active, the number of LDL receptors in the plasma membrane increases, and the liver removes more LDL-containing cholesterol from the blood. However, the lowered intracellular concentration of cholesterol also increases cholesterol biosynthesis by increasing the amount of HMG-CoA reductase. **Statins** may be administered in conjunction with bile acid sequestrants to counter this increase in cholesterol synthesis with greater use of cholesterol for bile acid synthesis.

**Monoclonal antibodies against PCSK9 (PCSK9 inhibitors)**, such as alirocumab and evolocumab, are approved for patients whose LDL cholesterol cannot be adequately controlled by diet and a statin drug. Alirocumab is injected once every 2 weeks and evolocumab once a month. When the amount of PCSK9 is reduced, there is increased survival of LDL receptors, which leads to greater removal of LDL from the blood (see Section 3.1).

## 6. COMBINED HYPERLIPIDEMIA

*Combined hyperlipidemia refers to elevated levels of triglycerides and cholesterol. Patients are at risk of coronary heart disease, and they may show tuberoeruptive xanthomas.*

### 6.1. Familial Combined Hyperlipidemia

Familial combined hyperlipidemia is a common heritable condition that manifests in elevated plasma triglycerides, elevated total cholesterol, or both of these abnormalities. In patients, these abnormalities may change over time. Laboratory values are often abnormal already in childhood. The cause of the disorder is not known; its prevalence in the general population is approximately 1 in 100, and 1 in 10 among persons who have coronary heart disease or a myocardial infarction before the age of 60 years.

Familial combined hyperlipidemia is primarily treated with diet, exercise, and a statin drug. Overweight or obese patients should lose weight.

### 6.2. Familial Dysbetalipoproteinemia

The disease is named based on the observation that there is an increased amount of apoB-containing lipoproteins. Total cholesterol and triglycerides are both elevated. The LDL cholesterol is low because LDL is produced at a reduced rate.

This disorder is due to homozygosity or compound heterozygosity for a variant apolipoprotein E that has a decreased affinity for its receptors. Homozygosity for **apolipoprotein E2**, seen in about 0.5% of the population, is the most common cause of familial dysbetalipoproteinemia, although penetrance often requires the presence of obesity, diabetes, high fat intake, high alcohol consumption, or another risk factor. The dyslipidemia is a result of the accumulation of chylomicron remnants and IDL because these cannot be removed efficiently by apolipoprotein E binding to LRP1 or LDL receptors. In the general population, there are three common isoforms of apolipoprotein E: E2, E3, and E4. Most people are homozygous for E3. E4 is a major risk factor for Alzheimer disease.

Patients who have familial dysbetalipoproteinemia often have premature **ASCVD** and tend to have **tuberoeruptive xanthomas** (see Fig. 29.14).

## SUMMARY

- Only foods derived from animals contain cholesterol.
- In the intestine, Niemann-Pick C1-like protein 1 (NPC1L1) transports sterols (including cholesterol) from the lumen into intestinal epithelial cells.
- Epithelial cells of the intestine, hepatocytes, steroid-producing cells, and macrophages can esterify cholesterol

with a fatty acid to produce cholesteryl esters, which they can store.

- The intestine exports cholesterol and cholesteryl esters in chylomicrons. Lipoprotein lipase removes triglycerides from chylomicrons, and the liver takes up the resulting cholesterol-rich chylomicron remnants (apoprotein E on the remnants binds to the low-density lipoprotein (LDL) receptor-related protein (LRP) receptor on hepatocytes).

- The liver plays a central role in cholesterol homeostasis in that it acquires dietary cholesterol, synthesizes cholesterol and cholesteryl esters and releases these into the blood in very-low-density lipoprotein (VLDL), takes up a large fraction of (cholesterol-rich) LDL, acquires cholesterol from high-density lipoprotein (HDL), secretes cholesterol into bile, and converts cholesterol into bile salts.

- PCSK9 facilitates the destruction of LDL receptors.

- HDL are formed from apolipoprotein A-I. HDL accept cholesterol from peripheral cells. LCAT on HDL receives cholesterol from a variety of cells and esterifies it for storage inside HDL. HDL transfers cholesterol to the liver.

- Cholesteryl ester transfer protein (CETP) exchanges triglycerides and cholesteryl esters between VLDL and HDL. Hepatic lipase removes triglycerides from such HDL and generates lipid-poor particles that are degraded. These processes account for the low plasma HDL cholesterol that is typical of patients who have hypertriglyceridemia.

- The liver synthesizes bile salts and secretes them into the bile canaliculi. The amount of bile salt secretion determines bile flow. Bile is stored in the gallbladder, which empties in response to dietary fat and protein. In the intestine, bile salts emulsify lipids and form mixed micelles with cholesterol and other lipids. An absence of bile salts causes lipid malabsorption. The ileum takes up bile salts for recirculation to the liver.

- Cholesterol gallstones may be caused by excessive secretion of cholesterol from the liver or by deficient secretion of bile salts.

- Cholestasis often causes pruritus, perhaps due to the accumulation of bile salts. It is treated with certain bile acid sequestrants.

- A lipid panel includes measuring total cholesterol, HDL cholesterol, and triglycerides. From these values, non-HDL cholesterol and LDL cholesterol can be calculated.

- A high concentration of plasma LDL cholesterol is associated with atherosclerosis and cardiovascular disease. Patients with very high LDL cholesterol also have xanthomas.

- Familial hypercholesterolemia can be caused by mutations in the genes for the LDL receptor, apoB-100, and PCSK9.

- Approaches to lowering an elevated LDL cholesterol include weight loss; a diet low in fat and cholesterol but high in fiber and plant sterols; a diet that contains a reasonable amount of unsaturated fatty acids; and drugs such as statins, ezetimibe, PCSK9 inhibitors, and bile acid sequestrants. All currently used drugs have in common that they lead to increased expression of LDL receptors on hepatocytes.

- Statin drugs inhibit HMG-CoA reductase, the enzyme that controls the rate of cholesterol de novo synthesis. This leads to increased expression of LDL receptors and, consequently, a lowering of plasma LDL cholesterol.

- Plant sterols compete with cholesterol for uptake via the NPC1L1, and ezetimibe inhibits transport via the NPC1L1.

- Inhibitors of PCSK9 increase the number of LDL receptors and thus lower the concentration of LDL cholesterol in the plasma.

- Bile acid sequestrants prevent the enterohepatic recirculation of bile acids, thereby increasing the use of cholesterol for bile acid synthesis.

- Low HDL cholesterol (most often due to hypertriglyceridemia) is associated with an increased risk of coronary artery disease (CAD).

## FURTHER READING

- Ferdinand KC, Nasser SA. PCSK9 inhibition: discovery, current evidence, and potential effects on LDL-C and Lp(a). *Cardiovasc Drugs Ther.* 2015; 29:295-308.

- Goldstein JL, Brown MS. A century of cholesterol and coronaries: from plaques to genes to statins. *Cell.* 2015;161: 161-172.

- Rader DJ, deGoma EM. Approach to the patient with extremely low HDL cholesterol. *J Clin Endocrinol Metab.* 2012;97:3399-3407.

- Roma MG, Toledo FD, Boaglio AC, Basiglio CL, Crocenzi FA, Sánchez Pozzi EJ. Ursodeoxycholic acid in cholestasis: linking action mechanisms to therapeutic applications. *Clin Sci (Lond).* 2011;121:523-44.

- Zwicker BL, Agellon LB. Transport and biological activities of bile acids. *Int J Biochem Cell Biol.* 2013;45: 1389-1398.

# Review Questions

1. Provide a rationale as to why statins lower LDL cholesterol in patients with heterozygous familial hypercholesterolemia but have no or only a minimal effect in patients with the homozygous form of this disease.

2. Ezetimibe can lower LDL cholesterol in patients who consume a vegan diet because ezetimibe diminishes which one of the following?

   A. Absorption of cholesterol that was secreted into bile
   B. CETP-mediated exchange of cholesterol from HDL to VLDL
   C. HMG-CoA reductase activity
   D. PCSK9 activity
   E. Recirculation of bile salts

3. Which one of the following is a likely cause of low serum HDL cholesterol?

   **A.** CETP deficiency
   **B.** Cholelithiasis
   **C.** Deficiency of hepatic lipase
   **D.** Hypertriglyceridemia
   **E.** PCSK9 deficiency

4. A 25-year-old patient has a very high serum LDL cholesterol but normal values of plasma triglycerides and HDL cholesterol. Physical examination reveals tendon xanthomata. The patient's father had premature ASCVD. Heterozygosity for a loss-of-function mutation in the gene for which one of the following proteins is most compatible with these findings?

   **A.** CETP
   **B.** LDL receptor
   **C.** MTP
   **D.** NPC1L1
   **E.** PCSK9

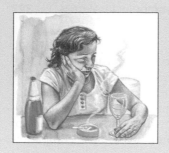

## SYNOPSIS

- Excessive alcohol consumption is a huge public health problem. Ethanol acutely impairs the function of the central nervous system; this gives rise to a high rate of accidental deaths and acute alcohol poisoning. Chronic high ethanol intake can lead to cancer, liver disease, heart disease, and the many problems associated with addiction.

- The liver metabolizes most of the dietary ethanol by first converting it to acetaldehyde and then to acetate. Various tissues then oxidize acetate to $CO_2$. Chronic alcohol consumption leads to increased expression of cytochrome P450 enzymes in the endoplasmic reticulum, which normally oxidize only a small portion of ethanol to acetaldehyde.

- Ethanol acutely suppresses gluconeogenesis and increases the production of triglycerides. In addition, it also increases the production of urate and thus increases the likelihood of an acute episode of gout.

- Alcoholism is a mental disorder with a hereditary component. Chronic high ethanol intake leads to damage of DNA and proteins, and it may induce fatty liver disease, cirrhosis, or cancer (especially of the upper aerodigestive tract). In pregnant women, chronic high ethanol intake may result in offspring with fetal alcohol syndrome; characteristics of this syndrome are abnormalities of the head and problems with behavior.

## LEARNING OBJECTIVES

*For mastery of this topic, you should be able to do the following:*

- Describe the metabolism of ethanol, including products, cellular location, and tissue distribution.
- List the major harmful effects of ethanol on the human body, and describe the known underlying biochemistry.
- Identify a range of alcohol consumption that is considered acceptable and a range that is indicative of abuse.
- Explain the increased toxicity of acetaminophen and procarcinogens in patients who habitually drink large quantities of alcohol.

## 1. EFFECTS OF ALCOHOL USE ON THE HEALTH OF THE PUBLIC

*Worldwide, excessive alcohol consumption is responsible for a large number of injuries and deaths through accidents, an increased prevalence of cancer and cancer-related deaths, disruptions of social interactions, and violence. Alcohol use is currently a far larger problem than the use of illicit psychoactive drugs.*

**Alcohol** is used here as a summary term for beverages that contain **ethanol**. Ethanol has the structural formula $CH_3CH_2OH$.

**Beer** often contains about 5% ethanol by volume (~860 mM ethanol), **wine** about 12% (~ 2,060 mM), and **vodka** about 40% (~ 6,900 mM; in the United States, 40% by volume is called 80 proof). An alcoholic beverage that contains 10% ethanol by volume contains about 8 g of ethanol per 100 mL of the drink.

Global per capita alcohol consumption (considering people aged 15 years or older) is approximately 6 L of pure alcohol per year, about half of which is consumed as spirits and about one-third as beer. Daily per capita consumption is thus about 275 mL of beer, or 35 mL of spirits, or 13 g of ethanol per day. Consumption is the highest in Europe and lowest in predominantly Muslim populations. In the United States, where per capita ethanol consumption is approximately 35% above the world average, 17% of the population aged 15 years or older binge drink (i.e., females consume ≥4 drinks and males consume ≥5 drinks within a 2-hour period) on at least one occasion per month. Among U.S. adults aged 26 years or older, men binge drink twice as frequently as women.

Ethanol depresses the activity of the cerebral cortex. After consumption of a small amount of alcohol on an empty stomach, the concentration of ethanol in the blood peaks within about 20 minutes; after a large dose, breath alcohol peaks within about 40 minutes. From the blood, ethanol readily diffuses through cell membranes without the need for a transporter; thus, it also readily passes through the blood-brain barrier. People who do not habitually drink alcohol eliminate about 10 g of alcohol per hour.

At low to moderate doses, ethanol exerts its effects on the central nervous system in part by enhancing the activity of certain γ-aminobutyric acid (GABA) receptors, which are chloride channels. At low concentrations of ethanol, increased activity of GABA receptors reduces anxiety; at high concentrations of ethanol, GABA receptor activity also induces sedation and anesthesia.

Alcohol is present in blood at relatively high concentrations. At an ethanol concentration above ~25 mg/dL blood (i.e., ~5 mM), a person's reaction time may be decreased and judgment impaired; in addition, the subject may feel that alcohol has taken effect. At an ethanol concentration of about 50 mg/dL (~11 mM), a person's reaction time, tracking ability, and vigilance are compromised. At a concentration of about 100 mg/dL (i.e., ~22 mM), balance is impaired. In an alcohol-naive person, at a concentration greater than ~300 mg/dL (i.e., ~65 mM), coma may set in. Moreover, at a concentration of approximately 400 mg or more of ethanol per dL blood (~80 mM), respiratory arrest and death may occur. In many countries, drivers who have a blood alcohol concentration more than 0.05% to 0.1% w/v (i.e., 50–100 mg/dL [11–22 mM]) are considered intoxicated and are forbidden from operating a vehicle.

In many countries, alcohol use leads to many more deaths than the use of illicit drugs. In the United States, an estimated 90,000 alcohol-attributable deaths occur per year; slightly more than 40% of these deaths occur due to acute intoxication. Each alcohol-attributable death reflects about 30 years of life lost. The most common reasons for death due to *acute* intoxication are motor vehicle accidents, suicides, falls, and being a victim of homicide or poisoning. The most common causes of premature death due to *chronic* alcohol abuse are liver disease, stroke, and cancer.

## 2. METABOLISM OF ETHANOL

*Ethanol is highly soluble in both water and the lipid phase of membranes. Hence, ethanol readily passes through membranes. Hepatocytes oxidize ethanol in two steps: first to acetaldehyde and then to acetate. The first step can occur in the cytosol or in the endoplasmic reticulum. The second step occurs mostly in mitochondria. The liver exports most of the acetate. Cardiac and skeletal muscles pick up acetate and oxidize it to acetyl-coenzyme A (CoA).*

### 2.1. Metabolism of Ethanol to Acetate

Ethanol is chiefly degraded by a combination of the stomach, intestine, and liver. The liver degrades virtually all of the ethanol that reaches the bloodstream. A low percentage of dietary ethanol is eliminated as ethanol via the urine or expired air. The concentration of ethanol in expired air is a reflection of the concentration of ethanol in blood.

Here, ethanol metabolism is described in three stages: (1) ethanol to acetaldehyde, (2) acetaldehyde to acetate, and (3) acetate to $CO_2$. The first two reactions occur primarily in the liver; they may also occur in the stomach. Blood vessel walls and cells of the upper digestive tract that are in contact with alcoholic beverages also carry out these reactions. Although this is of minor quantitative importance, it may be important in protecting these cells from the adverse effects of ethanol. The third reaction occurs mostly in muscle and brain.

The reaction ethanol → acetaldehyde is catalyzed independently by both alcohol dehydrogenase in the cytoplasm and by cytochrome P450 enzymes in the endoplasmic reticulum (Fig. 30.1), as follows.

**Alcohol dehydrogenase (ADH)** oxidizes the major portion of dietary ethanol to acetaldehyde in persons who drink alcohol occasionally. Humans synthesize several ADH isoenzymes and express them in a tissue-specific manner. These enzymes play a role in the oxidation of several different alcohols and other compounds (e.g., retinol). A *blood* ethanol concentration of 5 to 20 mM (~0.025-0.1% weight/volume) impairs a person's judgment and reaction time. ADH isoenzymes that play a physiologic role in removing ethanol have $K_m$ values ($K_m$ values are explained in Chapter 10) in the range 0.05 to 40 mM.

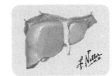

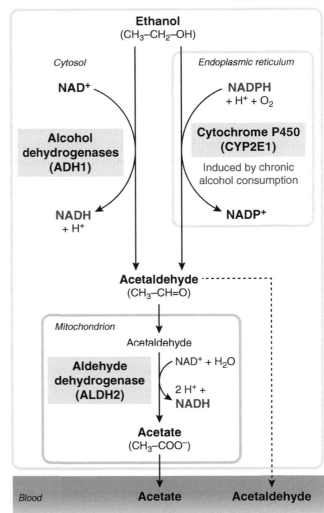

**Fig. 30.1** **Metabolism of ethanol to acetate in hepatocytes.**

Individuals may differ considerably in their ability to metabolize ethanol. Homodimers of the common **isoforms** of ADH in the liver exhibit $K_m$ values for ethanol that differ by a factor of greater than 100 and $V_{max}$ values that differ by a factor of greater than 30. **Women** and patients with **gastritis** (e.g., chronic alcohol abusers) express less ADH in the stomach than alcohol-abstaining **men**. Furthermore, aspirin and certain **histamine H2 blockers** (e.g., **cimetidine**) inhibit gastric ADH.

**Cytochrome P450 enzymes** also oxidize ethanol to acetaldehyde (see Fig. 30.1). The main contributor is **CYP2E1**; minor contributors are CYP1A2 and CYP3A4. Over a period of days to weeks, a persistent ethanol intake is accompanied by increased CYP2E1 activity, which contributes to ethanol tolerance. In habitual drinkers, CYP2E1 becomes the main enzyme that oxidizes ethanol.

**Aldehyde dehydrogenase (ALDH)** inside mitochondria oxidizes acetaldehyde to acetate. Akin to ADH, there are several isoenzymes for ALDH, which in turn oxidize various aldehydes. In the liver, ALDH1 is present in the cytosol and ALDH2 in mitochondria; the enzyme in mitochondria has a much higher affinity for acetaldehyde and oxidizes the lion's share of acetaldehyde.

Acetaldehyde, like ethanol, crosses membranes by diffusion (i.e., without the help of a transporter). Some acetaldehyde leaks from the liver into the blood.

Many persons of **East Asian** heritage (e.g., Japanese, Korean, or Han Chinese) do not efficiently metabolize acetaldehyde. These individuals are heterozygous or homozygous for a variant mitochondrial acetaldehyde dehydrogenase that has little enzymatic activity. As a consequence, the concentration of acetaldehyde in the blood is increased, causing nausea, headache, and flushing of the face and upper chest (flushing is due to temporary vasodilation).

**Disulfiram** (Antabuse) irreversibly inhibits both the mitochondrial and the cytosolic ALDH. Patients who take disulfiram and then drink alcohol experience flushing, nausea, and sufficient overall physical discomfort to stop drinking. For this reason, disulfiram can be used to keep alcohol-dependent patients from drinking alcohol (see also Section 4.3). However, unless someone ensures the patient takes the drug daily, compliance is low.

Acetaldehyde forms noxious adducts with proteins and DNA (see Section 4.2). These reactions contribute to the increased risk of certain types of cancer among people who consume alcohol.

In summary, the equation for the oxidation of ethanol by ADH and ALDH is:

$$\text{Ethanol} + 2\,NAD^+ + H_2O \rightarrow \text{Acetate}^- + 2\,NADH + 3\,H^+$$

The liver releases most of the **acetate** into the bloodstream; from there, it reaches other tissues for further metabolism.

## 2.2. Oxidation of Acetate to $CO_2$

Skeletal and cardiac muscle, the brain, and other tissues take up acetate from the blood and can oxidize it to $CO_2$ (Fig. 30.2). **Acetate-CoA ligase** (commonly called **acetyl-CoA synthetase**) inside mitochondria activates acetate to acetyl-CoA. This activation produces **adenosine monophosphate (AMP)** and can do so at a high rate (see Section 3.3).

## 3. ACUTE EFFECT OF ETHANOL ON PATHWAYS OF METABOLISM

*Ethanol metabolism affects the metabolism of other compounds largely through an increased ratio of NADH/NAD⁺ in the liver and an increased rate of AMP production from the activation of acetate in muscle. A moderate to large dose of ethanol thus inhibits gluconeogenesis, increases liver triglyceride stores, and increases urate production.*

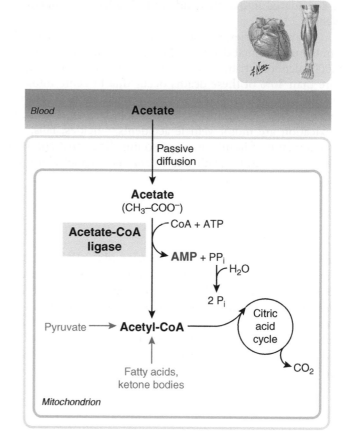

**Fig. 30.2** **Oxidation of acetate in skeletal and cardiac muscle.** The liver metabolizes ethanol to acetate and releases most of the acetate into the bloodstream (see Fig. 30.1).

## 3.1. Effect of Ethanol on Gluconeogenesis

After alcohol consumption, gluconeogenesis is suppressed significantly, which may cause **hypoglycemia**. For instance, in volunteers who fasted overnight and then imbibed 50 g of ethanol (equivalent to about 0.4 L of wine), gluconeogenesis, around noon, proceeded at approximately half the rate of individuals who had not consumed alcohol. However, glucose use also decreases (presumably due to the oxidation of ethanol and its metabolites), which dampens the expected decrease in blood glucose concentration. When patients who have **diabetes** or a **glycogen storage disease** who are **fasting** or consume few carbohydrate they cannot readily compensate for a decreased rate of gluconeogenesis with an increased rate of glycogenolysis. Hence, these patients are at greatest risk for alcohol-induced hypoglycemia.

The ethanol-induced decrease in gluconeogenesis is usually attributed to an altered **NADH/NAD⁺** ratio in hepatocytes that oxidize ethanol. As shown in Section 2, the degradation of 1 mol ethanol to acetate yields 2 mol of NADH from NAD⁺. The metabolism of ethanol is rapid enough that the NADH/NAD⁺ ratio changes substantially. In turn, this shifts the lactate/pyruvate equilibrium toward **lactate** and the dihydroxyacetone phosphate/glycerol 3-phosphate equilibrium toward glycerol 3-phosphate (Fig. 30.3). Pyruvate that is made

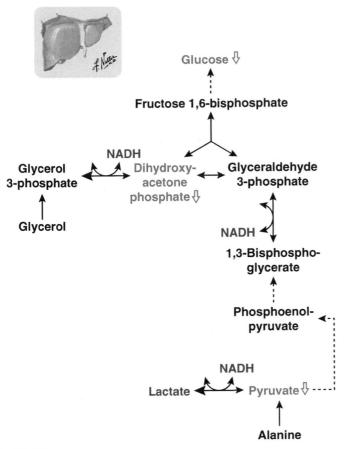

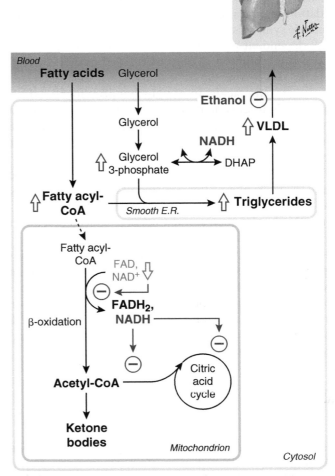

**Fig. 30.3**  **Effect of ethanol consumption on gluconeogenesis.** The rapid oxidation of ethanol in the liver leads to an increased concentration of NADH and a decreased concentration of NAD$^+$ (see Fig. 30.2). For more details on the reactions of gluconeogenesis, see Fig. 25.3.

from alanine is reduced to lactate instead of entering mitochondria. The lowered concentrations of pyruvate and dihydroxyacetone phosphate no longer support a normal rate of gluconeogenesis. A purely alcohol-induced **lactic acidosis** is usually mild and occurs only in a small fraction of patients who are hospitalized because of acute ethanol intoxication.

## 3.2. Effect of Ethanol on Fatty Acid Metabolism

Ethanol inhibits lipolysis and leads to a lowering of the concentration of free **fatty acids** in the plasma. The same effect can be achieved with acetate.

Ethanol inhibits **fatty acid β-oxidation** in the liver, perhaps via both the high NADH/NAD$^+$ ratio and the resulting low concentration of FAD (Fig. 30.4; see also Fig. 27.11).

Alcohol use also increases the **production of triglycerides**. This is commonly explained by the ready availability of fatty acids in the alcohol-intoxicated liver, combined with an elevated concentration of glycerol 3-phosphate and an increased amount of smooth endoplasmic reticulum (see Fig. 30.4). The concentration of glycerol 3-phosphate is high because alcohol raises the NADH/NAD$^+$ ratio, which shifts the equilibrium from dihydroxyacetone phosphate toward glycerol

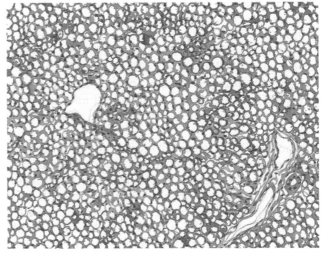

**Fig. 30.4**  **Effect of ethanol consumption on lipid metabolism in the fasting state.** Glycolysis is detailed in Fig. 19.2, gluconeogenesis in Fig. 25.3, β-oxidation in Fig. 27.11, the citric acid cycle in Fig. 22.6, synthesis of the ketone bodies acetoacetate and β-hydroxybutyrate in Fig. 27.14, and synthesis of triglycerides in Fig. 28.5.

3-phosphate. Alcohol use also induces a shift in the rate of transcription from genes that encode enzymes of fatty acid oxidation to genes that encode enzymes of fatty acid and triglyceride synthesis. In addition, alcohol use leads to a reduced AMP-dependent protein kinase (AMPK) activity, which can reduce the inhibition of acetyl-CoA carboxylase by AMPK, increase the formation of malonyl-CoA, and decrease the uptake of fatty acids into mitochondria for β-oxidation. Some alcohol-dependent patients have hypertriglyceridemia; however, this is not usually seen in patients who have liver cirrhosis because the livers of these patients has a reduced capacity for VLDL production.

In chronic alcoholics, **alcoholic ketoacidosis** may develop in the recovery phase after a period of intense binge drinking that is followed by nausea and vomiting. Ketone bodies are synthesized only when acetyl-CoA is produced at a high rate from the β-oxidation of fatty acids. For this to happen, the concentration of fatty acids in the blood must be relatively high. Since alcohol inhibits fatty acid β-oxidation, ketone production occurs only after ethanol has been removed from the blood. Since insulin would inhibit lipolysis, ketoacidosis is commonly seen in conjunction with mild hypoglycemia. Low food intake and vomiting increase the likelihood that an alcohol-abusing patient develops ketoacidosis.

## 3.3. Effect of Ethanol on the Production of Uric Acid

The metabolism of ethanol leads to increased production of **uric acid**. In muscle, activation of acetate to acetyl-CoA produces **AMP** (see Fig. 30.2). The concentration of AMP rises sufficiently to activate the degradation of AMP and guanosine monophosphate (GMP; GMP is in equilibrium with AMP) to urate (see Chapter 38). Indeed, after a moderate to large dose of ethanol, there is a mild increase in plasma urate and a more pronounced increase in urine uric acid. Chronic hyperuricemia increases the likelihood of an acute attack of **gout** (i.e., a very painful inflammation of one or more joints).

Alcohol also leads to a small increase in the concentrations of lactate and ketone bodies in the blood. Both lactate and ketone bodies decrease uric acid excretion by the kidneys (see Chapter 38). In the absence of **exercise**, these factors are minor. However, when alcohol is consumed after exercise (i.e., when the concentration of lactate in blood is markedly increased), there is a marked inhibition of uric acid excretion into the urine.

Consumption of *beer* or *liquor* at the world average of about 11 g of ethanol per day is associated with an increased concentration of urate in blood plasma, as well as an increased incidence of gout; this is not the case with a similar amount of alcohol consumed as *wine*. The reasons for these differences are not entirely clear, except that beer contains a significant amount of guanine, some of which is taken up and degraded to urate. Patients who have gout are advised to abstain from drinking beer or liquor.

## 3.4. Treatment of Acute Ethanol Intoxication in the Clinic

Patients who consume a very large amount of alcohol are at risk of severe hypoglycemia, respiratory arrest, sudden cardiovascular death, aspiration of vomit, and psychosis.

For the most part, ethanol-intoxicated patients receive supportive care. Hypoglycemic patients are given thiamine and glucose; thiamine is given to prevent Wernicke encephalopathy or cardiomyopathy (see Chapter 22). Patients who ingest a large amount of alcohol during the hour before treatment may be helped by gastric emptying. In addition, if needed, hemodialysis can be used to remove ethanol from the bloodstream.

# 4. EFFECTS OF CHRONIC ETHANOL INTAKE ON ORGAN FUNCTION

*Alcoholism is a common and partially hereditary mental disorder. Ethanol and its metabolites damage proteins, which in turn can cause organ damage (e.g., in the liver) and cancer (e.g., of the esophagus). In utero exposure to ethanol damages the central nervous system and leads to problems with behavior and sometimes also abnormalities of the face.*

## 4.1. General Comments About Alcohol Dependence Syndrome

Alcoholism is considered a **mental disorder**. The World Health Organization's latest International Statistical Classification of Diseases and Related Health Problems (ICD-10) uses the term **alcohol dependence syndrome**, which requires the presence of three of six listed risk factors (e.g., a strong desire to drink or exhibiting withdrawal symptoms) being present. The American Psychiatric Association's DSM-V5 uses the term **alcohol use disorder**, which can be mild, moderate, or severe depending on the number of 11 criteria that a person meets. In the United States in 2012, approximately 7% of people aged 18 years or older had alcohol use disorder.

In the United States, the National Institute on Alcohol Abuse and Alcoholism defines **binge drinking** as drinking that results in a blood alcohol content of 80 mg/dL or higher. Many adults reach this concentration by consuming four to five drinks during a 2-hour period. The same institution considers **low-risk** drinking as the consumption of fewer than 3 to 4 drinks in one day and fewer than 7 to 14 drinks per week (lower numbers are for women, higher numbers for men).

Chronic, excessive use of alcohol is associated with chronic disease, accidents, social problems, and increased domestic violence. Chronic effects of alcohol use are best predicted by a patient's average alcohol consumption. In the United States, alcohol-induced chronic disease is responsible for about half of all alcohol-attributable deaths and about one-third of alcohol-attributable potential life years lost.

Alcoholism is partly **hereditary**. Offspring of one alcohol-abusing parent are about five times more likely to abuse alcohol than offspring of nonabusing parents. Studies of twins show that genetic factors account for about 50% of the interindividual variation for alcoholism. Linkage studies implicate mutations that affect enzymes of ethanol metabolism and proteins that likely also play a role in neurotransmission.

People who experience **acetaldehyde-induced flushing** and nausea after alcohol consumption are least likely to become alcohol dependent. The concentration of acetaldehyde can be high for two main reasons: low acetaldehyde dehydrogenase activity or high ADH activity. The Glu487Lys variant of **mitochondrial acetaldehyde dehydrogenase** (also called the *ALDH2\*2* allele) has virtually no enzymatic activity. This variant is found almost exclusively in persons of East Asian heritage. Mitochondrial acetaldehyde dehydrogenase functions as a tetramer, and the Glu487Lys variant shows a dominant negative effect (see Chapter 5). Homozygotes have virtually no risk of becoming alcohol dependent, whereas heterozygotes have only about one-fourth the risk of patients with normal acetaldehyde dehydrogenase activity. High **ADH** activity is associated with the *ADH1B\*2* (Arg47His) allele. The *ADH1B\*2* allele provides some protection from alcohol dependence, but not as powerfully as the *ALDH2\*2* allele. After consumption of alcohol, this variant enzyme completes about 30 catalytic cycles in the time the normal enzyme completes one cycle.

Patients who chronically consume large quantities of alcohol often develop **malnutrition**. One gram of ethanol provides about 7 kcal (carbohydrates and proteins provide 4 kcal/g, and fat provides 9 kcal/g). One liter of vodka thus provides more calories than average daily meals. Many alcohol-dependent individuals consume only about half as much food as alcohol abstainers do. In addition, alcohol intake diminishes the absorption of **phosphate** and some **vitamins** in the intestine. Together, these effects may cause **hypophosphatemia** (see Chapter 19), **thiamine deficiency** (see Chapter 22), **folate deficiency** (see Section 7.1 in Chapter 36), **pyridoxal** (i.e., vitamin $B_6$) **deficiency**, or **pellagra** (i.e., niacin deficiency; see Section 1 in Chapter 19).

## 4.2. Effects of Ethanol and Acetaldehyde on Proteins and DNA

Ethanol and acetaldehyde can react with proteins and thus impair their function or make them immunogenic. Ethanol can give rise to **hydroxyethyl radicals** ($CH_3–C^•H–OH$, $CH_3–CH_2–O^•$, or $^•CH_2–CH_2–OH$) that react with proteins. These hydroxyethyl radicals are the result of hydroxyl radicals ($^•OH$) stealing an H from ethanol, and they can also be a by-product of CYP2E1 activity. Together with **malondialdehyde** ($O=CH–CH_2–CH=O$, a product of the peroxidation of polyunsaturated fatty acids), **acetaldehyde** can form hybrid protein adducts. Acetaldehyde adducts and mixed adducts of acetaldehyde and malondialdehyde are immunogenic. Ethanol consumption also leads to the acetylation of lysine residues in proteins.

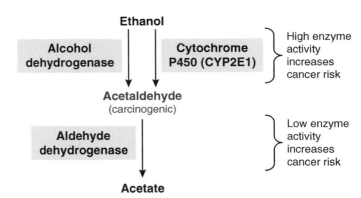

**Fig. 30.5** **Effect of variant enzymes on alcohol metabolism and cancer risk.**

The concentration of acetaldehyde in cells depends on the rates of its production and oxidation (i.e., on the activities of ADH, cytochrome P450 CYP2E1, and ALDH; Fig. 30.5). The alcohol-induced cancer risk thus depends on a person's genetic makeup for these enzymes. Patients who are heterozygous for the *2 allele of *ALDH2* (the gene for ALDH in mitochondria) have only about 40% of the normal ALDH activity. While severe, alcohol-induced flushing prevents *ALDH2\*2 homozygotes* from drinking alcohol, heterozygotes can become alcohol dependent. If so, they have an increased risk for cancer of the esophagus (see also Section 4.5 and Fig. 30.7).

Individuals who abuse ethanol regularly and therefore have increased P450 activity are at risk of a toxic reaction to the pain reliever **acetaminophen** (also called **paracetamol**). Normally, most acetaminophen is detoxified via glucuronidation or sulfation, and only about 15% is eliminated via the P450 system (Fig. 30.6), thereby generating NAPQI (N-acetyl-*p*-benzoquinoneimine). In alcohol-dependent individuals, due to higher activity of alcohol-metabolizing cytochromes P450, a much greater fraction of acetaminophen is detoxified through the P450 system. NAPQI is highly electrophilic and reacts with –SH and other groups. Reduced glutathione can react with NAPQI and thereby detoxify it. However, if the concentration of NAPQI exceeds that of reduced glutathione, NAPQI reacts with –SH groups of proteins.

Acetaldehyde forms adducts with DNA, such as with the amino group of guanine. At this time, the role of DNA adducts in alcohol-related tumorigenesis is not well understood. Furthermore, it is uncertain whether acetaldehyde modification of DNA methyltransferases, histones, and other proteins affects genome maintenance.

## 4.3. Drugs That Help Patients Free Themselves From Alcohol Dependence

Current treatment programs for alcohol-dependent patients are only moderately effective. A combination of psychosocial and drug therapy is commonly used. Most patients relapse within less than a year.

The major drugs used for the treatment of alcohol dependence are acamprosate, naltrexone, and disulfiram. Patients

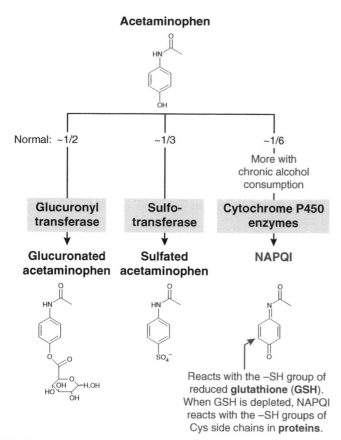

**Fig. 30.6** **Metabolism of acetaminophen (paracetamol).** NAPQI, N-acetyl-*p*-benzoquinoneimine.

who regularly abuse alcohol drink alcohol because it makes them feel better or because it alleviates symptoms of withdrawal. **Acamprosate**, through a yet unknown mechanism, helps maintain abstinence. **Naltrexone**, an opioid receptor antagonist, reduces the craving for alcohol and also diminishes the "elevated" feeling after alcohol. **Disulfiram**, an irreversible inhibitor of acetaldehyde dehydrogenase (see Section 2.1), has few effects by itself. However, when a disulfiram-treated patient consumes alcohol, headache, nausea, vomiting, chest pain, and other symptoms set in due to an excessive concentration of acetaldehyde; this discourages the patient from consuming more alcohol. A disulfiram-treated patient who nonetheless drinks a large quantity of alcohol risks severe pathologic effects. An extract of the root of **kudzu**, a traditional Chinese medicine, also inhibits alcohol consumption.

## 4.4. Effect of Ethanol on the Liver

Substantial intake of alcohol can lead to fatty liver, liver inflammation, and liver cirrhosis. All forms of liver disease together account for about one-fifth of all alcohol-attributable deaths and potential life years lost.

**Fatty liver (hepatic steatosis)** is an early and common consequence of chronic alcohol abuse (see Fig. 30.4). The steatosis is the result of increased production and decreased export of triglycerides (see Section 3.2). The triglycerides

accumulate in lipid droplets inside hepatocytes, particularly in the perivenous areas. These lipid droplets are visible by light microscopy. De novo fatty acid synthesis normally contributes only a minor portion of the fatty acids in triglycerides; this is also true for patients who consume excessive amounts of alcohol. With increasing lipid intake, the accumulation of triglycerides increases. With abstinence from alcohol, hepatic steatosis recedes.

Alcohol-induced **inflammation** of the liver (i.e., **alcoholic hepatitis**) and liver **cirrhosis** are the result of multiple pathogenic mechanisms. Thus alcohol and its metabolite acetaldehyde have direct toxic effects on proteins; they induce the expression of alcohol-metabolizing cytochromes P450 that generate free radicals, and they stimulate excessive synthesis of extracellular matrix components. In the absence of treatment, the combination of alcohol-induced fatty liver and inflammation is particularly dangerous; survival for more than 4 months is only approximately 70%.

**Stellate cells** (fat-storing cells, Ito cells, lipocytes) in the liver play a key role in the pathogenesis of ethanol-induced **fibrosis**. Stellate cells are normally the major producers of extracellular matrix in the liver, and they also store retinoic acid esters in lipid droplets. In response to alcohol and acetaldehyde, stellate cells morph into fibroblasts that store little retinoic acid and produce extracellular matrix at an increased rate.

## 4.5. Effect of Ethanol on Cancer Risk

Alcohol-attributable cancer accounts for roughly one-tenth of alcohol-attributable deaths and potential life years lost. Consumption of alcohol increases a person's risk of **cancer** of the mouth, pharynx, larynx, esophagus, liver, and breast (in women). The cancer risk increases with alcohol consumption. Fig. 30.7 shows examples; note that baseline risks for the disorders differ. In the upper digestive tract, particularly the esophagus, some resident microbes convert ethanol to acetaldehyde, which is mutagenic to epithelial cells.

Mechanisms that can potentially contribute to cancer risk include acetaldehyde-induced modification of DNA; increased production of free radicals from alcohol induction of cytochromes P450; decreased concentrations of antioxidants owing to their reaction with free radicals; increased conversion of procarcinogens to carcinogens by an increased quantity of cytochrome P450 CYP2E1; inflammation of tissues; low concentrations of folates owing to malnutrition; altered metabolism of retinol and its derivatives (see also Section 4.7); and an ethanol-induced reduction in the concentration of S-adenosylmethionine, which in turn leads to reduced methylation of DNA and proteins.

Approximately three-fourths of patients who abuse alcohol also **smoke**. Cancer risk from smoking and alcohol abuse is greater than the sum of the individual risks. The combination of **alcohol and smoking** is a particularly strong risk factor for the development of cancer of the oral cavity, pharynx, and esophagus. Procarcinogens in smoke converted to

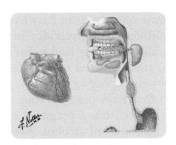

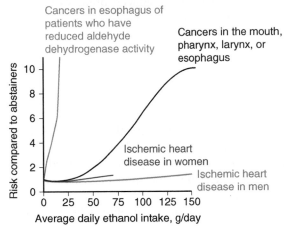

Cancers in esophagus of patients who have reduced aldehyde dehydrogenase activity

Cancers in the mouth, pharynx, larynx, or esophagus

Ischemic heart disease in women

Ischemic heart disease in men

Average daily ethanol intake, g/day

Risk compared to abstainers

**Fig. 30.7** **Epidemiological relationship between alcohol consumption and odds of upper aerodigestive tract cancer or ischemic heart disease.** The populations are as follows: gray line, Japan; black line, Italy and Switzerland; red and blue lines, meta-analysis of 51 studies in diverse countries. (Data from Yokoyama A, et al. Genetic polymorphisms of alcohol and aldehyde dehydrogenases and glutathione S-transferase M1 and drinking, smoking, and diet in Japanese men with esophageal squamous cell carcinoma. *Carcinogenesis.* 2002;23:1851-1859; Polesel J, et al. Estimating dose-response relationship between ethanol and risk of cancer using regression spline models. *Int J Cancer.* 2005;114:836; and Corrao G, et al. Alcohol and coronary heart disease: a meta-analysis. *Addiction.* 2000;95:1505.)

carcinogens by cytochromes P450 add to the carcinogenic activity of acetaldehyde from the metabolism of ethanol.

## 4.6. Effect of Ethanol on the Heart

Chronic consumption of large amounts of alcohol (≥70 g ethanol/day for ≥10 years) is associated with **hypertension** and **alcoholic heart muscle disease (alcoholic cardiomyopathy)**.

In epidemiological studies, consumption of small to moderate amounts of alcohol (compared with abstinence) is associated with a 15% to 20% reduction in the risk for **ischemic heart disease** (a decrease that is barely noticeable in Fig. 30.7). This association does not prove causality. It is unclear whether the association is due to a positive effect of alcohol on health or due to bias (e.g., abstinence due to a chronic illness). Due to a lack of reliable data and a risk of leading patients into alcohol abuse, patients are not advised to drink alcohol for protection against ischemic heart disease.

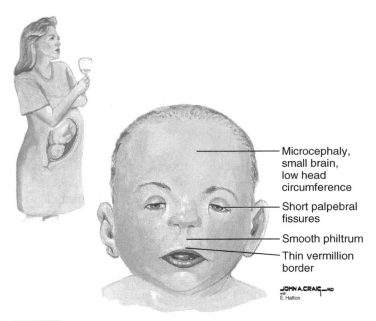

Microcephaly, small brain, low head circumference

Short palpebral fissures

Smooth philtrum

Thin vermillion border

**Fig. 30.8** **Features of newborns with fetal alcohol syndrome.**

## 4.7. Effect of Ethanol on the Fetus

**Fetal alcohol syndrome** is the consequence of a pregnant mother exposing her fetus to alcohol. Worldwide, fetal alcohol syndrome affects about 0.1% of all newborns. Less severe pathological effects of alcohol consumption are seen in about 1% of all newborns. Thus, ethanol is one of the most prevalent teratogens. Expression of the full fetal alcohol syndrome requires recurrent binge drinking (i.e., consumption of ≥75 g of alcohol per occasion) at least once a week. Yet, only a fraction of such alcohol-abusing mothers gives birth to a child with the complete fetal alcohol syndrome, most likely because genetic factors also play a role. Alcohol exposure early in pregnancy and in the last trimester (a period of extensive synaptogenesis) is especially damaging to the offspring. Whether there is a safe amount of alcohol that can be consumed during pregnancy is unknown.

In the fetus, alcohol leads to apoptosis of cranial neural crest cells as well as the abnormal migration of neurons and glial cells. Children who are affected with the most severe form of fetal alcohol syndrome have abnormal facial features (see Fig. 30.8), a growth deficit both in utero and after birth, cognitive deficits, and behavioral problems. Unfortunately, a high fraction of such persons spends time in prison or in a mental institution. Children who are only mildly affected by alcohol show only abnormal behavior.

The mechanisms by which alcohol causes neural crest cells to die by apoptosis are incompletely understood, but **retinoic acid** likely plays a role. Retinoic acid activates several transcription factors that play a role in development. Neural crest cells require retinoic acid for survival. Ethanol is expected to interfere with the oxidation of retinol (vitamin A) to retinoic acid by ADH and ALDH, as well as the degradation of retinoic acid by cytochrome P450 enzymes.

## SUMMARY

- The global daily per capita consumption of ethanol is about 13 g. In many countries, it is illegal for drivers to have a blood alcohol concentration of more than 50 to 100 mg/dL. A blood alcohol concentration more than 400 mg/dL in an alcohol-naive person can be lethal. A high concentration of alcohol leads to central nervous system depression, which may cause respiratory arrest.
- Worldwide, about equal numbers of people die from acute and chronic effects of alcohol. The major acute effects include accidents, suicide, homicide, and poisoning; the major chronic effects relate to liver disease and cancer.
- The liver metabolizes most of the consumed ethanol to acetate. In the liver, alcohol dehydrogenases (ADHs) and cytochrome P450 2E1 (CYP2E1) oxidize ethanol to acetaldehyde. In a person who does not habitually drink alcohol, CYP2E1 oxidizes only a small portion of the dietary ethanol. In a person who habitually drinks high amounts of alcohol, CYP2E1 oxidizes more ethanol than the ADHs. The increase in CYP2E1 activity also increases the rate of formation of toxic free radicals, a highly reactive degradation product (NAPQI) of the pain reliever acetaminophen, and carcinogens from certain procarcinogens.
- Aldehyde dehydrogenase (ALDH) in the mitochondria oxidizes acetaldehyde to acetate. Homozygotes for a deficient ALDH are common in East Asia. When such persons consume alcohol, an increased amount of acetaldehyde escapes into the blood and causes flushing of the face, nausea, and overall discomfort. Affected individuals are unlikely to become addicted to alcohol. In patients with normal ALDH activity, the inhibitor disulfiram causes a similar increase in blood acetaldehyde, flushing, and discomfort. Disulfiram is used to deter alcohol-dependent patients from consuming alcohol.
- In the liver, the oxidation of ethanol to acetate leads to a high NADH/NAD$^+$ ratio, which in turn shifts the lactate/pyruvate equilibrium toward lactate and the dihydroxyacetone phosphate/glycerol 3-phosphate equilibrium toward glycerol 3-phosphate. As a result, the concentration of substrates for gluconeogenesis is low, and the rate of gluconeogenesis is reduced. Furthermore, β-oxidation of fatty acids is inhibited, and the esterification of fatty acids with glycerol 3-phosphate is increased.
- Heart and skeletal muscle oxidize most of the acetate from ethanol metabolism to $CO_2$. The activation of acetate to acetyl-CoA yields AMP. If this reaction proceeds at a high rate, some of the AMP is degraded to urate. An increase in urate production increases a person's risk for gout.
- Hydroxyethyl radicals can modify proteins; these radicals stem from CYP2E1 activity and hydroxyl radicals reacting with ethanol. Acetaldehyde together with malondialdehyde forms adducts with proteins that are immunogenic and may impair protein function. Acetaldehyde also gives rise to adducts with DNA.
- Chronic alcohol abuse often leads to fatty liver (steatosis), owing to the deposition of triglycerides in intracellular lipid droplets. In addition, it may lead to inflammation of the liver (hepatitis) and increased production of extracellular matrix, thereby giving rise to cirrhosis.
- Ethanol is toxic to the developing nervous system. Fetal alcohol syndrome results from a pregnant mother's consumption of large quantities of alcohol. Affected persons (about 1 in 1,000) have reduced brain size, facial abnormalities, and problems with behavior.

## FURTHER READING

- Cederbaum AI. Alcohol metabolism. *Clin Liver Dis.* 2012;16:667-685.
- Hingson R, Rehm J. Measuring the burden: alcohol's evolving impact. *Alcohol Res.* 2013;35:122-127.
- Hurley TD, Edenberg HJ. Genes encoding enzymes involved in ethanol metabolism. *Alcohol Res.* 2012; 34:339-344.
- Lieber CS. Metabolism of alcohol. *Clin Liver Dis.* 2005; 9:1-35.
- McGuire LC, et al. Alcoholic ketoacidosis. *Emerg Med J.* 2006;23:417-420.
- Meadows GG, Zhang H. Effects of alcohol on tumor growth, metastasis, immune response, and host survival. *Alcohol Res.* 2015;37:311-322.
- Siler SQ, et al. The inhibition of gluconeogenesis following alcohol in humans. *Am J Physiol.* 1998;275:E897-E907.
- Siler SQ, et al. De novo lipogenesis, lipid kinetics, and whole-body lipid balances in humans after acute alcohol consumption. *Am J Clin Nutr.* 1999;70:928-936.
- World Health Organization: Global status report on alcohol and health 2014. Available at <http://www.who.int/substance_abuse/publications/global_alcohol_report/en/>.

# Review Questions

1. A 21-year-old college student is brought to the emergency department. He is unconscious after drinking large quantities of beer and liquor during a 4-hour period. The patient showed depressed respiration and was therefore intubated and mechanically ventilated. A blood sample showed glucose 144 mg/dL (8.0 mM) and alcohol 450 mg/dL. The urine was negative for ketones. Which of the following is the most appropriate additional care?

   A. Hemodialysis
   B. Infusion of disulfiram (an inhibitor of ALDH)
   C. Infusion of fomepizole (an inhibitor of ADH)
   D. Infusion of insulin
   E. Infusion of thiamine and glucose

2. In the emergency department, an alcohol-abusing patient is being treated for hypoglycemia. The treating physician decides to inject glucagon. However, within 10 minutes, glucagon has little or no effect on blood glucose. The most likely reason for the lack of effect is that the patient's liver contains which of the following?

   **A.** Too few glucagon receptors
   **B.** Too high a concentration of NADH to permit an adequate rate of gluconeogenesis
   **C.** Too little glycogen
   **D.** Too low a concentration of fatty acids to provide ATP for gluconeogenesis

3. A 50-year-old alcohol-addicted man has lost his job, family, and life savings. He sought help for his addiction and is being treated with disulfiram. If this patient drinks alcohol, the drug makes him feel very uncomfortable by inhibiting which one of the following processes?

   **A.** ADH-catalyzed oxidation of ethanol to acetaldehyde in the cytoplasm
   **B.** ALDH-catalyzed oxidation of acetaldehyde to acetic acid
   **C.** CYP2E1-catalyzed oxidation of ethanol to acetaldehyde in the endoplasmic reticulum

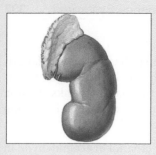

# Chapter 31
# Steroid Hormones and Vitamin D

## SYNOPSIS

- Steroids are synthesized from cholesterol.
- Steroids are membrane permeable and therefore cannot be stored inside cells. Thus they are synthesized on demand. Transport of cholesterol from the outer to the inner membrane of mitochondria is normally the rate-limiting step in the synthesis of steroids.
- During transport in the blood, steroids are bound to plasma proteins. Inside target cells, steroids bind to receptors that act as transcription factors and thus alter the rate of transcription of various genes. Steroids have a short life span.
- The brain regulates the synthesis of sex steroids. Abnormalities in sex steroid synthesis can affect the development of sex characteristics. Birth control pills reduce the stimulus from the brain to follicles in the ovaries, whereas the fertility drug clomiphene has the opposite effect. Patients with sex steroid–responsive tumors are often treated with drugs that impair sex steroid–dependent growth.
- The brain also regulates the synthesis of cortisol by the adrenal glands. Synthetic analogs of cortisol are widely used in medicine as antiinflammatory and immunosuppressive drugs. Long-term and high-dose use of these drugs or excess cortisol production leads to loss of muscle mass and changes in fat deposits.
- At low blood pressure, renin and angiotensin play a role in stimulating aldosterone synthesis in the adrenal cortex. Aldosterone then increases sodium and water retention by the kidneys, thereby increasing blood pressure.
- Vitamin D is formed in the skin on exposure to ultraviolet light. A low concentration of calcium in the blood leads to increased conversion of this precursor to calcitriol, which then leads to increased expression of proteins that participate in increasing the absorption of calcium in the intestine, the recovery of calcium in the kidneys, and the release of calcium form bone.

## LEARNING OBJECTIVES

*For mastery of this topic, you should be able to do the following:*
- Compare and contrast the mechanism of action of steroid hormones with that of peptide hormones.
- List the key steroids that are of physiological or pharmacological importance.
- Describe the female reproductive cycle and indicate points of pharmacological intervention for patients who have infertility or who use hormone-based birth control.
- Describe the mechanism of action of drugs that modulate steroid synthesis and thus have a beneficial effect on the development or treatment of breast cancer.
- Describe the regulation of blood pressure and pharmacological means of interfering with it in patients with hypertension.
- Describe the cause of Cushing syndrome. Compare and contrast the symptoms of Cushing syndrome with those of long-term corticosteroid treatment.
- Describe the synthesis of vitamin D, noting the effect of light.

## 1. GENERAL PROPERTIES AND SYNTHESIS OF STEROID HORMONES

*Steroid hormones are synthesized from cholesterol. In response to peptide hormones, the steroid acute regulatory (StAR) protein helps transport cholesterol to the inner mitochondrial membrane and thereby start steroid synthesis. Steroids are membrane permeable and are therefore synthesized on demand. Steroids exert their effects by binding to steroid receptors, which then bind to steroid response elements and thus affect the rate of transcription.*

### 1.1. Structure and Properties of Steroid Hormones

The physiologically important steroids derive from cholesterol. The core structure of steroids and the numbering of their rings and substituents is shown in Fig. 31.1.

The steroid hormones include glucocorticoids, mineralocorticoids, and the sex steroids. Vitamin D is a secosteroid; that is, a steroid with a cut cyclohexene ring (ring B in Fig. 31.1).

Steroids are membrane permeable and are therefore made to order rather than stored in membrane-enclosed secretory vesicles. In the blood, steroids bind to plasma proteins. In target cells, steroid hormones bind to receptors in the cytoplasm and nucleus of cells. Most of these receptors are transcription factors. The transcription factors bind to steroid response elements in promoters of genes. Thus steroid hormones affect the expression of certain genes.

### 1.2. Common Pathway of Steroid Hormone Synthesis

**Cholesterol** is the precursor of steroids. This cholesterol can derive from cholesteryl esters stored in intracellular droplets, from cholesterol retrieved from low-density lipoprotein (LDL) or high-density lipoprotein (HDL; see Section 3 in Chapter 29), and from de novo synthesis. Steroids are mainly synthesized in the adrenal glands, ovaries, and testes.

The first and rate-limiting step in steroid synthesis is the transport of cholesterol from the outer to the inner membrane of mitochondria (Fig. 31.2); this transport is controlled by the activity of the **steroidogenic acute regulatory (StAR) protein**. The mechanism of transport is not understood. StAR protein activity depends on intracellular signals from membrane receptors, such as cyclic adenosine monophosphate (**cAMP**) and **$Ca^{2+}$**, increased concentrations of which lead to increased

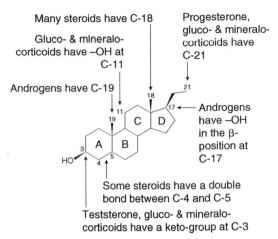

Many steroids have C-18

Gluco- & mineralo-
corticoids have –OH at
C-11

Androgens have C-19

Progesterone,
gluco- & mineralo-
corticoids have
C-21

Androgens
have –OH
in the β-
position at
C-17

Some steroids have a double
bond between C-4 and C-5

Teststerone, gluco- & mineralocorticoids have a keto-group at C-3

**Fig. 31.1** Some structural aspects of steroids.

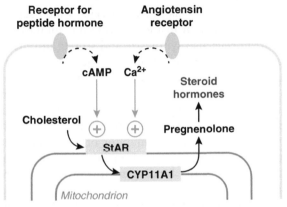

Receptor for
peptide hormone

Angiotensin
receptor

cAMP    Ca²⁺

Steroid
hormones

Cholesterol

Pregnenolone

StAR

CYP11A1

*Mitochondrion*

**Fig. 31.2** **Steroid acute regulatory (StAR) protein controls the synthesis of pregnenolone, the precursor of all steroid hormones.** StAR protein can be activated in two ways. cAMP, cyclic adenosine monophosphate.

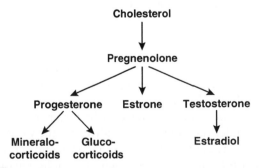

Cholesterol

Pregnenolone

Progesterone    Estrone    Testosterone

Mineralo-
corticoids

Gluco-
corticoids

Estradiol

**Fig. 31.3** **Overview of the synthesis of steroids from pregnenolone.**

transcription of the *STAR* gene, as well as increased activity of the StAR protein.

In the inner membrane of mitochondria, the **cholesterol side chain cleavage enzyme** (**CYP11A1**, **P450scc**) converts cholesterol to **pregnenolone** (see Fig. 31.2). Pregnenolone then leaves the mitochondrion.

Pregnenolone gives rise to progesterone, the mineralocorticoids, the glucocorticoids, estrone, testosterone, and estradiol (Fig. 31.3).

In steroid synthesis, specificity for a particular steroid is achieved by specific enzyme expression, and the specificity of regulation depends on the type of hormone receptor (e.g., receptor for luteinizing hormone, follicle-stimulating hormone, adrenocorticotropic hormone, or angiotensin) that leads to increased transcription of the *STAR* gene.

## 2. SEX STEROIDS

*In the brain, gonadotropin-releasing hormone (GnRH) stimulates the secretion of follicle-stimulating hormone (FSH) and luteinizing hormone (LH), which in turn stimulate the gonads to synthesize the sex steroids testosterone and estradiol. The testes produce testosterone, which gives rise to the more powerful dihydrotestosterone. Both testosterone and dihydrotestosterone bind to the androgen receptor. In the ovaries, developing follicles secrete 17β-estradiol, which binds to estrogen receptors. Hypogonadotrophic hypogonadism is due to insufficient signaling from the pituitary to the gonads. 46,XY disorders of sex development are due to a deficiency in synthesizing or sensing androgens. Birth control pills decrease FSH secretion from the pituitary. Patients who have androgen- or estrogen-dependent tumors are often treated with drugs that decrease sex steroid formation or signaling.*

### 2.1. Common Pathways for the Biosynthesis of Sex Steroids

Neurons in the hypothalamus secrete **gonadotropin-releasing hormone** (**GnRH, LHRH, FSH-RH**), which stimulates the anterior pituitary gland to secrete the **gonadotropins** FSH and **LH** (Fig. 31.4). FSH and LH then stimulate gonads to produce sex steroids. GnRH is a 10–amino acid peptide. FSH and LH are dimers that consist of a common α-subunit and a unique β-subunit; both subunits are peptides of ~100 amino acids. FSH and LH bind to G protein–coupled receptors, which then give rise to an increased concentration of **cAMP**, which in turn leads to increased synthesis of **StAR** protein (see Fig. 31.2).

The biosynthesis of sex steroids in men and women follows similar pathways (Fig. 31.5). In males and females, **estradiol** (produced from testosterone) activates the closure of the **epiphyseal growth plates** of the long bones.

**Hypogonadotropic hypogonadism** is due to deficient secretion of functional **GnRH**, **FSH**, or **LH**, deficient sensing of GnRH. The condition is most often acquired, and there are also many genetic causes for this disorder. Patients who have **Kallmann syndrome** have congenital hypogonadotropic hypogonadism and a reduced or absent sense of **smell** (**hyposmia** or **anosmia**).

The zona reticularis of the **adrenal cortex** produces **dihydroepiandrosterone** (**DHEA**) and **androstenedione** (see Figs. 31.5 and 31.15), which both have weak androgen activity. The function of these steroids is not well understood. Normally, they play little role in sex development. However, these steroids assume a major role when their production is

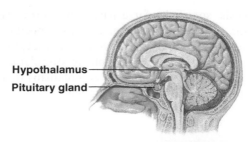

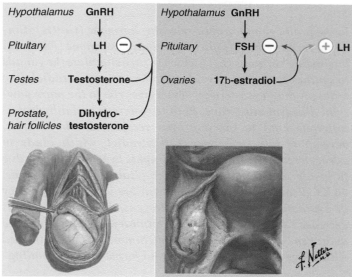

**Fig. 31.4** **Regulation of sex steroid synthesis in men and women.** FSH, follicle-stimulating hormone; GnRH, gonadotropin-releasing hormone; LH, luteinizing hormone.

increased due to a problem with glucocorticoid or mineralocorticoid synthesis in the other zones of the adrenal glands. DHEA in blood peaks at age ~20 years and then declines greatly until age ~65 years. **DHEA** is available as a supplement, but long-term safety and benefits to the general population are unclear.

## 2.2. Biosynthesis of Sex Steroids in Men

The primary sex steroids produced by men are **testosterone** and **dihydrotestosterone** (see Fig. 31.4). Testosterone synthesis occurs predominantly in the **Leydig cells** of the **testes** (Fig. 31.6) and is controlled by **LH**. When LH binds to the LH receptor, the concentration of cAMP inside Leydig cells rises, StAR protein is activated, more StAR protein is made, and the synthesis of testosterone increases. From the Leydig cells, testosterone reaches the blood. The **prostate** and **hair follicles** convert testosterone to dihydrotestosterone, which they release into the blood. Compared to testosterone, dihydrotestosterone has considerably higher affinity for the **androgen receptor**.

In the blood, both testosterone and dihydrotestosterone bind to **sex-hormone binding globulin** (**SHBG**). SHBG stems mainly from the liver. The concentrations of testosterone and dihydrotestosterone versus the concentration of SHBG determine the concentration of free testosterone and dihydrotes-

tosterone. In males, the concentration of SHBG is high during childhood and then drops to about one-third of that in puberty, thereby increasing the fraction of free testosterone and dihydrotestosterone.

**Androgen receptors** are found mostly in the cytosol of a variety of cells, where they are bound to a **heat-shock protein**. After binding dihydrotestosterone or testosterone, androgen receptors (without heat-shock protein) move into the nucleus and bind to an **androgen response element** in the promoter of various genes.

Activation of androgen receptors is required for normal development of the **prostate** and the male external **genitalia**, and later also for male pattern **baldness**.

Testosterone and dihydrotestosterone exert feedback inhibition on LH secretion from the pituitary gland such that the concentration of testosterone in the blood of adult men is maintained at ~6 ng/mL until andropause sets in.

In males, **FSH** stimulates **Sertoli cells**, which support the development of **sperm** inside seminiferous tubules (see Fig. 31.6). Sertoli cells also synthesize and secrete **inhibin**, which feedback inhibits FSH secretion from the pituitary gland.

Patients who have a **prostate cancer** that depends on androgens for growth (i.e., castration-sensitive prostate cancer) respond favorably to a reduction in circulating androgen (**androgen deprivation therapy**), which can be achieved in four ways: (1) use of an inhibitor of androgen synthesis, such as **abiraterone**; (2) use of an **antiandrogen**, that is, a drug that prevents the binding of dihydrotestosterone and testosterone to the androgen receptor, such as **bicalutamide, flutamide**, and **enzalutamide**; (3) use of a GnRH agonist, which leads to an initial surge in testosterone secretion that is 10 or more days later followed by depressed secretion; and (4) use of a GnRH antagonist, such as **degarelix**. After ~2 years of androgen deprivation therapy, most castration-sensitive tumors become castration insensitive.

## 2.3. 46,XY Disorder of Sex Development

At ~5 weeks, the fetus develops two **gonadal ridges** (Fig. 31.7). Along these ridges run a pair of **müllerian ducts** and a pair of **wolffian ducts**. At ~6 weeks, the fetus starts turning the gonads into **ovaries** or **testes**, which start to produce sex steroids. Under the influence of androgens, the wolffian ducts give rise to the epididymides, vas deferens, and seminal vesicles; under the influence of estrogens, the müllerian ducts give rise to the fallopian tubes, the uterus, and part of the vagina. The **sex steroids** regulate the development of the **external genitalia**. During puberty, androgens stimulate the growth of facial hair and a deepening of the voice, whereas estrogens stimulate the development of female breasts.

Patients who have a 46,XY karyotype and a **disorder of sex development** (DSD) fail to synthesize sufficient dihydrotestosterone or fail to respond normally to androgens. A number of these persons appear female at birth and are raised as females.

Among children and partially virilized women with 46,XY DSD, mutations occur in a number of genes, such as those

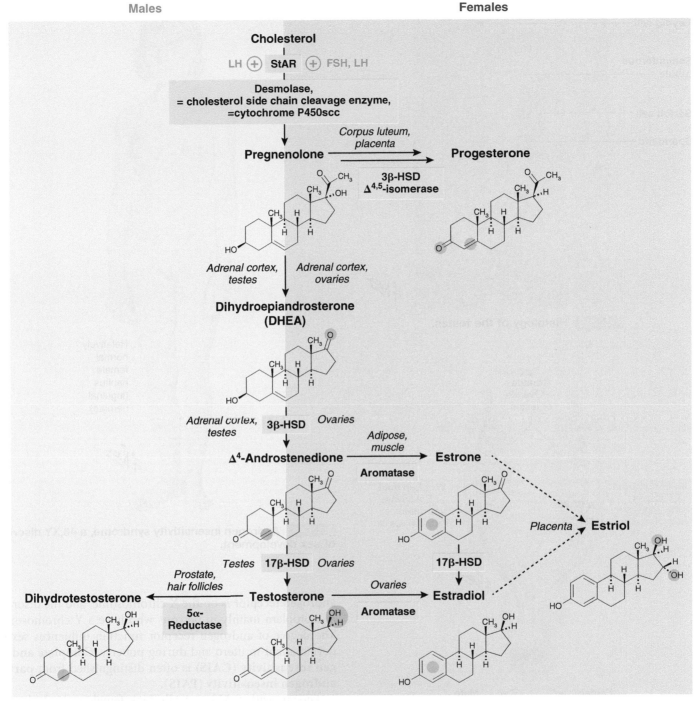

**Males**

**Females**

**Fig. 31.5** **Overview of the synthesis of sex steroids in men and women.** FSH, follicle-stimulating hormone; GnRH, gonadotropin-releasing hormone; HSD, hydroxysteroid dehydrogenase; LH, luteinizing hormone; StAR, steroid acute regulatory protein. 5α-Reductase is also called 3-oxo-5α-steroid 4-dehydrogenase (NADP⁺).

coding for **17β-hydroxysteroid dehydrogenase type 3, 5α-reductase,** or the **androgen receptor** (see Fig. 31.5). Many of these patients seek medical attention due to lack of onset of menstruation with puberty or due to infertility.

Depending on the severity of **5α-reductase deficiency,** newborns with a 46,XY karyotype may have male, ambiguous, or female external genitalia. After puberty, most of the persons who are raised as girls identify with the male gender.

Persons who have 46,XY DSD and a **deficiency** of **17β-hydroxysteroid dehydrogenase type 3** (the enzyme that synthesizes testosterone in the testes) often have female external genitalia at birth, are often raised as girls and then show virilization at puberty.

**Androgen insensitivity syndrome** (formerly called **testicular feminization**) is caused by a mutant **androgen receptor** with decreased function (Fig. 31.8). The gene for the

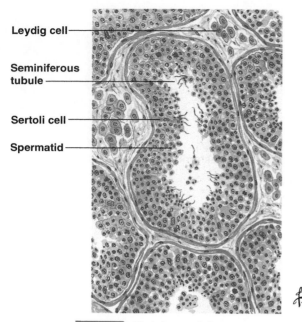

Leydig cell

Seminiferous tubule

Sertoli cell

Spermatid

**Fig. 31.6** **Histology of the testes.**

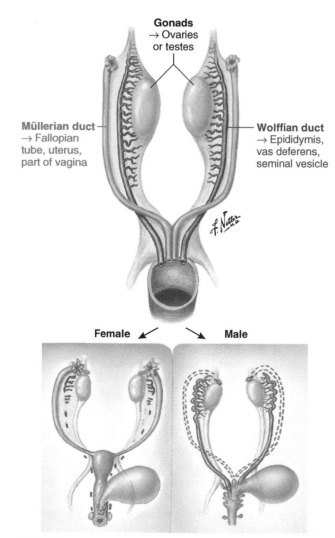

**Gonads**
→ Ovaries or testes

**Müllerian duct**
→ Fallopian tube, uterus, part of vagina

**Wolffian duct**
→ Epididymis, vas deferens, seminal vesicle

Female ↙      ↘ Male

**Fig. 31.7** **Development of female and male sex organs.**

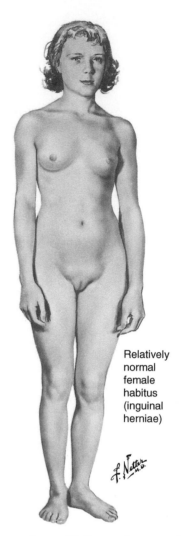

Relatively normal female habitus (inguinal herniae)

**Fig. 31.8** **Androgen insensitivity syndrome, a 46,XY disorder of sex development.**

androgen receptor is on the X chromosome, and the disorder is a problem mainly in persons who have a Y chromosome. The degree of androgen receptor function influences sexual development in utero and during puberty. **Complete androgen insensitivity** (**CAIS**) is often distinguished from **partial androgen insensitivity** (**PAIS**).

Persons with **CAIS** typically look female at birth, have a mildly enlarged clitoris, and lack a uterus. They have internal testes and are infertile. They are most often diagnosed around the time of puberty, because no menstruation occurs. The incidence is ~1 in 20,000 persons. During puberty, the testes produce excessive amounts of testosterone, which is then converted to estrogen and thus induces the development of breasts.

Persons with **PAIS** typically have hypospadias, a small penis, and a bifid scrotum at birth. Patients with the mildest form of PAIS look normal but are infertile.

Patients with CAIS or PAIS may have their gonads removed to reduce the risk of germ-cell tumors. Hormone replacement therapy is then instituted (typically estrogen to maintain female characteristics or testosterone to maintain male characteristics).

While several different loss-of-function mutations in the androgen receptor give rise to PAIS or CAIS, a pathogenic elongation of a **CAG trinucleotide repeat** in exon 1 of the androgen receptor gene gives rise to **spinal and bulbar muscular atrophy**. The normal CAG repeat length is ~20, and more than ~40 repeats are pathogenic. CAG encodes glutamine, and the CAG repeat length therefore determines the length of a glutamine tract in the androgen receptor. A pathogenic polyglutamine tract leads to the formation of protein aggregates in lower motoneurons in the brainstem and spinal cord. Around the age of 30 to 60 years, affected individuals can develop muscle cramps, muscle fasciculations during contractions, muscle weakness, difficulty speaking and swallowing, and inability to walk.

## 2.4. Biosynthesis of Sex Steroids in Women

In women, the physiologically produced estrogens include **estradiol, estriol,** and **estrone**, which differ in the substituents they carry on the D-ring (see Fig. 31.1). 17β-Estradiol is the most potent estrogen. Estriol is chiefly produced by the placenta during pregnancy. Estrone is the main estrogen in women after menopause.

In women (as in men), the hypothalamus secretes **GnRH**, which in turn stimulates the anterior pituitary to secrete **FSH** (see Fig. 31.4).

FSH stimulates **ovarian follicles** to produce and secrete **17β-estradiol**, as well as **inhibin**. As follicles are recruited and grow in size, the concentration of 17β-estradiol in the blood increases during a period of ~2 weeks (Fig. 31.9). 17β-Estradiol

feedback inhibits the secretion of GnRH and FSH (see Fig. 31.4). This inhibition in turn limits the number of active follicles in the ovaries. In an additional feedback loop, the follicles also produce inhibin, which decreases FSH secretion from the pituitary.

**Clomiphene**, a selective estrogen receptor modulator, is used in the treatment of **infertility** in women. Clomiphene impairs the estradiol-dependent feedback inhibition of GnRH secretion. As a result, more GnRH and FSH are secreted, and the ovaries produce more active follicles and more 17β-estradiol.

When the concentration of 17β-estradiol is high (>200 pg/mL) for at least 15 hours, it triggers the secretion of **LH** from the anterior pituitary. LH helps start ovulation; that is, the dominant follicle ejects its egg (Fig. 31.10). The less-developed follicles do not ovulate and atrophy.

After ovulation, follicular cells give rise to the **corpus luteum** (see Fig. 31.10), which synthesizes both 17β-estradiol and **progesterone** (see Fig. 31.5).

Progesterone inhibits the secretion of **LH** from the anterior pituitary. As the concentration of LH falls in the absence of a fertilized embryo (see Fig. 31.9), progesterone synthesis in the corpus luteum also ceases, and the corpus luteum dies. As the concentrations of progesterone and estradiol decrease, **menstruation** (Fig. 31.11) sets in. With menstruation, much of the inner lining of the uterus (endometrium) is degraded and expelled. However, if a **pregnancy** is established, the embryo produces **human chorionic gonadotropin** (hCG), which allows the corpus luteum to survive and synthesize progesterone for a while. Eventually, the placenta produces its own progesterone and the corpus luteum involutes. An increased concentration of progesterone promotes differentiation of the mammary glands. The placenta also produces both estradiol and **estriol**, which leads to a pronounced increase in the total concentration of estrogens as the pregnancy progresses.

The concentration of **hCG** in blood is commonly measured to screen for **pregnancy**.

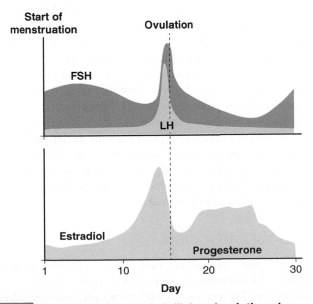

**Fig. 31.9** **Concentrations of follicle-stimulating hormone (FSH), luteinizing hormone (LH), estradiol, and progesterone during the menstrual cycle.** (Data from Häggström M. Reference ranges for estradiol, progesterone, luteinizing hormone, and follicle-stimulating hormone during the menstrual cycle. *WikiJournal of Medicine.* 2014;1[1].)

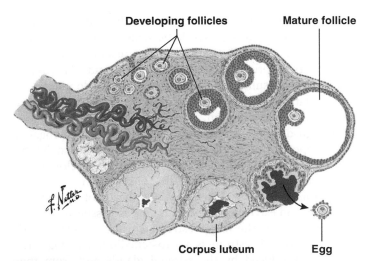

**Fig. 31.10** **Development of a dominant follicle and of a corpus luteum in an ovary during the menstrual cycle.** Development over time is shown clockwise. Many follicles develop at the same time, but one becomes the dominant follicle. The release of two eggs in one cycle, if fertilized, leads to a pregnancy with fraternal twins.

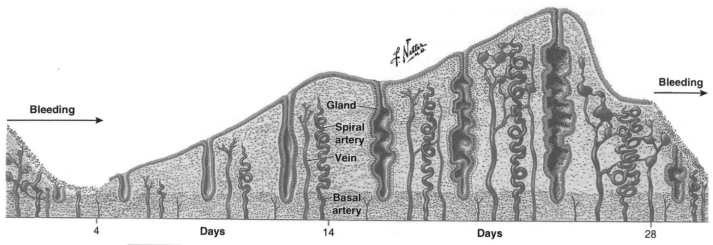

**Fig. 31.11** **Changes in the inner lining of the uterus during the menstrual cycle.**

In the second trimester of pregnancy, women are often screened for a fetus with neural tube defects, Down syndrome (trisomy 21), and Edward syndrome (trisomy 18). The **quad screen** contains measurements of α-fetoprotein, hCG, estriol, and inhibin A. The **penta screen** also contains a measurement of hyperglycosylated hCG. When the fetus has anencephaly, for example, the concentration of estriol in maternal blood is only ~10% of the normal concentration. When the fetus has Down syndrome (trisomy 21), the concentration of inhibin A is unusually high.

About 60% of patients with **polycystic ovary syndrome** (PCOS), a condition that affects ~5% to 15% of women of reproductive age (depending on criteria used), have an excess concentration of androgens (including testosterone and androstenedione; see Fig. 26.12). These patients are typically also insulin resistant and have reduced fertility. Besides PCOS, congenital adrenal hyperplasia (see Section 4.2), with its attendant high concentration of androgens, also gives rise to polycystic ovaries.

Oral **contraceptives** for women usually contain an **estrogen** and a **progestin** (a synthetic drug with progestational activity). The concentrations of these drugs in blood are high enough to suppress the secretion of FSH and LH from the brain. Without sufficient FSH, ovarian follicles do not develop and ovulation does not occur. Cessation of such a contraceptive leads to menstruation.

A high-dose **progestin** alone, such as medroxyprogesterone (Depo-Provera; injected every 3 months) also inhibits secretion of GnRH and FSH, thus inhibiting development of the follicles. The drug slso inhibits LH secretion.

In **postmenopausal women**, synthesis of estradiol is minimal, and **estrone** produced in adipose tissue and skeletal muscle becomes the major estrogen in the circulation. The precursor for this estrone is androstenedione (see Fig. 31.5), which is produced by the adrenal glands and from there reaches the bloodstream.

In obese patients, the increased mass of adipose tissue converts more androstenedione to estrone. In morbidly obese patients, the concentration of circulating estrone can be as much as 10-fold that in a lean person. Estrone stimulates the growth of the endometrial lining and thereby increases the chance of hyperplasia and cancer of the endometrium.

During and after menopause, exogenous estrogen (as part of **hormone therapy** after menopause) can sharply reduce the incidence of **hot flashes**. However, long-term oral estrogen plus progestin therapy increases a woman's risk for breast cancer and endometrial cancer.

**Selective estrogen receptor modulators** are used in the treatment of **osteoporosis** and as adjuvant treatment for **breast cancer**. The drugs used for this purpose have mixed activating and inhibitory effects on estrogen receptors in part because they do not induce the exact same conformational changes of the DNA- and protein-binding domains of estrogen receptors as does estrogen. **Tamoxifen** and **raloxifene** are both used to reduce the risk of breast cancer (chemoprevention) in women who are at high risk (these drugs are predominantly used for adjuvant therapy after surgery or radiation in women who had estrogen receptor–positive tumors). Raloxifene is also used in the treatment of osteoporosis (it has a weak estrogen-like effect on bone). **Toremifene** is used to treat estrogen receptor–positive metastatic breast cancer.

**Aromatase inhibitors** are used in the treatment of estrogen receptor–positive breast cancer. These tumors depend on activation of estrogen receptors for growth. Some of the currently used aromatase inhibitors (e.g., anastrozole, letrozole) show **competitive** inhibition of aromatase. Others, like exemestane, are **suicide** inhibitors of aromatase.

## 3. GLUCOCORTICOIDS

*In the brain, circadian and stress signals stimulate corticotropin-releasing hormone secretion, which in turn stimulates ACTH secretion, which then stimulates the adrenal cortex to synthesize the glucocorticoid cortisol. Cortisol exerts its effects by binding to a receptor that acts as a transcription factor. Synthetic glucocorticoids are widely used in medicine for their antiinflammatory and immunosuppressive effects. Cushing syndrome is due to excess endogenous cortisol production. Exogenous Cushing syndrome is induced by protracted use of exogenous glucocorticoid drugs.*

The term **glucocorticoid** derives from the words glucose (adrenal) cortex, and steroids. The main physiological glucocorticoid is **cortisol** (**hydrocortisone**).

The brain controls cortisol secretion (Fig. 31.12). The hypothalamus secretes **corticotropin-releasing hormone (CRH)**, which stimulates the pituitary gland to secrete **ACTH**. ACTH then stimulates the cortex of the adrenal glands to secrete **cortisol**. (The adrenal glands weigh about 4 g each.) Cortisol in turn feedback inhibits the secretion of CRH and ACTH. (The adrenal glands also produce DHEA and androstenedione, as well as aldosterone).

The concentration of cortisol in the blood changes markedly through the course of a day (Fig. 31.13). The **circadian clock** in the hypothalamus provides a cyclic, basal stimulus for the secretion of **CRH**. In addition, under conditions of **psychological stress**, neurons in the brain use the peptide hormone **pituitary adenylate cyclase-activating polypeptide** (PACAP) to further stimulate CRH secretion.

The synthesis of cortisol by the adrenal glands proceeds according to the reactions shown in Fig. 31.14. The cortex of the adrenal glands contains three different zones (Fig. 31.15) that produce cortisol, aldosterone, and DHEA plus androstenedione, respectively.

In the blood, glucocorticoids (and to a lesser degree progesterone and aldosterone) bind to **transcortin** (**corticosteroid-binding globulin**).

In cells, glucocorticoids bind to **glucocorticoid receptors** in the cytosol, which then translocate to the nucleus, where they bind to glucocorticoid response elements and thus stimulate transcription of certain genes (see Chapter 6); this in turn leads to the synthesis of proteins, which decrease inflammation, promote the export of amino acids from muscle and their import into the liver, stimulate gluconeogenesis and lipolysis, and decrease glucose use by muscle. Glucocorticoids also have an additional antiinflammatory effect that is mediated by the glucocorticoid receptor but does not require increased transcription.

A **deficiency** of glucocorticoids can lead to hypoglycemia, neurological problems, and failure to thrive. Patients with **Addison disease** show autoimmune destruction of the cortex of the adrenal glands, which causes a combined deficiency of glucocorticoids and mineralocorticoids (see Section 4). Many patients with the rare disease **familial glucocorticoid deficiency** have insufficient ACTH receptor function in the adrenal glands and hence diminished cortisol synthesis.

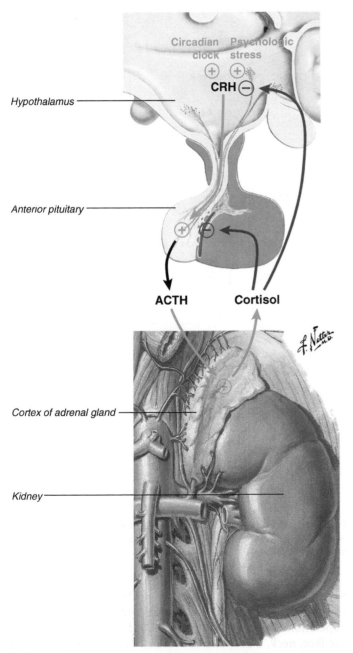

**Fig. 31.12** **Regulation of cortisol secretion.** ACTH, adrenocorticotropic hormone; CRH, corticotropin-releasing hormone.

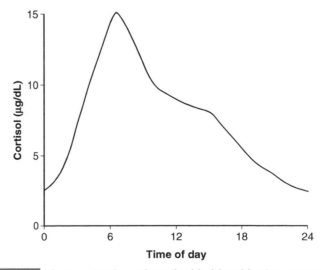

**Fig. 31.13** **Concentration of cortisol in blood in the course of a day.** (Data from Dimitrov S, Benedict C, Heutling D, et al. Cortisol and epinephrine control opposing circadian rhythms in T cell subsets. *Blood.* 2009;113:5134; and Hurwitz S, Cohen RJ, Williams GH. Diurnal variation of aldosterone and plasma renin activity: timing relation to melatonin and cortisol and consistency after prolonged bed rest. *J Appl Physiol.* 2004; 96:1406.)

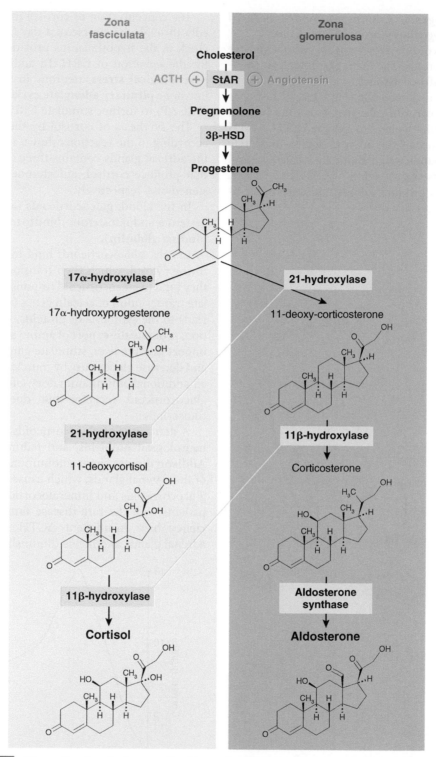

**Fig. 31.14** **Biosynthesis of glucocorticoids and mineralocorticoids in the adrenal glands.** Lines that link enzymes indicate that these enzymes are identical. ACTH, adrenocorticotropin hormone; HSD, hydroxysteroid dehydrogenase; StAR, steroid acute regulatory protein.

**Excessive** production of glucocorticoids gives rise to **Cushing syndrome** (Fig. 31.16). Cortisol secretion is excessive due to a pituitary tumor that secretes ACTH or a tumor in an adrenal gland that secretes cortisol. The excessive concentration of circulating cortisol causes degradation of muscle protein and an increase in the rate of gluconeogenesis.

Symptoms of Cushing syndrome include muscle weakness (limbs may show muscle wasting), wide purplish striae, fat deposition above the collar bone, and obesity (especially in the face, neck, trunk, and abdomen). The elevated concentration of glucocorticoids also leads to insulin resistance (the mechanism of this alteration remains unknown). Hence,

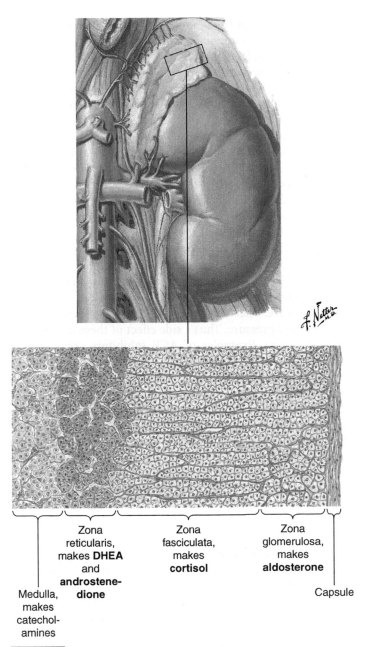

**Fig. 31.15** **Structure of the adrenal cortex.** DHEA, dihydro-epiandrosterone.

Zona
reticularis,
makes **DHEA**
and
**androstene-
dione**

Zona
fasciculata,
makes
**cortisol**

Zona
glomerulosa,
makes
**aldosterone**

Capsule

Medulla,
makes
catechol-
amines

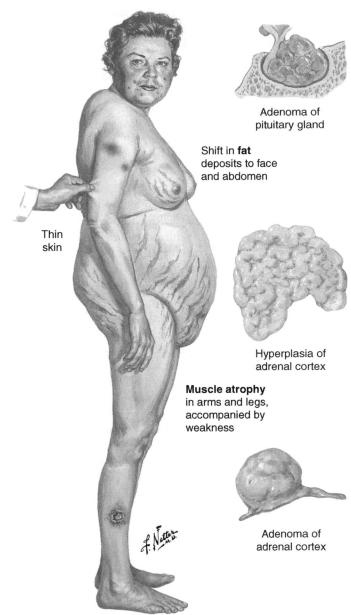

Adenoma of
pituitary gland

Shift in **fat**
deposits to face
and abdomen

Thin
skin

Hyperplasia of
adrenal cortex

**Muscle atrophy**
in arms and legs,
accompanied by
weakness

Adenoma of
adrenal cortex

**Fig. 31.16** **Cushing syndrome and its causes.**

patients with Cushing syndrome tend to be glucose intolerant and develop diabetes. Tumors of the pituitary are often resected (the cure rate is about 65%). Afterward, glucocorticoids must be given and eventually tapered (see below). Adrenalectomy with corticoid replacement is another option. Within several months, some of the disease-induced changes revert.

**Synthetic glucocorticoids** are used in supraphysiological concentrations in the treatment of allergies, rheumatoid arthritis, organ transplantation, ulcerative colitis, and multiple sclerosis. Examples include hydrocortisone, prednisone, dexamethasone, betamethasone, and triamcinolone. Long-term use of high-dose glucocorticoids leads to the same adverse effects as in Cushing syndrome, such as edema, muscle

wasting, shifting of fat depots, and osteoporosis. This syndrome is called **exogenous Cushing syndrome**. Glucocorticoids inhibit CRH and ACTH secretion and thus lead to atrophy of cortisol-producing cells in the adrenal glands that reverts only gradually. For instance, patients who receive more than 20 mg of prednisone per day for 3 weeks have depressed regulation of CRH secretion, ACTH secretion, and cortisol synthesis. To prevent dangerous hypocortisolism, patients are gradually "weaned" off the exogenous glucocorticoid (the drug is "tapered").

## 4. MINERALOCORTICOIDS

*Low blood pressure and a low concentration of Na⁺ in the blood stimulate the production of more angiotensin II and angiotensin III. These angiotensins stimulate the adrenal glands to synthesize and release aldosterone. Aldosterone in turn stimulates the synthesis of transporters in the kidneys that increase recovery of Na⁺ from the tubules in the kidneys. This recovery leads to an increase in blood pressure and in the concentration of Na⁺ in the blood. Drugs that are used to lower blood pressure incapacitate this regulatory system. Aldosterone deficiency leads to low blood pressure and aldosterone excess to high blood pressure.*

## 4.1. Synthesis of Aldosterone

Aldosterone plays a role in regulating blood pressure and the concentrations of $Na^+$ and $K^+$ in the blood. Aldosterone synthesis is regulated by the renin-angiotensin system. When **blood pressure** and the concentration of $Na^+$ in blood are too low or when the concentration of $K^+$ in blood is too high, angiotensin stimulates aldosterone synthesis.

The **renin-angiotensin system** works as follows (Fig. 31.17). **Renin** is a protease secreted from renal juxtaglomerular cells. At low blood pressure, high $[Na^+]$, or low $[K^+]$ in blood, the activity of renin in blood increases. (Note that renin secreted by the kidneys is a different enzyme from rennin in the stomach of ruminants that is used in the production of cheese.) Renin cleaves **angiotensinogen** (a 14-residue peptide and $\alpha$2-globulin) into **angiotensin I** (a 10-residue peptide) and another peptide (Fig. 31.18). **Angiotensin-converting enzyme (ACE)** in the blood cleaves angiotensin I into **angiotensin II** (an 8-residue peptide). Angiotensin II has a half-life of only 1 to 2 minutes. An aminopeptidase removes the N-terminal amino acid residue from angiotensin II, forming **angiotensin III** (a 7-residue peptide).

Both angiotensin II and angiotensin III bind to the **angiotensin receptor** on adrenal gland glomerulosa cells and activate the receptor. Receptor activation elicits an increase in the intracellular concentrations of inositol trisphosphate ($IP_3$) and diacylglycerol, which lead to increased synthesis of the StAR protein and thus increased synthesis of **aldosterone** via the pathway shown in Fig. 31.14. Aldosterone binds to the **mineralocorticoid receptor** in the kidneys and thus increases transcription of transport proteins in the renal tubules that take up $Na^+$ from the glomerular filtrate and transport it back into the blood. Secondarily, $Na^+$ uptake affects the transport of water and $K^+$, such that aldosterone favors excretion of $K^+$.

Angiotensin receptors are found not only in the adrenal glands but also throughout the vasculature; when activated in blood vessels, these receptors increase blood pressure via vasoconstriction (i.e., independent of aldosterone).

**ACE inhibitors**, **angiotensin receptor blockers** (ARBs), and **aldosterone antagonists** are used clinically to reduce blood pressure. These drugs impair the physiological regulation of blood pressure. Thus a side effect of these drugs is low blood pressure. Examples of ACE inhibitors are captopril, zofenopril, ramipril, and enalapril. Physiologically, ACE is not regulated or rate limiting, but in the presence of ACE inhibitors, less angiotensin II is formed. ARBs prevent the binding of angiotensins II and III to the angiotensin receptor in the adrenal glands. Examples of ARBs are losartan and irbesartan (the "sartans"). The aldosterone antagonists are the oldest drugs in this class and include spironolactone, eplerenone, and canrenone. These drugs prevent aldosterone from activating the mineralocorticoid receptor in the kidneys.

## 4.2. Disorders of Aldosterone Synthesis

**Primary aldosteronism** (**Conn syndrome**) is due to excessive production of aldosterone, which is most often due to a unilateral adenoma or bilateral hyperplasia of the aldosterone-producing zona glomerulosa (Figs. 31.15 and 31.19). The high concentration of circulating aldosterone leads to **secondary hypertension**. About 10% of all patients who have hypertension have primary aldosteronism. The **aldosterone/renin**

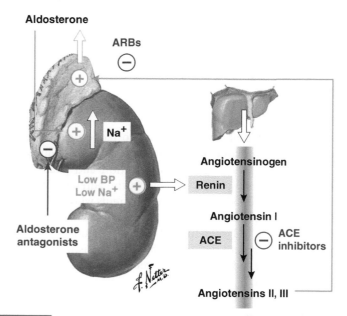

**Fig. 31.17** **Regulation of blood pressure (BP) and blood Na⁺ by the renin-angiotensin system and aldosterone.** Aldosterone is secreted from the adrenal glands. ACE, angiotensin-converting enzyme; ARBs, angiotensin receptor blockers.

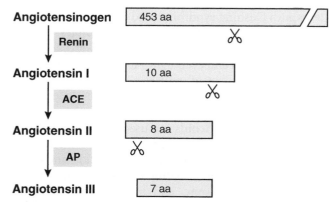

**Fig. 31.18** **Processing of angiotensinogen.** aa, amino acids; ACE, angiotensin-converting enzyme; AP, aminopeptidase.

The mutant channel leads to depolarization of the aldosterone-producing zona glomerulosa cells, influx of $Ca^{2+}$, increased transcription of the StAR protein, and thus increased aldosterone synthesis. Rare patients who are heterozygous for an inherited mutation in the *KCNJ5* gene have a type of **familial hyperaldosteronism** that is present from childhood.

**Congenital adrenal hyperplasia** is characterized by impaired production of both cortisol and aldosterone. Impaired production of cortisol leads to reduced feedback inhibition of ACTH secretion from the pituitary and hyperplasia of the adrenal glands in response to the increased concentration of ACTH. Both glucocorticoid and mineralocorticoid synthesis are impaired, because the two classes of steroids share precursors and steroid-producing enzymes. The most common cause of congenital adrenal hyperplasia is a deficiency of 21α-hydroxylase.

**21α-Hydroxylase (CYP21A2) deficiency** impairs the normal pathways of cortisol and aldosterone synthesis (see Fig. 31.14). The deficiency does not impair the synthesis of sex steroids. The severe, classic forms of this disorder are seen in ~1 in 15,000 newborns, whereas a less severe, nonclassic form occurs in ~1 in 1,000 newborns. In all forms, the increased ACTH secretion leads to an increased rate of cholesterol conversion to 17α-hydroxyprogesterone, which then accumulates. 17α-Hydroxylase catalyzes not only the introduction of a hydroxyl group at C-17 but also the cleavage of the side chain at C-17 with the formation of a ketone at C-17. For this reason, in patients who have a 21α-hydroxylase deficiency, 17α-hydroxylase converts 17α-hydroxyprogesterone to androstenedione, which then gives rise to excess testosterone. In the most severe 21α-hydroxylase deficiency, lack of aldosterone synthesis leads to salt wasting from birth, which needs to be treated immediately. In girls, this deficiency also leads to masculinization in utero and hence ambiguous genitalia at birth. In boys, the excess testosterone leads to premature virilization in childhood. In a less severe classic form of the disorder that does not entail salt wasting, there is similar masculinization in girls and boys. Finally, the mildest, nonclassic form of 21α-hydroxylase deficiency leads to early virilization in boys and to hirsutism and male pattern baldness in women. All forms of 21α-hydroxylase deficiency are inherited in autosomal recessive fashion. Newborn screening for 17α-hydroxyprogesterone allows the detection of babies who have a classic form of 21α-hydroxylase deficiency.

Patients who have the severe, salt-wasting form of 21α-hydroxylase deficiency are typically treated with fludrocortisone to restore blood pressure and the concentration of electrolytes in the blood. All patients who have classic 21α-hydroxylase deficiency are treated with a glucocorticoid, such as dexamethasone, in sufficient amounts to reduce the excessive testosterone production.

Less common causes of congenital adrenal hyperplasia are deficiencies in StAR protein activity, 3β-hydroxysteroid dehydrogenase, 17α-hydroxylase, or 11β-hydroxylase.

**Addison disease** (Fig. 31.20) develops over a period of months to years and leads to the destruction of the adrenal cortex and hence greatly reduced production of both cortisol

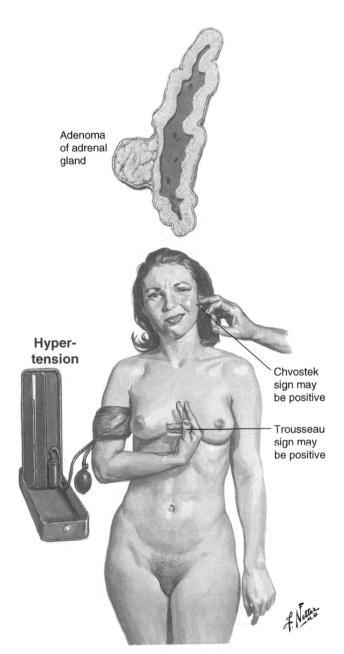

Adenoma of adrenal gland

**Hypertension**

Chvostek sign may be positive

Trousseau sign may be positive

**Fig. 31.19** **Primary aldosteronism.** The Chvostek sign indicates hyperexcitability of the facial nerve, which is due to hypokalemia. The Trousseau sign is observed after 3 minutes of occluding the brachial artery; it indicates hyperexcitability and is due to hypokalemia.

ratio in the blood serves as a screening tool for primary aldosteronism. The concentration of aldosterone is unusually high due to overproduction, whereas the activity of renin is unusually low due to the high blood pressure; that is, the renin-angiotensin system functions normally. As a consequence of persistent hyperaldosteronism, compensatory processes become active such that the concentration of $Na^+$ is high but still in the normal range, and the concentration of $K^+$ is normal or low.

Some 40% of patients who have a unilateral **adenoma** of the adrenal gland have a tumor that is heterozygous for a mutant *KCNJ5* gene, which encodes the Kir3.4 **$K^+$-channel**.

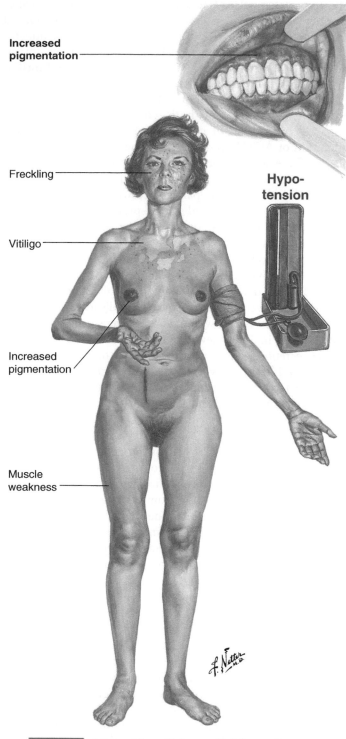

Increased pigmentation

Freckling

Vitiligo

Increased pigmentation

Muscle weakness

Hypo-tension

**Adrenal insufficiency (Addison disease).**

and androstenedione. In developed countries, the disease is most often due to an autoimmune reaction. Some of the antibodies are directed against 21-hydroxylase (the same enzyme that is missing in most individuals who have congenital adrenal hyperplasia; see Fig. 31.14). Like other autoimmune diseases, predisposition to Addison disease is linked to certain major histocompatibility alleles. The disease has a prevalence of ~1 in 20,000 persons. In other countries, tuberculosis is the

more common reason for the loss of the adrenal cortex. Patients show a multitude of symptoms, the more striking of which are low blood pressure, increased pigmentation (due to ACTH that is cleaved to produce $\alpha$-melanocyte stimulating hormone; see also Section 4.2 in Chapter 35), and muscle weakness. Treatment involves the use of a steroid with mineralocorticoid activity, such as fludrocortisone.

## 5. VITAMIN D

*Calciol (cholecalciferol), a form of vitamin D, is formed in the skin on exposure to ultraviolet (UV) light. Calciol can also be derived from a few types of food. Calciol gives rise to calcidiol, which is stored in blood and is the major storage form of vitamin D. In response to a low concentration of calcium or phosphate in the blood, calcidiol is hydroxylated to the biologically active calcitriol. Calcitriol stimulates transcription of certain genes with the effect of increasing the concentrations of calcium and phosphate in the blood. A deficiency of vitamin D causes demineralization of bone.*

Vitamin D is an umbrella term for several related compounds that play a role in calcium and phosphate homeostasis; the main biologically active compound is calcitriol. Vitamin D is not a steroid but rather a secosteroid; that is, a steroid with a broken ring (Figs. 31.1 and 31.21).

Vitamin D can be synthesized in the skin via a reaction that requires light or it can be obtained from the diet. **Vitamin D$_3$** (**calciol, cholecalciferol**) is synthesized from cholesterol in the skin and is also found in some animal products, such as oily fish, fish oil, or milk fortified with vitamin D. **Vitamin D$_2$** (**ergocalciferol**) is found in some plant foods, such as mushrooms. Ergocalciferol differs from cholecalciferol in the multicarbon substituent of the D-ring, but it seems to be as effective in humans as cholecalciferol.

The liver converts vitamin D$_3$ to **calcidiol** (**25-hydroxycholecalciferol, 25-hydroxyvitamin D$_3$**) and releases this into the blood, where it binds to **vitamin D–binding protein**. Calcidiol bound to vitamin D binding protein is the major storage form of vitamin D. A similar reaction occurs with vitamin D$_2$, but vitamin D$_3$ is commonly the predominant form of vitamin D. In many people, calcidiol is chiefly produced during the summer months. Measurement of bloodborne calcidiol is a common screening tool for vitamin D adequacy; this is typically done out of concern for fractures due to osteoporosis.

**Calcitriol** (**1,25-dihydroxycholecalciferol, 1,25-dihydroxyvitamin D$_3$**), the biologically active form of vitamin D$_3$, is produced in the kidney in response to low blood **calcium** or **phosphate** concentrations (see Fig. 31.21).

Calcitriol binds to a nuclear hormone receptor and increases transcription of certain genes (Fig. 31.22). To this end, calcitriol binds to the **vitamin D receptor (calcitriol receptor)**, a nuclear hormone receptor that forms a heterodimer with the **retinoid X receptor**. This heterodimer binds to a **vitamin D response element** in the promoter region of several genes, thereby favoring transcription of these genes. The mechanism of action of vitamin D resembles that of vitamin A in that both

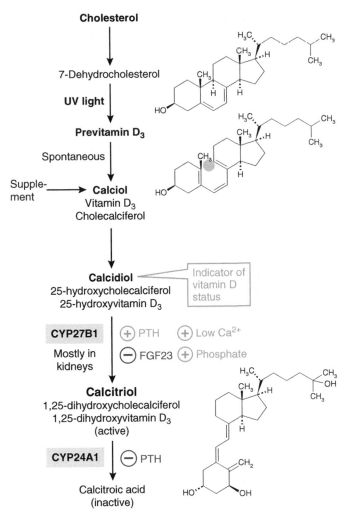

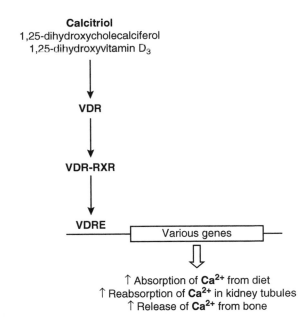

↑ Absorption of **Ca²⁺** from diet
↑ Reabsorption of **Ca²⁺** in kidney tubules
↑ Release of **Ca²⁺** from bone

**Fig. 31.22** **Mechanism of action of calcitriol in calcium homeostasis.** RXR, retinoid X receptor; VDR, vitamin D receptor; VDRE, vitamin D response element.

**Fig. 31.21** **Synthesis of vitamin D.** When the concentrations of calcium and phosphate in the blood are low, the pathway generates a higher concentration of circulating calcitriol. PTH, parathyroid hormone; UV, ultraviolet.

Vitamin D deficiency is mostly seen in the following groups of people: persons who have low exposure to sun, dark skin, or advanced age (decreased UV light–dependent synthesis of calciol), exclusively breastfed babies (low vitamin D content of breast milk), patients who have decreased absorption in the intestine (due to steatorrhea, celiac disease, or bariatric surgery), and patients who receive dialysis due to chronic kidney disease (decreased synthesis of calcitriol).

vitamins bind to a nuclear receptor that pairs with a retinoid X receptor to regulate gene expression.

Calcitriol leads to an increase in the concentrations of calcium and phosphate in the blood via increased absorption in the intestine, increased recovery in the kidneys, and, when a special need arises, increased release from hydroxyapatite in bone. These changes are a result of increased expression of transporters in the intestine and kidneys as well as increased activity of osteoclasts, which degrade bone.

**Vitamin D deficiency** (see Chapter 12) results in a low concentration of calcium and phosphate in the blood, which in turn leads to insufficient mineralization of bone with calcium phosphate. In children, vitamin D deficiency leads to **rickets**, a condition characterized by soft, pliable bones. In adults, vitamin D deficiency leads to **osteomalacia**, a condition in which bones are susceptible to fracture due to demineralization.

Vitamin D deficiency is also associated with increased rates of infection, cancer, muscle weakness, and skin disorders including psoriasis.

## SUMMARY

- Steroid hormones are synthesized from cholesterol as follows. Peptide hormones bind to membrane receptors which in turn increase the expression of the StAR protein. The StAR protein regulates the transfer of cholesterol to the inner mitochondrial membrane. This is the rate-limiting step in steroid hormone synthesis. Steroids are membrane permeable and bind to receptors that are transcription factors.

- In men and women, the hypothalamus secretes GnRH, which stimulates the secretion of FSH and LH from the anterior pituitary. Dihydrotestosterone, estradiol, and inhibin feedback inhibit the secretion of FSH and LH.

- The selective estrogen receptor modulator clomiphene is used to treat infertility. It prevents estradiol from inhibiting FSH secretion, which leads to increased FSH secretion and hence increased recruitment of follicles in the ovaries.

- Women of childbearing age produce estradiol in developing follicles in the ovaries. A persistently high concentration of estrogen induces LH secretion, which in turn stimulates ovulation.

- Most contraceptive drugs contain an estrogen and a progestin, which inhibit FSH secretion and the development of ovarian follicles.
- Hypogonadotropic hypogonadism is due to deficient secretion of functional GnRH, FSH, or LH, or deficient sensing of GnRH. If the hypogonadotropic hypogonadism is inherited and hyposmia or anosmia are present, the disorder is called Kallmann syndrome.
- Men produce testosterone in the Leydig cells of the testes. Testosterone is reduced to the more potent dihydrotestosterone. Men who have castration-sensitive prostate cancer often receive androgen deprivation therapy, which involves lowering GnRH secretion, inhibiting androgen synthesis directly, or preventing androgens from binding to the androgen receptor.
- Newborns who have a 46,XY disorder of sex development (DSD) often appear female and are raised as females, but then fail to menstruate at puberty and show unexpected virilization. The disorder is caused by an androgen receptor deficiency or an enzyme deficiency that leads to a low concentration of dihydrotestosterone.
- A pathogenic elongation of the CAG trinucleotide repeat in the androgen receptor leads to normal sex development but loss of motoneurons in men around the age of 30 to 60 years. The CAG sequence encodes glutamine. Androgen receptors with overly long glutamine repeats form aggregates in motoneurons.
- Tamoxifen and raloxifene are used as chemoprevention in patients at high risk of developing breast cancer. Tamoxifen is also used as an adjuvant in the treatment of estrogen receptor–positive breast cancer. Raloxifene is also used in the treatment and prevention of osteoporosis. Toremifene is used to treat metastatic breast cancer.
- Calcidiol (25-hydroxyvitamin $D_3$) is synthesized in sun-exposed skin and then in liver, followed by storage in blood; its concentration in blood is used as an indicator of vitamin D status. When the concentration of calcium or phosphate in the blood is low, the kidneys convert calcidiol to calcitriol. Calcitriol, acting via vitamin D receptors in the nucleus that stimulate transcription, increases the concentrations of calcium and phosphate in the blood via increased absorption in the intestine, increased recovery form the tubules in the kidneys, and increased degradation of bone.
- A deficiency of vitamin D leads to rickets in children and osteomalacia in adults. These diseases are characterized by insufficient mineralization of bone.

## FURTHER READING

- Husebye ES, Allolio B, Arlt W, et al. Consensus statement on the diagnosis, treatment and follow-up of patients with primary adrenal insufficiency. *J Intern Med.* 2014;275:104-115.
- Katzenwadel A, Wolf P. Androgen deprivation of prostate cancer: leading to a therapeutic dead end. *Cancer Lett.* 2015;367:12-17.
- Marsh M, Ronner W. *The Fertility Doctor: John Rock and the Reproductive Revolution.* Baltimore, MD: Johns Hopkins University Press; 2008.
- Olmos-Ortiz A, Avila E, Durand-Carbajal M, Díaz L. Regulation of calcitriol biosynthesis and activity: focus on gestational vitamin D deficiency and adverse pregnancy outcomes. *Nutrients.* 2015;7:443-480.

# Review Questions

1. The synthesis of aldosterone by the adrenal medulla is controlled primarily by the concentration of which one of the following hormones in the circulation?

   A. Androstenedione
   B. Angiotensin II
   C. Cortisol
   D. DHEA
   E. FSH

2. A 48-year-old woman has hypertension due to bilateral hyperplasia of the zona glomerulosa of the adrenal glands. This patient is best treated with which one of the following drugs?

   A. ACE inhibitor
   B. Aldosterone antagonist
   C. ARB
   D. Hydrocortisone
   E. Progestin

3. A 50-year-old woman has low blood pressure, extreme fatigue, decreased appetite, weight loss, and skin hyperpigmentation. A blood sample was taken and analyzed. A diagnosis of Addison disease would best be supported by which one of the following findings?

   A. Increased ACTH and increased renin
   B. Increased aldosterone and decreased angiotensin
   C. Increased FSH and increased LH
   D. Decreased GnRH and decreased CRH

4. A 40-year-old woman delivers a girl, although genetic testing had made her expect a boy. Which of the following could be a cause of the mismatch?

   A. Aldosterone synthase deficiency
   B. Aromatase deficiency
   C. Congenital adrenal hyperplasia due to 21α-hydroxylase deficiency
   D. Excessive secretion of ACTH from the pituitary
   E. Nonfunctional androgen receptor

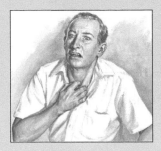

# Chapter 32    Eicosanoids

## SYNOPSIS

- Eicosanoids are short-lived 20-carbon lipids that generally play a role in local signaling. Most cells can produce eicosanoids. Examples of eicosanoids are prostaglandins, thromboxanes, leukotrienes, and lipoxins.
- Some eicosanoids are synthesized from the ω-6 fatty acid arachidonic acid and others from the ω-3 fatty acid eicosapentaenoic acid. These fatty acids are derived from the 18-carbon essential fatty acids linoleic acid and linolenic acid, respectively.
- Prostaglandins play a role in protecting the mucosa of the stomach and intestine, in ripening the cervix during pregnancy, and in regulating inflammation. A thromboxane favors aggregation of platelets at sites of vessel injury, whereas a prostaglandin opposes this effect.
- Nonsteroidal antiinflammatory drugs (NSAIDs), such as aspirin, acetaminophen, and ibuprofen, inhibit the synthesis of prostaglandins and thromboxanes. Prostaglandin analogs are used to protect the gastrointestinal mucosa from NSAID-induced damage and to ripen the cervix of pregnant women, if needed.
- Leukotrienes constrict the airways and promote the exit of white blood cells from blood vessels. Drugs that prevent leukotriene-induced bronchoconstriction play a role in the treatment of asthma.
- Lipoxins oppose the effect of leukotrienes and help resolve the inflammation.

## LEARNING OBJECTIVES

*For mastery of this topic, you should be able to do the following:*
- List good sources of ω-6 and ω-3 fatty acids, and discuss recommendations for daily intake of these essential fatty acids.
- Outline the synthesis of prostaglandins and thromboxanes, focusing on steps that are affected by drugs.
- Explain the role of prostaglandins in protecting the stomach mucosa, describe the effect of NSAIDs on prostaglandin synthesis in the stomach, and propose a treatment that protects the stomach mucosa in patients who use NSAIDs chronically.
- Explain the effect of low-dose aspirin on platelet activation.
- Outline the synthesis of leukotrienes and lipoxins.
- Explain the role of leukotrienes in asthma, and propose at least three different drugs that can be used in the prophylaxis or treatment of asthma.

## 1. EICOSANOID FAMILIES

*Many eicosanoids are made from the ω-6 fatty acid arachidonic acid, which in turn is derived from the essential ω-6 fatty acid linoleic acid. Another group of eicosanoids is made from the ω-3 fatty acid eicosapentaenoic acid (EPA), which in turn is derived from the essential ω-3 fatty acid linolenic acid. The eicosanoids derived from ω-3 fatty acids tend to* *have an opposite effect to eicosanoids derived from ω-6 fatty acids. Current diets are typically rich in vegetable oils and therefore provide plenty of ω-6 fatty acids. However, ω-3 fatty acids are scarce in most diets.*

Eicosanoids are made from 20-carbon polyunsaturated fatty acids, either ω-6 or ω-3. *Eicosa* means 20 in Greek. Eicosanoids are also called **icosanoids**.

**Omega-6 (ω-6, n-6)** and **omega-3 (ω-3, n-3) fatty acids** are **essential fatty acids** that we absorb from food. Humans cannot synthesize ω-6 or ω-3 fatty acids (see Section 3 in Chapter 27). The most basic ω-6 fatty acid is **linoleic acid** (C18:2), and the most basic ω-3 fatty acid is **linolenic acid** (C18:3). These essential fatty acids and their products are polyunsaturated. Polyunsaturated fatty acids react quite readily with oxygen, which can give food a rancid taste and generate oxidative stress in the human body.

We generally get plenty of ω-6 fatty acids but precious little ω-3 fatty acids. Plant oils are relatively rich in ω-6 fatty acids (Table 32.1). Flax seed and fish (especially oily ones, such as salmon) are relatively rich in ω-3 fatty acids.

Once linoleic acid (ω-6, C18:2) and linolenic acid (ω-3, C18:3) reach cells, cells convert some of these fatty acids to **arachidonic acid** (C20:4) and **eicosapentaenoic acid** (**EPA**, C20:5), respectively, using a combination of desaturation and elongation (Fig. 32.1). Elongation and desaturation occur as described in Chapter 27. Only a small fraction of linolenic acid is converted to EPA and even less to docosahexaenoic acid (DHA).

Cells store **arachidonic acid** and **EPA** in phospholipids in the endoplasmic reticulum and in the plasma membrane. Cells typically contain ~10 times more arachidonic acid than EPA, but an EPA-rich diet can raise the EPA content to ~70% that of arachidonic acid.

It is not clear what the optimal consumption of ω-6 fatty acids should be; current intake may be too high due to high consumption of vegetable oils. For example, more than 50% of the fatty acids of corn oil are ω-6 fatty acids and so are up to ~25% of the fatty acids of olive oil.

It is **recommended** that ω-3 fatty acids are consumed in an amount equivalent to ~0.5% of all calories (~1.4 g/day). **Flax-seed oil** contains mostly linolenic acid. By contrast, **fish oil** contains mainly EPA and DHA. Oil from **algae** contains DHA but almost no EPA.

A high intake of ω-3 fatty acids in the form of EPA and DHA lowers plasma triglycerides and the risk of death due to coronary heart disease. ω-3 fatty acids may exert their beneficial effects, for instance, by binding to proteins (e.g., PPAR-γ, a transcription factor), by giving rise to eicosanoids (see

**Table 32.1** **Essential Fatty Acids in Food**

| Food | ω-6 Fatty Acids (g/100 g Food) | ω-3 Fatty Acids (g/100 g Food) |
|---|---|---|
| Cod liver oil | 1.8 | 18.8 |
| Salmon | 0.5 | 1.7 |
| Canola oil | 18.6 | 9.1 |
| Corn oil | 53.2 | 1.2 |
| Olive oil | 9.8 | 0.8 |
| Walnuts | 0.3 | 10.6 |
| Flaxseed | 0.3 | 1.4 |
| Ground beef (30% fat) | 0.6 | 0.1 |

Based on data from the United States Department of Agriculture National Nutrient Database, release 28.

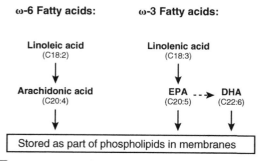

**Fig. 32.1** **Elongation and storage of ω-3 and ω-6 essential fatty acids.** EPA, eicosapentaenoic acid; DHA, docosahexaenoic acid.

Sections 2 and 3) and other lipid signals, and by lowering plasma triglycerides (see Section 8.1 in Chapter 28).

## 2. PROSTAGLANDINS AND THROMBOXANES

*Prostaglandins and thromboxanes are eicosanoids that are made from the ω-3 fatty acid EPA or from the ω-6 fatty acid arachidonic acid. These compounds act locally via G protein–coupled receptors. Prostaglandins play a role in inflammation, in protecting the stomach mucosa, and in ripening the cervix before delivery. Thromboxane A2 stimulates activation and aggregation of platelets near sites of vessel injury. The synthesis of prostaglandins and thromboxanes is inhibited by corticosteroids, phospholipase inhibitors, and NSAIDs.*

### 2.1. Synthesis of Prostanoids

**Prostanoids** is a summary term for **prostaglandins** and **thromboxanes**. This section discusses prostaglandins D, E, H,

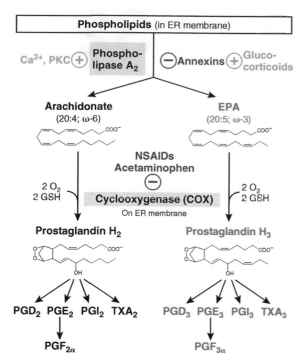

**Fig. 32.2** **Synthesis of prostaglandins.** EPA, eicosapentaenoic acid; ER, endoplasmic reticulum; GSH, reduced glutathione; NSAID, nonsteroidal antiinflammatory drug; PG, prostaglandin; PKC, protein kinase C; TX, thromboxane.

and I (prostaglandin I is also called **prostacyclin**), as well as thromboxane A (TXA).

In the rate-limiting step of eicosanoid synthesis, **cytosolic phospholipase A$_2$** (cPLA$_2$) moves onto the **endoplasmic reticulum membrane** and hydrolyzes phospholipids that contain EPA or arachidonic acid. cPLA$_2$ produces lysophospholipids and either eicosapentaenoic or arachidonic acid (Fig. 32.2). Physiologically, phospholipase A$_2$ activity is enhanced by an elevated concentration of **Ca$^{2+}$** in the cytosol and by increased activity of **protein kinase C**; on the other hand, **annexins (lipocortins)** inhibit cPLA$_2$.

**Glucocorticoids** indirectly reduce phospholipase A$_2$ activity by stimulating the transcription of **annexins (lipocortins)**, which then inhibit phospholipase A$_2$.

The **cyclooxygenase enzymes** (**COX-1** and **COX-2**) catalyze the synthesis of **prostaglandin H$_2$** (PGH$_2$) from arachidonic acid and the synthesis of **prostaglandin H$_3$** (PGH$_3$) from EPA (see Fig. 32.2). COX-1 is expressed in most tissues at all times, whereas COX-2 is mostly induced during inflammation, typically over a period of hours. The rate of synthesis of eicosanoids from arachidonic acid is generally substantially greater than that from EPA.

PGH$_2$ and PGH$_3$ give rise to the prostaglandins PGD, PGE, PGF, and PGI as well as TXA. PGH$_2$ has a half-life of ~2 min.

Prostanoids are identified with a **subscript** that denotes the number of **double bonds**, e.g., PGE$_2$. Arachidonic acid (ω-6, C20:4) gives rise to prostanoids with two double bonds, whereas EPA (ω-3, C20:5) gives rise to prostanoids with three double bonds (see Fig. 32.2). Prostaglandin F has an additional subscript of $\alpha$ or $\beta$ that indicates the configuration at carbon-9.

As a rule of thumb, $\omega$-6 fatty acids give rise to **proinflammatory eicosanoids**, whereas $\omega$-3 fatty acids give rise to **antiinflammatory eicosanoids** or to eicosanoids that resolve inflammation.

Eicosanoids are generally **short lived** and exert their effects **locally**, near their place of origin. Most cells can produce eicosanoids. The half-life of eicosanoids is on the order of seconds to a few minutes. Secreted eicosanoids induce changes in nearby cells (**paracrine** effect) or in the cell that secreted it (**autocrine** effect). The short lifespan of eicosanoids is due to inherent lability, uptake into cells, and degradation by enzymes.

## 2.2. Prostanoid Receptors

Prostaglandins and thromboxane act via **G protein–coupled receptors** (GPCRs; see Section 2 in Chapter 33) that are named after their ligands (e.g., receptors for prostaglandin $E_2$ [$PGE_2$] are called EP receptors).

Some prostaglandins bind to several types of prostaglandin receptor. For example, there are four different $PGE_2$ receptors: EP1, EP2, EP3, and EP4. $PGE_2$ is the most abundantly and most ubiquitously synthesized of all prostanoids. The diversity of EP receptors accounts for some of the variety of $PGE_2$ effects. The other prostanoids have only one receptor.

Prostaglandin receptors fall into three major categories: some receptors (DP1, EP2, EP4, and IP) raise the concentration of **cyclic adenosine monophosphate (cAMP)** in the cytosol, whereas one receptor (EP3) can decrease it. Activation of other receptors (EP1, FP, and TP) can lead to an increase in the concentration of $Ca^{2+}$ in the cytosol. Diversity in signaling is further increased via alternative splicing of mRNA (see Fig. 6.13 and Section 3.4 in Chapter 6), via homodimerization and heterodimerization, and via promiscuous coupling to $G\alpha$ proteins.

The biological effects of prostaglandins and thromboxanes of the 3 series (PGE3, TXE3, etc.) are poorly understood. It seems that these prostanoids are partial agonists; they bind to the same receptors as the 2 series prostanoids. However, they induce a smaller effect and thereby prevent more effective signaling via 2 series prostanoids.

## 2.3. Physiological Roles of Prostaglandins D$_2$, E$_2$, and F$_2$

**Prostaglandins** play a role in inflammation. Prostaglandin production is low in uninflamed tissue but rises rapidly during the onset of inflammation, preceding the arrival of white blood cells. As part of the innate immune system, **toll-like receptors (TLRs)** and **pattern recognition receptors (PRRs)** on mast cells and macrophages recognize **pathogen-associated molecular patterns (PAMPs)**. PAMPs are found in double-stranded RNA, lipopolysaccharides, glycans, glycoconjugates, and endotoxins. In response, mast cells and macrophages secrete $PGE_2$. Some of the incoming white blood cells produce

$PGD_2$, $PGE_2$, and $TXA_2$. During the resolution phase of inflammation, the number of white blood cells in the tissue returns to normal, in large part through apoptosis.

$PGE_2$ causes pain, induces vasodilation, and increases the permeability of the vessel wall. Pain can be induced peripherally, in the spinal cord, and in the brain. The vasodilation causes redness. The increased permeability of the vessel wall leads to the flow of blood plasma into the extracellular space and thus causes edema.

In the **stomach** and **duodenum**, an acid-sensing pathway fosters the release of $PGE_2$. $PGE_2$ lowers the exposure of epithelial cells to **acid** by increasing bicarbonate secretion and mucus production.

**NSAIDs** and acetaminophen inhibit the COX enzymes and may lead to damage of the mucosa of the stomach and intestine. These drugs are the first-line treatment for common musculoskeletal disorders such as back pain, osteoarthritis, and rheumatoid arthritis.

**Nonselective NSAIDs** such as aspirin (acetylsalicylic acid), ibuprofen, ketoprofen, naproxen, diclofenac, and indomethacin inhibit prostaglandin $E_2$ synthesis in the gastric mucosa. The decrease in $PGE_2$ synthesis leads to decreased bicarbonate secretion and decreased mucus production. This increases the risk of symptomatic **ulcers** in the stomach. Nonselective NSAIDs are even more damaging to the lower gastrointestinal tract, where they may cause bleeding or perforation. Perforation of the intestine requires emergency surgery.

Although **enteric-coated aspirin** (an NSAID) passes through the stomach intact, it still acts systemically and therefore still impairs $PGE_2$-mediated protection of the mucosa.

Compared with nonselective COX inhibitors (used with or without a proton pump inhibitor), **selective COX-2 inhibitors** reduce the risk of perforation, obstruction, or bleeding in the gastrointestinal tract of long-term users. The only selective COX-2 inhibitor in current use is **celecoxib**.

COX-2 is overexpressed in most premalignant and malignant colorectal tumors, and both nonselective NSAIDs and NSAIDs that selectively inhibit COX-2 can have a chemopreventive effect, to some extent independent of COX inhibition. The benefits and risks of such drug treatment are complex.

**Misoprostol** (a $PGE_1$ analog) is used clinically to protect the mucosa of the stomach and duodenum during long-term NSAID therapy.

$PGE_2$ and $PGF_{2\alpha}$ soften the **cervix** during pregnancy, and they also favor contraction of the uterus. **Misoprostol** (a $PGE_1$ analog) and **dinoprostone** ($PGF_{2\alpha}$) are used for **ripening** the **cervix** so that induction of labor with the peptide oxytocin is more likely to be successful.

## 2.4. Roles of Thromboxane A$_2$ and Prostacyclin

Activated **platelets** produce and release thromboxane $A_2$ (**TXA$_2$**), which in turn activates other nearby platelets via TP receptors and leads to **platelet aggregation**. Platelet activation occurs preferentially at sites of vessel injury. The short half-life of $TXA_2$ and the rapid dilution of $TXA_2$ in the bloodstream help confine platelet activation to the site of injury. Activated platelets then display a receptor that binds fibrinogen. Fibrinogen is a prevalent, threadlike protein in blood plasma that links platelets in a process called aggregation.

TXA$_2$ from activated platelets also binds to TP receptors on **smooth muscle cells** in the vessel wall, and thereby leads to an elevated concentration of Ca$^{2+}$ in the cytosol, which stimulates smooth muscle contraction. The resulting **vasoconstriction** reduces blood loss.

TXA$_2$ is degraded to the inactive **TXB$_2$**.

**Prostaglandin I$_2$ (PGI$_2$, prostacyclin)** released from endothelial cells and smooth muscle cells in vessel walls, acting via IP receptors, inhibits platelet aggregation and promotes vasodilation. PGI$_2$ release increases in response to hypoxia or vessel injury.

Via inhibition of COX, the antiplatelet drugs **aspirin** and **sulfinpyrazone** inhibit the synthesis of TXA$_2$ to a greater extent than the synthesis of prostacyclin (see also Fig. 32.2). Aspirin irreversibly inactivates COX in a number of tissues such that the synthesis of PGH$_2$ is impaired. Platelets contain only a small amount of cytoplasm (including granules) and plasma membrane. Platelets therefore do not have the means to synthesize new COX. By contrast, endothelial cells and smooth muscle cells can synthesize new COX. The net effect is that aspirin and sulfinpyrazone inhibit platelet activation.

**Iloprost** is an analog of PGI$_2$ that is used to decrease blood pressure in the pulmonary artery. Thereby, PGI$_2$ also has mild antiplatelet activity.

## 3. LEUKOTRIENES AND LIPOXINS

*Like prostanoids, leukotrienes and lipoxins are synthesized from arachidonic acid or EPA. Leukotrienes constrict bronchi and facilitate extravasation of leukocytes. Lipoxins antagonize the action of leukotrienes and help resolve inflammation. The synthesis of lipoxins starts in one type of cell and ends in a second type of cell in a process termed transcellular synthesis.*

### 3.1. Leukotrienes

**Macrophages, mast cells,** and **leukocytes** such as neutrophils, eosinophils, and monocytes synthesize leukotrienes from arachidonic acid (Fig. 32.3).

In mast cells and macrophages, leukotriene synthesis is stimulated by antigens that combine with immunoglobulin E on the cell surface. The IgE-antigen complex activates a receptor that in turn causes PLA$_2$ and 5-lipoxygenase to become active.

Liberation of arachidonic acid from a phospholipid in the endoplasmic reticulum membrane is the first and rate-limiting step of leukotriene synthesis (see Fig. 32.3), just as it is in the synthesis of prostaglandins and TXA (see Fig. 32.2).

**Leukotriene A$_4$ (LTA$_4$)** is inactive; however, it gives rise to the active **LTB$_4$** and **LTC$_4$** (see Fig. 32.3). LTC$_4$ is formed by conjugation with **glutathione** (γ-Glu-Cys-Gly; see also Fig. 21.5 and Section 2.2 in Chapter 21). Stepwise removal of the

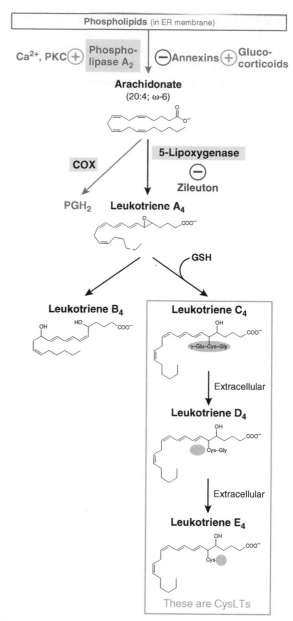

**Fig. 32.3** **Synthesis of leukotrienes of the 4 series.** The same enzymes also catalyze the synthesis of leukotrienes of the 5 series from eicosapentaenoic acid. COX, cyclooxygenase; CysLT, cysteine-containing leukotriene; ER, endoplasmic reticulum; GSH, reduced glutathione; PG, prostaglandin; PKC, protein kinase C;

Glu and Gly residues gives rise to **LTD$_4$** and **LTE$_4$**. LTC$_4$, LTD$_4$, and LTE$_4$ all contain a cysteine residue and are called **cysteinyl leukotrienes.** In general, LTC$_4$ and LTD$_4$ have higher proinflammatory activity than LTE$_4$.

LTB$_4$ attracts neutrophils, dendritic cells, and T cells. Leukotriene B$_4$ binds to **LTB4R** receptors. Neutrophils contain LTB4R receptors and use them to home in on the source of LTB$_4$. Once they meet a higher concentration of LTB$_4$, neutrophils activate secretion of their granules.

Leukotriene C$_4$ (LTB$_5$) increases the permeability of postcapillary venules.

There are two receptors for cysteine-containing leukotrienes, **CYSLTR1** and **CYSLTR2**. In airway smooth muscle cells, activation of CYSLTR1 leads to constriction of the **bronchi**. In blood vessels, CYSLTR1 affects cell junctions between endothelial cells so that it is easier for leukocytes and small molecules to leave the bloodstream (termed **extravasation**).

In the bronchi and bronchioles of the lungs (Fig. 32.4), GPCRs (see Section 2 in Chapter 33) coupled to $G\alpha_q$ stimulate contraction of smooth muscle, whereas GPCRs coupled to $G\alpha_s$ inhibit contraction. $G\alpha_q$ become active when the leukotrienes $LTC_4$, $LTD_4$, or $LTE_4$ bind to CYSLTR1 receptors. Similarly, $G\alpha_s$ become active when epinephrine or norepinephrine activate $\beta_2$-adrenergic receptors.

**Asthma** is due to an inflammation of the bronchi and bronchioles that leads to contraction of smooth muscle in these airways, as well as recruitment of leukocytes (Fig. 32.5). In the long term, asthma also leads to hypertrophy of smooth muscle and the glands that produce mucus.

**Zileuton**, an inhibitor of 5-lipoxygenase (see Fig. 32.3), and the CYSLTR1 antagonists **montelukast** and **zafirlukast** are used in the prophylaxis and chronic treatment of asthma. The CYSLTR1 antagonists diminish activation of $G\alpha_q$.

**Short-acting $\beta_2$-adrenergic receptor agonists**, such as **albuterol** and **levalbuterol**, and **long-acting $\beta_2$-adrenergic receptor agonists**, such as **salmeterol** and **formoterol**, are used to dilate the bronchi in patients with asthma via activation of $G\alpha_s$. (These $\beta_2$-adrenergic agonists stimulate the heart only moderately.)

**Glucocorticoids** reduce inflammation and are used for both short- and long-term control of asthma.

## 3.2. Lipoxins

While leukotrienes (see Section 3.1) are proinflammatory, lipoxins play a role in the **resolution of inflammation**. Lipoxins inhibit activation of neutrophils and eosinophils, and they stimulate macrophages to phagocytose dead white blood cells.

Lipoxins can be synthesized from **leukotrienes** or from **15(S)-hydroxyeicosatetraenoic acid (15-HETE)**. In both cases, synthesis is split into two so that it starts in one type of cell and ends in another type of cell; this is called **transcellular synthesis**. The requirement for two different locations for lipoxin synthesis helps delay the action of lipoxins.

One pathway for the synthesis of lipoxins depends on the availability of $LTA_4$ (Fig. 32.6). For example, leukocytes produce $LTA_4$ (see Fig. 32.3). Nearby platelets convert $LTA_4$ to the isomers **lipoxin $A_4$ ($LXA_4$)** and **lipoxin $B_4$ ($LXB_4$)**.

A second pathway for the synthesis of lipoxins depends on the availability of 15-HETE (see Fig. 32.6). For example, endothelial cells produce 15-HETE. Nearby leukocytes convert 15-HETE to lipoxin $A_4$ and lipoxin $B_4$. (Leukocytes cannot produce lipoxins on their own, because they lack 12-lipoxygenase to convert $LTA_4$ to lipoxins, and they lack 15-lipoxygenase to synthesize 15-HETE as a precursor for lipoxins.)

In line with their antiinflammatory effect, $LXA_4$ and $LXB_4$ have the following two effects: They antagonize signaling by cysteinyl leukotrienes via CYSLTR1 and CYSSLTR2 (see Section 3.1) and thereby prevent the activation of neutrophils. On the other hand, $LXA_4$ and $LXB_4$ bind to the **formyl peptide receptor 2 (FPR2)**, and to **GPCR32**, both of which are GPCRs.

**Aspirin** relieves pain not only by inhibiting prostaglandin synthesis (see Section 2.3), but also by acetylating COX-2, which then makes **epi-$LXA_4$**. Like $LXA_4$ and $LXB_4$,

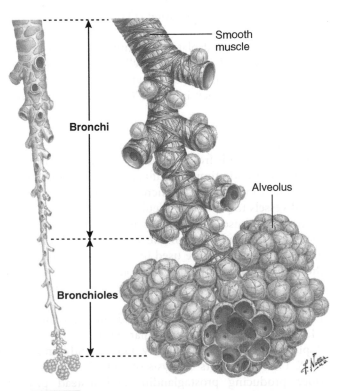

**Fig. 32.4** Bronchioles and bronchi of the lungs.

Smooth muscle

Bronchi

Bronchioles

Alveolus

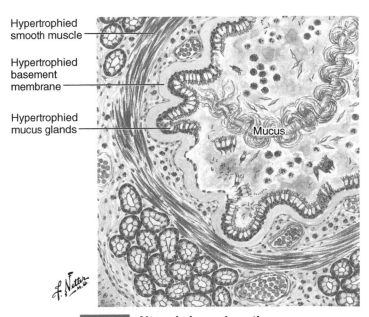

**Fig. 32.5** Altered airway in asthma.

Hypertrophied smooth muscle

Hypertrophied basement membrane

Hypertrophied mucus glands

Mucus

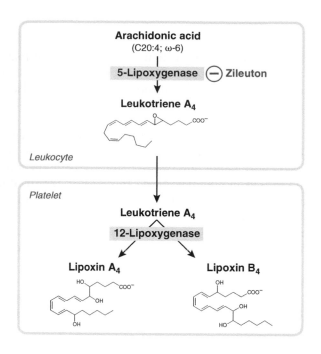

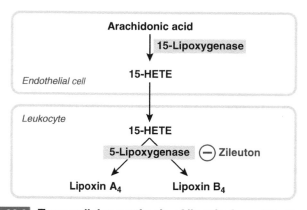

**Fig. 32.6  Transcellular synthesis of lipoxin $A_4$ and $B_4$.** The two lipoxins are isomers. 15-HETE, 15(S)-hydroxyeicosatetraenoic acid.

epi-lipoxin $A_4$ binds to the FPR2 and therefore has an antiinflammatory effect.

The ω-3 fatty acid **DHA** (C22:6) gives rise to **D-series resolvins**, some of which also act on FPR2 and GPR32. Similar to lipoxins, resolvins terminate inflammation.

## SUMMARY

- We take in ω-3 fatty acids mainly by consuming fats from plant seeds, nuts, algae, or fish. A small amount of linolenic acid (C18:3) is converted to eicosapentaenoic acid (EPA, C20:5) and docosapentaenoic acid (DHA, C22:6). Fat from algae or fish are the only good sources of EPA and DHA. Linolenic acid, EPA, and DHA are incorporated into membrane phospholipids. The recommended intake of ω-3 fatty acids is an amount equivalent to 0.5% of all calories.

- Current Western diets are rich in plant oils, which in turn provide plenty of ω-6 fatty acids. Linoleic acid (C18:2) is converted to arachidonic acid (C20:4) and incorporated into membrane phospholipids.

- Phospholipase $A_2$ catalyzes the production of EPA or arachidonic acid from phospholipids in the endoplasmic reticulum membrane. This is the rate-limiting step in eicosanoid biosynthesis. The eicosanoids include prostanoids, thromboxanes, leukotrienes, and lipoxins.

- EPA and arachidonic acid can give rise to prostanoids (prostaglandins and thromboxanes), leukotrienes, and lipoxins. Eicosanoids have a short life span and act locally. Prostaglandins of the 2 series (derived from arachidonic acid) are generally proinflammatory, whereas prostaglandins of the 3 series (derived from EPA) are generally antiinflammatory.

- COX-1 and COX-2 convert EPA and arachidonic acid to $PGH_3$ and $PGH_2$, respectively. COX-1 is present in most cells at all times. COX-2 is predominantly synthesized only in response to inflammation. COX-2 is also found in many tumor cells.

- Eicosanoids exert their effects via GPCRs, which in turn either alter the concentration of cAMP or $Ca^{2+}$ in the cytosol.

- In the stomach and duodenum, $PGE_2$ protects the mucosa by enhancing the secretion of mucus and bicarbonate. Nonselective NSAIDs inhibit $PGE_2$ synthesis and raise the risk of ulcers and perforation of the mucosa. Compared with nonselective NSAIDs, celecoxib, a selective COX-2 inhibitor, is associated with a lower risk of perforation or bleeding in the gastrointestinal tract. Misoprostol, a $PGE_1$ analog, protects the stomach mucosa in long-term NSAID users.

- Misoprostol and dinoprostone ($PGF_{2\alpha}$) are used to ripen the cervix.

- $TXA_4$ from activated platelets stimulates platelet aggregation, whereas $PGI_2$ from endothelial cells inhibits platelet aggregation. Aspirin and sulfinpyrazone have an antiplatelet effect because they inhibit $TXA_4$ synthesis more than $PGI_2$ synthesis.

- The $PGI_2$ analog iloprost is used to decrease blood pressure in patients who have pulmonary hypertension.

- Leukotrienes made from arachidonic acid induce bronchoconstriction and stimulate inflammation, thereby attracting white blood cells and increasing the permeability of blood vessels to plasma and leukocytes.

- Asthma is caused by prostaglandin- and leukotriene-mediated inflammation of the bronchi and bronchioles. The following agents are used in the treatment of asthma: the 5-lipoxygenase inhibitor zileuton, the CysLTR1 antagonists montelukast and zafirlukast, β2-adrenergic receptor agonists, and glucocorticoids.

- Lipoxins are antiinflammatory and are generated from $LTA_4$ or 15-HETE via transcellular synthesis.

- Aspirin acetylates and thereby permanently inactivates COX-1 while it alters catalysis of COX-2 so that COX-2 stops producing prostaglandins and instead produces lipoxins, which are antiinflammatory.

## FURTHER READING

- Capra V, Bäck M, Barbieri SS, Camera M, Tremoli E, Rovati GE. Eicosanoids and their drugs in cardiovascular diseases: focus on atherosclerosis and stroke. *Med Res Rev.* 2013;33:364-438.
- Lenaeus MJ, Hirschmann J. Primary care of the patient with asthma. *Med Clin North Am.* 2015;99:953-967.
- Patrício JP, Barbosa JP, Ramos RM, Antunes NF, de Melo PC. Relative cardiovascular and gastrointestinal safety of non-selective non-steroidal anti-inflammatory drugs versus cyclo-oxygenase-2 inhibitors: implications for clinical practice. *Clin Drug Investig.* 2013;33:167-183.
- Ricciotti E, FitzGerald GA. Prostaglandins and inflammation. *Arterioscler Thromb Vasc Biol.* 2011;31:986-1000.
- Serhan CN, Chiang N, Dalli J. The resolution code of acute inflammation: novel pro-resolving lipid mediators in resolution. *Semin Immunol.* 2015;27:200-215.
- Theron AJ, Steel HC, Tintinger GR, Gravett CM, Anderson R, Feldman C. Cysteinyl leukotriene receptor-1 antagonists as modulators of innate immune cell function. *J Immunol Res.* 2014;2014:608930.

# Review Questions

1. By weight, which one of the following oils contains the highest fraction of a fatty acid that can be converted to PGE$_3$?

   A. Algae oil
   B. Cod liver oil
   C. Flaxseed oil
   D. Olive oil

2. The antiplatelet effect of aspirin is ascribed to inhibition of the synthesis of which one of the following?

   A. Arachidonic acid
   B. LTB$_4$
   C. LXB$_4$
   D. PGI$_2$
   E. TXA$_2$

3. Which one of the following drugs is most suitable to inhibit the synthesis of leukotrienes and lipoxins, but not the synthesis of prostaglandins or thromboxanes?

   A. Albuterol
   B. Celecoxib
   C. Dinoprostone
   D. Montelukast
   E. Zileuton

4. A 67-year-old woman takes NSAIDs chronically to treat rheumatoid arthritis. Which one of the following drugs is best suited to prevent the formation of ulcers?

   A. Cortisol
   B. Misoprostol
   C. Salmeterol
   D. Zafirlukast
   E. Zileuton

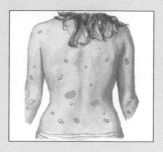

# Chapter 33  Signaling

## SYNOPSIS

- After binding a ligand, such as epinephrine, G protein–coupled receptors (GPCRs) activate heterotrimeric G proteins, a subunit of which then favors or inhibits the formation of a second messenger, such as cyclic adenosine monophosphate (cAMP). cAMP in turn activates protein kinase A, which then phosphorylates a variety of substrates.
- Many growth factor receptors have tyrosine kinase activity and activate the RAS/RAF/MEK/ERK pathway, which leads to changes in the activity of many transcription factors.
- The RAS/RAF/MEK/ERK pathway is overly active in Noonan syndrome, neurofibromatosis type 1, and in many tumor cells.

## LEARNING OBJECTIVES

*For mastery of this topic, you should be able to do the following:*
- Describe how adrenergic receptors with epinephrine or norepinephrine bound to them activate intracellular signaling pathways.
- Compare and contrast the signaling pathways of adrenergic receptors with those of activated glucagon receptors and glucagon-like peptide-1 receptors.
- List molecular events that terminate signaling via GPCRs and heterotrimeric G proteins.
- Describe the RAS/RAF/MEK/ERK signaling pathway, and list hormones and their receptors that use this pathway.
- Explain how the causes of Noonan syndrome and neurofibromatosis type 1 relate to a signaling pathway.

## 1. PRINCIPLES OF SIGNALING

*Chemical signaling takes place over short (cell to cell) and long distances (via blood). Signaling pathways often generate a concentration wave of a signaling molecule because there are mechanisms for both starting and ending a signal. Phosphorylation/dephosphorylation and associated changes in protein conformation are a common occurrence in intracellular signaling pathways.*

Many signaling pathways involve the conversion of an extracellular signal into an intracellular signal, amplification of the intracellular signal, and both stimulatory and inhibitory interactions with other pathways.

**Endocrine** signaling typically involves the secretion of a hormone into the bloodstream and the recognition of that hormone in a distant tissue. Accordingly, **endocrine secretion** refers to secretion of a substance into the blood, whereas **exocrine secretion** refers to secretion of a substance into the lumen of the gastrointestinal tract, the airways, the urinary tract, the environment, and so forth. For instance, exocrine

cells of the pancreas secrete enzymes into the pancreatic ducts that digest food; endocrine cells of the pancreas secrete insulin and glucagon into the bloodstream to control the concentration of glucose in the blood.

The term **autocrine** signaling refers to secretion of a substance into the extracellular space by a cell whereby the secreting cell is also the one that responds to the secreted product. The term **paracrine signaling** refers to secretion of a substance into the extracellular space by a cell whereby a nearby cell responds to the secreted product. In paracrine signaling, the signal is typically short lived, such as in eicosanoid signaling (see Chapter 32).

For almost every pathway that leads to an **increase** in output, there is at least one reaction that leads to a **decrease** in output. For instance, binding of epinephrine to a GPCR leads not only to an increased intracellular signal in the form of cAMP but also to the temporary or permanent removal of the receptor from the plasma membrane. Activation occurs more quickly than inactivation and thus generates a time-limited signal.

**Protein phosphorylation** is commonly involved in signal transduction. **Protein kinases** typically add a phosphate group, and **protein phosphatases** remove a phosphate group. Phosphorylation can render an enzyme or protein active or inactive. Most kinases react a phosphate with the hydroxyl group of a **serine** or **threonine** side chain. A smaller group of kinases react a phosphate with the hydroxyl group of a **tyrosine** side chain.

## 2. G PROTEIN–COUPLED RECEPTOR SIGNALING

*GPCRs sense many peptide hormones, neurotransmitters, and chemokines; they are also involved in smell, taste, and sight. Ligand binding to the extracellular portion of the receptor leads to a change in conformation of the cytosolic portion, which in turn activates a heterotrimeric G protein. The activated heterotrimeric G protein often produces a change in the concentration of a second messenger. Common second messengers are cAMP, inositol trisphosphate (IP$_3$), and diacylglycerol (DAG). The second messenger in turn triggers changes in metabolism or gene expression.*

The **GPCRs** form a large class of receptors that respond to extracellular water-soluble signals, such as hormones, neurotransmitters, odorants, or light. Humans have ~800 genes that encode GPCRs.

A large number of drugs in current use target GPCRs. For example, angiotensin receptor 1 blockers (e.g., losartan) lower blood pressure (see Fig. 31.17 and Section 4.1 in Chapter 31). Histamine H2-receptor antagonists (e.g., cimetidine) lower acid production in the stomach (see Fig. 34.2 and Section 1 in Chapter 34). Epinephrine and a variety of drugs that act on adrenergic receptors can be used for control of hypersensitivity reactions, bleeding, asthma, and blood pressure.

The description of GPCRs in this section is limited to GPCRs that play a role in the biochemistry discussed in this book; that is, glucagon receptors, glucagon-like peptide-1 (GLP-1) receptors, adrenergic receptors, angiotensin receptors, and histamine receptors (Table 33.1).

When a GPCR is activated by a ligand (e.g., epinephrine), it acts as a **guanine nucleotide exchange factor (GEF)** that exchanges a guanosine diphosphate (GDP) for a guanosine triphosphate (GTP) bound to a **heterotrimeric G protein** (Fig. 33.1). GTP binding to a heterotrimeric G protein activates the G protein. Certain GPCRs bind a heterotrimeric G protein with GDP bound to it before they bind a hormone, whereas others bind the G protein only after they have been activated by a hormone.

**Heterotrimeric G proteins** consist of an $\alpha$-, a $\beta$-, and a $\gamma$-subunit (see Fig. 33.1). The $\alpha$- and the $\gamma$-subunits are each anchored in the plasma membrane (on the cytosolic side) with myristic acid and either palmitic acid or a prenyl group (see Fig. 11.9 and Section 1.5 in Chapter 11). The $\alpha$-subunit binds GDP or GTP. When inactive—that is, when bound to GDP—the $\alpha$-, $\beta$-, and $\gamma$-subunits form a trimeric complex. When activated by GTP binding, the $\alpha$ subunit separates from the dimeric $\beta\gamma$-complex and assumes a new conformation. The $\alpha$-subunit is active until GTP is hydrolyzed to GDP (see below); the activated $\alpha$-subunit has the features of a timer.

The GTP-activated $\alpha$ subunit has intrinsic GTPase activity, and a **GTPase-activating protein (GAP)** can often greatly increase this GTPase activity, thus rendering the $\alpha$-subunit inactive (see Fig. 33.1).

The membrane-bound **$\beta\gamma$-complex** also acts as a signal and activates certain ion channels or phospholipases, effects that are not discussed further here.

There are several isoforms of **$\alpha$-subunits** that differ in their effects (Fig. 33.2). The $\alpha$-subunits are membrane bound and alter the activity of membrane-bound enzymes. Activated $\alpha_s$-subunits activate **adenylyl cyclase** and thus increase the concentration of cAMP. Activated $\alpha_i$-subunits inhibit adenylyl cyclase and thus decrease the concentration of cAMP.

**Table 33.1  Some G Protein–Coupled Receptors**

| Receptor | Relevant Ligands | Type of G$\alpha$, Second Messenger, and Effect |
|---|---|---|
| Glucagon receptor | Glucagon | G$\alpha_s$ activates an adenylyl cyclase, which produces cAMP. cAMP activates protein kinase A. |
| GLP-1 receptor | GLP-1 | |
| $\alpha_1$-Adrenergic receptor, subtypes A, B, D | Epinephrine, norepinephrine. Agonists such as phenylephrine are used as decongestants | G$\alpha_q$ and G$\alpha_{11}$ activate a phospholipase C, which hydrolyzes PIP2 to IP$_3$ and DAG. IP$_3$ increases cytosolic Ca$^{2+}$. DAG activates protein kinase C. |
| $\alpha_2$-Adrenergic receptor, subtypes A, B, C | Epinephrine, norepinephrine. The agonist clonidine is used to reduce blood pressure and to relieve pain via epidural administration | G$\alpha_i$ inhibits adenylyl cyclases |
| $\beta_1$-Adrenergic receptor | Epinephrine, norepinephrine | G$\alpha_s$ activates an adenylyl cyclase, which produces cAMP. cAMP activates protein kinase A. |
| $\beta_2$-Adrenergic receptor | Epinephrine, norepinephrine. The agonist albuterol is used to prevent or treat bronchospasm | |
| $\beta_3$-Adrenergic receptor | Epinephrine, norepinephrine | |
| Angiotensin II receptor type 1 | Angiotensin II, angiotensin III | G$\alpha_q$ or G$\alpha_{11}$ activate a phospholipase C, which hydrolyzes PIP2 to IP$_3$ and DAG. IP$_3$ increases cytosolic Ca$^{2+}$. DAG activates protein kinase C. |
| Histamine H2 receptor | Histamine. The antagonist cimetidine reduces acid production in the stomach | G$\alpha_s$ activates an adenylyl cyclase, which produces cAMP. cAMP activates protein kinase A. |
| Prostanoid EP2 and EP4 receptors | Prostaglandin E$_2$ | G$\alpha_s$ activates an adenylyl cyclase, which produces cAMP. cAMP activates protein kinase A. |
| Cysteinyl leukotriene receptors CYSLTR1 and CYSLTR2 | Leukotrienes LTC$_4$, LTD$_4$, LTE$_4$ | G$\alpha_q$ and G$\alpha_{11}$ activate a phospholipase C, which hydrolyzes PIP2 to IP$_3$ and DAG. IP$_3$ increases cytosolic Ca$^{2+}$. DAG activates protein kinase C. |

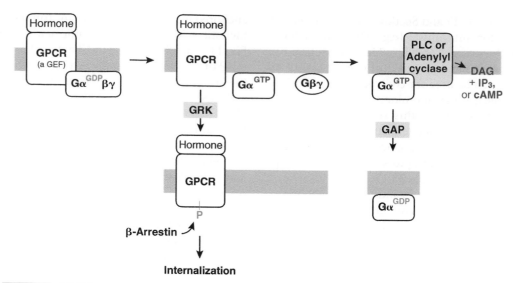

**Fig. 33.1** **GPCR activation of heterotrimeric G proteins.** DAG, diacylglycerol (a lipid); GEF, guanine nucleotide exchange factor; GPCR, G protein–coupled receptor; GRK, GPCR kinase; GAP, GTPase activating protein; IP₃, inositol trisphosphate (a sugar); P, phosphate group; PLC, phospholipase C.

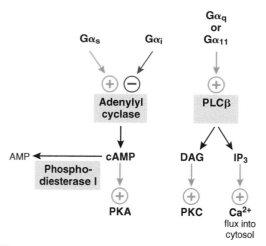

**Fig. 33.2** **Signaling pathways activated by activated Gα-subunits.** DAG, diacylglycerol; PKA, protein kinase A; PKC, protein kinase C; PLC, phospholipase C.

Activated $\alpha_q$- or $\alpha_{11}$-subunits activate phospholipase C, which hydrolyzes phosphatidylinositol bisphosphate (PIP2), which leads to an increase in the concentrations of **IP₃** in the cytosol and **DAG** in the membrane. Activated $\alpha_t$-subunits activate guanylyl cyclase and thus increase the concentration of **cGMP**.

During prolonged stimulation, GPCRs undergo appreciable **downregulation**. Once activated by a ligand, a GPCR becomes a target for phosphorylation by a **GPCR kinase**. This is followed by binding of β-**arrestin** to the GPCR, which thereby prevents the GPCR from activating another G protein. Furthermore, the β-arrestin-GPCR complex binds to clathrin-coated pits and is internalized via endocytosis. Some of these GPCRs eventually return to the plasma membrane; others are degraded.

The **glucagon receptor** is found mostly in the liver, where protein kinase A activity leads to phosphorylation of glycogen synthase and glycogen phosphorylase and thus increases glycogen degradation (see Figs. 24.5 and 24.7, Sections 1.3 and 2.2 in Chapter 24, and Fig. 26.9). Furthermore, cAMP and protein kinase A activity increase the rate of gluconeogenesis via increased activity of phosphoenolpyruvate carboxykinase, fructose 1,6-bisphosphatase, and glucose 6-phosphatase (see Fig. 25.7 and Section 3 in Chapter 25).

**GLP-1 receptors** work essentially in the same fashion as glucagon receptors, raising the intracellular concentration of cAMP. Note that cAMP has different effects on different cells. For instance, in hepatocytes, a glucagon-induced increase in the concentration of cAMP enhances glycogenolysis and gluconeogenesis, whereas in pancreatic β-cells a GLP-1–induced increase in cAMP enhances insulin secretion.

**Adrenergic receptors** bind the physiological ligands epinephrine or norepinephrine, and receptor diversity accounts for tissue-specific effects. In pancreatic β-cells, $\alpha_2$-adrenergic receptors inhibit insulin secretion. In hepatocytes, β-adrenergic receptors stimulate glycogenolysis and gluconeogenesis. In adipose tissue, $\beta_3$-adrenergic receptors stimulate lipolysis (see Section 5.1 in Chapter 28).

## 3. GROWTH FACTOR RECEPTORS THAT ARE RECEPTOR TYROSINE KINASES

*Insulin and other growth factors such as epidermal growth factor (EGF) bind to receptors, which, when activated, have a tyrosine kinase that phosphorylates both the receptor and adaptor proteins. The adaptor proteins activate two different signaling pathways: the PI3K/AKT pathway and the RAS/RAF/MEK/ERK pathway. The PI3K/AKT pathway is chiefly responsible for the effects of insulin on metabolism, and the RAS/RAF/MEK/ERK pathway accounts for the effects of insulin on cell proliferation and differentiation. The RAS/RAF/MEK/ERK pathway has abnormal activity in neurofibromatosis type 1, in Noonan syndrome, and in Cowden syndrome.*

## 3.1. Normal Receptor Tyrosine Kinase Signaling

Growth factors, such as insulin, insulin-like growth factor 1 (IGF-1), and EGF, bind to membrane-embedded receptors, which subsequently undergo a conformational change that activates a tyrosine kinase on the cytoplasmic face of the receptor; accordingly, these receptors are called **receptor tyrosine kinases.** Humans have more than 50 genes that encode receptor tyrosine kinases.

The insulin receptors and the IGF-1 receptor are always present as an α$_2$β$_2$ complex, whereby the α-subunits form an extracellular high-affinity hormone binding site, and the β-subunits each have a tyrosine kinase domain in the cytosol. (As will be shown below, there are two different isoforms of the insulin receptor, but for now this does not matter.) Upon binding of insulin, the tyrosine kinase domains in the insulin receptor β-subunits phosphorylate each other in a process called **trans-autophosphorylation.**

After trans-autophosphorylation, the tyrosine kinases of the receptors for insulin and IGF-1 phosphorylate a membrane-associated **insulin receptor substrate (IRS)** protein, of which there are four varieties (Fig. 33.3). Phosphorylated IRS protein can activate both the PI3K/AKT pathway and the RAS/RAF/MEK/ERK pathway. The PI3K/AKT pathway is especially important for insulin control of glucose transport, glucose metabolism, and protein synthesis, whereas the RAS/RAF/

MEK/ERK pathway is particularly important for regulating transcription, cell division, and cell differentiation.

Phosphorylated IRS activates the **PI3K/AKT signaling pathway** by binding to **phosphatidylinositol-4,5-bisphosphate 3-kinase (PI3K, phosphoinositide 3-kinase,** of which there are multiple isozymes), thereby activating it (see Fig. 33.3). PI3K then phosphorylates the phospholipid **PIP2** to **PIP3** (phosphatidylinositol trisphosphate). PIP3 then serves as a binding site for **PDPK1** (phosphoinositide-dependent protein kinase 1, also called PDK1) and **AKT2,** whereby PDPK1 phosphorylates and thus activates AKT2. Active AKT2 in turn generates a signal that leads to the insertion of **GLUT-4 glucose transporters** into the plasma membrane and to activation of **glycogen synthase kinase (GSK3),** which in turn activates **glycogen synthesis** (GSK3 also plays a role in many other signaling pathways). (The PI3K/AKT pathway was mentioned in Fig. 8.3 and Section 1.1 of Chapter 8. There are two AKTs, AKT1 and AKT2; AKT1 mostly plays a role in growth, whereas AKT2 is more important for glucose homeostasis.)

**PTEN** is a phosphatase that attenuates PI3K/AKT signaling by degrading PIP3.

Phosphorylated IRS also activates the **RAS/RAF/MEK/ERK signaling pathway** by binding to **GRB2,** which then binds **SOS.** SOS is a guanine nucleotide exchange factor (GEF; see Section 1) for the membrane-bound **RAS;** that is, it forces RAS to release bound GDP. Thereafter, RAS binds the more abundant GTP and thus becomes active. Thus active RAS functions like the active α-subunit of a heterotrimeric G

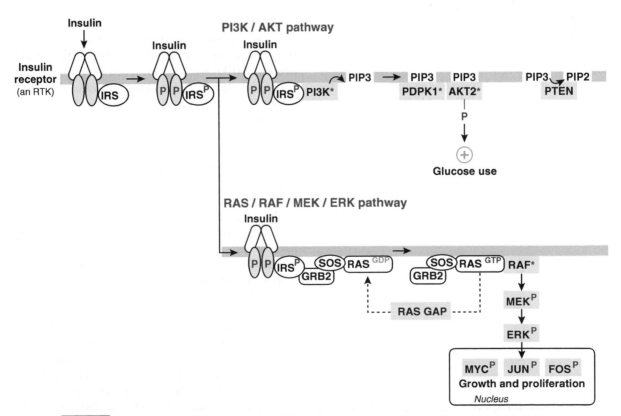

**Fig. 33.3**  **Insulin receptor signaling pathways.** P, phosphate. See text for other abbreviations.

protein (see Section 1). RAS is actually a member of the family of **small GTPases**. Active RAS binds to and thereby activates **RAF**, which is then also membrane bound. RAS has inherent GTPase activity to hydrolyze GTP, which renders RAS inactive. **GTPase activating proteins** (**GAPs**) enhance the intrinsic GTPase activity of RAS (GAPs also stimulate hydrolysis of GTP bound to the α-subunit of heterotrimeric G proteins; see Section 1). Thus SOS activates RAS, and RAS, enhanced by a RAS GAP, inactivates itself.

The kinase RAF starts a cascade of phosphorylation in the sequence RAF → MEK → ERK, whereby the signal is amplified at each step, and ERK can travel from the cytosol to the nucleus. The RAF → MEK → ERK kinase cascade is sometimes called the **MAP kinase cascade**. Phosphorylated ERK can move into the nucleus and affect transcription by phosphorylating a variety of transcription factors (e.g., MYC, JUN, FOS, CREB; see also Fig. 8.6). ERK also helps end signaling by phosphorylating RAF in a way that inhibits RAF activity.

Three different receptor tyrosine kinases bind **insulin**, **IGF-1**, and **IGF-2** (Fig. 33.4). Due to alternative splicing of mRNA from a single gene, there are two insulin receptor isoforms. **IR-B** contains all 22 exons, whereas **IR-A** lacks exon 11, which encodes 12 amino acids. IR-A and IR-B are each synthesized as a prorecptor protein that is then cleaved to give rise to an α- and a β-subunit. These subunits form an $\alpha_2\beta_2$ complex, which is stabilized by multiple disulfide bonds. IR-A is most common in fetal tissues and tumor cells, and IR-B is most common in differentiated cells. There is only a single form of the IGF-1 receptor.

The insulin receptors and the IGF-1 receptor can each bind multiple ligands (see Fig. 33.4). To complicate matters, IR-A, IR-B, and IGF-1R can form hybrid receptors. Furthermore, although insulin, IGF-1, and IGF-2, for example, each bind to IR-A, they have different effects on the conformation of the cytosolic portion of the receptor; the reason for this is unclear.

As shown above, the insulin receptor can activate both the PI3K/AKT pathway and the RAS/RAF/MEK/ERK pathway. The balance of activity in these pathways is in part tissue dependent.

Due to the structure of the signaling network, IGF-2 affects glucose metabolism, and insulin affects both carbohydrate metabolism and the cell cycle. Large solid tumors sometimes produce enough IGF-2 to cause hypoglycemia. In the development of insulin analogs for the treatment of diabetes, a reasonable balance has to be found between effects on glucose homeostasis and on growth (which could be tumorigenic).

An adaptor protein binds insulin-activated insulin receptors to budding clathrin-coated pits, and the insulin receptors then end up in **endosomes**, where a phosphotyrosine phosphatase dephosphorylates them (and thus inactivates them). This is a common mechanism for downregulation of other ligand-activated receptor tyrosine kinases and GPCRs (see Section 2), although the adaptor proteins differ.

Activation of the RAS/RAF/MEK/ERK pathway is observed in many **tumors**, as explained in Section 1.1 of Chapter 8.

The **EGF receptor** (**EGFR**) and **HER2** (human EGF receptor-2, NEU) are receptor tyrosine kinases that are monomers in the inactive state and dimers in the active state. The EGFR (encoded by *EGFR* gene) can be activated by EGF and by transforming growth factor-α (TGF-α). *EGFR* is a proto-oncogene, and activating mutations in one allele are frequently observed in tumors, such as breast cancer and adenocarcinoma of the lung (see Section 3 in Chapter 8). The tyrosine kinase activity of EGFRs can be inhibited with lapatinib, erlotinib, or afatinib. HER2 is encoded by the *ERBB2* gene. There is no known hormone that activates HER2. Perhaps HER2 is constitutively active, or it forms heterodimers with EGFRs. Activating mutations in one *ERBB2* allele are frequently seen in invasive breast tumors. The HER2 kinase activity can be inhibited with a kinase inhibitor (lapatinib, afatinib) or a monoclonal antibody (trastuzumab, pertuzumab).

## 3.2. Neurofibromatosis, Noonan Syndrome, and Cowden Syndrome

**Neurofibromatosis type 1** (**von Recklinghausen disease**) is a heritable tumor syndrome caused by heterozygous loss of function of **neurofibromin 1** (**neurofibromatosis-related protein, NF1**), which is encoded by the *NF1* gene. NF1 is a RAS GAP; that is, a protein that activates the intrinsic GTPase activity of RAS and thereby inactivates RAS. There are ~1,500 known pathogenic mutations in *NF1*, most of which lead to a truncated protein. As in other heritable cancer syndromes (see Chapter 8), some somatic cells lose the function of the remaining normal NF1 allele and thus are more likely to give rise to a neoplasm.

The prevalence of neurofibromatosis type 1 is ~1 in 3,000 births, and ~50% of affected persons have a de novo mutation that in turn most likely occurred in the germline of one parent.

The diagnosis of neurofibromatosis type 1 involves meeting at least two of the following seven criteria (see also Fig. 33.5): café-au-lait macules, skin-fold freckling, neurofibromas, Lisch nodules (in the irises), optic pathway tumor, bone dysplasia, or a family history of the disorder. Virtually all affected persons develop symptoms before age 8 years.

Most persons who have neurofibromatosis type 1 develop benign neurofibromas of the skin. About half of all patients have congenital plexiform neurofibromas, which may be superficial or inside the body, be disfiguring, or impair the function of an organ. Plexiform neurofibromas sometimes

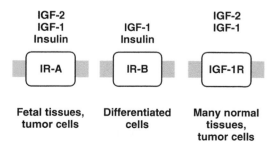

**Fig. 33.4** **Physiological stimuli of insulin receptors (IR) and insulin-like growth factor (IGF) receptors.**

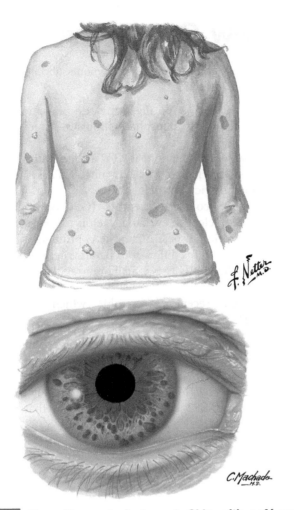

**Fig. 33.5** **Neurofibromatosis type 1: Skin with café-au-lait spots and neurofibromas, iris with Lisch nodules.** The neurofibromas have the appearance of nodules. Many affected persons also have scoliosis.

turn malignant. About 15% of affected children develop an optic glioma by 6 years of age (rarely later). Optic gliomas sometimes impair vision. In adulthood, malignancies arise mostly in the central nervous system, in the gastrointestinal system (especially the small intestine), and in the genitourinary tract.

**Noonan syndrome** is frequently associated with a congenital heart defect, failure to thrive during childhood that causes short stature, a dysmorphic face, and abnormalities of the skeleton. Subtypes of Noonan syndrome are caused by heterozygosity for gain-of-function mutations in the RAS/RAF/MEK/ERK signaling pathway, specifically in the following genes: *PTPN11* (encoding an adaptor protein of poorly understood function), *SOS1*, *KRAS*, *NRAS*, *RIT1* (encoding a small GTPase of the RAS family), *BRAF*, and *RAF1*.

Noonan syndrome has a prevalence of ~1 in 1,500 births. About 60% of the observed mutations are de novo, and the mutations are inherited in autosomal dominant fashion.

Some of the criteria for a diagnosis of Noonan syndrome are facial dysmorphology, pulmonary valve stenosis or hyper-

trophic cardiomyopathy, height less than the third percentile, intellectual disability, cryptorchidism, and a first-degree relative with the syndrome.

**Cowden syndrome**, a hereditary cancer syndrome, is caused by a loss-of-function mutation in *PTEN* (see Section 1.1 in Chapter 8). PTEN normally catalyzes the reaction PIP3 → PIP2 and thereby prevents the activation of PI3K and the PI3K-AKT signaling pathway.

## SUMMARY

- Glucagon, glucagon-like peptide, epinephrine, norepinephrine, angiotensin II, histamine, prostaglandin E2, and the cysteinyl leukotrienes signal via G protein–coupled receptors (GPCRs), which are coupled to membrane-bound heterotrimeric G proteins. The activated GPCR acts as a guanine nucleotide exchange factor (GEF) so that the $G\alpha$-subunit releases GDP and binds GTP, which activates the $G\alpha$-subunit. The main families of the $G\alpha$-subunit discussed in this chapter are $G\alpha_s$, $G\alpha_i$, $G\alpha_q$, and $G\alpha_{11}$. Active $G\alpha_s$ stimulates the activity of adenylyl cyclase (which produces cAMP), whereas active $G\alpha_i$ inhibits adenylyl cyclase. $G\alpha_q$ and $G\alpha_{11}$ are very similar proteins, which activate phospholipase C (PLC). PLC hydrolyzes phosphatidyl inositol bisphosphate (PIP2) into diacyl glycerol (DAG) and inositol trisphosphate (IP$_3$). DAG activates protein kinase C (PKC), whereas IP$_3$ stimulates the flow of $Ca^{2+}$ into the cytosol.

- After GPCR kinase phosphorylates a GPCR, β-arrestin binds to the GPCR and prevents further activation of G proteins. β-Arrestin also induces the endocytosis of these GPCRs via clathrin-coated pits.

- GTPase activating proteins (GAPs) stimulate the intrinsic GTPase activity of $G\alpha$-subunits and thereby inactivate $G\alpha$.

- After binding a ligand, the IR-A and IR-B insulin receptors, the IGF-1 receptor, the EGF receptor, and other receptor tyrosine kinases activate the RAS-RAF-MEK-ERK pathway. The receptor tyrosine kinases trans-autophosphorylate and then phosphorylate IRS on tyrosine. Phosphorylated IRS binds GRB2, which activates SOS, which in turn activates the membrane-bound small G protein RAS by facilitating the exchange of GTP for GDP. RAS with GTP bound to it activates the kinase RAF. RAF is the first member of a kinase cascade with the sequence RAF → MEK → ERK. Phosphorylated ERK phosphorylates the transcription factors MYC, JUN, FOS, and CREB, with the effect of increasing cell growth and proliferation.

- Noonan syndrome is caused by a variety of mutations that activate the RAS/RAF/MEK/ERK pathway and is characterized by congenital heart defects, short stature, and abnormalities of the skeleton.

- Neurofibromatosis type 1 is caused by a loss-of-function mutation in the *NF1* gene, which encodes a RAS GAP. Benign and malignant tumors form as a result of somatic loss of the remaining normal NF1 allele.

## FURTHER READING

- Bhambhani V, Muenke M. Noonan syndrome. *Am Fam Physician*. 2014;89:37-43.
- Kang DS, Tian X, Benovic JL. Role of β-arrestins and arrestin domain-containing proteins in G protein-coupled receptor trafficking. *Curr Opin Cell Biol*. 2014;27:63-71.
- Karnik SS, Unal H, Kemp JR, et al. International Union of Basic and Clinical Pharmacology. XCIX. Angiotensin receptors: interpreters of pathophysiological angiotensinergic stimuli. *Pharmacol Rev*. 2015;67:754-819.
- Panula P, Chazot PL, Cowart M, et al. International Union of Basic and Clinical Pharmacology. XCVIII. Histamine Receptors. *Pharmacol Rev*. 2015;67:601-655.
- Tatulian SA. Structural dynamics of insulin receptor and transmembrane signaling. *Biochemistry*. 2015;54:5523-5532.

# Review Questions

1. Which one of the following statements about G protein signaling is correct?

   A. Activated $G\alpha_s$ typically activates phospholipase C, which converts phosphatidylinositol to cAMP and PIP2.

   B. $G\beta\gamma$-subunits function as GTPase activating proteins (GAPs) that facilitate the intrinsic GTPase activity of heterotrimeric G proteins.

   C. G protein–coupled receptors (GPCRs) function as guanine nucleotide exchange factors (GEFs) to promote the activation of heterotrimeric G proteins.

   D. Small G proteins differ from heterotrimeric G proteins in that their activity is usually not regulated by GAPs.

2. β-Adrenergic receptors resemble which one of the following?

   A. $\alpha_1$-Adrenergic receptors in that they are coupled to $G\alpha_i$

   B. Angiotensin II type 1 receptors in that they are coupled to $G\alpha_q$ or $G\alpha_{11}$

   C. Glucagon receptors in that they are coupled to $G\alpha_s$

   D. Prostanoid EP2 and EP4 receptors in that they are coupled to $G\alpha_i$

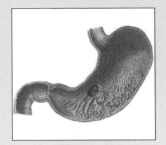

# Chapter 34

# Digestion of Dietary Protein and Net Synthesis of Protein in the Body

## SYNOPSIS

- In the stomach, proteins are denatured at low pH and then degraded into polypeptides. The stomach epithelium protects itself with mucus and bicarbonate secretion against the proteases and acid in the lumen of the stomach. *Helicobacter* bacteria and nonsteroidal inflammatory drugs impair this protection and can lead to ulceration of the mucosa.
- In the intestine, enzymes secreted by the pancreas and enzymes anchored to the surface of epithelial cells of the intestine degrade polypeptides into amino acids and small peptides. These digestive processes are impaired in patients who secrete too little or too much acid in the stomach, and in patients who secrete an insufficient amount of proteases from the pancreas.
- Epithelial cells of the intestine take up tripeptides, dipeptides, and amino acids from the lumen of the intestine. They then hydrolyze the peptides into amino acids. The epithelial cells release amino acids into the bloodstream, and other cells take up amino acids from the blood.
- Amino acids are transported across cell membranes by a large number of different transporters, some of which pump amino acids by using an electrical gradient or a concentration gradient for $Na^+$; others facilitate passive transport or catalyze an exchange of amino acids.
- Patients with cystinuria cannot recover cystine from the glomerular filtrate. As a consequence, they form cystine stones in the kidneys. Patients with Hartnup disease have symptoms of niacin deficiency due to deficient transport of tryptophan.
- The human body can synthesize many amino acids from intermediates of glycolysis or the citric acid cycle, provided that nitrogen can be transferred from another amino acid. However, the essential amino acids (i.e., Arg, His, Ile, Leu, Lys, Met, Phe, Thr, Trp, Val) must be part of the diet.
- Inside cells, protein synthesis occurs mostly after a meal, whereas protein degradation occurs mostly in the fasting state.

## LEARNING OBJECTIVES

*For mastery of this topic, you should be able to do the following:*
- Describe the digestion of protein in the stomach and intestine, including the contribution of the pancreas to this process.
- Explain the mechanism of action of currently used drugs that interfere with acid secretion by the stomach.
- List and explain the major causes of peptic ulcers in the stomach.
- List the major causes of pancreatitis, and explain the role of proteases in the pathogenesis of pancreatitis.
- Explain the pathogenesis of cystinuria and Hartnup disease.
- Explain why some amino acids are essential.

## 1. DIGESTION OF PROTEIN IN THE STOMACH

*In the lumen of the stomach, a low pH denatures proteins, and pepsins digest most proteins into shorter polypeptides.*

*Reduced acid secretion impairs digestion of proteins. If the normal defenses of the mucosa against the acid and pepsins break down locally, the mucosa can form a necrotic hole (i.e., a peptic ulcer). Acid secretion from the stomach can be pharmacologically inhibited with histamine $H_2$ receptor antagonists or with proton pump inhibitors.*

In the stomach, proteins from the diet are denatured and partially hydrolyzed. In the upper portion of the stomach (i.e., the **fundus** and **corpus**; Fig. 34.1) **parietal cells** secrete **hydrochloric acid** (HCl) so that the pH of the stomach contents is about 1 to 2. At this low pH, most proteins denature; that is, they lose their normal three-dimensional structure (see Section 7 in Chapter 9). Also in the upper portion of the stomach, **chief cells** secrete **pepsinogens A** and **C**. At a low pH, pepsinogens A and C become active and cleave themselves to **pepsins A** and **C**. Pepsins cleave denatured proteins more readily than native proteins. Thus, a low pH in the stomach is important for protein digestion in two ways: to denature dietary proteins and to activate the pepsinogens. Parietal cells also secrete intrinsic factor, and they are destroyed in the autoimmune disease **pernicious anemia** (see Section 7.2 in Chapter 36); persons who have pernicious anemia secrete a reduced amount of HCl.

A layer of **mucus** protects the entire stomach epithelium from the low pH and the pepsins of the lumen. The mucosa of the stomach is punctuated by **gastric pits** (see Fig. 34.1) that lead down to the neck region of the mucosa and provide an outlet for the secretions of deeper lying glands. Cells of the glands secrete into canaliculi, which drain into the pits (three to seven canaliculi per pit). The neck region contains stem cells and progenitor cells that renew the tissue bidirectionally; that is, toward the base and toward the lumen of the stomach. A firmly adhering, 0.1- to 0.5-mm-thick layer of mucus covers all epithelial cells. By pumping bicarbonate ($HCO_3^-$) under this layer of mucus, the cells maintain a pH of about 7 at the extracellular face of their plasma membrane. In addition, epithelial cells between the neck region of the mucosa and the lumen (see Fig. 34.1) produce a *loose* layer of mucus that covers the walls of the stomach. Epithelial cells between the neck region of the mucosa and the lumen live for several days before sloughing off, while the cells between the neck region and the base of the gland live for a year or longer.

The lower portion of the stomach (the **antrum**) predominantly secretes hormones that regulate the secretion of HCl and pepsinogens (Figs. 34.1, 34.2, and 34.3). Thus, **G-cells** secrete **gastrin**, which leads to increased secretion of both HCl and pepsinogens. In both the lower and the upper portions of the stomach, as a type of feedback regulation, **D-cells** secrete

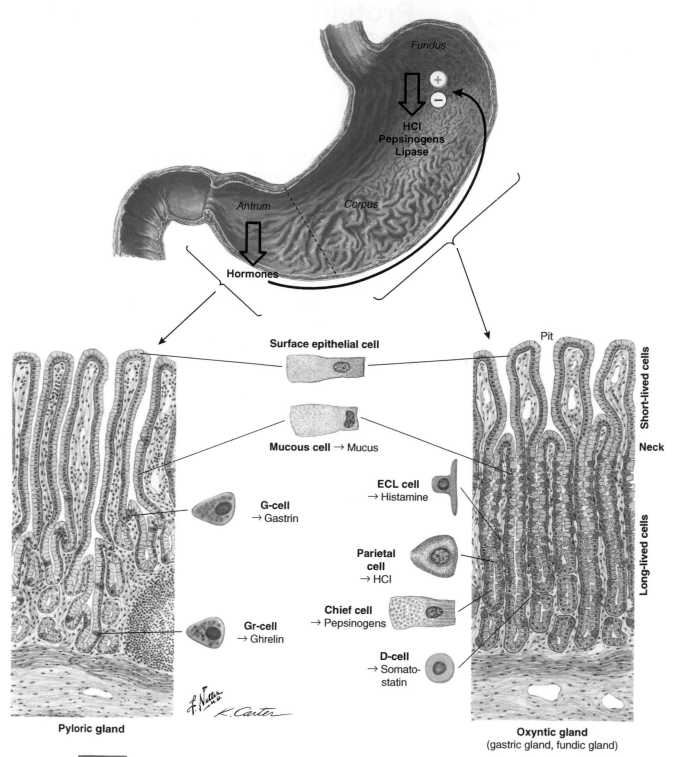

**Fig. 34.1** **Pyloric and oxyntic glands in the stomach.** The fundus and corpus mainly contain oxyntic glands, in which parietal cells secrete HCl and chief cells secrete pepsinogens A and C. The antrum mainly contains pyloric glands that secrete gastrin and somatostatin, which regulate acid secretion from oxyntic glands. ECL, enterochromaffin-like.

**somatostatin** when the pH is especially low; somatostatin then inhibits HCl secretion. Postganglionic neurons that receive input from the **vagus nerve** and secrete acetylcholine stimulate secretion of HCl and pepsinogens.

Adequate digestion of proteins in the stomach is needed to kill **pathogens** and minimize the chance of an **allergic**

**reaction** to proteins in food. The larger a peptide is in the intestine, the more likely it will elicit an allergic reaction.

Patients who have **hypochlorhydria** (deficient secretion of HCl in the stomach, e.g., due to **atrophic gastritis**) or **achlorhydria** (lack of secretion of HCl) are prone to infections of the intestine, as well as "bacterial overgrowth," which is the growth

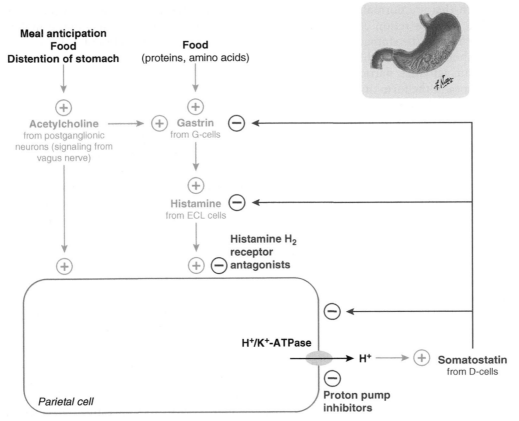

**Fig. 34.2** **Regulation of acid secretion in the stomach.** In the basal state, somatostatin inhibits acid secretion at three levels: $H^+$-secreting parietal cells, gastrin-secreting G-cells, and histamine-secreting enterochromaffin-like (ECL) cells. After a meal, neural signaling via acetylcholine increases gastrin secretion, which stimulates histamine secretion, which in turn stimulates $H^+$ secretion. The mechanisms by which the stomach detects food are poorly understood.

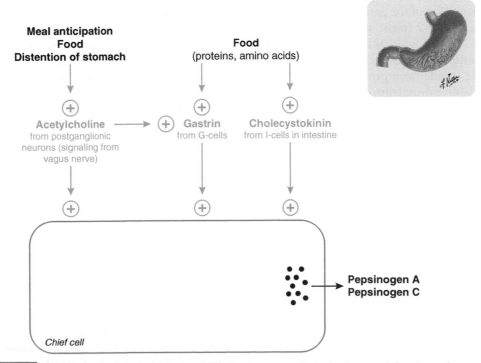

**Fig. 34.3** **Regulation of pepsinogen secretion in the stomach.** In the lumen of the stomach, pepsinogens are cleaved to form enzymatically active pepsins. Secretion of cholecystokinin is described in Section 2.1.

of bacteria in the stomach that are normally present only in the lower small intestine. Acid secretion can be assessed by measuring the pH of the fluid in the stomach.

In patients with an inherent vulnerability of the mucosa, HCl secretion and pepsin activities participate in forming necrotic holes in the mucosa in the form of **ulcers** (Fig. 34.4). The vulnerability commonly arises from infection with *Helicobacter pylori* or from chronic use of nonsteroidal antiinflammatory drugs (NSAIDs; see below). As part of the treatment of these patients, acid secretion can be inhibited with an oral **histamine H₂ receptor antagonist** (e.g., cimetidine), which prevents histamine from stimulating parietal cells, or with a **proton pump inhibitor** (e.g., omeprazole), which irreversibly inhibits the H⁺ pump (H⁺/K⁺-ATPase) in parietal cells. To the extent that these drugs inhibit degradation of proteins from the diet, they lead to an increased concentration of antibodies to common food allergens.

More than half of the world's population is currently infected with the flagellated bacterium **H. pylori**, which moves through the mucus of the stomach, attaches itself to the epithelium, and causes chronic gastritis. The bacterium can also colonize the duodenum. If untreated, the infection can lead to ulcers of the stomach or duodenum (see Fig. 34.4). In patients with ulcers in the duodenum or antrum, the secretion of both acid and pepsinogens is elevated and contributes to ulceration. Conversely, patients with ulcers exclusively in the oxyntic mucosa usually have decreased acid secretion and fewer parietal cells. Gastric ulcer due to infection with *Helicobacter* is associated with an increased risk for **stomach cancer** and gastric mucosa–associated **B-cell lymphoma**. *Helicobacter* can be eradicated with antibiotics.

Chronic use of **NSAIDs** (e.g., aspirin, naproxen, ibuprofen) leads to erosion and ulceration of the gastric mucosa. NSAIDs inhibit cyclooxygenase-1 and -2 (prostaglandin H synthase-1 and -2; see Section 2.1 in Chapter 32), which catalyze the synthesis of **prostaglandin H2** from arachidonic acid (see Fig. 32.2). Prostaglandin E2 (made from prostaglandin H2) plays an important role in adaptive protection of the mucosa, as well as in the healing of damage to the mucosa. As part of this protective effect, prostaglandins stimulate mucus and bicarbonate production and inhibit the secretion of HCl.

## 2. DIGESTION OF PROTEIN IN THE INTESTINE

*In the lumen of the intestine, proteases from the pancreas hydrolyze polypeptides to short peptides. Peptidases on the intestinal epithelial surface hydrolyze the short peptides to tripeptides, dipeptides, and amino acids. Decreased acid denaturation of proteins in the stomach and decreased secretion of proteases from the pancreas each lead to an inadequate digestion of protein in the intestine. When the pancreas is inflamed, proteases in the pancreas become unduly active and destroy cells in the pancreas.*

### 2.1. Normal Protein Digestion in the Intestine

Acidified, partially digested food, called **chyme**, travels from the stomach through the pyloric canal to the duodenum. At the juncture with the common bile duct, **bicarbonate** from the pancreas raises the pH of the luminal contents to about 7. **Bile salts** (see Section 4.1 in Chapter 29) from the gallbladder solubilize and emulsify lipids (see Section 2.2 in Chapter 28), and digestive enzymes from the pancreas hydrolyze starches, lipids, nucleic acids, proteins, and peptides. (Pepsin from the stomach becomes inactive when the pH is near 7.)

The exocrine **pancreas** synthesizes and stores *enzymes* and *enzyme precursors* (zymogens) inside secretory granules (Fig. 34.5). Pancreatic acinar (exocrine) cells secrete the protease precursors **trypsinogen** 1 (cationic trypsinogen), trypsinogen 2 (anionic trypsinogen), trypsinogen 3 (meso-trypsinogen), **chymotrypsinogen, proelastase, procarboxypeptidase** A, and procarboxypeptidase B (Table 34.1). Pancreatic duct cells secrete a fluid that is rich in sodium bicarbonate (NaHCO₃). The **cystic fibrosis transmembrane regulator** (CFTR; the *CFTR* gene is mutated in patients who have cystic fibrosis) is essential for this fluid secretion. The pancreatic fluid flushes the precursor proteases into the intestine.

Upon arrival in the small intestine, the protease zymogens from the pancreas become active proteases (see Table 34.1). Brush border membranes of epithelial cells in the duodenum contain the integral membrane protein **enteropeptidase** (enterokinase). Enteropeptidase becomes active when **bile acids** (secreted from the gallbladder) are present. Active enteropeptidase cleaves trypsinogen to **trypsin**. Trypsin can also cleave trypsinogen to trypsin. Trypsin proteolyzes the other zymogens to produce **chymotrypsin, carboxypeptidases** A and B, and **elastase**.

Trypsin, chymotrypsin, elastase, and the carboxypeptidases differ in their substrate specificity. Together, they degrade most proteins in the diet, although some of these proteins are longer lived than others. A small amount of dietary proteins and peptides normally passes through the gastrointestinal tract without being absorbed.

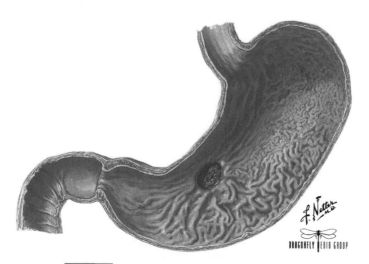

**Fig. 34.4**  **Ulceration of the stomach mucosa.**

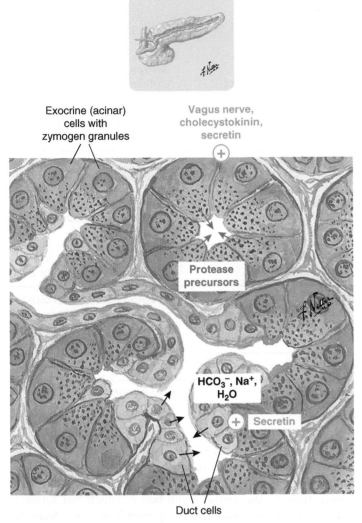

**Fig. 34.5** **Structure of a pancreatic acinus.** The exocrine pancreas consists of numerous acini, which drain into a tree-like system of ducts.

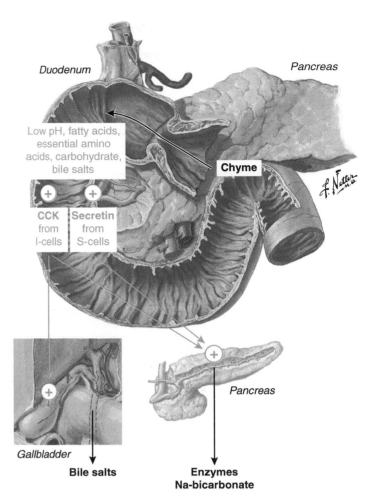

**Fig. 34.6** **Regulation of exocrine secretion from the gallbladder and pancreas.** I-cells and S-cells in the small intestine secrete cholecysto-kinin and secretin, respectively, into the bloodstream. Cholecystokinin (CCK) also affects neurons in the brain and thereby induces satiety.

During an overnight fast, the pancreas continuously secretes enzymes, and after a regular meal, the rate of secretion readily increases to a plateau of about four times this value. This high rate of secretion then lasts until nutrient flow into the duodenum abates. Chronic ingestion of a high-fat diet elicits greater pancreatic enzyme secretion (both after a meal and between meals) than a chronic high-carbohydrate diet. The exact proportion of enzymes that degrade carbohydrates, lipids, and proteins, changes slightly with the composition of a meal and also with dietary habits.

**Secretin** and **cholecystokinin** are the major controllers of enzyme secretion from the pancreas and bile secretion from the gallbladder (Fig. 34.6). Secretin and cholecystokinin are both peptide hormones. **S-cells** in the duodenum and jejunum secrete secretin when they encounter a low pH, carbohydrates, fatty acids, essential amino acids, or bile salts. **I-cells** in the intestine secrete cholecystokinin in response to amino acids, triglycerides, and glucose.

In the clinic, secretin is used in diagnostic tests of the function and shape of the **exocrine pancreas**, and sometimes also

in the diagnosis of gastrin-secreting tumors (gastrinomas, see below).

In the small intestine, proteins are degraded into amino acids, dipeptides, and tripeptides. This protein derives mainly from the diet and, to a lesser extent, from enzymes secreted by the pancreas, and from sloughed-off intestinal epithelial cells. Pancreatic proteases degrade about two-thirds of the polypeptides to two- to six-residue peptides, and about one-third to amino acids. The peptides and amino acids diffuse through the layer of mucus that lines the epithelium to the brush border membrane of epithelial cells. There, membrane-bound **aminopeptidases** cleave single amino acids from the N-termini of these short peptides to produce tripeptides, dipeptides, and amino acids. Two examples of these amino-peptidases are glutamyl aminopeptidase (also called aspartate aminopeptidase or aminopeptidase A) and membrane alanyl aminopeptidase (also called aminopeptidase N or amino-oligopeptidase). As detailed in Section 3, a peptide transporter transports tripeptides and dipeptides into intestinal epithelial cells; similarly, many different amino acid transporters transport amino acids into intestinal epithelial cells.

**Table 34.1**  **Enzymes Secreted by the Pancreas**

| Secreted Protein | Active Enzyme | Mode of Activation | Role in Digestion |
|---|---|---|---|
| Trypsinogen | Trypsin | Proteolysis by enteropeptidase (anchored to brush border membrane of epithelial cells of duodenum; activated by bile salts) | Activates all other protease precursors. Degrades proteins, producing peptides |
| Chymotrypsinogen | Chymotrypsin | Proteolysis by trypsin | Degrades proteins, producing peptides |
| Proelastase | Elastase | Proteolysis by trypsin | Degrades proteins, producing peptides |
| Procarboxypeptidases A and B | Carboxypeptidases A and B | Proteolysis by trypsin | Degrade proteins from C-terminus, producing amino acids |
| Pancreatic lipase | Pancreatic lipase | Colipase | Hydrolyzes triglycerides and diglycerides (see Chapter 28) |
| Prophospholipase $A_2$ | Phospholipase $A_2$ | Proteolysis by trypsin | Degrades glycerophospholipids |
| Amylase | Amylase | None needed | Degrades starches and dietary glycogen (see Chapter 18) |
| Deoxyribonuclease | Deoxyribonuclease | None needed | Degrades DNA |
| Ribonuclease | Ribonuclease | None needed | Degrades RNA |

## 2.2. Diseases Associated With Impaired Digestion of Protein

Malabsorption of protein is called **creatorrhea**, which means flesh (undigested muscle fibers) in the stools. Creatorrhea becomes apparent when protease activity is but a small fraction of the normal. Protease activity may be deficient due to an abnormality of the stomach, small intestine, or pancreas, as outlined below.

**Celiac disease** (**celiac sprue**) is caused by an allergic reaction to certain gliadin proteins in **gluten**, which is found in wheat, barley, and rye. The disorder has a strong genetic component. Individuals who have the *HLA-DQ2* or *HLA-DQ8* alleles of the major histocompatibility complex are especially likely to develop celiac disease, which has a prevalence of ~1 in 200. Persons who have active disease show atrophy of the villi in the small intestine and may have malabsorption, diarrhea, a blistering skin rash, and ataxia. These symptoms can usually be corrected with a lifelong gluten-free diet.

Patients with **achlorhydria** (a lack of gastric HCl secretion, most commonly due to destruction of parietal cells in autoimmune gastritis) lack an adequate nutrient *stimulus* for secretin secretion from S-cells in the intestine; this can be corrected with acidic drinks, such as orange juice. Patients with hypochlorhydria or achlorhydria are at an increased risk of protein and lipid malabsorption, infections of the intestine, and cobalamin deficiency (see Chapter 36).

Patients who have **severe pancreatic insufficiency** due to chronic pancreatitis or pancreatic cancer malabsorb protein and other nutrients; consequently, they have diarrhea. Before creatorrhea sets in, abnormal results are typically found for leaked pancreatic enzymes in serum (amylase, lipase, trypsin, and carboxypeptidase B, which was formerly referred to as pancreas-specific protein), and for fecal fat, cobalamin status, and blood glucose (due to impairment of islet β-cells). In addition, the response to diagnostic stimulation with secretin may be abnormal (due to pancreatic dysfunction).

**Pancreatitis**, an inflammation of the pancreas, is often caused by **alcohol dependence syndrome** (see Section 4.1 in Chapter 30) or blockage of pancreatic secretions by **gallstone disease** (see Section 4.2 in Chapter 29); it is also a consequence of severe **hypertriglyceridemia** (see Section 8.1 in Chapter 28 and Section 4.2 in Chapter 29). Occasionally, pancreatitis is caused by an **invasive procedure** that leads to ischemia of the pancreas or blockage of the common bile duct. Factors that play a role in the diagnosis of pancreatitis are the type of pain, high serum lipase or amylase activity, and imaging studies. Acute pancreatitis is of two types: **interstitial edematous pancreatitis** (Fig. 34.7), which generally resolves within a week, and **necrotizing pancreatitis,** in which necrosis develops over several days. It is currently hypothesized that nonhereditary pancreatitis is triggered by an event that produces more active trypsin inside acinar cells than can be inactivated by trypsin inhibitor. This trypsin then activates other zymogens, and the inappropriately active digestive enzymes destroy pancreatic cells. About 10% of the patients who have pancreatitis die from this disease, often due to a generalized

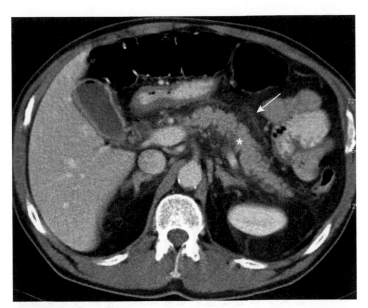

**Fig. 34.7** **Interstitial pancreatitis**. Computed tomographic image of a swollen pancreas (*asterisk*). Fat stranding is seen around the pancreas (*arrow*). (From Bollen TL. Acute pancreatitis: international classification and nomenclature. *Clin Radiol.* 2016;71:121-133.)

inflammatory response and sepsis that lead to multiorgan failure.

Every episode of acute pancreatitis leads to some permanent damage of the pancreas. Recurrent episodes of acute pancreatitis, when combined with persistent inflammation and ongoing fibrosis of the pancreas, often lead to chronic pancreatitis. Chronic pancreatitis in turn can lead to the destruction of the pancreas. Hence, the prevention of episodic pancreatitis is important.

Prematurely active **trypsin** normally **autolyzes** inside pancreatic exocrine cells. Inside cells, the concentration of calcium ($Ca^{2+}$) is generally low, whereas it is high in the lumen of the intestine. A high concentration of calcium in the lumen is needed for trypsin to remain active and activate trypsinogen. Conversely, at the low concentration of calcium inside pancreatic exocrine cells, trypsin destroys itself (autolyzes). Abnormalities in autolysis can give rise to pancreatitis (see below).

**Hereditary causes of pancreatitis** shed light on the pathogenesis of nonhereditary forms of pancreatitis. Patients who are heterozygous or homozygous for a mutant **trypsinogen 1** (encoded by the *PRSS1* gene) that lacks the Arg site for cleavage by another trypsin molecule develop chronic pancreatitis as children. The pathogenic mutant trypsins typically become excessively active inside pancreatic exocrine cells, and their activity is then also abnormally stable. Trypsin inhibitor cannot inhibit all intrapancreatic trypsin because there is normally only about one molecule of trypsin inhibitor per five molecules of trypsin (although this ratio improves during pancreatitis).

Patients who are homozygous (and, in some cases, heterozygous) for an inactivating mutation in **pancreatic secretory trypsin inhibitor** (encoded by the *SPINK1* gene) develop

chronic pancreatitis as young adults. Many of these mutant trypsin inhibitors do not effectively bind to trypsin.

Patients who have **cystic fibrosis** do not express an adequate amount of CFTR. These patients are homozygous or compound heterozygous for a mutation in the *CFTR* gene. Hundreds of mutations are known that cause disease of varying severity. Thus, some patients present with acute pancreatitis in the absence of overt airway disease. CFTR transports chloride ions across the apical plasma membrane of pancreatic duct cells; chloride in turn exchanges for bicarbonate via an additional transporter. CFTR plays additional roles in the regulation of fluid secretion, but the mechanisms have not been well elucidated. Without active CFTR in the luminal membrane, pancreatic duct cells do not secrete an adequate amount of bicarbonate and water to flush digestive enzymes into the intestine (a somewhat similar situation is found in patients who have a temporarily blocked common bile duct). Severe forms of cystic fibrosis are associated with chronic pancreatitis from infancy and loss of pancreatic function before birth as well as within the first few years of life; acinar cells are lost early on, endocrine cells only later. Since the pancreas does not secrete enough bicarbonate, patients with cystic fibrosis also do not effectively neutralize HCl in the intestine. This can be counteracted with antacids and inhibitors of HCl secretion from the stomach.

Patients who have severe pancreatitis are treated in part by withholding all oral food to diminish the stimuli for synthesis of enzymes in the pancreas.

Patients who have **Zollinger-Ellison syndrome**, a rare syndrome caused by a **gastrinoma**, secrete too much acid from the stomach, so that a low pH in the intestinal lumen leads to damage of the intestinal mucosa and inactivity of pancreatic enzymes. These patients typically have gastroesophageal reflux disease, ulcers in the duodenum, and diarrhea (from malabsorption). Most gastrinomas are in the duodenum or pancreas and are malignant. Diagnosis commonly entails demonstration of fasting hypergastrinemia despite a low pH in the stomach (a low pH normally attenuates the secretion of gastrin). If this test is not diagnostic, a secretin test is used. In this test, patients are infused with the hormone secretin. While secretin normally inhibits gastrin secretion, it increases gastrin secretion from gastrinomas.

Zollinger-Ellison syndrome can also be a manifestation of **multiple endocrine neoplasia-1**. If so, patients may not only have a gastrinoma but also a tumor of the pituitary gland or of the parathyroid gland.

## 3. TRANSPORT OF AMINO ACIDS AND SMALL PEPTIDES

*In the intestine, transporters in the epithelial cell membranes move tripeptides, dipeptides, and amino acids into the cytosol. There, peptidases cleave most intracellular tripeptides and dipeptides into amino acids. The epithelial cells of the intestine then release amino acids into the bloodstream. Patients who have cystinuria cannot remove cystine from the tubules of the kidneys and therefore develop kidney stones. Patients who have Hartnup disease are deficient for a transporter of neutral amino acids and, as a result, have a deficit of tryptophan and nicotinamide.*

### 3.1. Normal Transport of Amino Acids in the Intestinal Epithelium and in Other Cells

About 90% of the amino acids of the protein in a mixed diet are absorbed into the epithelial cells of the small intestine. This is the result of efficient proteolysis and uptake of amino acids and short peptides into cells.

Epithelial cells of the small intestine express a **peptide transporter** (**PEPT1**, encoded by the *SLC15A1* gene) that accepts dipeptides and tripeptides of virtually any amino acid sequence. The peptide transporter uses an inwardly directed $H^+$ gradient to drive the uptake of peptides (although the lumen of the intestine is alkaline, the surface of the intestinal brush border membrane has an acid microclimate). Intracellular peptidases cleave dipeptides and tripeptides into amino acids.

PEPT1 also transports drugs such as **aminocephalosporins**, **aminopenicillins**, some **angiotensin-converting enzyme inhibitors** (e.g., captopril, enalapril), and amino acid–conjugated nucleosides that are used as **antiviral agents** (e.g., valacyclovir). Another transporter releases these drugs from the epithelial cells into the bloodstream.

The brush border membrane of the intestinal epithelial cells has several **transporters for amino acids**, most of which transport several different amino acids. Some of these transporters are $Na^+$:amino acid cotransporters that use the inward-directed concentration gradient of $Na^+$ to pump amino acids into the epithelial cells (the same cells also contain a $Na^+$:*glucose* cotransporter; see Section 3.1 in Chapter 18). Other transporters use the membrane potential to pump positively charged amino acids into epithelial cells, and still others exchange intracellularly accumulated amino acids for other amino acids in the lumen of the intestine.

The total **concentration of amino acids in the blood** is ~3 mM. Glutamine and alanine are the largest contributors (Fig. 34.8), amounting to about 35% of the total. With a weight-maintaining, typical Western diet, the total concentration of amino acids in the blood changes by less than ~20%.

### 3.2. Diseases Due to Deficiencies of Amino Acid Transporters

**Cystinuria** is caused by a deficiency of the transport of **cystine** out of the proximal tubules of the kidneys into epithelial cells; this transport deficiency gives rise to **kidney stones** composed primarily of cystine (Fig. 34.9). Cystine forms by the spontaneous oxidation and condensation of two cysteine molecules. Inside cells, an enzyme uses glutathione to reduce virtually all cystine to cysteine (for glutathione, see Chapter 21). However, in blood plasma, the concentration of cystine is about six times higher than that of cysteine. Normal kidneys recover both cysteine and cystine from the glomerular filtrate. Kidneys

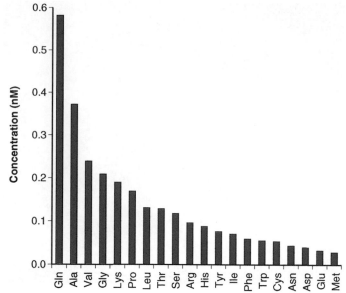

**Fig. 34.8** **Concentration of individual amino acids in human blood plasma.** (Data from Cynober LA. Plasma amino acid levels with a note on membrane transport: characteristics, regulation, and metabolic significance. *Nutrition.* 2002;18:761-766; Nakamura H, Jinzu H, Nagao K, et al. Plasma amino acid profiles are associated with insulin, C-peptide, and adiponectin levels in type 2 diabetic patients. *Nutr Diabetes.* 2014;4:e133; Lewis AM, Waterhouse C, Jacobs LS. Whole-blood and plasma amino acid analysis: gas-liquid and cation-exchange chromatography compared. *Clin Chem.* 1980;26:271-276; and Nasset ES, Heald FP, Calloway DH, Margen S, Schneeman P. Amino acids in human blood plasma after single meals of meat, oil, sucrose, and whiskey. *J Nutr.* 1979;109:621-630.)

of patients with cystinuria fail to recover cystine. Cystine in the renal tubular fluid crystallizes when its concentration exceeds the limit of solubility. The crystals then aggregate into stones.

Almost all patients who have cystinuria carry mutations in the *SLC3A1* or the *SLC7A9* gene, which encode the two subunits of the rBAT/B^0,+AT transporter. This protein complex transports cystine, other dibasic amino acids (i.e., lysine, arginine, and ornithine), and neutral amino acids. The transporter is embedded in the brush border membrane of the epithelia of the kidney tubules. In general, the disease shows an **autosomal recessive** pattern of inheritance.

In England, Spain, and the Eastern Mediterranean region, cystinuria is found in ~1 in 2000 newborns; in other populations, the disorder is somewhat less common. On average, about 10% of all children who present with kidney stones have cystinuria. Most patients develop symptomatic stones by the end of their teen years.

In patients who have cystinuria due to a mutant *SLC3A1* or *SLC7A9* gene, the rBAT/B^0,+AT basic amino acid transporter is also deficient in the brush border membranes of the epithelium of the *small intestine*. However, this is not pathogenic, most likely because essential basic amino acids (i.e., lysine and arginine) enter in sufficient amounts as part of dipeptides and tripeptides (see Section 3.1).

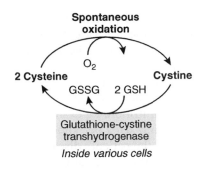

**Spontaneous oxidation**

2 Cysteine $\xrightarrow{O_2}$ Cystine

GSSG    2 GSH

Glutathione-cystine transhydrogenase

*Inside various cells*

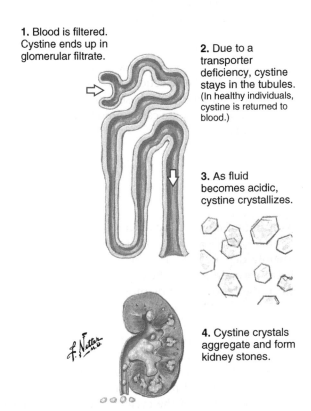

**1.** Blood is filtered. Cystine ends up in glomerular filtrate.

**2.** Due to a transporter deficiency, cystine stays in the tubules. (In healthy individuals, cystine is returned to blood.)

**3.** As fluid becomes acidic, cystine crystallizes.

**4.** Cystine crystals aggregate and form kidney stones.

**Fig. 34.9** **Spontaneous formation of cystine and pathogenesis of cystinuria.** *GSH*, reduced glutathione; *GSSG*, oxidized glutathione (see Chapter 21).

Cystinuria is treated by alkalinizing the urine with oral potassium **citrate** (at a higher pH, cystine is more soluble) and by maintaining a large **flow** of urine (to lower the concentration of cystine). Patients are also advised against consuming a lot of protein or salt; protein contains cysteine, and salt increases the excretion of cystine for unknown reasons. If these measures do not provide satisfactory results, patients can often be given **penicillamine** (a degradation product of penicillin), **meso-2,3-dimercaptosuccinic acid**, or **α-mercaptopropionyl glycine** (also called thiopronin). These drugs contain –SH groups that react with cystine to form mixed drug-cysteine disulfides that are very soluble in urine.

A homozygous or compound heterozygous deficiency in the SLC6A19 (B⁰AT1) transporter, which transports neutral amino acids across the brush border membrane of the intestinal and renal epithelial cells, leads to **Hartnup disorder** and possibly **Hartnup disease**. (Hartnup is the name of the family, members of which had a severe form of this disease and were first described in a scientific publication in 1956.) Patients with Hartnup *disorder* have documented neutral amino-aciduria but no symptoms. The disorder occurs in ~1 in 30,000 persons. About 10% of these patients show symptoms and therefore have Hartnup *disease* (its incidence is thus ~1 in 300,000 persons). The symptoms arise from a deficiency of **tryptophan**, and some of the symptoms resemble those of pellagra (a deficiency of nicotinic acid; see Fig. 19.5 in Chapter 19). Tryptophan is an essential amino acid that is required for the synthesis of nicotinic acid (see Section 1 in Chapter 19) and the neurotransmitter serotonin (see section 4.2 in Chapter 35). Affected patients are susceptible to photodamage starting in early childhood. Later, they may have intermittent cerebellar ataxia (lasting a few days), emotional lability, and psychosis. Episodes are often triggered by poor nutrition, diarrhea, fever, or sun exposure. Symptomatic patients are treated with nicotinamide. Those patients who have a low concentration of amino acids in the blood should also consume a high-protein diet. The reasons that a deficiency of the SLC6A19 (B⁰AT1) transporter does not have more serious pathologic effects are that a fraction of amino acids reach the epithelial cells of the intestine as dipeptides and tripeptides via the peptide transporter, and that there are other transporters for neutral amino acids.

## 4. SYNTHESIS OF BODY PROTEIN

*Of the 21 amino acids needed for translation, humans can synthesize about half; they must consume the remainder with the diet. Net synthesis of body protein occurs in the postprandial state.*

### 4.1. Daily Turnover of Body Protein

In a healthy adult, daily protein synthesis and degradation amount to about 400 g, or 3% of the total protein content of the body (Fig. 34.10). Humans must consume a minimum of about 50 g of protein per day because an equivalent amount of amino acids is oxidized or used for the synthesis of nonprotein compounds. The term nitrogen balance is a measure of the difference between protein intake and nitrogen loss (see Section 5 in Chapter 35). Synthesis and degradation of body protein affect the nitrogen balance.

### 4.2. Essential and Nonessential Amino Acids

Humans cannot synthesize His, Ile, Leu, Lys, Met, Phe, Thr, Trp, or Val; therefore, these amino acids are called **essential** (or **indispensable**) **amino acids**. For growing children, this list has to be expanded; they must consume Arg because they commonly do not produce enough of it in the urea cycle (see Section 2.5 in Chapter 35) and Cys because they do not make enough of it from methionine (see Sections 4.1 and 9 in Chapter 36). Gln, Tyr, Gly, Pro, and ornithine are

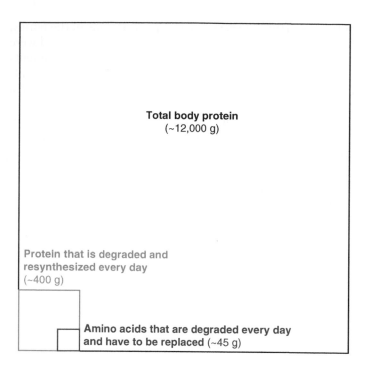

Total body protein
(~12,000 g)

Protein that is degraded and
resynthesized every day
(~400 g)

Amino acids that are degraded every day
and have to be replaced (~45 g)

☐ Amino acids that are used daily for synthesis of
creatine, nucleotides, heme, etc. (~5 g)

▫ Amino acids that are circulating in the blood (~1 g)

**Fig. 34.10** **Protein and amino acid content and turnover in a healthy adult.**

conditionally essential amino acids; that is, they are essential in certain disease conditions.

In protein synthesis, the translation of mRNA stops if an amino acid is not available (see Chapter 7). Hence, a deficiency in a *single* amino acid leads to deficient synthesis of proteins.

Sources of dietary protein can be rated for their **quality**, or how well they match the needs of the human body. For instance, gelatin (as contained in Jell-O) is a very low-quality protein because it consists mostly of collagen, which contains mostly glycine, proline (some of it as hydroxyproline), and alanine (see Chapter 12). In contrast, human breast milk is a source of very high-quality protein for infants because the amino acid composition of milk proteins closely matches the requirements. Since the body can synthesize *nonessential* amino acids, the protein quality of a meal depends largely on its content of *essential* amino acids. For people who eat mostly a vegan diet, methionine is usually the limiting essential amino acid.

Adults should consume a minimum of about 50 g of protein per day. For adults, the World Health Organization (WHO) recommends a minimum intake of 0.75 g of protein per kilogram of body weight per day; this protein should have a good balance of amino acids. Individuals who eat a high-protein diet consume as much as 3 g of protein per kilogram of body weight per day (i.e., ~200 g of protein per day). In North and South America, as well as in Australia, **meat** usually contrib-

utes 30% to 40% of all protein in the diet. In Europe, this fraction is 20% to 30%; in Africa, it is 0% to 30%; and in Asia, it is generally 10% to 20%. Children, pregnant women, and patients who are recovering from surgery or trauma need more protein in the diet than the World Health Organization recommends for healthy people. Hospitalized patients who receive parenteral nutrition, for example, are commonly given 0.8 to 2.0 g of amino acids per kilogram of body weight per day, depending on the patient's disease.

Humans can synthesize about half of all amino acids. For this, they need nitrogen from other amino acids. Humans can synthesize Ala, Asp, Asn, Gln, Glu, Pro, and Ser starting with intermediates of glycolysis and the citric acid cycle (Fig. 34.11), and they can obtain Tyr from Phe (see Section 4.2 in Chapter 35), Arg via the urea cycle (see Section 2.5 in Chapter 35), and Cys from Met (see Sections 4.1 and 9 in Chapter 36). Because humans can synthesize these amino acids and do not need them in the diet, they are called **nonessential** or **dispensable amino acids**.

## 4.3. Regulation of the Concentration of Amino Acids in Blood and of Protein Synthesis

The concentration of amino acids in the blood is the result of flux of amino acids *into* and *out of* the blood. Flux *into* the blood mainly depends on intestinal uptake of amino acids from dietary protein and on the degradation of body protein. Flux *out of* the blood depends mostly on protein synthesis, gluconeogenesis, and oxidation of amino acids for production of energy in the form of ATP. After a meal, the major users of amino acids are the intestine, liver, and muscle (Fig. 34.12). In the fasting state, muscle is the major producer of amino acids, and the liver is the major user. It is not clear which proteins participate in this cycle of protein synthesis and protein degradation; the regulation of the cycle is likewise incompletely understood. Known major regulators of amino acid flux are the concentrations of leucine, insulin, glucagon, and cortisol in the blood, as well as the activity of the protein complex mTORC1 inside cells.

Activated **mTORC1** stimulates protein synthesis (Fig. 34.13). The complex is activated by growth factors and amino acids, especially leucine. The complex is inhibited when a cell is hypoxic or has impaired production of adenosine triphosphate, as sensed by adenosine monophosphate–dependent protein kinase (AMPK). Metformin, a drug used to inhibit gluconeogenesis as part of the treatment of type 2 diabetes, leads to the activation of AMPK. The mTORC1 inhibitor **rapamycin** (also called **sirolimus**) is an immunosuppressant that is used after organ transplantation.

**Leucine** appears to serve as a signal of the influx of dietary protein. Accordingly, leucine stimulates protein synthesis and inhibits protein degradation postprandially. In the fasting state, when muscle protein is degraded, leucine is transaminated within muscles and only the resulting keto acid is released into the blood (the same is true of the other branched-chain amino acids, isoleucine and valine).

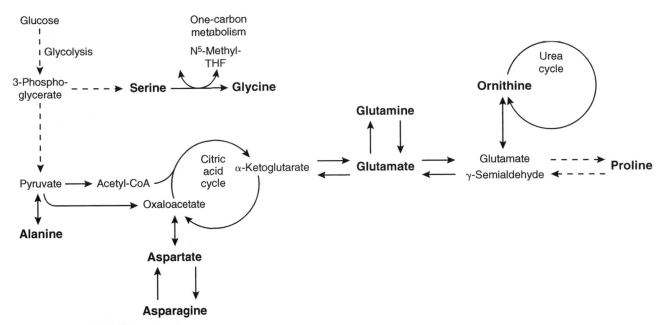

**Fig. 34.11** **Biosynthesis of serine, glycine, alanine, aspartate, asparagine, glutamate, glutamine, ornithine, and proline from intermediates of glycolysis and the citric acid cycle.** The pathway for glycolysis is shown in Fig. 19.2, that of the citric acid cycle in Fig. 22.6, and that of the urea cycle in Fig. 35.7.

**A.** After a meal: net protein synthesis

**Food**

↓

**Intestine:**
uses Gln, Glu, Asp; releases remaining amino acids

↓

**Liver:**
uses ~75% of most amino acids but very little Ile, Leu, Val

↓

**Muscle:**
uses most remaining amino acids

**B.** During fasting: net protein degradation

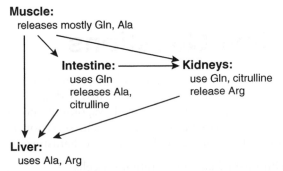

**Muscle:**
releases mostly Gln, Ala

**Intestine:** → **Kidneys:**
uses Gln         use Gln, citrulline
releases Ala,    release Arg
citrulline

**Liver:**
uses Ala, Arg

**Fig. 34.12** **Major flux of amino acids in the fed and fasting state.** Flux of amino acids is controlled by insulin, glucagon, cortisol, and leucine. Protein degradation is detailed in Chapter 35.

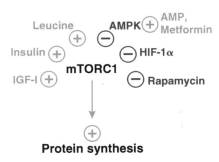

**Fig. 34.13** **Role of mTORC1 in the regulation of protein synthesis.** *AMPK,* adenosine monophosphate–activated protein kinase.

**Insulin** stimulates *transcription* via the mitogen-activated protein kinase pathway and *translation* via mTORC1 and eukaryotic initiation factor 2 phosphorylation, pathways that are present in virtually every cell (see Fig. 33.3 and Section 3 in Chapter 7). After a meal, the pancreatic islets secrete insulin in response to glucose and presumably an increase in the concentrations of leucine, glutamine, and arginine (details are not certain; see Section 3.3.2 in Chapter 26). Protein synthesis lowers the concentrations of branched-chain and other essential amino acids in blood plasma.

**Insulin-like growth factor-I (IGF-I)** stimulates muscle protein synthesis. IGF-I occupation of receptors for IGF-I leads to activation of protein kinase B and mTORC1, which in turn stimulate the translation of mRNA into protein.

**Glucagon** stimulates gluconeogenesis in the liver and in the kidneys (see Section 3 in Chapter 25), which lowers the concentration of amino acids in the blood. In the fasting state, the pancreas secretes glucagon in response to epinephrine and a lower concentration of glucose. Note that muscle does not have appreciable numbers of glucagon receptors and hence does not respond to glucagon.

**Cortisol** stimulates degradation of muscle protein, oxidation of branched-chain amino acids in muscle, and use of the released amino acids in gluconeogenesis by the liver and the kidneys. The adrenal medulla secretes cortisol in a diurnal fashion so that the concentration of cortisol in the blood is highest in the early morning and lowest in the early evening (see Fig. 31.13). Fasting and intense exercise both increase cortisol secretion. Patients who are treated with high doses of glucocorticoids and patients who have a high concentration of circulating cortisol due to Cushing syndrome both show muscle wasting (see Section 4.2.3 in Chapter 25 and Section 3 in Chapter 31).

## SUMMARY

- In the fundus and corpus of the stomach, parietal cells secrete HCl and chief cells secrete pepsinogens. In the acidic lumen of the stomach, pepsinogens autocatalytically activate to become active pepsins, which cleave dietary proteins.
- The vagus nerve works via acetylcholine, gastrin, and histamine to *stimulate* HCl secretion from parietal cells. Physiologically, pH-sensing D-cells throughout the stomach *inhibit* HCl secretion. Pharmacologically, HCl secretion can be inhibited with histamine $H_2$ receptor antagonists or with proton pump inhibitors.
- The pancreas secretes bicarbonate, which raises the pH of chyme in the duodenum to a value greater than 7. The pancreas also secretes digestive enzymes into the small intestine. Among these is trypsinogen. Enterokinase on the surface of the intestinal brush border membranes, when activated by bile salts, cleaves trypsinogen to produce trypsin. Trypsin in turn cleaves other pancreas-derived zymogens to active chymotrypsin, elastase, and carboxypeptidases A and B.
- Pancreatitis is associated with activation of trypsin and other digestive enzymes inside the pancreas. In most cases, pancreatitis is due to blockage of the common bile duct or due to the alcohol dependence syndrome. In patients with cystic fibrosis, inadequate flushing of zymogens out of the pancreas into the intestine causes pancreatitis and loss of pancreatic function. Patients who express mutant trypsinogen or mutant pancreatic trypsin inhibitor develop pancreatitis at a young age.
- The brush border membrane of the epithelium of the small intestine contains aminopeptidases that hydrolyze single amino acids from the N-terminus of oligopeptides. The brush border membrane also contains a peptide transporter (PEPT1) that facilitates uptake of dipeptides and tripeptides into intestinal epithelial cells; in addition, the membrane contains a variety of transporters for amino acids.

- A large number of different transporters facilitate amino acid transport from the intestinal epithelium into the blood, from the blood into peripheral cells, and from the renal glomerular filtrate into tubular cells and from there to the blood. Patients who have cystinuria cannot efficiently remove cystine from the glomerular filtrate and form cystine stones in the kidneys. Patients with Hartnup disease show symptoms of tryptophan deficiency that is caused by deficient transport of neutral amino acids into the intestinal and renal epithelial cells.
- Humans must consume certain amino acids in their diet because they cannot synthesize them. These amino acids are called essential amino acids and comprise Arg, His, Ile, Leu, Lys, Met, Phe, Thr, Trp, and Val. Humans can synthesize nonessential amino acids from intermediates of glycolysis or the citric acid cycle, and from the nitrogen of other amino acids.
- Net protein synthesis occurs after consuming a protein-containing meal. Insulin and leucine, working through mTORC1 and an initiation factor for translation, are the principal stimuli of this protein biosynthesis.

## FURTHER READING

- For approximately yearly brief updates on the state of knowledge of gastrointestinal function and related diseases, see the journal *Current Opinions in Gastroenterology*.
- Brandsch M. Drug transport via the intestinal peptide transporter PepT1. *Curr Opin Pharmacol*. 2013;13: 881-887.
- Hunt RH, Camilleri M, Crowe SE, et al. The stomach in health and disease. *Gut*. 2015;64:1650-1668.
- Saravakos P, Kokkinou V, Giannatos E. Cystinuria: current diagnosis and management. *Urology*. 2014;83:693-699.
- Yandrapu H, Sarosiek J. Protective factors of the gastric and duodenal mucosa: an overview. *Curr Gastroenterol Rep*. 2015;17:24.

# Review Questions

1. Before histamine $H_2$-antagonists (and proton pump inhibitors) were available, patients who had a duodenal ulcer were often treated surgically with vagotomy and antrectomy. These procedures decreased acid secretion in part through which one of the following mechanisms?

   A. Diminished gastrin secretion (G-cells)
   B. Increased histamine secretion
   C. Reduced somatostatin secretion
   D. Removal of parietal cells
   E. Removal of chief cells

2. After an overnight fast, an adult patient with atrophic gastritis was prepared for continuous aspiration of stomach fluids via a nasogastric tube. At 15-minute intervals, fluid volume and acid content were determined. Samples were taken before and after parenteral administration of pentagastrin, an analog of gastrin. This test is a measure of which of the following?

   **A.** Acetylcholine stimulation of acid output
   **B.** Function of parietal cells
   **C.** Histamine stimulation of somatostatin secretion
   **D.** Infection with *Helicobacter pylori*
   **E.** Mass of mucus-producing cells

3. Apart from a gastrinoma, which of the following can be expected to increase the concentration of gastrin in the blood?

   **A.** Abnormally high concentration of somatostatin
   **B.** Abnormally high concentration of histamine
   **C.** Abnormally low pH in the lumen of the stomach
   **D.** Treatment with a proton pump inhibitor

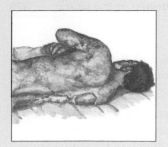

## Chapter 35

# Protein Degradation, Amino Acid Metabolism, and Nitrogen Balance

## SYNOPSIS

- Degradation of proteins is an important part of maintaining a set of normal proteins, providing amino acids for synthesis of new proteins during illness or injury, and synthesizing glucose via gluconeogenesis (see Chapter 25).
- The cytosol and the nucleus contain proteasomes, which are large protein complexes that degrade proteins into short peptides and amino acids. Hundreds of different enzymes conjugate proteins with ubiquitin (a small, conserved polypeptide) to mark them for degradation by proteasomes. The cytosol also contains lysosomes; these organelles provide an acidic milieu for the degradation of a variety of compounds (including proteins). Lysosomes acquire proteins both from the extracellular space and from within the cell.
- Amino acids are mostly used for protein synthesis. The degradation of amino acids yields nitrogen and carbon compounds. Nitrogen in these compounds is eliminated largely as urea or ammonium ions; the carbon compounds are used for the production of energy.
- The kidneys can excrete ammonium ions ($NH_4^+$) into the urine and simultaneously release bicarbonate into the blood. This process plays an important role in bicarbonate homeostasis of the blood.
- Patients who have severe liver disease can develop hepatic encephalopathy, which is often accompanied by hyperammonemia (a high concentration of $NH_4^+$ in the blood). Hyperammonemia impairs the function of the central nervous system.
- Deficient conversion of phenylalanine to tyrosine causes phenylketonuria. Lifelong treatment with a low-phenylalanine diet prevents intellectual disability.
- Tyrosine gives rise to dopamine, norepinephrine, and epinephrine, which act as neurotransmitters and hormones (see Chapters 26 and 33). Tyrosine also gives rise to melanin, which is responsible for the pigmentation of skin and hair.
- Tryptophan gives rise to serotonin (a transmitter in the central and enteric nervous system), melatonin (a hormone that plays a role in the sleep/wake cycle), and $NAD^+$ and its relatives (see Chapters 19 and 22).
- The term "nitrogen balance" refers to the amount of nitrogen gained with food intake (mostly as protein) versus the amount lost (mostly as urea and $NH_4^+$ in urine).

## LEARNING OBJECTIVES

*For mastery of this topic, you should be able to do the following:*
- Explain how intracellular proteins are degraded to peptides and amino acids and how this process is regulated.
- Explain how tissues produce ammonia, how the liver removes ammonia from the blood, and how the kidneys excrete ammonia.
- Explain how a deficiency of any one of the components of the urea cycle causes hyperammonemia.
- Describe the symptoms and treatment of hyperammonemia.
- Describe the newborn screening, pathogenesis, and treatment of phenylketonuria.
- Describe the factors that influence the pigmentation of the skin, hair, eyes, and parts of the brain and describe the bases of the common pigmentation disorders.
- Devise a plan to estimate the nitrogen balance of a patient who has extensive burns and receives parenteral nutrition.

## 1. DEGRADATION OF BODY PROTEIN

*For the most part, damaged proteins are not repaired; rather, proteins in the body undergo ongoing degradation and de novo synthesis. During fasting, protein degradation increases and amino acids are used for gluconeogenesis. Protein degradation increases to a much greater degree during illness, trauma, or burns. Inside cells, proteins are degraded in proteasomes or lysosomes.*

### 1.1. General Comments

There is ongoing degradation of proteins in the body. Protein degradation provides a cell with a means of adjusting its set of proteins to its needs. Some proteins are degraded as part of the regulation of the cell cycle and metabolic pathways, while others are normally produced in excess and then degraded to match true needs (e.g., globins for hemoglobin, apoproteins for lipoprotein particles); others are detected, marked, and degraded when they are misfolded, modified, or damaged; and still others are degraded as part of a general increase in protein degradation during fasting or illness.

As explained below, proteins are degraded largely by *proteasomes* in the cytosol and nucleus and by proteases in *lysosomes*. Certain amino acid sequences determine the lifetime of proteins. In addition, hormones regulate protein degradation. Section 4 in Chapter 34 provides a brief overview of whole-body protein synthesis and degradation.

Amino acids derived from the degradation of proteins (whether by proteasomes or lysosomes) are reused for the synthesis of proteins (see Section 4.1 in Chapter 34), released into the bloodstream, used for the synthesis of other molecules, or degraded. Overall, most amino acids are used for resynthesis of proteins, and only a small portion is degraded (see Fig. 34.10).

### 1.2. Degradation of Proteins by Proteasomes

Proteasomes play a role in the degradation of proteins as part of the following: the feeding/fasting cycle, regulation of metabolism and the cell cycle (see also Chapter 8), presentation of short peptides on major histocompatibility complex (MHC) class 1 proteins to passing cytotoxic T-cells, and degradation of misfolded or damaged proteins (see also Chapter 7).

Most protein degradation in cells proceeds via the proteasome pathway. A lesser amount of protein is degraded in lysosomes and a still smaller amount in the cytosol by calcium-activated calpains and caspases, which play roles mostly in regulation.

Proteasomes are in the cytosol and nucleus of all types of cells. Enzymes in these compartments mark certain proteins for degradation by conjugating them with ubiquitin (see below). Proteasomes recognize these proteins and hydrolyze them into peptides of six to nine amino acids. Cellular peptidases then degrade these peptides into individual amino acids. Ubiquitin from the polyubiquitin tail is *reused* to mark other proteins for degradation.

Four types of enzymes, E1 through E4, are used to mark proteins with **ubiquitin** to target them for hydrolysis by proteasomes (Fig. 35.1). Ubiquitin is a 76-residue protein. The C-terminal glycine of ubiquitin is linked to a lysine residue of the target protein. Further ubiquitin residues are then added to Lys-48 of the preceding molecule of ubiquitin to yield a polyubiquitinated protein. Conjugation with four or more Lys-48–linked ubiquitins is equivalent to a kiss of death because such conjugated proteins are degraded inside proteasomes. (In contrast, monoubiquitination, conjugation with multiple single ubiquitins to multiple amino acids in a protein, and polyubiquitination via linkages other than Lys-48 serve other purposes inside cells.)

Note that the E3 component of the ubiquitin conjugating system is an entirely different protein from the E3 component of dehydrogenases, such as pyruvate dehydrogenase and α-ketoglutarate dehydrogenase (Chapter 22).

Several of the E3 ubiquitin protein ligases are associated with disease.

The **papilloma virus** (the cause of **warts** and **cervical cancer**) encodes the protein E6, which activates the E3 ligase **E6AP** that ubiquitinates the tumor suppressor p53; inappropriate destruction of p53 paves the way to tumorigenesis (see Chapter 8).

Lack of a functional, maternally inherited **E6AP ubiquitin-protein ligase** causes **Angelman syndrome**, which is associated with severe motor dysfunction and intellectual disability.

Patients who are homozygous or compound heterozygous for mutations that inactivate the E3 ligase **Nedd4** have impaired Na$^+$ transport in the kidneys; this leads to a form of **hereditary, salt-sensitive hypertension**.

**VHL-factor (von Hippel–Lindau factor)** is an E3 ligase that regulates the ubiquitination of HIFα and hence the production of erythropoietin (see Section 1.4 in Chapter 16). Mutations in the *VHL* gene give rise to **von Hippel-Lindau disease**, and affected persons have an unusually high tendency to develop neoplasms. VHL factor is frequently mutated in clear-cell renal cell carcinomas.

Among patients with **hereditary Parkinson disease**, the disease is most commonly due to a mutation in **parkin**. Parkin

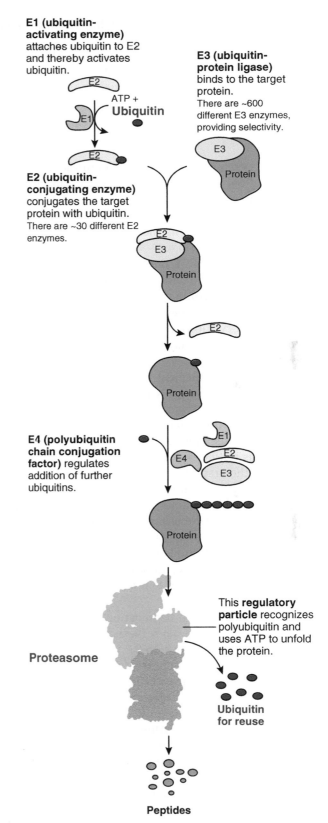

**E1 (ubiquitin-activating enzyme)** attaches ubiquitin to E2 and thereby activates ubiquitin.

ATP + **Ubiquitin**

**E3 (ubiquitin-protein ligase)** binds to the target protein. There are ~600 different E3 enzymes, providing selectivity.

**E2 (ubiquitin-conjugating enzyme)** conjugates the target protein with ubiquitin. There are ~30 different E2 enzymes.

**E4 (polyubiquitin chain conjugation factor)** regulates addition of further ubiquitins.

**Proteasome**

This **regulatory particle** recognizes polyubiquitin and uses ATP to unfold the protein.

**Ubiquitin for reuse**

**Peptides**

**Fig. 35.1** **The proteasome pathway of protein degradation.**

is a ubiquitin E3 ligase that seems to be important for long-term survival of dopamine neurons.

Some proteins are degraded by the catalytic portion of proteasomes without a need for ubiquitination. These proteins often have an inherently disordered structure.

## 1.3. Regulation of Protein Degradation via Proteasomes

The lifetime of proteins depends on their amino acid sequence, their conformation, covalent modifications of amino acids, and the concentrations of both hormones and free amino acids (see Section 4.3 in Chapter 34). The **E3 ubiquitin protein ligases** play a crucial role in the selection of proteins for degradation.

Proteins containing **PEST motifs**, that is, regions rich in proline (single amino acid code P; see Chapter 9), glutamate (E), serine (S), and threonine (T), are degraded particularly rapidly, often by proteasomes. **Posttranslational modification** (e.g., phosphorylation), binding of ions (e.g., $Ca^{2+}$), and binding of other proteins may affect the recognition of PEST motifs for protein degradation.

The **N-terminal amino acid** influences the lifetime of a protein; this is reflected in the **N-end rule**. The E3 ubiquitin-protein ligases bind to an N-terminal amino acid and an internal lysine residue. If the N-terminal amino acid side chain is either positively charged (as in Arg, Lys, or His) or hydrophobic and bulky (as in Phe, Tyr, Trp, Ile, or Leu), the protein is ubiquitinated rather rapidly. By contrast, the E3 ubiquitin-protein ligases usually do not accept proteins with Ser, Gly, Val, or Met at their N-terminus, resulting in slow turnover of such proteins. The N-terminal amino acid of a protein may be altered after translation; this may modify the lifetime of the protein. For instance, deamidation of Asn to Asp or Gln to Glu (by N-terminal amidohydrolases), or arginylation of Asp, Glu, or Cys (by Arg-tRNA-protein transferase) shortens the lifetime of a protein.

**Fasting** enhances protein degradation. Most amino acids are glucogenic; that is, they can serve as substrates for gluconeogenesis (for details, see Section 2.2 in Chapter 25 and Fig. 25.5). Gluconeogenesis is important for the provision of glucose to the brain, red blood cells, and other cells during an extended fast. Protein degradation is maximal after a brief fast. Then, as tissues use more fatty acids and ketone bodies, protein degradation declines. After about 1 week of fasting, protein degradation amounts to less than protein degradation in the course of a day with adequate consumption of protein and calories. In the fasting state, a relatively low concentration of **insulin** and **leucine** permits degradation of protein, a rising concentration of **cortisol** stimulates protein degradation in muscle, and an elevated concentration of **glucagon** enhances the use of amino acids in the liver for gluconeogenesis.

**Infection**, **postpartum recovery**, major **trauma**, and **burn injury** stimulate whole-body protein degradation more than starvation does. These conditions are associated with a large increase in the concentration of **cytokines**, such as **tumor** necrosis factor-α (TNF-α) and **interleukins** (IL) **1**, **2**, **6**, and **8**. The cytokines are released by endothelial cells and white blood cells, such as neutrophils, lymphocytes, macrophages, and monocytes. Particularly high concentrations of cytokines in the blood are seen in patients who have sepsis, pancreatitis, graft versus host disease (most commonly seen in response to transplanted cells from bone marrow), or burn injuries.

**Proteasome inhibitors** are used in the treatment of **multiple myeloma**, a malignancy of antibody-producing cells in the bone marrow. **Bortezomib** is an analog of a dipeptide, and **carfilzomib** is an analog of a tetrapeptide; both drugs have to be injected.

The balance of protein synthesis and degradation is discussed in Section 5 below.

## 1.4. Degradation of Proteins by Lysosomes

Lysosomes are intracellular organelles, which contain many different hydrolases that degrade proteins, lipids, carbohydrates, or nucleic acids. The hydrolases are synthesized in the endoplasmic reticulum, move through the Golgi complex, leave the *trans* face of the Golgi complex inside vesicles, and then reach the lysosomes.

Lysosomes acquire material to be digested both from extra- and intracellular sources. Extracellular and plasma membrane-bound proteins enter lysosomes via **endocytosis**, **pinocytosis**, or **phagocytosis**. Intracellular organelles and cytosol enter lysosomes via autophagosomes. **Autophagy** (the cell's "eating" of some of its components) represents a means of producing amino acids from cellular proteins when these amino acids are not available from the bloodstream. Autophagy also plays an important role in removing misfolded proteins, aggregated proteins, and pathogens from the cytosol. Importantly, autophagy generally has tumor suppressor activity, whereas *inhibition* of autophagy usually promotes tumorigenesis. In antigen-presenting cells, some of the peptides produced by phagolysosomes are loaded onto MHC class II proteins for display on the cell surface to passing helper T-cells.

Lysosomes acidify and hydrolyze acquired compounds, and they release products through transporters into the cytosol. The lumen of lysosomes is acidic (pH ~5). Lysosomes contain several different **cathepsins**, which are acid-activated proteases. Amino acids, monosaccharides, oligosaccharides, and nucleotides are transported across the membranes of lysosomes and released into the cytosol.

Deficiencies of enzymes in lysosomes that degrade components of the extracellular matrix are described in Chapter 13.

## 2. ELIMINATION OF AMINO ACID NITROGEN

*When amino acids are degraded, their nitrogen can be released into the blood as part of ammonium ions, glutamine, or alanine. Nitrogen from these compounds can then enter the urea cycle and become part of urea, which is excreted in the urine. Ammonium ions are also excreted directly into the urine, especially during acidosis.*

## 2.1. Production of Ammonium Ions From Amino Acids

The nitrogen of some amino acids can be released as an ammonium ion ($NH_4^+$; Fig. 35.2). Ammonium ions are in chemical equilibrium with ammonia ($NH_3$; equation: $NH_4^+ \leftrightarrow NH_3 + H^+$). Ammonia diffuses across plasma membranes; in the kidneys, a transporter may enhance transport. Ammonium ions can move through various channels, including many potassium channels.

The kidneys can excrete ammonium ions into the urine (see Section 2.2). Many cell types can incorporate nitrogen into biological molecules by reacting ammonium ions with α-ketoglutarate to produce glutamate and then with glutamate to form glutamine, which is nontoxic and can be transported between organs (see Section 2.3). The liver and the intestine can convert ammonium ions to carbamoylphosphate for the eventual elimination as urea (see Section 2.5).

## 2.2. Excretion of Ammonium Ions Into the Urine

A small portion of excess nitrogen is excreted into the urine as ammonium ions (see Fig. 35.11). In a healthy person who consumes protein, the daily rate of ammonium ion production stays fairly constant (meanwhile, the rate of *urea* production fluctuates and adjusts to the rate of degradation of amino acids, see Section 2.5).

Exhalation of $CO_2$ via the lungs is the body's *prime* defense against acidosis, and production of ammonium ions and bicarbonate from glutamine by the kidneys is a lower-capacity, *secondary* defense as well as a means of supplying the blood with bicarbonate (Fig. 35.3). Bicarbonate in the blood is the primary buffer for $H^+$, and it gets depleted when there is a greater influx of acid into the blood than efflux from the blood. The acid is typically lactic acid or the ketone bodies acetoacetic acid and β-hydroxybutyric acid but can also be formic acid.

To produce bicarbonate and ammonium ions, the kidneys convert glutamine to phosphoenolpyruvate (see Fig. 35.3). $NH_3$ can diffuse into the tubule, perhaps via both passive and facilitated diffusion. The Na:$H^+$ antiport pumps $H^+$ from $H_2CO_3$ (carbonic acid) into the tubules to generate $NH_4^+$. $HCO_3^-$ is then exported into the blood.

During **acidosis**, the kidneys increase the rate of ammonium ion excretion into the urine, and muscle increases glutamine output (see Fig. 35.3). In patients who have metabolic acidosis due to **chronic kidney disease**, sufficient muscle protein is degraded to lead to muscle weakness.

The maximal rate of bicarbonate production by the kidneys is much lower than the maximal rate of $CO_2$ loss via the lungs. Hence, patients who have an inordinately high rate of acid release into the blood (because of hypoxia or a deficiency in

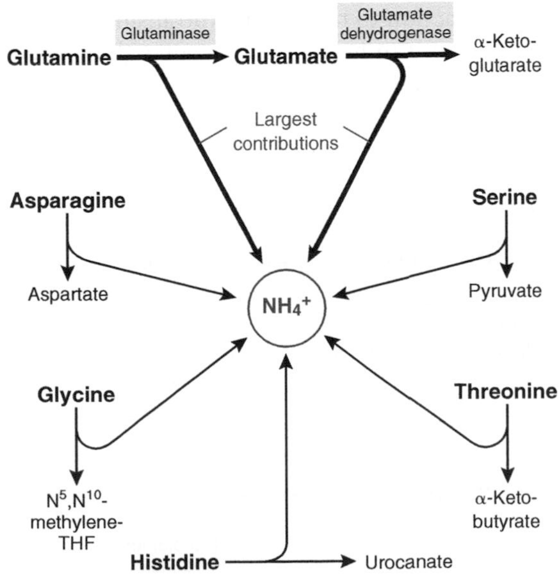

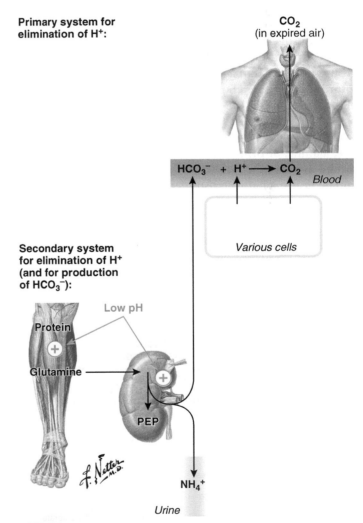

**Fig. 35.3 Role of ammonium excretion in the defense against acidosis.** As the kidneys take up glutamine from the blood, excrete $NH_4^+$ into the urine, and release $HCO_3^-$ into the blood, they remove $H^+$ from the blood and supply $HCO_3^-$ to the blood. PEP, phosphoenolpyruvate.

**Fig. 35.2 Deamination of some amino acids yields ammonium ions.** The deamination of glycine is also described in Section 2.1 in Chapter 36.

metabolism) usually also have an abnormally low concentration of bicarbonate in the blood.

## 2.3. Transamination

The amino group of many amino acids can be transferred to an α-keto acid, thereby forming a different amino acid. This is a way to conserve nitrogen for the biosynthesis of nonessential amino acids, which helps minimize the need for daily protein consumption. The transfer of an amino group is called transamination. There are many different amino acid–specific **transaminases** (**aminotransferases**) that catalyze transaminations (Fig. 35.4). Transaminases use **pyridoxal phosphate** as a prosthetic group and cofactor. Pyridoxal phosphate derives from pyridoxine (one form of vitamin $B_6$; well over 100 different enzymes use this cofactor). α-**Ketoglutarate** is the most common and frequent *acceptor* of amino groups, and it forms glutamate. Another common acceptor is **pyruvate**, which forms alanine. The amino acid that *loses* its amino group becomes an α-keto acid. These keto acids are degraded or, in liver and kidneys, used for gluconeogenesis (see Fig. 25.5).

Transaminations play a major role in the interorgan transport of nitrogen in the form of glutamine and alanine. When muscle, for instance, degrades protein, it transfers amino groups of the resulting amino acids to pyruvate and glutamate to produce alanine and glutamine, which it releases into the blood (see Fig. 35.10).

For the biosynthesis of **nonessential amino acids, glutamate** can donate its nitrogen for the synthesis of serine, aspartate, alanine, or ornithine, and the entire glutamate molecule can be used for the synthesis of proline (see Fig. 34.11). Glutamate is also a neurotransmitter. Presumably for this reason,

glutamate is largely confined to the cell interior. Many tissues do not efficiently transport glutamate across their plasma membranes, and the concentration of glutamate in the blood is low. Instead of glutamate, *glutamine* is transported among organs. To this end, glutamate is aminated to produce glutamine; then, glutamine is deaminated to produce glutamate (see Fig. 34.11).

The activities of **aspartate transaminase (AST)** and **alanine transaminase (ALT)** in blood serum are frequently measured to gauge tissue damage, especially of the liver. AST catalyzes the reaction aspartate + α-ketoglutarate ↔ glutamate + oxaloacetate; ALT catalyzes the reaction alanine + α-ketoglutarate ↔ glutamate + pyruvate. Damaged cells lose more of these enzymes into the bloodstream than do healthy cells. In the blood, AST and ALT have half-lives of about 1 to 4 days. In blood, neither AST nor ALT is known to play a physiological role.

## 2.4. Role of Glutamine in Nitrogen Metabolism

Glutamine is synthesized from glutamate and an ammonium ion with the help of **glutamate-ammonia ligase** (also called **glutamine synthetase**) via the following reaction: glutamate + $NH_4^+$ + ATP → glutamine + ADP + $P_i$.

Physiologically important sites of glutamate-ammonia ligase expression are muscle, liver, and brain;

- When muscle degrades amino acids (particularly branched-chain amino acids), it exports their nitrogen as part of glutamine (and also as part of alanine; see Fig. 35.10).
- In the liver, perivenous hepatocytes use the glutamate-ammonia ligase–catalyzed reaction to remove $NH_4^+$ (which is neurotoxic) from the blood (see Fig. 35.9); in patients with hyperammonemia, the concentration of glutamine in blood thus rises with the concentration of ammonium ions.
- In the brain, astrocytes use the glutamate-ammonia ligase–catalyzed reaction to remove neurotransmitter and recycle a precursor of it to neurons as part of a glutamate/GABA-glutamine cycle (Figs. 35.5 and 35.6). Some neurons use

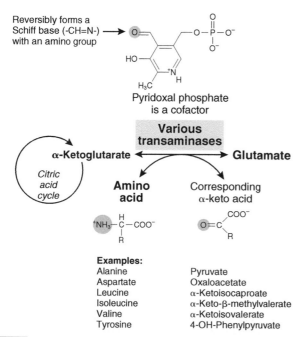

**Fig. 35.4** **Transamination of some amino acids yields glutamate.** The transaminases use pyridoxal phosphate, a derivative of the vitamin pyridoxine (vitamin $B_6$).

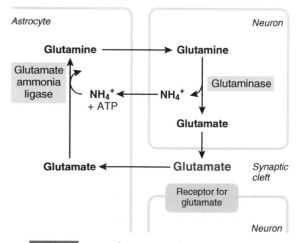

**Fig. 35.5** **The glutamate-glutamine cycle.**

and release glutamate or GABA (γ-aminobutyric acid) as a neurotransmitter. Astrocytes remove most of these neurotransmitters from the extracellular space and convert them to glutamine, which they release into the extracellular space. Neurons take up glutamine and use it to synthesize glutamate and GABA.

Glutamine is used for a wide variety of reactions, including biosynthetic reactions and energy production. The synthesis of asparagine, IMP (see Fig. 38.3), orotate (see Fig. 37.2), CTP (see Fig. 37.4), and all amino sugars (e.g., sialic acid; see Chapters 11 and 13) requires glutamine as a source of nitrogen. Neutrophils, macrophages, and lymphocytes use a large amount of glutamine for energy generation. Indeed, in some of the patients who degrade endogenous protein at a high rate, an intravenous infusion of glutamine reduces the rate of infection and the length of hospital stay. Many cancer cells have been found to use large amounts of glutamine for a variety of processes.

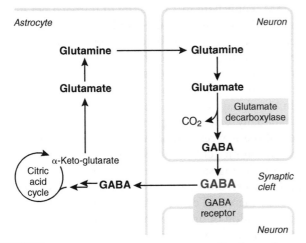

**Fig. 35.6** The γ-aminobutyric acid (GABA)-glutamine cycle.

## 2.5. Elimination of Nitrogen via the Urea Cycle

The urea cycle provides a means for excreting excess nitrogen as urea. This is the main path for nitrogen excretion.

Urea contains two nitrogen atoms; one of these stems from $NH_4^+$ and the other from aspartate (Fig. 35.7). $NH_4^+$ is produced by deamination of amino acids (see Fig. 35.2), whereas aspartate nitrogen arises predominantly from transamination reactions (see Figs. 35.4 and 35.7). The summary reaction of the urea cycle is: $NH_4^+ + HCO_3^- + aspartate + 3\ ATP \rightarrow urea + fumarate + 2\ ADP + AMP + 4\ P_i$.

The activity of the urea cycle is regulated short term via the formation of **N-acetylglutamate** (see Fig. 35.7) and, in addition, long term via the rate of **synthesis** of all enzymes of the cycle. Arginine activates the synthase that catalyzes the

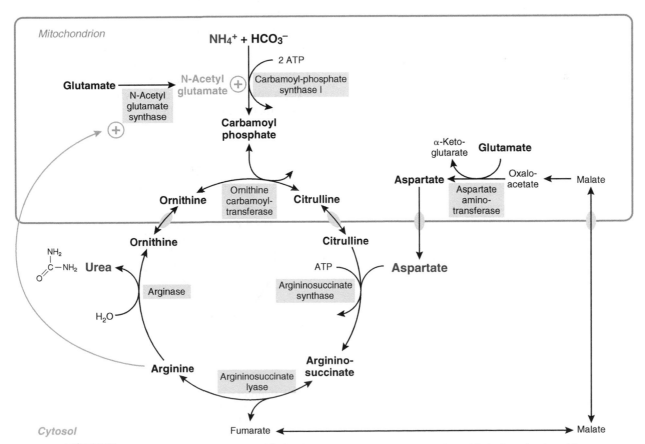

**Fig. 35.7** **Reactions of the urea cycle.** While carbamoyl-phosphate synthase I is in the mitochondria and works as an accessory to the urea cycle, a second enzyme, carbamoyl-phosphate synthase II, is in the cytosol and catalyzes a reaction in the de novo synthesis of pyrimidine nucleotides (see Fig. 37.2).

formation of N-acetylglutamate; this in turn allosterically activates carbamoyl-phosphate synthase I. The quantity of urea cycle enzymes in a healthy person reflects that person's long-term protein intake. **Protein intake** in turn is regulated and limited such that the need for nitrogen elimination can be met by existing enzyme capacities.

Only the *liver* contains significant amounts of *all* enzymes of the urea cycle; however, the *intestine* and the *kidneys* each express enzymes for a portion of the urea cycle (Fig. 35.8). The intestine converts glutamine to ornithine, condenses ornithine with carbamoylphosphate to form citrulline, and exports citrulline into the bloodstream. The kidneys, and to a much smaller extent other organs, take up citrulline and convert it to arginine, which they release into the bloodstream. The liver cleaves the majority of this arginine into ornithine and urea, whereas various tissues use a small fraction of arginine for protein synthesis.

In the liver, cells that receive portal and arterial blood first use the urea cycle to produce urea, whereas cells that receive this blood last use glutamate-ammonia ligase (glutamine synthase) to convert any remaining $NH_4^+$ to glutamine (Fig. 35.9). The peri*portal* hepatocytes are close to incoming blood and convert $NH_4^+$ and alanine to urea. These cells can also use pyruvate, the carbon skeleton of alanine, for gluconeogenesis (see Fig. 25.3). Downstream, the peri*venous* hepatocytes remove any remaining $NH4^+$ by synthesizing glutamine, which they release into the blood. The intestines convert this glutamine to citrulline (Figs. 35.8 and 35.10).

Antibodies against **carbamoyl-phosphate synthase I** and **arginase** are used in immunohistochemical analysis to distin-guish **hepatocellular carcinomas** from other adenocarcinomas. Thereby, carbamoyl-phosphate synthase is commonly called **HepPar-1**, a name created at a time when the nature of the antigen was unknown. Both normal epithelial cells of the intestine and normal hepatocytes show HepPar-1 immunoreactivity (see also Fig. 35.8).

Fig. 35.10 provides a summary of the major traffic of amino acids and ammonia among muscle, intestine, kidneys, and liver.

In **blood**, urea is normally present at a concentration of 1.2 to 3.0 mM (equivalent to 7 to 18 mg of nitrogen per dL). The acronym **BUN** is commonly used for blood urea nitrogen. The concentration of urea in the blood depends on protein intake; the feeding/fasting cycle; and the presence of injuries, stress, or illness. In a person who eats three meals per day and for which protein intake just covers needs, the concentration of urea in blood stays constant throughout the day. In a person who habitually eats more protein than needed, the larger portion of these excess amino acids is degraded, but some of the excess amino acids are used for extra protein synthesis; then, in the fasting state, there is also some extra protein degradation. As a result, a person with this diet ends up having a persistently increased concentration of urea in the blood, and the concentration of urea is as much as 30% higher in the fed state than in the fasting state.

The term **azotemia** refers to an increase in the concentration of nitrogen in the blood; often, this is an increased value for BUN.

The term **uremia** can mean an excess of the concentration of urea in the blood (i.e., an elevated BUN) or it can refer to a *syndrome* of which an elevated concentration of urea is a hallmark. (Note that the term *hyperuricemia* refers to an excess concentration of urate, which is a different molecule from urea; see Chapter 38.)

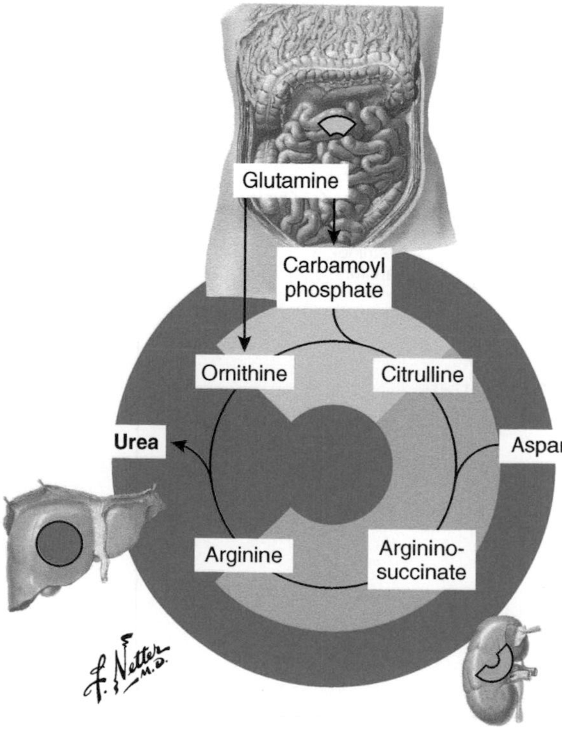

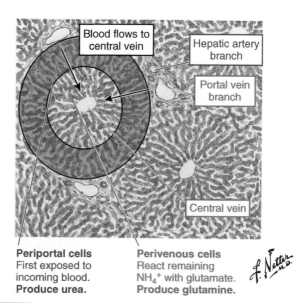

**Fig. 35.8** **Tissue location of the urea cycle.** Only the liver contains the entire urea cycle. The intestine and the kidneys carry out selected steps. Citrulline and arginine are transported through the blood.

**Fig. 35.9** **Compartmentation of the urea cycle in the liver.** The cells that produce urea also perform gluconeogenesis (see Figs. 25.2 and 25.3).

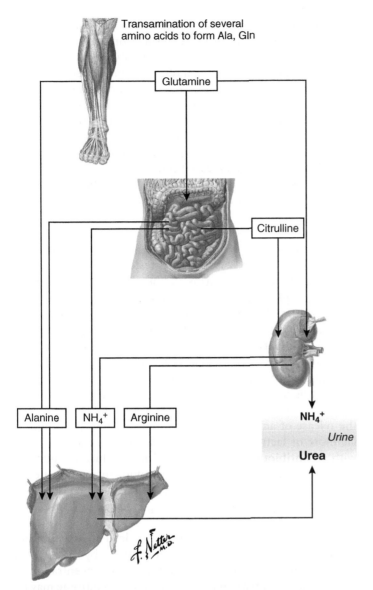

Fig. 35.10 **Interorgan nitrogen flux in the elimination of excess amino acid nitrogen.**

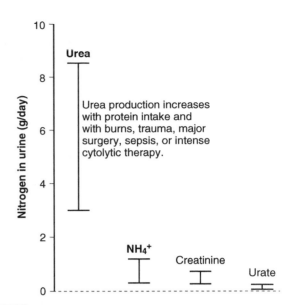

Fig. 35.11 **Normal ranges of daily amounts of nitrogen-containing compounds in urine.**

A patient who has **severe liver disease** may have a reduced capacity to make urea and may therefore have an unusually low BUN. Conversely, a patient who has **kidney failure** may have a reduced capacity to excrete urea and may therefore have an unusually high BUN and uremia or the uremic syndrome.

Physicians commonly use the **BUN/serum creatinine ratio** to interpret abnormalities of nitrogen metabolism. The concentration of creatinine in the blood is a function of the balance of production and excretion of creatinine (more information on creatinine can be found in Section 1.5 in Chapter 23). Creatinine production tends to be fairly similar from person to person (although increased muscle mass and exercise increase creatinine production). Hence, an increased concentration of creatinine in the blood often indicates a decrease in filtration by the kidneys. The kidney tubules do not reabsorb creatinine, but they can reabsorb urea. In a healthy patient, the BUN/creatinine ratio (each expressed in mg/dL) is 10 to 20. If this ratio is less than 10, the patient likely has **kidney damage** (this reduces uptake of filtered urea) and if it is more than 20, the patient is likely to be **dehydrated** (this reduces filtration).

Urea normally contributes the largest amount of nitrogen to **urine** (Fig. 35.11), whereas $NH_4^+$, creatinine (a useless product of accidental cyclization of creatine and phosphocreatine, see Section 1.5 in Chapter 23), and uric acid (see Section 2 in Chapter 38) contribute lesser amounts. Urea is one of the major solutes of urine and plays a vital role in the concentration of urine beyond the osmolarity of plasma.

## 3. DEFICIENCIES OF NITROGEN ELIMINATION

*Impairment of the urea cycle causes hyperammonemia, which may be life threatening. Impairment of the urea cycle and hyperammonemia are most commonly seen in patients who have severe liver dysfunction, often as a result of alcohol abuse, metabolic syndrome, cancer, or infection with hepatotropic viruses. Hyperammonemia may also be due to an inborn deficiency of an enzyme or transporter that is important to the function of the urea cycle. Patients who have a severe deficiency of a urea cycle enzyme develop life-threatening hyperammonemia during the first few days of life. Patients who have a mild deficiency experience symptoms only during periods of high nitrogen excretion, such as after high-protein meals, during extended fasts or illness, after delivery of a baby, or after appreciable tissue injury. Treatment options for all urea cycle deficiencies include minimizing protein intake, avoiding states of intense protein degradation, and using oral drugs that remove nitrogen as glycine or glutamine conjugates.*

## 3.1. General Comments

Problems converting nitrogen to urea cause **hyperammonemia**, which impairs the function of the central nervous system (CNS) and can be life threatening. The pathogenesis of hyperammonemia is explained below. The most common cause of deficient urea formation is **liver** failure. Much less commonly, deficient urea formation is due to an inherited deficiency of an enzyme or transport protein.

Measurements of **"ammonia"** in blood are not part of routine laboratory studies; they are only prompted by clinical suspicion. **Respiratory alkalosis** is usually the earliest sign of hyperammonemia (hyperammonemia stimulates breathing). The reported concentration of ammonia refers to the sum of $NH_3$ and $NH_4^+$ (at a physiological pH, $NH_4^+$ is by far the major contributor). Measurements vary appreciably with the analytical method used. Concentrations more than ~3 times the upper limit of normal are usually associated with changes in mentation; coma and seizures can also be seen. Patients with blood ammonia concentrations greater than ~20 times the upper normal limit often become severely ill, and those with "ammonia" concentrations of ~50 times the upper limit usually do not survive the episode.

Hyperammonemia is preceded and accompanied by **hyperglutaminemia**. Hyperammonemia stimulates glutamate-ammonia ligase (glutamine synthetase) in perivenous hepatocytes and in astrocytes. In both tissues, glutamine serves as a buffer against hyperammonemia. In patients with hyperammonemia from a urea cycle disorder, the concentration of glutamine in the blood rises with the concentration of "ammonia," and it is usually at least 10 times higher than that of "ammonia."

Hyperammonemia primarily affects CNS function by causing swelling of **astrocytes**. Astrocytes contain a significant amount of glutamate-ammonia ligase (glutamine synthetase). With an increasing concentration of $NH_4^+$ in the blood, astrocytes synthesize more glutamine, which is osmotically active. In patients who have *persistent* mild hyperammonemia, compensatory degradation of other osmolytes (e.g., myo-inositol, N-acetyl-aspartate, creatine, and phosphocreatine) inside astrocytes essentially eliminates swelling; still, over time, Alzheimer-like damage to astrocytes occurs. In patients who show acute, *steadily increasing* concentrations of $NH_4^+$ (and hence of glutamine), the rate of degradation of osmolytes is too low to maintain a near-normal cell volume. Eventually, swollen tissue in the brainstem restricts the blood supply to the brain.

Patients who are in a coma due to severe hyperammonemia are treated with **hemodialysis** and assisted ventilation.

## 3.2. Nitrogen Elimination in Patients With Liver Failure or Kidney Failure

A severe impairment of liver function leads to **hyperammonemia** and a syndrome called **hepatic encephalopathy** (i.e., encephalopathy due to impaired liver function). Hepatic encephalopathy is commonly seen in a setting of portal hypertension (increased blood pressure in the portal vein). In developed countries, the portal hypertension is usually caused by cirrhosis, which in turn can result from many disorders, including virus infection (most commonly hepatitis B or C), alcoholic liver disease, or metabolic syndrome. Metabolic syndrome is defined in various ways; a common definition used in the United States is three of the following five abnormalities: hypertension, hypertriglyceridemia, low high-density lipoprotein cholesterol, abdominal obesity, and impaired glucose homeostasis. Patients with hyperammonemia have **respiratory alkalosis** and an increased concentration of glutamine in the cerebrospinal fluid. The blood of these patients may also contain other substances that would normally be removed by the liver and are toxic to the brain.

Patients who have hepatic encephalopathy often have **asterixis**, an impaired ability to maintain position due to brain dysfunction. Asterixis is typically tested for by asking the patient to stretch out the arms and bend the hands upward. If asterixis is present, the patient's hands display a repetitive, nonrhythmic "flapping" relaxation of wrist dorsiflexion.

Patients who have chronic hepatic encephalopathy can be treated with **lactulose** [*galactose-β(1→4)-fructose*] or **lactitol** [*galactose-β(1→4)-sorbitol*], a sugar and sugar alcohol that are not digested by human enzymes but only by bacteria in the gut. Acting as laxatives, lactulose and lactitol increase excretion of nitrogen compounds via the feces, and they also reduce the release of ammonia from the intestine into the blood. If lactulose or lactitol are not tolerated, patients can be treated with an **antibiotic**, such as **rifaximin**, to reduce the number of $NH_4^+$-producing bacteria in the colon. In many patients, degradation of blood from gastrointestinal bleeding is a major cause of ammonia in blood; bleeding is usually stopped with invasive procedures.

Severe loss of **kidney** function can lead to **uremia** and **uremic syndrome**, which are characterized by an elevated concentration of **urea** in the blood. A high concentration of urea per se is not particularly toxic. Uremic syndrome may be associated with headache, dementia, seizures, or coma. In the uremic syndrome, as opposed to hepatic encephalopathy, the CNS dysfunction is due to inadequate removal of toxic substances by the kidneys rather than the liver. There is no thorough understanding yet of the many pathogenic processes that harm the CNS; however, the offending compounds in the blood can be removed with hemodialysis. Protein restriction minimizes symptoms.

## 3.3. Inborn Deficiencies That Affect the Urea Cycle

Inborn deficiencies of urea cycle enzymes are rare. Collectively, they occur in ~1:10,000 to ~1:50,000 newborns. Deficiencies in all enzymes of the cycle have been described. **Ornithine carbamoyltransferase (ornithine transcarbamoylase)** deficiency is the most common urea cycle disorder. This disorder is inherited in X-linked fashion, whereas all other urea cycle disorders are inherited in an autosomal recessive fashion. Depending on residual enzyme activity, a urea cycle disorder manifests between the newborn period and a period of extreme amino acid degradation in adults. A classic example of the latter is a woman who is heterozygous for X-linked ornithine carbamoyltransferase deficiency and shows symptoms in the postpartum period, a time of tremendous tissue degradation and remodeling.

A deficiency of nitrogen excretion via the urea cycle is usually discovered because of an acute attack that is characterized by progressive lethargy, vomiting, seizures, and coma. As mentioned above, respiratory alkalosis is an early sign of hyperammonemia. **Diagnosis** of a specific urea cycle defect generally requires measurements of ornithine, citrulline, argininosuccinate, arginine, and homocitrulline in blood, and orotate in urine. Homocitrulline structurally resembles citrulline but has an aliphatic chain that is longer by one $-CH_2-$ group. Homocitrulline may derive from the condensation of carbamoyl phosphate with lysine. Orotate results from leakage of excess carbamoyl phosphate from mitochondria into the cytosol (see Section 1 in Chapter 37). Fig. 35.12 provides an overview of known deficiencies and metabolite abnormalities.

The **hyperammonemia** associated with the deficiency of an enzyme of the urea cycle is due to decreased removal of ammonium ions, either because of a primary or secondary carbamoyl-phosphate synthase I deficiency (see Fig. 35.12). Secondary carbamoyl-phosphate synthase I deficiency is due to inadequate activity of N-acetyl glutamate synthase, either because of mutation or arginine deficiency. Arginine deficiency is observed in all urea cycle disorders that originate in defective enzymes or transporters between the synthesis of carbamoyl phosphate and the formation of arginine from argininosuccinate.

The **treatment** of urea cycle disorders aims to diminish the need for nitrogen elimination and to establish alternate routes of nitrogen elimination. Nitrogen elimination is minimized by limiting **protein intake** to the amount needed to maintain growth in children and protein homeostasis in adults (see also the discussion of nitrogen balance in Section 5). A long fast should be avoided because it increases breakdown of body protein. Illness causes degradation of body protein and often precipitates a hyperammonemic crisis that requires hospitalization. Supplemental arginine or citrulline is given to patients who are otherwise deficient in **arginine**. Citrulline is an effective precursor for arginine in patients who have normal argininosuccinate synthase and argininosuccinate lyase activity. A normal concentration of arginine normalizes protein synthesis and optimizes performance of the urea cycle

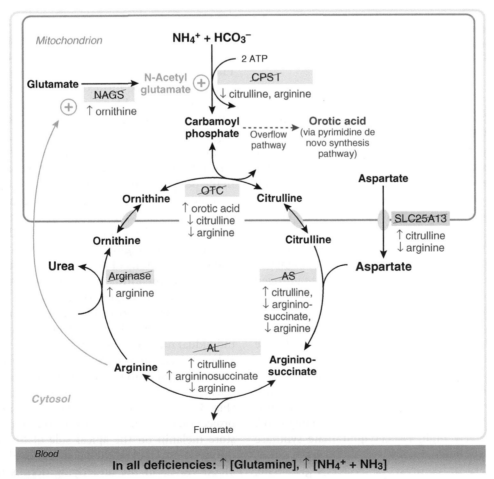

**Fig. 35.12** **Characteristic metabolite abnormalities of patients with impaired function of the urea cycle.**

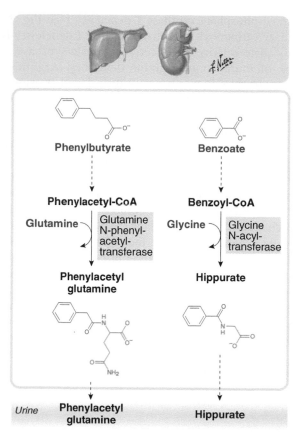

**Fig. 35.13** Phenylbutyrate and benzoate remove nitrogen from the body because they are excreted in the urine as conjugates with glutamine and glycine, respectively.

(via stimulation of N-acetylglutamate synthase). **Carglumic acid (N-carbamyl-glutamate)** is used as an analog of N-acetyl-glutamate for patients who are deficient in N-acetylglutamate synthase. Oral **sodium phenylbutyrate** removes nitrogen via conjugation of its metabolite with glutamine (Fig. 35.13). Oral **sodium benzoate** works similarly (see Fig. 35.13) but is not used as frequently. In hospitals, a mixture of sodium phenyl-acetate (which is also conjugated with glutamine) and sodium benzoate is often infused intravenously; the blood of patients with severe hyperammonemia is also depleted of ammonia by **hemodialysis**. **Liver transplantation** can normalize nitrogen excretion.

In patients who have an elevated concentration of **propionyl-CoA**, the urea cycle has low activity owing to insufficient activation of carbamoyl phosphate synthase I. The elevated concentration of propionyl-CoA may be a result of insufficient activity of **propionyl-CoA carboxylase** (this includes problems of **biotin** metabolism) or **methylmalonyl-CoA mutase** (this includes problems of cobalamin metabolism; see Chapter 36). When the concentration of propionyl-CoA in the liver is excessively high, N-acetylglutamate synthase produces N-*propionyl*-glutamate instead of N-*acetyl*-glutamate (see Fig. 35.7). In contrast to N-acetyl-glutamate, N-propionyl-glutamate is an *inhibitor* of carbamoyl phosphate synthase and thus causes hyperammonemia.

## 4. SUMMARY OF THE METABOLISM OF AMINO ACIDS

*The degradation of amino acids is a vast and complex field that is covered in several chapters of this book; a summary and references are provided here. A deficiency in converting phenylalanine to tyrosine gives rise to phenylketonuria, which is treatable with a low-phenylalanine diet. A deficiency in the conversion of tyrosine to melanin leads to hypopigmentation of the skin, hair, and eyes. A deficiency in the degradation of tyrosine leads to tyrosinemia or alkaptonuria. Tryptophan gives rise to serotonin, melatonin, and nicotinamide adenine dinucleotides. Maple syrup disease is due to a deficiency in the degradation of the branched-chain amino acids Leu, Val, and Ile; it is best treated with a diet that is especially low in leucine.*

### 4.1. Overview

Table 35.1 provides an overview of the coverage of the metabolism of amino acids in this book. Deamination and transamination reactions, as well as the excretion of amino acid nitrogen, are described in Section 2 above.

### 4.2. Normal Metabolism of Phenylalanine, Tyrosine, and Tryptophan

**Phenylalanine** is used for protein synthesis. The remainder of phenylalanine is hydroxylated to form **tyrosine** (Fig. 35.14). Phenylalanine is an essential amino acid, but tyrosine is not, as long as it can be formed from phenylalanine.

**Tyrosine** is used for protein synthesis and the synthesis of **catecholamines** and **melanins**; excess tyrosine is mostly degraded in the liver (see Fig. 35.14). Among the catecholamines, dopamine and epinephrine serve as neurotransmitters in the brain, norepinephrine serves as a neurotransmitter in the peripheral nervous system, and epinephrine also serves as a blood-borne hormone for the regulation of metabolism (see Sections 2.3, 3.4, and 4.4 in Chapter 26; Section 5.1 in Chapter 28; and Section 2 in Chapter 33).

Melanins are pigments that are found in skin, hair, retina, and certain regions of the brain. There are three categories of melanins: **eumelanins**, which are brown to black; **pheomelanins**, which are yellow to red-brown; and **neuromelanins**, which are brown to black. Melanins are synthesized inside intracellular organelles called **melanosomes**. In the skin, an individual melanosome synthesizes only one type of melanin, either eumelanin or pheomelanin; however, a melanocyte can contain one or both types of melanosomes. In the epidermis of the skin, ~10% of cells are melanin-synthesizing melanocytes (Fig. 35.15). Each melanocyte transfers melanin via dendritic projections to about 3 dozen keratinocytes. Keratinocytes store melanin on the apical side of the nucleus. Eumelanin thus protects DNA in the nuclei of keratinocytes and heme in blood vessels of the underlying dermis from photodamage. Pheomelanin, on the other hand, generates reactive oxygen radicals that are potentially damaging. Differences in skin

| Table 35.1 | **Overview of the Degradation of Amino Acids** | |
|---|---|---|
| **Amino Acid** | **Pathway for Degradation** | **Relevant Figure** |
| Alanine | Transamination yields pyruvate | Figs. 27.3 and 34.11 |
| Arginine | Hydrolysis yields urea and ornithine | Fig. 35.7 |
| Asparagine | Deamination yields aspartate | Figs. 35.2 and 34.11 |
| Aspartate | Entry into urea cycle yields fumarate in the citric acid cycle<br>Transamination yields oxaloacetate in the citric acid cycle | Fig. 35.7<br>Fig. 34.11 |
| Cysteine | Degradation includes transamination and yields mostly pyruvate | Fig. 36.16 |
| Glutamate | Deamination or transamination yields $\alpha$-ketoglutarate in the citric acid cycle | Figs. 34.11 and 35.2 |
| Glutamine | Deamination yields glutamate | Figs. 34.11 and 35.2 |
| Glycine | Deamination yields $CO_2$ and $N^5,N^{10}$-methylene-THF | Figs. 35.2 and 36.3 |
| Histidine | Deamination, followed by hydrolysis and transfer of a formimino-group to THF, yields glutamate | Fig. 36.3 |
| Isoleucine | Transamination yields $\alpha$-keto-$\beta$-methylvalerate, which is converted to acetyl-CoA and propionyl-CoA (which gives rise to succinyl-CoA) | Fig. 35.21 |
| Leucine | Transamination yields $\alpha$-ketoisocaproate, which is degraded to acetyl-CoA and acetoacetate | Fig. 35.21 |
| Lysine | Transfer of side chain N to $\alpha$-ketoglutarate; transamination of resulting $\alpha$-aminoadipate to $\alpha$-ketoglutarate, yielding $\alpha$-ketoadipate, which is degraded to acetoacetyl-CoA | Not shown |
| Methionine | Forms S-adenosyl-methionine in the activated methyl group cycle and from there gives rise to cysteine | Figs. 36.6 and 36.15 |
| Phenylalanine | Hydroxylation yields tyrosine | Fig. 35.14 |
| Proline | Oxidation gives rise to glutamate $\gamma$-semialdehyde, which can be oxidized to glutamate or give up an amino group to generate ornithine | Fig. 34.11 |
| Serine | Deamination yields pyruvate<br>Loss of a one-carbon group yields glycine and $N^5,N^{10}$-methylene-THF | Fig. 35.2<br>Figs. 34.11 and 36.3 |
| Threonine | Oxidation to $\alpha$-amino-$\beta$-ketobutyrate gives rise to either pyruvate or acetyl-CoA + glycine<br>Deamination generates $\alpha$-ketobutyrate, which is oxidatively decarboxylated to propionyl-CoA and then gives rise to succinyl-CoA | Not shown<br>Fig. 35.2 for first step; rest not shown |
| Tryptophan | Can be used for the synthesis of serotonin and melatonin or degraded to yield numerous products, including a precursor for $NAD^+$ | Fig. 35.16 |
| Tyrosine | Can be used for the synthesis of catecholamines, melanins, and thyroid hormone or degraded to yield fumarate in the citric acid cycle and acetoacetate | Fig. 35.14 |
| Valine | Transamination yields $\alpha$-ketoisovalerate, which is degraded to propionyl-CoA, which gives rise to succinyl-CoA | Fig. 35.21 |

pigmentation reflect differences in melanin synthesis, as well as the size and distribution of melanosomes in keratinocytes.

After **UV irradiation**, keratinocytes release endothelin-1, $\alpha$-melanocyte stimulating hormone ($\alpha$-MSH, $\alpha$-melanocortin), and fibroblast growth factor, whereas melanocytes express an increased number of MSH receptors. In response, the number of melanocytes increases, as do melanin synthesis and transfer of melanosomes to keratinocytes.

The hormones $\alpha$-MSH, $\beta$-MSH, and **adrenocorticotropic hormone** (**ACTH**) all stimulate melanin production and a

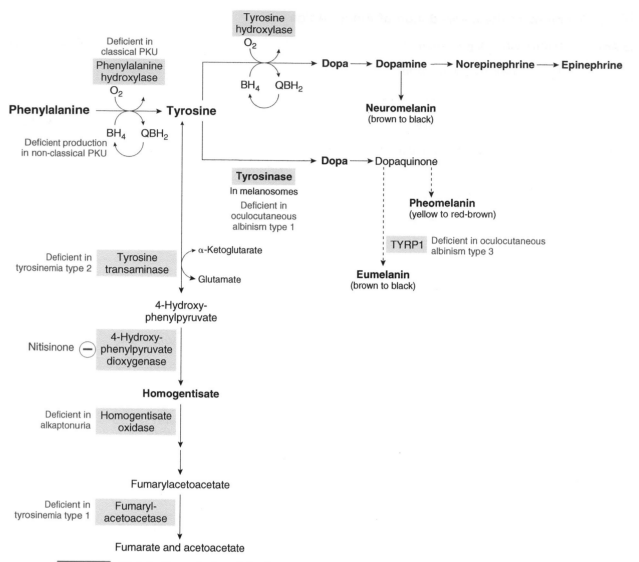

**Fig. 35.14** **Metabolism of phenylalanine and tyrosine.** Humans synthesize BH4 from GTP in three steps (not shown). BH$_4$, tetrahydrobiopterin (see also Fig. 35.17); QBH$_2$, quinonoid dihydrobiopterin.

switch from the synthesis of pheomelanins toward eumelanins. Patients who have an increased concentration of ACTH in the blood, such as those with **Addison disease** (see Section 4.2 in Chapter 31), show increased pigmentation, particularly in areas that are exposed to sunlight. Conversely, patients who produce mutant MSH or receptors for MSH (melanocortin 1 receptor, MC1R) have decreased pigmentation, and pheomelanin production is favored over eumelanin production. Most people who have **red hair** have a variant melanocortin receptor 1; they are fair skinned, do not tan well after exposure to sunlight, and have an increased risk of melanoma.

Melanins bind **metals** such as copper, iron, mercury, lead, and cadmium; the daily shedding of melanins in hair and skin plays a role in the removal of these metals from the body.

In the retina, melanin reduces light-scatter and photo damage. In the brain, only catecholamine-synthesizing neurons make melanin (**neuromelanin**), mainly from dopamine (tyrosinase is not needed). The largest amounts of neuromelanin are found in dopaminergic neurons of the substantia

nigra and in noradrenergic neurons of the locus coeruleus. The neuromelanins act as a sink of both toxic metals and excess dopamine. Neuromelanin deposits in these areas of the brain increase with age. When neuromelanin-containing neurons die, the pigment is released into the extracellular space, where it may remain for a long time and elicit inflammation.

**Tryptophan** is the precursor for the neurotransmitter serotonin and also for melatonin (see Fig. 35.16). **Serotonin** (5-hydroxytryptamine, 5-HT) is synthesized in some neurons in the brainstem, in serotonin-containing enterochromaffin cells of the gastrointestinal mucosa, and in neurons of the enteric nervous system. Like the synthesis of tyrosine and the synthesis of catecholamines from tyrosine, the synthesis of serotonin from tryptophan includes a hydroxylation reaction that requires tetrahydrobiopterin (BH$_4$, THB; see Fig. 35.17). Transporters take up serotonin from the extracellular space and thus end its signaling effect. **Amphetamines** and **selective serotonin reuptake inhibitors** decrease the rate of serotonin

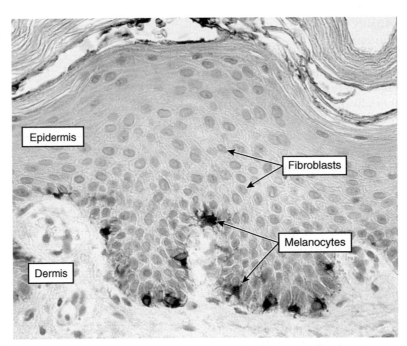

**Fig. 35.15** **Melanocytes in the skin.** Melanosomes containing melanin travel from melanocytes to fibroblasts. The skin surface is at the top of the image. Melanin was detected with an antibody, which was used to give rise to a brown stain.

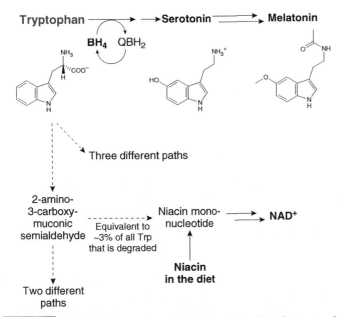

**Fig. 35.16** **Use of tryptophan for the synthesis of serotonin, melatonin, and NAD⁺.** $BH_4$, tetrahydrobiopterin.

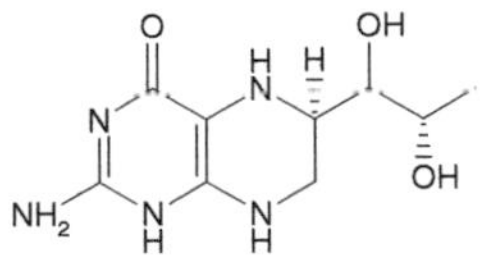

**Fig. 35.17** **Tetrahydrobiopterin (also called BH₄, THB, or sapropterin).**

removal from the extracellular space and thus enhance the effects of serotonin. **Melatonin** plays a role in the regulation of the sleep/wake cycle. The pineal gland in the brain synthesizes melatonin in cyclical fashion, with a peak in the middle of the night.

Tryptophan can be degraded via several pathways (Fig. 35.16). A small yet physiologically important fraction of tryptophan gives rise to about half of the **niacin mononucleotide** that is required for the synthesis of $NAD^+$ and $NADP^+$. (The

other half of the niacin mononucleotide is made from niacin in the diet; see Section 1 in Chapter 19.)

## 4.3. Hyperphenylalaninemias (Including Phenylketonuria)

Hyperphenylalaninemia is commonly defined as a concentration of phenylalanine in the blood in excess of 120 $\mu$M (the mean normal concentration is about 60 $\mu$M). About 1 in 10,000 to 15,000 newborns in Western countries develops hyperphenylalaninemia. Mutations in **phenylalanine hydroxylase** (the enzyme that transforms Phe to Tyr; see Fig. 35.14) are the most common cause of hyperphenylalaninemia (this is also the most common disease of amino acid metabolism). Patients with pathogenic hyperphenylalaninemia due to mutant phenylalanine hydroxylase are said to have **classic phenylketonuria** (**PKU**; phenylketones, such as phenylpyruvate, appear in the urine when the concentration of phenylalanine in the blood is high). Patients who do not synthesize an adequate amount of the cofactor **tetrahydrobiopterin** (**BH₄, THB, sapropterin;** Fig. 35.17) for phenylalanine hydroxylase are said to have **resistant** or **nonclassic PKU**. This group of patients accounts for 1% to 2% of hyperphenylalaninemic patients. Some patients have only mildly elevated plasma phenylalanine, and this abnormality is sometimes referred to as **non-PKU hyperphenylalaninemia**.

After birth, a few days are needed for hyperphenylalaninemia to develop in an affected infant. Phenylalanine passes through the placenta. Thus if the fetus fails to metabolize phenylalanine, a healthy mother's liver metabolizes the fetus's excess phenylalanine. In newborns with PKU, the blood phenylalanine concentration keeps rising after birth. To reach adequate sensitivity and accuracy with the screening test, a blood sample is typically collected 24 to 48 hours after birth.

Modern screening tests for PKU use tandem mass spectrometry to measure the ratio of the concentrations of phenylalanine to tyrosine in spots of dried blood. All patients who have hyperphenylalaninemia are also tested for urine biopterin to determine whether they have nonclassic PKU due to a $BH_4$ deficiency.

Classic PKU is inherited in an autosomal recessive fashion. Affected patients typically show complete or near-complete deficiency of phenylalanine hydroxylase, often due to an unstable mutant enzyme. There are more than 500 known mutations of phenylalanine hydroxylase that result in PKU. Individual mutations are sufficiently infrequent that most affected patients are compound heterozygotes. Consequently, patients show a spectrum of phenylalanine hydroxylase activities.

A high concentration of phenylalanine is damaging to the brain. At a few months of age, untreated patients with classic PKU regress in their development, and their brains show a decreased amount of **myelin**. The most likely reason for the damage is that a high concentration of phenylalanine in the blood competes with other neutral amino acids for the same amino acid transporter and thereby reduces the uptake of other amino acids into the brain. As a consequence, a low concentration of one or more amino acids may limit the synthesis of protein or neurotransmitters. Untreated patients also show decreased pigmentation, owing to deficient synthesis of melanins (see Fig. 35.14).

Patients who have marked hyperphenylalaninemia need to be treated with a **low-phenylalanine diet** as soon as possible. The treatment goal is to lower the concentration of phenylalanine in the blood sufficiently that patients achieve normal development and function of brain and body. The concentration of phenylalanine in the blood is measured at least monthly and is used to guide the diet. Patients with classic PKU typically tolerate only 200 to 400 mg of phenylalanine per day. As a rule of thumb, one gram of protein in meats, fowl, or fish contains 50 mg of phenylalanine. Some vegetables and fruits contain as little as 15 mg of phenylalanine per gram of protein (Table 35.2). In practice, patients with PKU cannot eat high-protein foods, such as meat, fowl, fish, dairy, legumes, or regular grain products. They also avoid **aspartame**-sweetened diet drinks because the metabolism of aspartame yields phenylalanine. Affected patients eat special low-protein grain products, as well as vegetables and fruits that contain little phenylalanine. They consume most of their protein as a phenylalanine-free mixture of synthetic amino acids (in solid or liquid form). Optimization of these mixtures is still ongoing. A supplement of amino acids that is rich in amino acids that

**Table 35.2    Phenylalanine Content of Various Foods**

| Food | mg of Phe/100 g edible portion |
| --- | --- |
| Cheese, cheddar | 1,310 |
| Hamburger | 810 |
| Couscous, prepared | 320 |
| Peas | 190 |
| Milk (whole) | 160 |
| Cauliflower | 90 |
| Broccoli | 76 |
| Banana | 45 |
| Potatoes, boiled | 44 |
| Lettuce | 40 |
| Tomato, raw | 21 |
| Carrots | 15 |
| Onions, raw | 14 |
| Mango | 14 |
| Pineapple | 10 |
| Orange juice | 7 |
| Tapioca | Trace |

use the same amino acid transporter as phenylalanine (e.g., tyrosine, tryptophan) appears to be effective in lowering the concentration of phenylalanine in the brain. Patients should also receive supplements of vitamin $B_6$ and cobalamin because their normal diet does not contain enough of these vitamins. A patient with PKU who receives adequate lifelong diet treatment can expect near-normal health and development; still, subtle brain abnormalities are the rule.

All the patients with nonclassic PKU, and about half of the patients with classic PKU, benefit from supplementation with **tetrahydrobiopterin**. The rare patients who have nonclassic PKU also should be treated for deficiencies in the synthesis of catecholamines and serotonin.

Phenylalanine in the blood is derived both from the diet and the degradation of body proteins. Degradation is increased during infection or trauma or if intake of any one of the essential amino acids is insufficient.

### 4.4. Disorders of Pigmentation

Decreased melanin production is observed in patients who have vitiligo, albinism, or piebaldism.

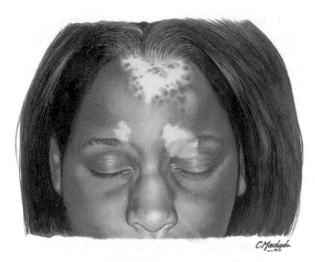

C. Machado

**Fig. 35.18**  **Vitiligo.**

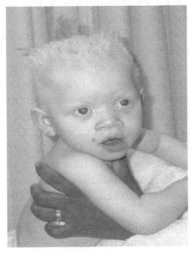

**Fig.35.19**  **Oculocutaneous albinism type 2 in a 17-month-old African-American girl, held by her mother.** This patient also has Angelman syndrome, which causes developmental delay and microcephaly. (From Saadeh R, Lisi EC, Batista DA, McIntosh I, Hoover-Fong JE. Albinism and developmental delay: the need to test for 15q11-q13 deletion. *Pediatr Neurol.* 2007;37:299-302.

**Vitiligo** is a condition of patchy loss of skin pigmentation (Fig. 35.18), which is seen in 1% to 2% of the population. It is due to an absence of melanin-producing cells and may be due to an inflammatory process. Serum of patients who have vitiligo contains antibodies to melanocytes, including antibodies to tyrosinase. Vitiligo is sometimes treated with a psoralen (see Section 4.2 in Chapter 2).

**Oculocutaneous albinism** is an autosomal recessively inherited condition of decreased or absent pigmentation of the eyes, skin, and hair. Affected patients have impaired clarity of vision, in part due to an improperly formed fovea and misrouted optic neurons. There are three known causes of oculocutaneous albinism (OCA; see Fig. 35.14):

- In type 1 OCA, which occurs in ~1:10,000 to 70,000 whites (it is much less common in others), both **tyrosinase** alleles carry a harmful mutation.

- In type 2 OCA (Fig. 35.19), which occurs in up to 1:1,000 black Africans and ~1:2,000 people among the Navajo Native Americans (but much less commonly in white or Japanese people), both alleles of the *OCA2* gene carry a mutation. The OCA2 protein appears to be an integral membrane protein of melanosomes, but its function is not well understood. (Many patients with Prader-Willi or Angelman syndrome have altered expression of several genes near the *OCA2* gene and also show reduced pigmentation.)

- In type 3 OCA, which occurs mostly in blacks, both alleles for tyrosinase-related protein 1 (TYRP1) carry a mutation; this protein has an oxidase activity that is needed for the synthesis of eumelanin.

There are many other hereditary diseases of skin pigmentation, which generally also impair vision. Some of these diseases, such as **piebaldism** (a hereditary condition marked by patches of decreased pigmentation), **Waardenburg syndrome**, and **dyschromatosis symmetrica hereditaria**, are due to impaired population of the skin with melanoblasts that are derived from the neural crest. Others, such as **Hermansky-Pudlak syndrome** and **Chédiak-Higashi syndrome**, are due to impaired formation of melanosomes. In Puerto Rico, up to ~1 in 2,000 persons have Hermansky-Pudlak syndrome. Patients with this disorder have oculocutaneous albinism, abnormal blood clotting, and damage to lungs and kidneys due to impaired function of lysosomes and lysosome-related organelles. Patients who have Chédiak-Higashi syndrome have severe immune deficiency. Finally, **Griscelli syndrome** is due to impaired transfer of melanosomes from melanocytes to keratinocytes.

Excessive melanin production due to melanocortin-1 receptor variants is observed in patients who have **freckles**. Exposure to sunlight enhances freckling.

## 4.5. Disorders of Tyrosine Degradation

**Tyrosinemia type 1**, also called **hepatorenal tyrosinemia,** is due to **fumarylacetoacetase deficiency** (see Fig. 35.14). This disorder shows autosomal recessive inheritance and has a worldwide incidence of about 1 in 100,000; however, it is much more common in parts of Finland and Canada (e.g., 1:2,000 in a region of Quebec province). Presumably due to mutagenic effects of fumarylacetoacetate, the deficiency causes liver disease in infancy or childhood. Without treatment, patients have a very high long-term risk of **hepatocellular carcinoma**. The concentration of tyrosine in the blood is only mildly elevated (mechanism unclear) and not pathogenic. Affected patients are treated with a diet low in phenylalanine and tyrosine as well as with the drug **nitisinone**, a synthetic inhibitor of the upstream enzyme 4-hydroxyphenylpyruvate dioxygenase (see Fig. 35.14) that reduces the concentration of fumarylacetoacetate. Liver transplantation is used for patients who do not respond to nitisinone therapy or who develop liver cancer.

**Tyrosinemia type 2** (**oculocutaneous tyrosinemia, Richner-Hanhart syndrome**) is due to a deficiency of **tyrosine**

**transaminase**, an enzyme that is expressed predominantly in the liver (see Fig. 35.14). This disorder shows autosomal recessive inheritance. It is rare but most common among persons with ancestry in the Mediterranean (especially Italy) or on the Arabian peninsula. Affected persons show intellectual disability (cause unknown), a very high concentration of tyrosine in the blood, deposition of tyrosine crystals in the cornea, and painful hyperkeratosis patches on palms and soles (due to tyrosine crystals and an inflammatory reaction to them). Current treatment is by a low-protein, phenylalanine- and tyrosine-restricted diet.

**Alkaptonuria** is due to a near-complete deficiency of homogentisic acid oxidase (see Fig. 35.14). Alkaptonuria occurs in 1 of about 500,000 people; in Slovakia, the prevalence is ~1 in 20,000 persons. The urine of patients with alkaptonuria sometimes turns black on standing. The cartilage and some tendons of affected patients accumulate black pigment that derives from homogentisic acid; this pigmentation is called **ochronosis**. The pigment has an adverse effect on the mechanical properties of various tissues (Fig. 35.20). Adult patients have debilitating arthritis, degenerative changes in the spine, problems with heart valves, coronary artery calcification, and kidney stones.

## 4.6. Maple Syrup Disease and the Degradation of Branched-Chain Amino Acids

The branched-chain amino acids Val, Leu, and Ile make up about 22% of body protein. All of these amino acids are essential (see Chapter 34).

For degradation, branched-chain amino acids first undergo transamination to form **branched-chain keto acids** (Fig. 35.21). These transamination reactions mostly take place in muscle and adipocytes, and to a lesser extent in the liver. Muscle releases most branched-chain keto acids into the blood.

The liver oxidizes the branched-chain keto acids that are formed inside the liver, as well as most of those that are released by muscle. A single enzyme, **branched-chain keto acid dehydrogenase**, oxidatively decarboxylates the three branched-chain keto acids (see Fig. 35.21). This step is irreversible and constitutes the first committed step in the degradation of branched-chain amino acids.

**Maple syrup disease** (also called maple syrup *urine* disease) is the consequence of a deficiency of branched-chain keto acid dehydrogenase (see Fig. 35.21). This disease is inherited in autosomal recessive fashion. Worldwide, it occurs in ~1 in 200,000 newborns; however, it has a prevalence of ~1 in 200 births among Mennonite communities in the United States. In affected patients, branched-chain amino acids and branched-chain keto acids accumulate in the blood and urine. One of the branched chain keto acids, α-keto-β-methylvalerate (derived from isoleucine) imparts the smell of maple syrup; this smell is noticeable with ear wax and to a lesser extent with urine. The maple syrup smell of ear wax is the earliest specific sign of the disease.

Patients who have the classic (severe) form of maple syrup disease develop an encephalopathy a few days after birth. Without treatment, myelination of the brain is reduced, and patients have mental retardation and premature death. The neuropathology is most closely related to the concentration of leucine in blood. In a setting of hyponatremia, a high concentration of leucine causes cerebral edema and encephalopathy. Leucine is believed to outcompete other amino acids for uptake into cells; as a result, there is a deficit of other amino acids inside cells. However, the exact pathogenesis of the encephalopathy is still a mystery. Patients should be treated by about 3 days of age. The aim of treatment is to normalize the concentration of branched-chain amino acids in the blood and to provide enough protein for growth. The concentration of leucine in the blood is minimized by facilitating the use of leucine in protein synthesis; this can often be achieved with infusions of valine and isoleucine. Since branched-chain amino acids are ubiquitous, patients with maple syrup disease must consume a low amount of regular dietary protein and a supplement of an artificial **amino acid cocktail** that is free of

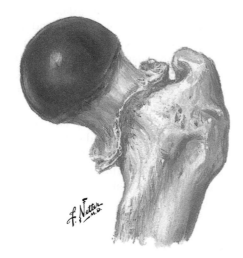

Fig. 35.20   **Ochronosis due to alkaptonuria.**

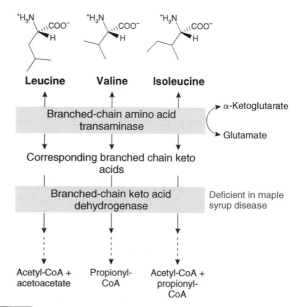

Fig. 35.21   **Degradation of the branched-chain amino acids.**

**Table 35.3** | Nitrogen Balance in Adults

| | In | Out |
|---|---|---|
| **Actual** | N in dietary protein (~100% of all gains) | Urea, NH₃, creatinine, and uric acid in urine (~85% of all losses) <br> Feces and miscellaneous (~15% of all losses) |
| **Estimate** | N in dietary protein (weight of amino acids in g/6.25) | Method I: N as part of urea in urine in g; add 4 g for baseline amount of other N losses <br> Method II: (N as part of urea in urine in g) × 1.25 |

For more information about creatinine, see Section 1.5 in Chapter 23. For more information about uric acid, see Section 2 in Chapter 38. Fig. 35.11 shows the normal ranges of the contributions of urea, NH₃, creatinine, and uric acid to nitrogen losses via the urine.

branched-chain amino acids. Some patients respond favorably to extra **thiamine**, which is a cofactor of branched-chain keto acid dehydrogenase. Illnesses are challenging to manage because of increased degradation of body protein. Patients who are effectively treated show normal physical and mental development. Liver transplantation can normalize the concentrations of branched-chain amino acids in the blood and enable patients to eat a normal amount of protein in their diet.

Newborns can be screened for maple syrup disease by measuring the concentration of leucine (or the ratio of the concentrations of leucine and alanine) or the concentration of alloisoleucine (a diastereomer of leucine) in blood. This screening is commonly performed using chromatography or tandem mass spectrometry.

**Isovaleric acidemia** is caused by a deficiency of **isovaleryl-CoA dehydrogenase** in the pathway for leucine degradation. The disease is inherited in an autosomal recessive fashion and occurs in ~1 in 60,000 births in Germany and ~1 in 250,000 births in the United States. Some affected patients develop encephalopathy and severe acidosis in the newborn period, whereas others show episodes of vomiting, lethargy, coma, and acidosis only later on. These acute attacks are accompanied by hyperammonemia and ketosis. During episodes of major protein catabolism, the concentration of isovaleric acid in blood plasma may rise to as much as 5,000 µM (normal: <10 µM). During these episodes, patients exude an odor of sweaty feet. Isovaleric acidemia is primarily treated with carnitine and glycine supplementation to enhance the conversion of isovaleryl-CoA to isovalerylcarnitine and isovalerylglycine, which are excreted in the urine.

## 5. NITROGEN BALANCE

*Nitrogen balance is the difference between nitrogen intake (in the form of protein) and nitrogen losses (mostly via the urine). If losses exceed intake, the balance is negative. A negative nitrogen balance is seen with starvation and to a much greater extent after delivery of a fetus, during sepsis, after trauma, or days after extensive burns.*

### 5.1. Concept of Nitrogen Balance

Nitrogen balance is defined as nitrogen intake minus nitrogen losses. Table 35.3 provides an overview of individual contribu-

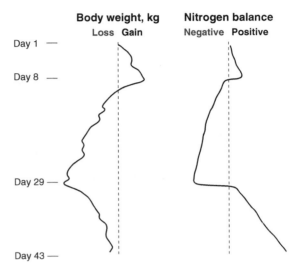

**Fig. 35.22** **Nitrogen balance with weight gain and weight loss.** A total of 32 nonobese men consumed too many or too few calories in a prescribed pattern to change their body weight. Maximum weight loss was ~4 kg, and maximum positive nitrogen balance was ~0.14 g/day. Changes in weight are largely due to changes in the amount of body fat in the form of triglycerides. (Data from Müller MJ, Enderle J, Pourhassan M, et al. Metabolic adaptation to caloric restriction and subsequent refeeding: the Minnesota Starvation Experiment revisited. *Am J Clin Nutr.* 2015;102:807-19.)

tors to the nitrogen balance sheet. In the clinic, *estimates* of nitrogen balance are usually based only on protein intake and loss of urea in urine (see Table 35.3). The nitrogen balance is most commonly measured in patients who receive enteral or parenteral nutrition because they cannot consume regular food. Parenterally fed patients cannot be infused with protein; rather, they are infused with a mixture of purified synthetic amino acids.

The nitrogen balance is normally **positive** in patients who increase the amount of protein in their body as, for example, in growing children and pregnant women. The nitrogen balance is **negative** during acute illness, trauma, sepsis, burns, and malnutrition as well as after delivery of a fetus. As these latter patients improve, they eventually develop a positive nitrogen balance and finally a zero balance when they are fully recovered. Fig. 35.22 illustrates the effects of excess and insufficient food intake on nitrogen balance.

## 5.2. Nitrogen Balance in Health and Illness

Consumption of a diet that is adequate in calories but deficient in protein for a protracted time leads to a major loss of protein mostly from visceral organs, such as the liver. Muscle protein is somewhat spared due to insulin secretion in response to meals. The condition is sometimes called **kwashiorkor** (a term from Ghana that refers to the disease a child gets who is displaced from breastfeeding). An affected person has a markedly protuberant abdomen and some loss of muscle mass. Children who have kwashiorkor often weigh only 60% to 80% of their recommended weight. The protein and amino acid deficit leads to decreased synthesis of proteins in the liver that are secreted into the blood, such as clotting factors, transferrin, and albumin. Hypoalbuminemia leads to edema, particularly of the abdomen. In addition, patients with kwashiorkor develop an enlarged, fatty liver due to inadequate synthesis of apoprotein B-100 for VLDL particles, which leads to retention of triglycerides. Low concentrations of albumin and transferrin (measured as total iron-binding capacity) in the blood can be used as indicators of protein depletion in visceral organs. Finally, persons who have kwashiorkor also develop atrophy of the villi and microvilli of the small intestine, leading to disaccharidase deficiency, impaired carbohydrate uptake, and diarrhea (see Chapter 18).

In persons who have a combined deficiency of calories and protein, there is a marked loss of muscle and fat mass, usually without a protuberant abdomen. This condition is often called **protein-energy malnutrition**. Protein loss is marked in both skeletal and cardiac muscle, whereas the visceral organs are somewhat spared. Muscle protein is degraded to support gluconeogenesis. The concentration of albumin in the blood is normal or nearly normal. However, affected persons are often anemic, and they are readily infected because they are immune deficient.

In Western countries, about 0.5% of all young women have **anorexia nervosa** (Fig. 35.23), a disease that is characterized by very low body weight. In the United States, a body mass index (BMI) of 16 to 17 kg/m² is indicative of moderate anorexia and one of 15 to 16 kg/m² is indicative of severe anorexia. The low BMI is the result of pathologically restricted food intake and often also excessive exercise. The disease is rare among men. Anorexia nervosa is an example of protein-energy malnutrition. Some patients have anemia and leukopenia. About 10% of affected patients die of the disease, often due to complications of a decreased mass of the heart.

**Cachexia** is an illness-induced loss of body weight in an individual who has access to food and is not trying to lose weight. Diagnostic signs include unexplained recent weight loss in excess of 5%, or a BMI less than 20 to 22 kg/m² (depending on age). There is wasting of both skeletal muscle and adipose tissue. The wasting is a result of a combination of decreased food intake and increased degradation of body protein due to an elevated concentration of **cytokines** in the blood. The cytokines (e.g., interleukins-1 and -2, interferon-γ, tumor necrosis factor-α) stimulate proteasome-mediated **proteolysis** of muscle protein (see Section 1).

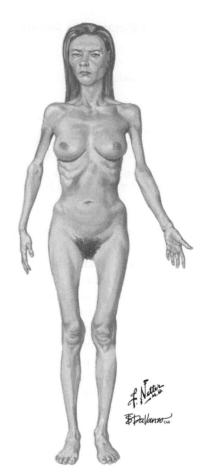

**Fig. 35.23** **Anorexia nervosa, an example of protein-energy malnutrition.**

Cachexia is most commonly seen in patients who have a malignancy, a chronic inflammatory condition, or a degenerative disease; examples are chronic obstructive pulmonary disease; heart failure; acquired immunodeficiency syndrome; or cancer of the pancreas, stomach, colon, or lungs (Fig. 35.24). Cachexia is marked by general weakness, anemia, and a low concentration of albumin in blood plasma. Cachectic patients are immune deficient (a general feature of malnutrition) and commonly die of pneumonia.

Patients who have extensive **burns** (Fig. 35.25) exhibit some of the highest rates of proteolysis seen in hospitalized patients. For example, burns affecting about two-thirds of the body surface area double the basic energy expenditure and almost double the rate of degradation of muscle protein. Some of the resulting amino acids are used within muscle for resynthesis of protein and some are transported to other tissues for wound healing. In wounds, protein synthesis far exceeds protein degradation. While a healthy individual needs about 0.8 to 1.0 g of protein per kilogram of body weight per day to achieve zero nitrogen balance, patients with appreciable burns need about 2.0 to 2.5 g of protein per kilogram body weight per day. Provision of a relatively large amount of protein and calories to patients with burns greatly improves their rate of recovery. Estimates of nitrogen balance are routinely used to

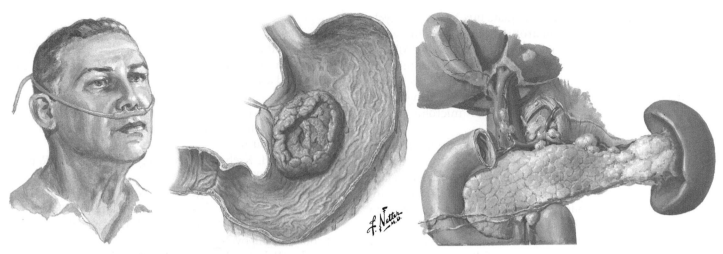

**Fig. 35.24** Some conditions often associated with cachexia: chronic obstructive pulmonary disease, cancer of the stomach, and cancer of the pancreas.

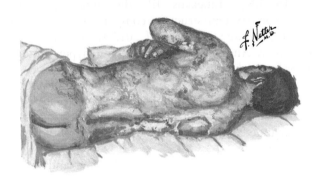

**Fig. 35.25** Extensive burn injuries are associated with a very high rate of nitrogen loss.

guide nutrition during their hospital stay. Increased degradation of muscle protein in patients with burns is in part due to elevated concentrations of cortisol and cytokines.

After major burns or moderate to severe traumatic brain injury, it takes months for the basal rate of metabolism to return to normal.

## SUMMARY

- Proteasomes recognize proteins that are conjugated with 4 or more ubiquitin polypeptides (linked via Lys-48) and degrade them into short peptides, thereby liberating ubiquitin for reuse. Peptidases in the cell then degrade the peptides into amino acids. The concentrations of leucine, insulin, cortisol, and various cytokines (Il-1, IL-1, IFγ, and TNF-α) determine the overall rate of protein degradation in proteasomes. Within cells, the lifetime of proteins depends in part on the N-terminal amino acid sequence, the presence of a PEST motif, protein conformation, and posttranslational modifications.

- Aberrant ubiquitination is caused by altered E6AP ubiquitin-protein ligase activity following papilloma virus infection and also in patients who have Angelman syn-

drome, by mutant von Hippel Lindau (VHL)-factor in VHL disease and in many clear-cell renal carcinomas, and by altered ubiquitin E3 ligase activity of parkin in a form of hereditary Parkinson disease.

- Lysosomes have an acidic pH; cathepsins inside lysosomes degrade proteins in acquired extracellular material and in intracellular material obtained via autophagy.

- Degradation of amino acids requires disposal of nitrogen. This disposal occurs primarily via excretion of urea and secondarily via excretion of $NH_4^+$ into the urine. The full urea cycle is present in the liver, and portions of it are present in the intestine and in the kidneys. The urea cycle converts $NH_4^+$ and the nitrogen from aspartate into urea. The $NH_4^+$ stems mostly from the deamination of Gln and Glu. Almost all amino acids can participate in transamination, thereby giving rise to glutamate, glutamine, and aspartate. Transaminases (aminotransferases) that catalyze these reactions use pyridoxal phosphate as a cofactor and temporary acceptor of an amino group.

- Nitrogen is transported between tissues primarily in the form of glutamine and alanine. Muscle mainly releases alanine and glutamine. The intestine converts glutamine to alanine and citrulline. The kidneys convert citrulline to arginine. The liver uses alanine and some of the arginine. Ammonia is toxic and normally is present in blood at concentrations well below 0.1 mM.

- Periportal hepatocytes convert ammonia (principally $NH_4^+$) to urea, and perivenous hepatocytes incorporate any remaining ammonia into glutamate, thereby forming nontoxic glutamine, which they release. For this reason, hyperglutaminemia precedes and accompanies hyperammonemia. The concentrations in the blood of glutamine and ammonia are not measured routinely. However, respiratory alkalosis is an early sign of hyperammonemia, and abnormal cognition (or even coma) is seen at higher concentrations of ammonia.

- Patients who have severe liver disease may develop hepatic encephalopathy, which is accompanied by hyperammonemia due to inadequate flux in the urea cycle. Besides ammonia, other neurotoxic substances likely play a role in the pathogenesis of the encephalopathy. Affected patients can be treated with the disaccharides lactulose or lactitol or with the antibiotic rifaximin to decrease the concentration of ammonia in the blood via a change in gut pH and an effect on metabolism of microbes in the intestine.

- Some patients have hyperammonemia due to an inherited deficiency of an enzyme of the urea cycle. The deficiency may cause symptoms a few days after birth or later, such as after a high-protein meal, during an extended fast, during illness or sepsis, or following major trauma or burns. Many women who are heterozygous for a deficient allele of the X-linked ornithine carbamoyltransferase develop their first episode of severe hyperammonemia following delivery of a fetus. The more severely affected patients with a urea cycle deficiency have to chronically limit protein intake and take oral phenylbutyrate daily to remove nitrogen as phenylacetyl glutamine.

- Treatment options for patients who are hospitalized due to hyperammonemia include dialysis and treatment with IV phenylacetate and benzoate to remove nitrogen by conjugation with glutamine and glycine.

- Classic phenylketonuria is due to homozygosity for deficient phenylalanine hydroxylase, which can be detected by newborn screening. Treatment with a low-phenylalanine diet prevents intellectual disability caused by altered amino acid transport into the brain. All phenylketonuria patients should be tested for a deficiency of tetrahydrobiopterin production.

- Maple syrup disease is due to homozygosity for deficient branched-chain keto acid dehydrogenase, which can be detected by newborn screening. Treatment with a low leucine diet reduces intellectual disability from altered amino acid transport into the brain.

- Oculocutaneous albinism can be caused by mutant tyrosinase, OCA2 protein, or tyrosinase-related protein 1, all of which impair melanin production and lead to impaired clarity of vision.

- Vitiligo is an inflammatory disease that leads to patchy loss of melanocytes in the skin.

- Patients with tyrosinemia type 1 accumulate the mutagen fumarylacetate and have a very high risk of developing hepatocellular carcinoma. Treatment with nitisinone inhibits an upstream enzyme and thereby reduces the formation of fumarylacetate.

- Alkaptonuria is due to a deficiency of homogentisic acid oxidase that causes ochronosis and debilitating joint pain in adults.

- The nitrogen balance is positive when there is a net gain of body protein.

- A prolonged, severe deficiency of protein in the diet can lead to impaired protein synthesis, edema, and immune deficiency.

- The rate of protein degradation is particularly high after delivery of a baby and after major burns.

## FURTHER READING

- Centerwall SA, Centerwall WR. The discovery of phenylketonuria: the story of a young couple, two retarded children, and a scientist. *Pediatrics.* 2000;105:89-103. This is an excellent account of the relevant history.
- Hooley E. PKU and me. *Arch Dis Child.* 2006;91:711, This is a brief first-hand account of a 13-year-old with phenylketonuria.
- Kornberg H. Krebs and his trinity of cycles. *Nat Rev Mol Cell Biol.* 2000;1:225-228.
- Strauss KA, Puffenberger EG, Morton DH. Maple syrup urine disease. In: Pagon RA, Adam MP, Ardinger HH, et al, editors. *GeneReviews.* 2006. Available at www.ncbi.nlm.nih.gov/NBK1319/.
- Tomko RJ Jr, Hochstrasser M. Molecular architecture and assembly of the eukaryotic proteasome. *Annu Rev Biochem.* 2013;82:415-445.
- Tsakiri EN, Trougakos IP. The amazing ubiquitin-proteasome system: structural components and implication in aging. *Int Rev Cell Mol Biol.* 2015;314:171-237.
- Walker V. Ammonia metabolism and hyperammonemic disorders. *Adv Clin Chem.* 2014;67:73-150.
- Weetch E, Macdonald A. The determination of phenylalanine content of foods suitable for phenylketonuria. *J Hum Nutr Dietetics.* 2006;19:229-236. This publication contains an expanded list of the phenylalanine content of fruits and vegetables.
- Weiner ID, Mitch WE, Sands JM. Urea and ammonia metabolism and the control of renal nitrogen excretion. *Clin J Am Soc Nephrol.* 2015;10:1444-1458.

# Review Questions

1. A 3-day-old boy was in the intensive care unit and received mechanical ventilation. Analysis of his blood revealed the following:

| | |
|---|---|
| Ammonia | 3,500 µM (normal: 0–59 µM) |
| Glutamine | 6,400 µM (normal: 420–705 µM) |
| Citrulline | 0 µM (normal: 17–43 µM) |
| Ornithine | 1,100 µM (normal: 8–26 µM) |

Analysis of his urine revealed the following:

Orotate  1,700 µmol/g creatinine (normal: 8–26 µmol/g creatinine)

This boy most likely has a deficiency of which one of the following enzymes?

A. Argininosuccinate lyase
B. Argininosuccinate synthase
C. Carbamoyl-phosphate synthase I
D. N-Acetylglutamate synthase
E. Ornithine carbamoyltransferase

2. A 34-year-old morbidly obese woman underwent a gastric bypass procedure. During the ensuing 8 months, she was almost continuously hospitalized for various medical problems. Her presurgery weight was 400 lb; 8 months after surgery she weighed 160 lb. At the current admission, she displayed uncontrolled status epilepticus. The concentration of ammonia in her serum was 440 μM (normal: 20–50 μM). Appropriate acute treatment of this patient is which of the following?

   **A.** Hemodialysis, IV citrulline
   **B.** Hemodialysis, IV phenylacetate and benzoate
   **C.** IV essential amino acids, IV phenylbutyrate
   **D.** IV glutamate, IV ornithine
   **E.** Total parenteral nutrition

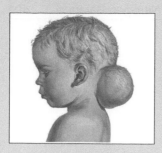

## Chapter 36

# One-Carbon Metabolism, Folate Deficiency, and Cobalamin Deficiency

## SYNOPSIS

- One-carbon metabolism refers to reactions that involve one-carbon groups such as methyl-, methylene, methenyl, and formyl groups. These groups can be carried by tetrahydrofolic acid, which is derived from folic acid, a vitamin.
- Tetrahydrofolic acid is required for the detoxification of methanol.
- Folate-linked one-carbon metabolism feeds one-carbon groups into the synthesis of purine and pyrimidine nucleotides as well as into the activated methyl group cycle.
- The activated methyl group cycle uses S-adenosylmethionine as a methyl group donor in the synthesis of creatine and catecholamines, as well as in the methylation of DNA, RNA, lysine side chains, and arginine side chains. The activated methyl group cycle can drain into the transsulfuration pathway, yielding cysteine.
- Patients with a folate deficiency have impaired thymine nucleotide synthesis and hence impaired DNA replication; this causes diarrhea and megaloblastic anemia.
- Cobalamin (derived from vitamin $B_{12}$) is needed for the transfer of a methyl group from tetrahydrofolates to the activated methyl group cycle. Patients with a cobalamin deficiency may show the same symptoms as those with a primary folate deficiency. In addition, they have impaired peripheral nerve conduction and suffer damage to the central nervous system.
- Cobalamin is also needed for converting propionyl-CoA to succinyl-CoA (an intermediate of the citric acid cycle). Patients with a cobalamin deficiency cannot properly convert propionyl-CoA to succinyl-CoA and thus have an increased concentration of methylmalonic acid in their blood and urine. This is used clinically to distinguish between a primary folate deficiency and a secondary folate deficiency caused by cobalamin deficiency.

## LEARNING OBJECTIVES

*For mastery of this topic, you should be able to do the following:*
- Define folates and list folate-rich foods.
- Describe the absorption of folates in the intestine and the transport to peripheral tissues.
- Describe the body's use of folates.
- Describe the pathobiochemistry and treatment of methanol poisoning.
- List cobalamin-rich foods.
- Describe the absorption of cobalamin.
- Describe the enzyme-catalyzed reactions that require cobalamin.
- Describe the synthesis of S-adenosylmethionine and its role in methylation reactions.
- Explain how a cobalamin deficiency can lead to a secondary folate deficiency.
- Interpret laboratory data (e.g., serum folic acid, cobalamin, and methylmalonic acid) to distinguish between a primary and a secondary folate deficiency.

- Select laboratory tests that contribute to a diagnosis of pernicious anemia.
- Explain the treatment of folate deficiency and cobalamin deficiency.

## 1. SOURCES AND ABSORPTION OF DIETARY FOLATES

*The human body cannot synthesize folic acid. Folic acid is a vitamin that gives rise to tetrahydrofolic acid, which can carry a one-carbon group, such as a methyl group. Folic acid and its derivatives are found primarily in legumes, green leafy vegetables, and grains. The intestine releases mostly $N^5$-methyl-tetrahydrofolic acid into the blood.*

### 1.1. Structure of Folates

**Folic acid**, sometimes called **vitamin $B_9$**, is absorbed and then reduced to **dihydrofolic acid** (**DHF**) and finally **tetrahydrofolic acid** (**THF**; Fig. 36.1 and Section 1.2).

Tetrahydrofolates can carry a methyl ($-CH_3$), methylene ($-CH_2-$), methenyl (also called methylidene; $=CH-$), formyl ($-CH=O$), or formimino group ($-CH=NH$; see Fig. 36.1). Inside peripheral cells, tetrahydrofolate **monoglutamates** can be extended with glutamate to produce tetrahydrofolate **polyglutamates**.

The term **folates** customarily includes all folate compounds regardless of one-carbon group or number of glutamate residues. Folates are present in the body only in sub-$\mu$M concentrations.

### 1.2. Absorption of Folates in the Intestine and Transport in the Blood

Folates are contained in grains, citrus fruit, legumes, and green leafy vegetables (Table 36.1).

Folic acid is commonly used in supplements and food fortification. Natural foods mostly contain folates other than folic acid, principally $N^5$-methyl-tetrahydrofolate. Through oxidation and enzymatic deconjugation (i.e., removal of the polyglutamate tail) by glutamate carboxypeptidase II in the intestine, these folates give rise to folic acid monoglutamate.

The intestine takes up supplementary folic acid about twice as efficiently as natural folates. The main reasons for this difference appear to be the enclosure of natural folates inside cells and the longer polyglutamate tail of natural folates that has to be removed before uptake. The measure **"dietary folate equivalents"** (**DFE**) was introduced to account for differences in the

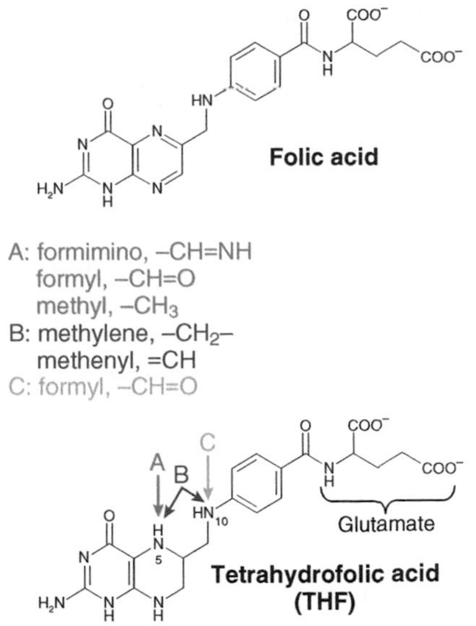

**Fig. 36.1** **Folic acid and tetrahydrofolates.** THF carries one-carbon groups at $N^5$, $N^{10}$, or both $N^5$ and $N^{10}$. Inside cells, THF mostly has a polyglutamate tail; here, only one glutamate residue is shown.

**Table 36.1** **Folate Content of Various Foods**

| Food | Folates ($\mu$g/100 g Edible Portion) |
|---|---|
| Lentils | 181 |
| Asparagus | 147 |
| Spinach | 146 |
| Bread, white, fortified* | 140 |
| Pasta, cooked, fortified* | 120 |
| Broccoli | 50 |
| Peas | 32 |
| Orange juice | 30 |
| Ground beef | 11 |
| Potato, boiled | 9 |
| Milk | 5 |
| Ice cream | 5 |
| Apple | 3 |

*In the United States and Canada, enriched cereal grain products must be fortified with folic acid.

efficiency of uptake: 1 $\mu$g of *natural folates* in food is worth 1 $\mu$g of DFE, and 1 $\mu$g of *supplemental folic acid* is worth 1.7 $\mu$g of DFE if taken with food but 2 $\mu$g of DFE if taken on an empty stomach.

The recommended daily folate allowance for healthy children 1 to 3 years old is 150 $\mu$g of DFE, for people 14 years of age and older it is 400 $\mu$g of DFE, and for pregnant women it is 600 $\mu$g of DFE. Patients who have increased tissue turnover (e.g., due to chronic **hemolytic disease**) need more folates than the recommended dietary amount.

The Food and Nutrition Board of the Institute of Medicine in the United States recommends that adults not take more than 1,000 $\mu$g of *supplemental* folic acid per day. The intake of folates from the *diet* is not limited. The major concern over a high intake of folic acid is that it may allow a cobalamin-deficient patient to not develop megaloblastic anemia, to not seek medical attention, and then unknowingly experience slowly progressive nerve damage (see Section 7.2 below).

Most **folate absorption** occurs in the duodenum and jejunum via the **proton-coupled folate transporter** (**PCFT**, **SLC46A1**). Folates produced by bacteria in the colon are also absorbed but correspond to only about 10% of the folate absorption in the small intestine if the diet contains adequate folates.

Patients who have **hereditary folate deficiency** are homozygous or compound heterozygous for a nonfunctional PCFT. The PCFT transports folates both from the lumen of the intestine into the epithelium and from the blood into the central nervous system. Accordingly, the serum and spinal fluid of affected patients have an abnormally low folate concentration. Without supplementary folate treatment, the defect causes severe anemia, as well as abnormal development of the brain, which may be associated with seizures. The disease is very rare.

Inside enterocytes, dihydrofolate reductase reduces folic acid first to **dihydrofolic acid** (**DHF**) and then to **THF**. THF is methylated to form $N^5,N^{10}$-**methylene-THF**, which is reduced to $N^5$-methyl-THF (Fig. 36.2). The intestinal epithelial cells then release $N^5$-methyl-THF into the bloodstream.

Efflux of folate from intestinal epithelial cells into the extracellular space and blood is at least partially mediated by **multidrug resistance-associated proteins** (**MRPs**).

In the bloodstream, about half of the $N^5$-methyl-THF is free; the rest is bound to albumin or a **soluble folate receptor** (see Fig. 36.2). Protein binding of folates reduces losses of folates by filtration in the kidneys. The proximal tubules in the kidneys express transport systems and receptors for the reuptake of free folates, albumin, and folate-binding protein.

The uptake of folates into peripheral cells occurs via the **reduced folate carrier** (**RFC**), also called **SLC19A1**. The RFC has a higher affinity for reduced folates, such as $N^5$-methyl-THF, than for folic acid. RFC transports folates into cells, probably in exchange for transporting organic phosphates into the extracellular space. Both thiamine phosphate and thiamine pyrophosphate can exit cells via the RFC (thiamine enters cells through other transporters, SLC19A2, and SLC19A3). The PCFT facilitates the transfer of folates from the blood to the central nervous system. Membrane-bound **folate receptors** (FR$\alpha$ and FR$\beta$), which contain a glycosyl phosphatidyl inositol anchor and are endocytosed, are used for some of the folate uptake by hematopoietic cells, macrophages, and epithelial cells in the kidneys.

Endocytosis of a folate receptor is followed by the release of $N^5$-methyl-THF in endosomes. Cells liberate THF from

$N^5$-methyl-THF in a single step of the activated methyl group pathway.

Most **antifolate drugs**, which resemble folates but oppose their effects, are transported by the PCFT and/or the RFC. Antifolates are used against tumors and certain autoimmune diseases. Examples are **methotrexate** and **pemetrexed** (see Chapter 37).

A **tetrahydrofolate synthase** (also called **folylpolyglutamate synthase**) adds glutamate residues to THF

monoglutamate. Compared with folyl*mono*glutamates, folyl*poly*glutamates are less likely lost from cells by diffusion (owing to increased charge), less likely transported out of the cell by membrane transporters, and have a greater affinity to many of the enzymes that are involved in folate metabolism.

Folates are **stored** in the liver and the kidneys.

Several drugs have an adverse effect on folate uptake or cellular folate content. The antifolate **methotrexate**, which is used in the treatment of rheumatoid arthritis and moderate to severe psoriasis, traps cellular folates as dihydrofolates (see Chapter 37). The antibiotic **trimethoprim** and the antimalarial **pyrimethamine** inhibit the dihydrofolate reductase of humans less than that of bacteria, plasmodia, or *Toxoplasma gondii*. These drugs are contraindicated in patients who are anemic due to a folate deficiency, and they are used cautiously in patients who are at risk of folate deficiency. Many antiepileptic drugs (e.g., **phenytoin**, **phenobarbital**) lead to low folate status, and patients treated with these drugs often need supplemental folate. Supplementation is especially important in women of child-bearing age (see neural tube defects in Section 8.1).

## 2. LOADING TETRAHYDROFOLATES WITH ONE-CARBON GROUPS

*Serine and glycine are the main sources of one-carbon groups that are added to THF, giving rise to $N^5,N^{10}$-methylene-THF. $N^5,N^{10}$-methylene-THF in turn can give rise to other one-carbon THFs. The detoxification of methanol yields formate (HCOO⁻), which is toxic and must form $N^{10}$-formyl-THF before it can be disposed of as $CO_2$. $N^5$-formyl-THF, also called leucovorin, is an injectable folate that rapidly becomes part of the pool of one-carbon tetrahydrofolates.*

### 2.1. Glycine and Serine as Sources of One-Carbon Groups

Fig. 36.3 provides an overview of the reactions that *add* one-carbon groups to THFs.

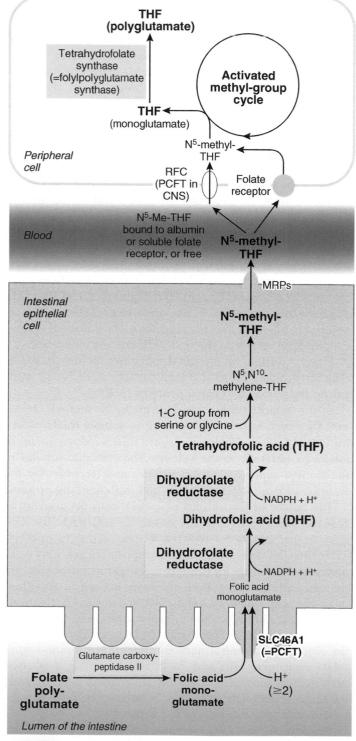

Fig. 36.2 **Uptake of folates into the intestine and transport to peripheral tissues (bottom to top).**

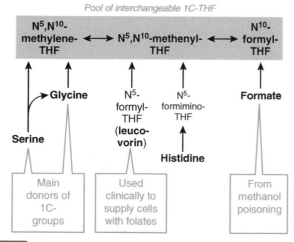

Fig. 36.3 **Overview of reactions that donate one-carbon groups to tetrahydrofolic acid.**

The majority of one-carbon groups loaded onto THF stems from **serine**, and a lesser amount from **glycine** (see Fig. 36.3). There is a limitless supply of serine because serine can readily be made de novo from an intermediate of glycolysis/gluconeogenesis (see Figs 19.11 and. 34.11). Removal of a one-carbon group from serine yields glycine. Glycine can also donate a one-carbon group to THF. For example, when intestinal enterocytes take up folic acid and export $N^5$-methyl-THF as discussed above (see Section 1.2 and Fig. 36.2), the one-carbon groups stem chiefly from serine and glycine.

## 2.2. Other Sources of One-Carbon Groups and Folates

Minor amounts of one-carbon groups on THF normally arise from the degradation of **formic acid** and **histidine**. The degradation of **formic acid** plays a crucial role in methanol detoxification (see Section 3.4). The degradation of **histidine** yields formiminoglutamate, which forms $N^5$-formimino-THF and glutamate (see Fig. 36.3).

Several one-carbon group–containing folates can readily be converted to other one-carbon group–containing folates (Fig. 36.4). The three folates $N^5,N^{10}$-methylene-THF, $N^5,N^{10}$-methenyl-THF, and $N^{10}$-formyl-THF form a pool of reversibly convertible folates. In an irreversible reaction, $N^5,N^{10}$-methylene-THF from this pool gives rise to $N^5$-methyl-THF; this reaction is important in understanding the induction of a secondary folate deficiency by a cobalamin deficiency (see Section 7.2).

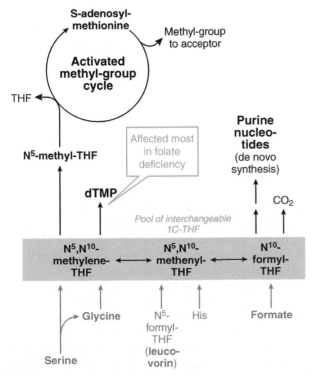

**Fig. 36.4** **Overview of the use of one-carbon groups from folates.**

## 3. USE OF ONE-CARBON GROUPS ON TETRAHYDROFOLATES

*Physiologically, most one-carbon groups are used for the synthesis of purine nucleotides (chiefly adenosine triphosphate) and the pyrimidine nucleotide deoxythymidine triphosphate. A lesser amount of one-carbon groups is fed into the activated methyl group cycle. $N^{10}$-formyl-THF can release its one-carbon group as $CO_2$; this plays a role in the detoxification of methanol.*

### 3.1. Overview

Fig. 36.4 provides an overview of the reactions that *use* one-carbon groups from folates.

$N^{10}$-formyl-THF can give off its one-carbon group as $CO_2$ (see Fig. 36.4). This reaction can be viewed as a way to bleed excess one-carbon groups from a pool of one-carbon-THF compounds. This reaction becomes important in the detoxification of methanol (see 3.4).

### 3.2. Synthesis of Inosine Monophosphate and Deoxythymidine Monophosphate

The major use of one-carbon groups is in the synthesis of inosine monophosphate (**IMP**), a precursor for the **purine nucleotides** adenosine monophosphate (AMP) and guanosine monophosphate (GMP; see Fig. 36.4 and Chapter 38). However, a dietary folate deficiency (see Section 7.1) does not impair this pathway to a medically relevant extent.

One-carbon groups are also used for the synthesis of **thymidine** monophosphate (deoxythymidine monophosphate, dTMP; see Chapter 37). The synthesis of dTMP is impaired in folate-deficient and in cobalamin-deficient patients (see Section 7), as well as in patients who receive chemotherapy with certain antifolates. The synthesis of dTMP is unique in that it produces dihydrofolate, which has to be reduced to tetrahydrofolate before it can carry a one-carbon group. Chemotherapy of tumors exploits this situation as well as the dTMP need of fast-growing cells.

### 3.3. Transfer of Methyl Groups to the Activated Methyl Group Cycle

For most methylation reactions, the methyl group on $N^5$-methyl-THF is not sufficiently reactive. The methyl group of $N^5$-methyl-THF is transferred into the activated methyl group cycle. There, S-adenosyl-methionine carries a much more reactive methyl group (see Section 4).

### 3.4. Detoxification of Methanol

The basic reactions of oxidizing **methanol** to the corresponding aldehyde and acid are similar to those of the degradation of ethanol (Fig. 36.5; see also Chapter 30).

**Methanol poisoning** leads to a transient high concentration of **formate** in cells and blood (see Fig. 36.5). Catalyzing

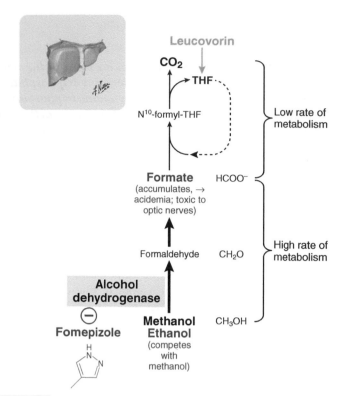

**Fig. 36.5** **Detoxification of methanol.** Fomepizole or ethanol, as well as leucovorin, may be a part of treatment.

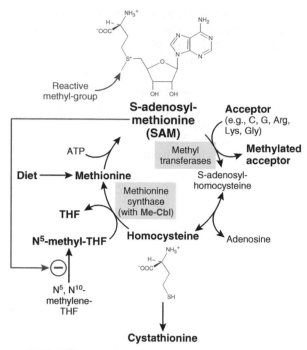

**Fig. 36.6** **The activated methyl group cycle.**

sequential reactions, alcohol dehydrogenase, and formaldehyde dehydrogenase oxidize methanol to formate at a high rate. However, formate reacts with folates only at a comparatively low rate. Thus, formate can accumulate to millimolar concentrations; this leads to acidosis and damage to the optic nerve (mechanism unknown).

In the treatment of methanol poisoning, it is important to prevent the concentration of formate in the blood from rising into the toxic range. Soon after ingestion, gastrointestinal lavage can diminish the absorption of methanol. Conversion of methanol to formate can be slowed either with **ethanol** (which competes with methanol as a substrate of alcohol dehydrogenase) or with **fomepizole** (which inhibits alcohol dehydrogenase and is also used in the treatment of **ethylene glycol poisoning**; ethylene glycol is used in cars to prevent freezing or cooling of water). Patients can be injected with **leucovorin** (also called folinic acid, $N^5$-formyl-THF) to ensure an optimal concentration of folates for removing formate.

## 4. THE ACTIVATED METHYL GROUP CYCLE

*The activated methyl group cycle produces S-adenosylmethionine, which is used for a large number of methylation reactions that involve DNA, RNA, or proteins. In addition, S-adenosylmethionine is used for the synthesis of creatine, epinephrine, and phosphatidylcholine.*

### 4.1. Reactions of the Activated Methyl Group Cycle

The activated methyl group cycle is found in most cells, but it is most active in the liver, kidneys, intestine, and pancreas.

The activated methyl group cycle produces **S-adenosylmethionine** (**SAM**), which can donate a methyl group for methylation reactions (Fig. 36.6). Demethylation of SAM yields S-adenosylhomocysteine, which is nearly in equilibrium with **homocysteine**. On average, **methionine synthase** remethylates about half of the homocysteine to methionine, whereas the other half is converted to cystathionine and thus enters the transsulfuration pathway (see Section 9). After a high-protein meal, more homocysteine enters the transsulfuration pathway, whereas in the fasting state, more homocysteine stays in the activated methyl group cycle. Methionine synthase activity depends on two vitamins: $N^5$-**methyl-THF** and **cobalamin**.

In the liver and the brain, homocysteine can also be methylated to methionine by a second reaction catalyzed by **betaine-homocysteine S-methyltransferase**. This reaction uses **glycine betaine** (=trimethylglycine, $(CH_3)_3N^+-CH_2-COO^-$) as a one-carbon group donor. The reaction does not depend on either folates or cobalamin.

The concentration of SAM is regulated. If the concentration of SAM is low, there is increased conversion of $N^5$-$N^{10}$-methylene-THF to $N^5$-methyl-THF (see Fig. 36.6), which can then give rise to more SAM. If the concentration of SAM in the liver is high, SAM stimulates glycine N-methyltransferase, which methylates **glycine** to **sarcosine**. Sarcosine dehydrogenase then demethylates sarcosine to yield glycine and

$N^5,N^{10}$-methylene-THF. This net transfer of a one-carbon group from the activated methyl group cycle to the THF pool also becomes active when there is an **excess of methionine in the diet.**

A buildup of S-adenosylhomocysteine product inhibits the activity of many SAM-dependent methyltransferases.

## 4.2. Use of Methyl Groups From the Activated Methyl Group Cycle

SAM is used in the biosynthesis of creatine, phosphatidylcholine, plasmenylcholine, and epinephrine; it is also used to methylate DNA, RNA, and proteins.

In muscle, the **phosphocreatine**/creatine pair participates in moving high-energy phosphate compounds from the site of ATP production in the mitochondria to the site of ATP consumption by the contractile machinery (see Fig. 23.5). In the brain, creatine phosphate presumably serves mostly as a reservoir of high-energy phosphate groups during periods of impaired ATP production.

Phosphocreatine spontaneously and irreversibly cyclizes to **creatinine** (Fig. 23.6), which is lost in the urine. On average, an adult excretes about 500 mg of creatinine per day (see Fig. 35.11). This requires de novo synthesis of creatine.

The synthesis of **creatine** requires the transfer of a methyl group from SAM to guanidino acetate. This reaction uses about half of all SAM. The liver releases creatine into the bloodstream; brain and muscles pick it up from there.

Creatine in the *diet* also reaches the bloodstream and is taken up into muscle. Some people consume a daily **supplement** of creatine in an effort to improve their physical performance. Creatine supplements may benefit patients with

neurologic disorders that are caused by impaired energy production.

After the synthesis of creatine, the synthesis of **phosphatidylcholine** and **plasmenylcholine** requires the second-highest daily amount of SAM. SAM is used to methylate phosphatidylethanolamine threefold to produce **phosphatidylcholine** and, similarly, plasmenylethanolamine to produce **plasmenylcholine** (see Figs. 11.1 and 11.2).

The synthesis of **epinephrine** from norepinephrine also requires a methyl group from SAM (see Fig. 35.14).

**DNA** contains methyl cytosine (Fig. 36.7; see also Fig. 1.1). The methylation of cytosine occurs to inactivate retrotransposons (a class of movable genetic elements), the second X chromosome in females, imprinted regions of the genome (to silence select maternal or paternal genes; see Chapter 5), and gene expression at various stages of development (see Chapter 6).

The 5′-ends of **mRNAs** contain a **7-methyl-guanosine** cap (see Fig. 36.7; also see Fig. 6.8), while the 5′-ends of some tRNAs and snRNAs in the spliceosomes contain a **trimethyl-guanosine** cap.

**Proteins** (e.g., histones; see Chapter 6) can be methylated on **lysine** or **arginine** side chains (see Fig. 36.7). The amino group of the side chain of lysine residues can be methylated up to threefold, and the guanidino group of the side chain of arginine residues up to twofold (yielding up to three different isomers).

## 5. ABSORPTION OF COBALAMIN

*We take in generous amounts of cobalamin when we eat meats, fowl, fish, or dairy. The stomach secretes intrinsic*

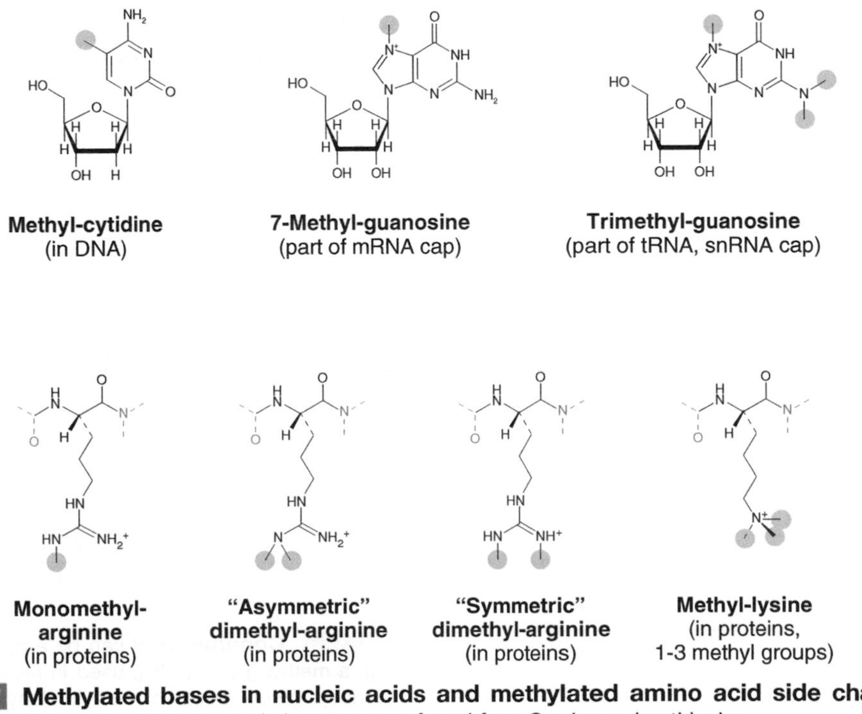

**Methyl-cytidine**
(in DNA)

**7-Methyl-guanosine**
(part of mRNA cap)

**Trimethyl-guanosine**
(part of tRNA, snRNA cap)

**Monomethyl-arginine**
(in proteins)

**"Asymmetric" dimethyl-arginine**
(in proteins)

**"Symmetric" dimethyl-arginine**
(in proteins)

**Methyl-lysine**
(in proteins, 1-3 methyl groups)

**Fig. 36.7** **Methylated bases in nucleic acids and methylated amino acid side chains in proteins.** Pink circles highlight methyl groups transferred from S-adenosylmethionine.

*factor, and an intrinsic factor-cobalamin complex is taken up after binding to the cubam receptor in the distal portion of the ileum. The ileum then secretes a complex of cobalamin and transcobalamin II into the blood.*

Cobalamin is a vitamin principally acquired from eating foods that are derived from animals. Only bacteria can make cobalamin; animals acquire their cobalamin from bacteria. Table 36.2 states the cobalamin content of various foods.

The U.S. Institute of Medicine **recommended daily allowance** of cobalamin for people aged 14 years or older is 2.4 μg; for pregnant and breastfeeding women it is 2.6 and 2.8 μg, respectively. No tolerable upper intake level for cobalamin is set because no adverse effects have been reported in healthy persons. Since there is a high prevalence of maldigestion among older adults, the Institute further recommends that **adults older than 50 years** receive the recommended amount of cobalamin mainly from fortified foods or cobalamin supplements.

Because of their diet, strict **vegans** need to take a supplement of cobalamin; this is especially important for pregnant women and nursing mothers to avoid cobalamin deficiency in their infants (see also Section 7.2).

The structure of cobalamin is shown in Fig. 36.8. Cobalamin contains a substituted corrin ring with a cobalt ($Co^{3+}$) ion in its midst. This $Co^{3+}$ can bind to a methyl, 5′-deoxyadenosyl, hydroxyl, or cyano group. Cyanocobalamin is also called **vitamin $B_{12}$**. Cyanocobalamin is the most commonly used form of cobalamin in fortified foods and vitamin supplements. The human body converts cyanocobalamin to the cofactors methylcobalamin and 5′-deoxyadenosylcobalamin (see below).

Efficient uptake of cobalamin requires a stomach that secretes acid, pepsin, and intrinsic factor; a pancreas that

secretes proteases; and an ileum that expresses cubam. As a low pH and proteases in the stomach free dietary cobalamin from the food matrix, **haptocorrin**, secreted by salivary glands and the gastric mucosa, binds to cobalamin. Parietal cells in the stomach secrete **intrinsic factor**. In the small intestine, as chyme reaches a near-neutral pH, proteases from the pancreas degrade haptocorrin, and cobalamin leaves haptocorrin and instead binds to intrinsic factor (shown in abbreviated form in Fig. 36.9). In the terminal portion of the ileum, the intrinsic factor-cobalamin complex binds to **cubam** (a heterodimer of **cubilin** and **amnionless**); this binding requires $Ca^{2+}$, which is normally supplied by the pancreas. The cubam-intrinsic factor-cobalamin complex is taken up via endocytosis. In the lysosomes, proteolysis of the complex liberates cobalamin, which then binds to **transcobalamin** II, a protein. Cubam is also liberated and recycled to the plasma membrane. Intrinsic factor is degraded.

Cubam is also expressed in the proximal tubules of the **kidneys** for the reabsorption of multiple proteins. Cubilin in cubam has multiple different binding sites. These enable cubilin to bind not only the intrinsic factor-cobalamin complex but also **albumin**, **vitamin D–binding protein**, **transferrin**, and **apolipoprotein A1**.

The cobalamin-transcobalamin II complex, which circulates in the blood, is commonly called **holotranscobalamin II**.

Cells take up holotranscobalamin II via receptor-mediated endocytosis. Lysosomes degrade transcobalamin II and thereby liberate cobalamin. Cobalamin is then either methylated or 5′-deoxyadenosylated to become methylcobalamin or 5′-deoxyadenosylcobalamin, respectively.

Of all the cobalamin in the blood, only about one quarter is bound to transcobalamin II, while about three-fourths are bound to **transcobalamin I** (also called **haptocorrin** or **R binder**, the same protein that the stomach secretes into its lumen). About 1% of patients who have a low serum cobalamin have a **deficiency of transcobalamin I**.

| Table 36.2 | Cobalamin Content of Various Foods | |
| --- | --- |
| **Food** | **Cobalamin (μg/100 g Edible Portion)** |
| Salmon | 5.8 |
| Ground beef | 2.7 |
| Lamb, leg | 2.6 |
| Cheese (mozzarella) | 2.3 |
| Eggs (boiled) | 1.1 |
| Milk | 0.4 |
| Ice cream | 0.4 |
| Chicken breast | 0.3 |
| Potato, boiled | 0.0 |
| Broccoli | 0.0 |
| Bread, fortified* | 0.0 |

*Fortification with folic acid and other vitamins but not cobalamin.

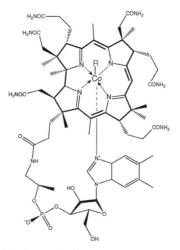

**Fig. 36.8** **Cobalamin.** R can be a cyano group (–CN, as in vitamin $B_{12}$), a methyl group (–$CH_3$, used in methionine synthase), a 5′-deoxyadenosyl group (used in methylmalonyl-CoA mutase), or a hydroxyl group (–OH; in hydroxocobalamin, used in cyanide poisoning).

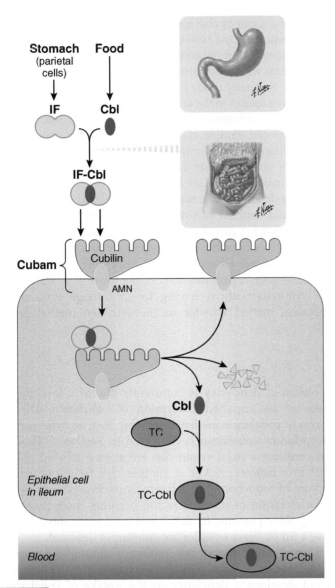

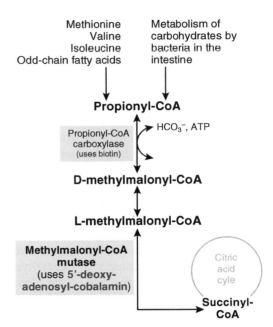

**Fig. 36.10** Role of cobalamin in converting propionyl-CoA to succinyl-CoA.

## 6.2. Methylmalonyl-CoA Mutase

Methylmalonyl-CoA mutase requires 5'-deoxyadenosyl-cobalamin and catalyzes a reaction in the conversion of propionyl-CoA to succinyl-CoA. Propionyl-CoA arises from the metabolism of methionine (Fig. 36.10), the branched-chain amino acids valine and leucine (see Fig. 35-21), and odd-chain fatty acids (see Section 4 in Chapter 27). Succinyl-CoA is an intermediate of the citric acid cycle (see Fig. 22.6). A cobalamin deficiency leads to an increase in the concentration of methylmalonic acid in the blood, which is useful for a diagnosis (see Section 7.2).

## 7. MEGALOBLASTIC ANEMIA DUE TO FOLATE DEFICIENCY OR COBALAMIN DEFICIENCY

*A folate deficiency impairs dTMP production. This impairs replication of rapidly dividing cells and thus leads to megaloblastic anemia and diarrhea. Cobalamin deficiency leads to a largely irreversible destruction of the myelin sheaths of the nervous system; in addition, by inactivating methionine synthase, a cobalamin deficiency may lead to a secondary folate deficiency.*

### 7.1. Folate Deficiency

Folate deficiency is most common in countries without folic acid food fortification, among people who eat few foods of high folate content, and among persons who have a high rate of tissue turnover. We generally consume about as many folates as we need. Furthermore, normal folate stores (which are mainly in the liver) equal only a few weeks of folate needs. Persons who are at the highest risk of a folate deficiency are

**Fig. 36.9** **Absorption of cobalamin.** AMN, amnionless; Cbl, cobalamin; IF, intrinsic factor; TC, transcobalamin II.

## 6. ENZYMES THAT USE COBALAMIN AS A COFACTOR

*Cobalamin is a cofactor for two enzymes: methionine synthase in the activated methyl group cycle and methylmalonyl-CoA mutase in the pathway that feeds propionyl-coenzyme A (proprionyl-CoA) into the citric acid cycle.*

### 6.1. Methionine Synthase

Methionine synthase, the enzyme that transfers a methyl group from $N^5$-methyl-THF to homocysteine in the activated methyl group cycle, requires the cofactor **methylcobalamin** (see Figs. 36.6 and 36.8). As shown in Section 7.2, the rate of the cobalamin-dependent methyl transfer to homocysteine is abnormally low in patients who have a cobalamin deficiency.

those who consume a folate-deficient diet, regularly abuse alcohol, take certain drugs (e.g., methotrexate, trimethoprim, pyrimethamine; see Section 1.2), or produce new cells at a high rate (e.g., children, pregnant women, patients with rapid tumor growth, and patients who have persistent hemolysis or moderate to severe psoriasis).

A shortage of cellular folates affects primarily the synthesis of **dTMP** (Fig. 36.11; see also Fig. 37.6) and hence DNA replication. This means that a folate deficiency affects rapidly dividing tissues; other tissues do not need to make a substantial amount of the thymidine nucleotides. In turn, this explains the principal effects of folate deficiency on the body: **megaloblastic anemia** (also called **macrocytic anemia**; see Fig. 36.13) and diarrhea. Any inhibition of DNA replication yields unusually large (megaloblastic, macrocytic), red blood cells (see Chapter 16). An inadequate supply of deoxythymidine triphosphate (dTTP) also limits the rate of red blood cell production and leads to cells of highly variable size, many of which are destroyed in the bone marrow instead of being released into the bloodstream (hence the anemia). Anemia makes patients fatigue early and experience shortness of breath with minor physical activity. A decrease in the number of absorptive epithelial cells in the intestines leads to malabsorption, increased metabolism of remaining nutrients by bacteria, and **diarrhea** when a significant amount of osmotically active compounds reaches the colon (see Chapter 18). There is no solid evidence that a folate deficiency impairs the synthesis of **purine nucleotides** in vivo (see Chapter 38).

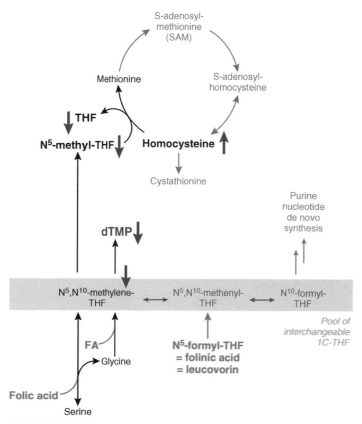

**Fig. 36.11** **Effects of folate deficiency on one-carbon metabolism.** Treatment options are shown in blue. FA, folic acid.

A folate deficiency also leads to a decreased rate of methylation of **homocysteine** (see Fig. 36.11) and hence an increase in the concentration of homocysteine in the blood.

In patients with megaloblastic anemia, a **diagnosis** of folate deficiency is usually made based on finding a decreased concentration of folates in the serum. When necessary, the plasma concentration of homocysteine is also measured, but this test requires special sample handling. Whenever a folate deficiency is found, a cobalamin deficiency must be ruled out by findings of normal serum concentrations of cobalamin and/or methylmalonic acid (see Section 7.2).

A folate deficiency can readily be treated with a supplement of **folic acid**. Instead of folic acid, $N^5$-**formyl-THF** (**folinic acid, leucovorin**) can also be used, either orally or by injection, but this is typically done only in conjunction with antifolate therapy (see Chapter 37). When $N^5$-formyl-THF enters peripheral cells, it becomes part of the folate pool for thymidine synthesis without having to go through cobalamin-dependent methyl transfer to the activated methyl group cycle.

## 7.2. Cobalamin Deficiency

A cobalamin deficiency is commonly due to a low dietary intake or an impaired absorption of cobalamin. Dietary sources of cobalamin are listed in Table 36.2, and the normal absorption of cobalamin is described in Section 5. Patients who consume a strict **vegan** diet are at an increased risk of cobalamin deficiency. **Age** is another risk factor, as malabsorption of food-bound cobalamin, sometimes due to insufficient secretion of intrinsic factor, becomes more prevalent among older persons. In developed countries, about 5% of those aged 60 years or older are cobalamin deficient.

Normal **cobalamin stores** amount to about 2 to 3 years of the recommended daily intake of cobalamin. Hence, if a patient develops a deficiency in the uptake of cobalamin, symptoms generally appear only on a scale of months to years later.

The release of cobalamin from the diet is decreased in patients who secrete an abnormally low amount of **hydrochloric acid** (HCl) in their stomach. For example, patients who take a **proton pump inhibitor** (e.g., omeprazole) for the long-term treatment of gastroesophageal reflux disease (GERD) release an abnormally low fraction of cobalamin from their diet. After several years of drug use, these patients may develop cobalamin deficiency. Long-term use of $H_2$-**receptor antagonists** (e.g., cimetidine, famotidine, and ranitidine) does not cause a cobalamin deficiency, probably because these drugs are less effective at blocking acid secretion. A deficiency in acid secretion does not impair absorption of supplemental cobalamin.

The absorption of cobalamin into the intestinal epithelium is impaired in patients who do not produce a sufficient amount of **intrinsic factor**. This occurs in patients whose parietal cells are under attack, either because of **atrophic gastritis** (a chronic inflammation of the stomach mucosa) or **pernicious anemia** (an autoimmune disease of the stomach);

both diseases are most prevalent among the elderly. Tests for pernicious anemia typically involve measurement of antibodies to intrinsic factor. Patients who have undergone **bariatric surgery** to reduce the size of their stomach also secrete less intrinsic factor.

The uptake of the cobalamin-intrinsic factor complex in the **ileum** is impaired in patients who have **chronic ileitis, Crohn disease, sprue** (often also called celiac disease, a disease of marked intolerance to gluten) or **tropical sprue** (probably due

to infection), or whose ileum has been resected. **Imerslund-Gräsbeck syndrome** (also called megaloblastic anemia type I) is recessively inherited, rare, and caused by mutant cubam (mutation either in the *CUBN*/cubilin or *AMN*/amnionless gene). Affected patients often show signs of cobalamin deficiency at 2 to 4 years of age.

Patients who for several years take **metformin** to treat type 2 diabetes (see Chapter 39) have a decreased concentration of cobalamin in serum.

The symptoms of cobalamin deficiency include damage to the nervous system and symptoms of a primary folate deficiency. A cobalamin deficiency leads to demyelination of the nervous system; the mechanism for this is unclear. Impaired peripheral nerve conduction can be tested with a **tuning fork** held to the sole of a patient's foot. Demyelination of the central nervous system manifests itself as a gradual onset of **dementia**.

By slowing the rate of methyl group transfer from $N^5$-methyl-THF to homocysteine, a cobalamin deficiency induces a **secondary folate deficiency**. Because this leads to a low concentration of SAM, methylene-THF reductase becomes more active, thereby funneling folates into the formation of an excessive amount of $N^5$-methyl-THF (Fig. 36.12). This process is often referred to as the **folate trap** or folate trap hypothesis (the hypothesis is now thought to be correct). Hence, a patient with a cobalamin deficiency not only has a damaged nervous system but may also have a **megaloblastic anemia** (Fig. 36.13) and **diarrhea**.

The laboratory-based diagnosis of cobalamin deficiency relies on a decreased concentration of **total cobalamin** and/or an elevated concentration of **methylmalonic acid** in the serum. The serum cobalamin assay is a screening test that may be diagnostic. The more expensive methylmalonic acid test is definitive. Decreased activity of methylmalonyl-CoA mutase leads to an accumulation of methylmalonyl-CoA (see Fig. 36.12B) and subsequently, an increased concentration of methylmalonic acid in the blood and urine. As in a primary folate deficiency, the concentration of homocysteine in the plasma is elevated due to decreased activity of methionine synthase.

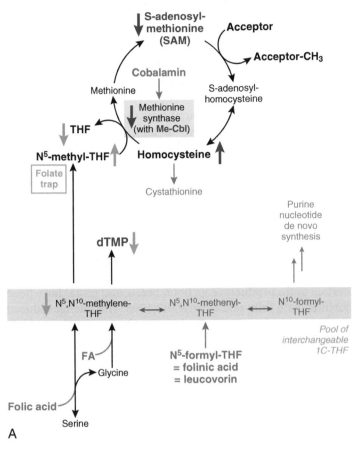

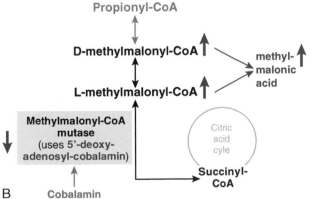

**Fig. 36.12** **Effects of cobalamin deficiency on one-carbon metabolism and propionyl-CoA metabolism.** (A) Cobalamin deficiency often induces a secondary folate deficiency and changes in metabolite concentrations (brown arrows). (B) Cobalamin deficiency leads to an elevated concentration of methylmalonic acid in the blood and urine.

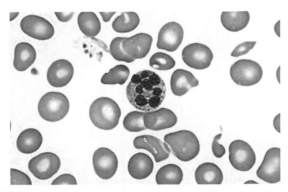

**Fig. 36.13** **Macrocytosis and hypersegmentation of neutrophils in secondary folate deficiency due to a cobalamin deficiency.** Blood smears of primary and secondary folate deficiency are indistinguishable.

A cobalamin deficiency can be treated with supplementary cobalamin. This is obvious in the case of patients whose *diet* is cobalamin deficient. Patients who have a deficiency in cobalamin *uptake* can either be injected intramuscularly with cobalamin approximately monthly, or they can be treated with very large daily oral doses of cobalamin because ~1% of oral cobalamin is absorbed via a process that does not depend on intrinsic factor and cubam.

There are several rare inborn errors of cobalamin metabolism. These disorders are named cblA through cblG. **cblA** and **cblB** both diminish synthesis of 5′-deoxyadenosyl-cobalamin, the cofactor of methylmalonyl-CoA mutase, causing methylmalonic aciduria. **cblC**, **cblD**, and **cblF** all diminish the synthesis of both methyl-cobalamin and 5′-deoxyadenosyl-cobalamin, the cofactors of methionine synthase and methylmalonyl-CoA mutase, causing both homocystinuria and methylmalonic aciduria. **cblE** and **cblG** are associated with impaired activity of methionine synthase, causing homocystinuria.

## 8. OTHER DISEASES LINKED TO FOLATES

*A low folate status around the time of conception and early pregnancy is associated with an increased risk of neural tube defects, conotruncal heart disease, cleft lip, and cleft palate. In all adults, low folate status increases the risk of tumorigenesis, yet many tumors grow faster at a high folate status.*

### 8.1. Neural Tube Defects and Other Folate-Dependent Congenital Anomalies

Failure of the neural tube to close during embryogenesis gives rise mainly to **spina bifida** or **anencephaly** (Fig. 36.14). To date, it is unclear how an absolute or relative folate deficiency leads to neural tube defects. In most countries, neural tube defects occur in about 1 in 300 to 1 in 1,700 newborns. Any part of the neural cord may fail to close in the first 3 to 4 weeks of pregnancy, a time when women often do not know that they are pregnant.

In many developed countries, at about 16 to 18 weeks of gestation, the serum concentration of **α-fetoprotein (AFP)** of most women is determined to screen for developmental disorders of the fetus. α-Fetoprotein is produced by the liver of the fetus, and some of it crosses into the maternal bloodstream. The concentration of AFP depends on the gestational age of the fetus. An abnormal concentration of AFP is commonly followed by ultrasound examination of the fetus, repeat determination of AFP, and, if needed, determination of the concentration of AFP in the fluid of the amnion. For neural tube defects, the AFP screening test has approximately 80% sensitivity.

Some newborns with neural tube defects die shortly after birth, and others may have lifelong paralysis. Surgery in utero, shortly after birth, or later can reduce the degree of disability.

Congenital neural tube defects are partially preventable with **supplemental folic acid**. Epidemiological studies revealed that 30% to 70% of the neural tube defects can be prevented with supplements of folic acid given to women who contemplate pregnancy or who have just become pregnant. Accordingly, some countries require that grain products be **enriched with folic acid**. In the United States and Canada, certain grain products (e.g., flour, bread, and pasta) have been fortified with folic acid since about 1998. This change reduced the birth prevalences of spina bifida and anencephaly by about 30% in the United States and by about 45% in Canada. The U.S. Food and Nutrition Board recommends that all women of childbearing age, particularly those who contemplate pregnancy, take a daily supplement of 400 μg of folic acid. Women who are pregnant are given a daily supplement of 600 μg folic

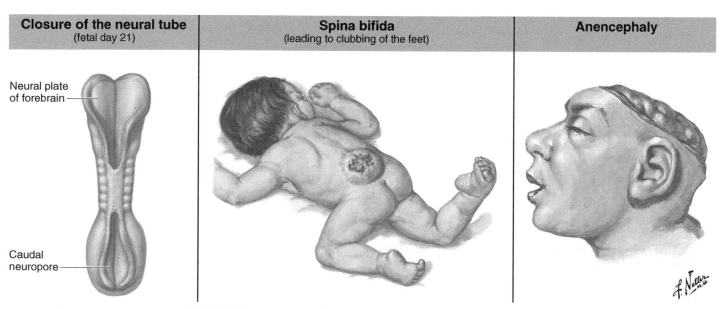

| Closure of the neural tube (fetal day 21) | Spina bifida (leading to clubbing of the feet) | Anencephaly |
|---|---|---|

Neural plate of forebrain

Caudal neuropore

**Fig. 36.14** Normal and abnormal closure of the neural tube.

acid to accommodate the needs for tissue production in the mother and fetus.

Mothers who are homozygous for the C677T mutation of **$N^5,N^{10}$-methylenetetrahydrofolate reductase** (the enzyme that reduces $N^5,N^{10}$-methylene-THF to $N^5$-methyl-THF) are somewhat more likely to have a child with a neural tube defect. Fetuses who are homozygous for 677T likewise are at an increased risk of a neural tube defect. Among studied populations, 10% to 25% of individuals are homozygous for 677T. The C677T mutation results in an Ala → Val substitution, which renders the enzyme less stable. When folate intake is low, this mutant enzyme is associated with an increased concentration of homocysteine in the blood.

A low intake of folic acid early in pregnancy is also associated with an increased incidence of **conotruncal heart defects**, **cleft lip**, and **cleft palate**. Cells for the lips and palate arise from the same cells as the neural tube.

Although in the United States a complete **cobalamin deficiency** is rare among pregnant women, women who have a low concentration of cobalamin are more likely to have a child with a neural tube defect, perhaps because of trapping of $N^5$-methyl-THF (see Section 7.2).

## 8.2. Folates and Cancer

In normal tissues, a low concentration of folates presents an increased risk of neoplastic transformation. In contrast, once a tumor has developed, folate deficiency has the beneficial effect of slowing the replication of cells (this is the basis of the effect of methotrexate and other antifolate chemotherapeutic agents; see Chapter 37). The beneficial effect of normal folate status before tumorigenesis may relate to normal concentrations of deoxyribonucleotides and SAM, which allow normal DNA replication and repair, as well as normal methylation of DNA and associated proteins.

## 9. TRANSSULFURATION PATHWAY AND METABOLISM OF CYSTEINE

*The transsulfuration pathway is most active in the liver and converts homocysteine to cysteine. Cysteine, in turn, is used for the synthesis of glutathione, taurine, and conjugated bile salts. Catabolism of cysteine yields sulfate, some of which is conjugated with xenobiotics and drugs.*

The transsulfuration pathway commonly refers to the conversion of homocysteine to cysteine (Fig. 36.15). The pathway is most active in the liver and, to a lesser extent, the kidneys, intestines, and pancreas.

The enzymes that convert homocysteine to cystathionine and then cysteine require pyridoxal phosphate (a derivative of vitamin $B_6$). For yet unknown reasons, **cystathionine** is present in the brain at millimolar concentrations and is needed for the proper function of the brain.

A **cystathionine β-synthase deficiency** is the cause of classical **homocystinuria**; patients with this disease have severe hyperhomocysteinemia, mental retardation, osteoporosis in

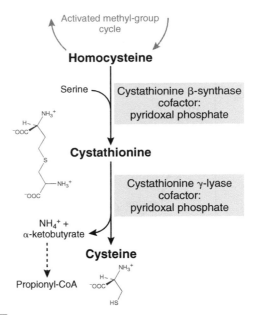

**Fig. 36.15** **Transsulfuration pathway.** Cystathionine γ-lyase is also called cystathioninase or cystathionase. The metabolism of propionyl-CoA to succinyl-CoA is described in Section 6.2 and Fig. 36.10.

childhood, thromboembolisms in their teens and twenties, subluxation of their lenses before age 30 years, and a reduced life span. The disease is inherited in autosomal recessive fashion and occurs in 1 of about 50,000 newborns. In addition to homocysteine, the concentrations in the blood of methionine, SAM, S-adenosylhomocysteine, and sarcosine are also elevated. Most patients are treated with a low-methionine diet and given a supplement of cystine. Some patients respond to large doses of vitamin $B_6$, which gives rise to pyridoxal phosphate, the cofactor of cystathionine β-synthase. Many patients who do not respond to extra vitamin $B_6$ do respond to supplemental betaine; betaine helps methylate homocysteine to methionine in a reaction that occurs parallel to the one that is catalyzed by methionine synthase.

**Cysteine** plays a central role in the metabolism of sulfur-containing compounds (Fig. 36.16). Free cysteine is used for the synthesis of **glutathione**, an antioxidant and radical scavenger (see Chapter 21). Many cells contain millimolar concentrations of glutathione, and glutathione also serves as a reservoir for cysteine. The concentration of cysteine is the rate-limiting factor in the synthesis of glutathione.

Free cysteine itself, together with iron, forms toxic free radicals, and the intracellular concentration of cysteine is kept relatively low (~<0.2 mM). To this end, cysteine is degraded into cysteine sulfinate, which is either degraded further or used for the synthesis of **taurine** (see Fig. 36.16). Taurine is an amino acid with which bile acids are conjugated to increase their hydrophilicity (see Chapter 29). Some cells produce taurine to compensate for extracellular hyperosmolality. Otherwise, the degradation of cysteine yields sulfate, which can react with ATP to form **3'-phosphoadenosine 5'-phosphosulfate** (**PAPS**). PAPS can be used to sulfate proteins (see Chapters 7 and 13), steroids, or xenobiotics, thereby making them more water soluble.

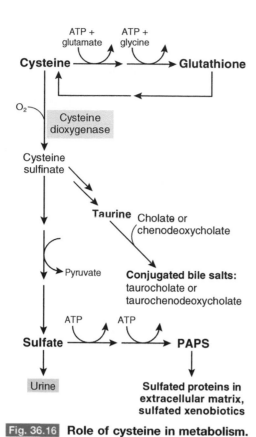

**Fig. 36.16** Role of cysteine in metabolism.

## SUMMARY

- The term *folates* includes folic acid, dihydrofolic acid (DHF), tetrahydrofolic acid (THF), $N^5$-methyl-THF, $N^5,N^{10}$-methylene-THF, $N^5,N^{10}$-methenyl-THF, $N^5$-formyl-THF, $N^{10}$-formyl-THF, and $N^5$-formimino-THF, regardless of the length of the polyglutamate tail.

- Folates are found in legumes, green leafy vegetables, citrus fruit, and grains. In some countries, grain products are fortified with folic acid, a vitamin. Folic acid enters the intestine via the proton-coupled folate transporter (PCFT). DHF reductase then reduces folic acid to THF. THF is loaded with a one-carbon group from serine or glycine and exported as $N^5$-methyl-THF.

- Peripheral cells take up $N^5$-methyl-THF via the RFC or endocytosis of folate receptors. The PCFT is involved in transporting folates from the blood into the brain. Once inside a cell, $N^5$-methyl-THF must donate its methyl group to homocysteine in the activated methyl group cycle; the resulting THF receives a polyglutamate tail and can then accept a one-carbon group and become part of the general one-carbon-THF pool.

- The methyl transfer from $N^5$-methyl-THF to homocysteine is catalyzed by methionine synthase, which uses methylcobalamin as a cofactor. In cobalamin-deficient patients, this reaction is impaired such that cells have a reduced capacity to gain THF from $N^5$-methyl-THF in the bloodstream. Hence, cobalamin deficiency often leads to a secondary folate deficiency.

- One-carbon loaded THFs are primarily required for the de novo synthesis of inosine monophosphate (IMP, from which AMP and GMP are made) and the conversion of deoxyuridine monophosphate (dUMP) to dTMP. In folate-deficient patients, only the synthesis of dTMP is decreased in a pathogenic manner, thereby slowing the replication of cells in the bone marrow and intestinal epithelium; this causes megaloblastic anemia and diarrhea.

- Patients who have megaloblastic anemia most often have a primary or secondary folate deficiency. Laboratory data that support a primary folate deficiency include a low concentration of folate and a normal concentration of cobalamin and methylmalonic acid in the serum. A secondary folate deficiency can be caused by a cobalamin deficiency via decreased activity of methionine synthase and the trapping of most folates as $N^5$-methyl-THF. Laboratory data that support a cobalamin deficiency are a low concentration of cobalamin and an elevated concentration of methylmalonic acid in the serum. Because a cobalamin deficiency damages the nervous system and high doses of folates can cure the megaloblastic anemia, it is important that folate-deficient patients be tested for cobalamin deficiency and given cobalamin if needed. A folate deficiency is treated with oral folic acid or with oral or injected leucovorin.

- Several conditions can lead to cobalamin deficiency: decreased acid secretion by the stomach (which leads to decreased liberation of dietary cobalamin) due to the chronic use of a proton pump inhibitor for gastroesophageal reflux disease; reduced numbers of intrinsic factor–secreting parietal cells owing to atrophic gastritis, pernicious anemia, or bariatric surgery; and impaired absorption of the cobalamin-intrinsic factor complex via cubam in the ileum due to chronic inflammation or surgical resection of the ileum.

- The activated methyl group cycle generates S-adenosylmethionine (SAM), which is used as a methyl donor for almost all methylation reactions in the body. Most of the SAM is needed for the synthesis of creatine (to make up for the loss of creatinine), phosphatidylcholine, and plasmenylcholine. The remaining SAM is used for the synthesis of epinephrine from norepinephrine, and by numerous enzymes that methylate lysine or arginine residues in proteins, cytosine bases in DNA, or guanine bases in RNA.

- The degradation of methanol by alcohol dehydrogenase and formaldehyde dehydrogenase yields formate, which must be removed via $N^{10}$-formyl-THF. Methanol poisoning causes the transient accumulation of millimolar concentrations of formate in the blood, which can cause severe metabolic acidosis as well as severe damage to the optic nerve. The accumulation of formate can be prevented with fomepizole (an inhibitor of alcohol dehydrogenase) or with ethanol (another substrate of alcohol dehydrogenase). In patients poisoned with ethylene glycol, fomepizole or ethanol are used in a similar manner.

- The transsulfuration pathway converts homocysteine to cysteine. This pathway is most active in the liver.

■ Free cysteine is toxic. Cysteine is needed for the synthesis of glutathione, which is used for diverse redox reactions. Degradation of glutathione yields cysteine, and glutathione thus also serves as a reservoir for cysteine. When cysteine is metabolized, it can give rise to taurine, which serves as an intracellular osmolyte and which the liver conjugates with bile acids. The degradation of cysteine yields sulfate, which can be activated to 3′-phosphoadenosine 5′-phosphosulfate (PAPS) for the sulfation of xenobiotics or extracellular matrix proteins.

## FURTHER READING

■ Devalia V, Hamilton MS, Molloy AM, on behalf of the British Committee for Standards in Haematology. Guidelines for the diagnosis and treatment of cobalamin and folate disorders. *Br J Haematol.* 2014;166:496-513.

■ Quadros EV. Advances in the understanding of cobalamin assimilation and metabolism. *Br J Haematol.* 2010;148: 195-204.

■ Visentin M, Diop-Bove N, Zhao R, Goldman ID. The intestinal absorption of folates. *Annu Rev Physiol.* 2014; 76:251-274.

# Review Questions

1. A 2½-year-old child is treated for methanol poisoning. She is given an intravenous infusion of ethanol. In addition, intravenous administration of which one of the following would be most appropriate to prevent damage to her optic nerve?

   A. Biotin
   B. Cobalamin
   C. Leucovorin
   D. Niacin
   E. Thiamine

2. An anemic patient is found to have a low serum folate level and a serum cobalamin level that is inconclusive. A common test to distinguish primary folate deficiency from cobalamin-induced secondary folate deficiency involves measuring which of the following?

   A. Red blood cell folate
   B. Serum antibodies to haptocorrin (R-binder)
   C. Serum homocysteine
   D. Serum methylmalonic acid

3. Many patients who have type 2 diabetes are treated with the drug metformin. Based on preliminary data, investigators hypothesized that cobalamin deficiency is a side effect of metformin treatment. Serum of metformin-treated and untreated control diabetic patients was analyzed. A significantly elevated concentration in metformin-treated patients of which one of the following metabolites would be the strongest indication that the hypothesis is correct?

   A. Homocysteine
   B. Methionine
   C. Methylmalonate
   D. S-adeonosylmethionine

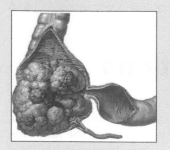

## SYNOPSIS

■ A pyrimidine nucleotide contains a uracil (U), cytosine (C), or thymine (T) base and a ribose or deoxyribose.

■ A person needs to synthesize about half a gram of pyrimidine nucleotides per day. The main clinical interest in pyrimidine nucleotides is derived from the fact that DNA replication and repair are the only processes that depend on the production of deoxythymidine triphosphate (dTTP).

■ Persons who are folate deficient synthesize an inadequate amount of deoxythymidine monophosphate (dTMP) and dTTP (see Chapter 36).

■ One way of inhibiting the growth of a tumor is to deprive its cells of dTTP (see Fig. 37.1). This can be achieved by inhibiting the enzyme that makes dTMP with 5F-deoxyuridine monophosphate (5F-dUMP) or with pemetrexed. It can also be achieved by inhibiting the reduction of dihydrofolate (DHF) to tetrahydrofolate (THF) with the antifolate methotrexate.

■ The deoxyribonucleotides deoxyuridine diphosphate (dUDP), deoxycytidine diphosphate (dCDP), deoxyadenosine diphosphate (dADP), and deoxyguanosine diphosphate (dGDP) are made from the respective ribonucleotides by a single enzyme (see Fig. 37.1). This enzyme can be inhibited by hydroxyurea or the active metabolite of gemcitabine. Gemcitabine and hydroxyurea are used for the treatment of a variety of cancers. Hydroxyurea is also used to reduce the frequency of sickle cell crises in patients who have a sickle cell disease.

■ Pyrimidine nucleotides are also used in the synthesis of RNAs, phospholipids, and glycogen, as well as for glucuronidation (a detoxification reaction). For the most part, nucleotides used in these processes are recycled.

## LEARNING OBJECTIVES

*For mastery of this topic, you should be able to do the following:*

■ Describe the biosynthesis of pyrimidine nucleotides with emphasis on the key regulated steps.

■ Explain the relationship between folates and thymidine synthesis.

■ Describe the ribonucleotide reductase reaction and its regulation, and explain its role in cancer chemotherapy with hydroxyurea or gemcitabine.

■ Compare and contrast the effects of 5-fluoruracil, pemetrexed, and methotrexate on the synthesis of thymidine, paying special attention to the mechanisms of action.

## 1. DE NOVO SYNTHESIS OF URIDINE MONOPHOSPHATE, A PRECURSOR FOR ALL PYRIMIDINE NUCLEOTIDES

*De novo synthesis of a precursor for all pyrimidine nucleotides, uridine monophosphate (UMP), takes place mainly in the liver and in dividing cells. Use of a ribose from the pentose phosphate pathway yields phosphoribosylpyrophosphate (PRPP). Synthesis of a pyrimidine base starts with bicarbonate and yields orotate. PRPP and orotate then give rise to UMP. The liver converts UMP to uridine and releases uridine into the blood. From there, other cells can pick up uridine and phosphorylate it to UMP.*

The synthesis of pyrimidine nucleotides involves the following steps: (1) synthesis of PRPP; (2) synthesis of the base orotate; (3) the combination of PRPP and orotate to form the nucleotide UMP; (4) conversion of UMP to cytidine triphosphate (CTP); (5) the reduction of ribonucleotides to deoxyribonucleotides; and (6) the conversion of dUMP to dTMP. This section deals only with the synthesis of UMP.

Pyrimidine nucleotides are needed for the synthesis of **DNA, RNA, phospholipids,** and **glycogen,** as well as for **glycosylation** and **glucuronidation** reactions. DNA replication and repair require dCTP and dTTP (see Chapters 2 and 3). RNA synthesis requires UTP and CTP (see Chapter 6). Phospholipid de novo synthesis needs CTP. Glycogen synthesis, glycosylation reactions, and glucuronidation reactions require UTP (see Chapters 7, 14, and 24). DNA is degraded only at a low rate and yields dCMP and dTMP, which can be reused (see Section 6). Similarly, RNA degradation yields CMP and UMP, which can be reused (see Section 6).

Most pyrimidine nucleotide synthesis takes place in the **liver** and in **dividing cells,** such as intestinal epithelial cells, erythropoietic cells in the bone marrow, and tumor cells. The liver provides a service to other cells by synthesizing uridine and releasing it into the blood. Other cells then take up uridine and phosphorylate it to UMP. Total daily pyrimidine nucleotide synthesis amounts to about 0.5 g per day, comparable to the de novo synthesis of purine nucleotides (see Chapter 38).

**PRPP** is a phosphorylated ribose that plays a role in the production of all nucleotides and that cells synthesize only when they have normal energy production (see Fig. 37.3). **PRPP synthetase** makes PRPP from ribose 5-phosphate, an intermediate of the pentose phosphate pathway (see Chapter 21). PRPP synthetase is active when the concentration of **phosphate** is near normal and that of **ADP** is low. PRPP is also used for the salvage of purine bases and the de novo synthesis of purine nucleotides (see Chapter 38).

**Orotate** is synthesized mostly in response to a need for **DNA replication** or **repair** (Fig. 37.2). The rate-limiting enzyme for orotate synthesis is the carbamoyl-phosphate synthase II moiety of CAD, a trifunctional enzyme. PRPP feed forward activates carbamoyl-phosphate synthase activity. At

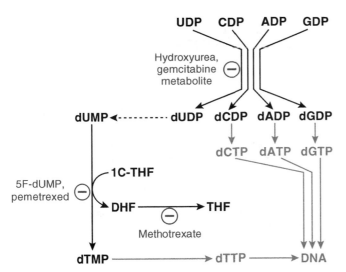

**Fig. 37.1** Overview of clinical interference with pyrimidine nucleotide metabolism.

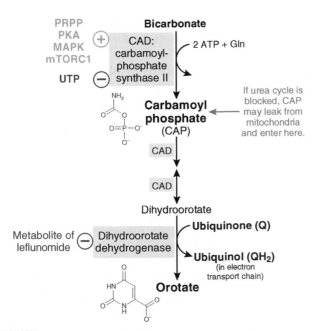

**Fig. 37.2** **Synthesis of orotate.** CAD, carbamoyl-phosphate synthase II/aspartate carbamoyl-transferase/dihydroorotase (a trifunctional enzyme); Gln, glutamine; MAPK, mitogen-activated protein kinase; PKA, protein kinase A; PRPP, phosphoribosylpyrophosphate. Ubiquinone is also called coenzyme Q. Leflunomide is used in the treatment of rheumatoid arthritis.

rest (in the $G_0$ phase of the cell cycle), orotate synthesis is mostly limited by feedback inhibition from UTP. When cells synthesize DNA, active protein kinase A (PKA), MAP kinase (MAPK), and mTORC1 (see Chapters 8 and 34) lead to the phosphorylation of CAD. Phosphorylated CAD is less sensitive to UTP feedback, allowing for increased production of orotate and hence pyrimidine nucleotides.

The carbamoyl-phosphate synthase II moiety of CAD carries the number II because a different carbamoyl-phosphate synthase (I) was first discovered in mitochondria. Carbamoyl-phosphate synthase I produces carbamoylphosphate (CAP) for the urea cycle (see Chapter 35).

In patients who have a disease of the **urea cycle** (see Fig. 35.12 and Section 3.3 in Chapter 35) that leads to the accumulation of CAP, CAP leaks from the mitochondria into the cytosol. This leaked CAP bypasses the regulation of the activity of carbamoyl phosphate synthase II. Leaked CAP therefore gives rise to excess **orotate** via the reactions shown in Fig. 37.2. The excess orotate spills into the blood and the urine. The concentration of orotate in the urine is used to determine the cause of urea cycle defects.

The early steps in orotate synthesis take place in the **cytosol** and **nucleus**, but the final step takes place in the intermembrane space of **mitochondria**. **Dihydroorotate dehydrogenase** is an integral protein of the inner mitochondrial membrane that oxidizes dihydroorotate in the intermembrane space. Thereby, the enzyme reduces ubiquinone in the membrane to ubiquinol, which is part of the electron transport chain (see Fig. 23.3). This reaction is not an important contributor to oxidative phosphorylation.

**Leflunomide** is used as a disease-modifying antirheumatic drug (DMARD) for the treatment of the autoimmune disease **rheumatoid arthritis** (see Fig. 37.10 and Section 5.3). In the body, leflunomide is metabolized to teriflunomide, which inhibits dihydroorotate dehydrogenase and thus leads to a deficiency of pyrimidine nucleotides, particularly in lymphocytes.

**UMP synthase** joins **PRPP** with **orotate** to generate **UMP** (Fig. 37.3). UMP synthase is found both in the cytosol and in the nucleus. A hereditary **deficiency** of UMP synthase, which is rare, causes an orotic aciduria (also compare to the above discussion of urea cycle defects). The deficiency can be treated with uridine supplementation.

The liver dephosphorylates UMP to **uridine** and releases uridine into the bloodstream; from there, peripheral cells take up uridine (see Fig. 37.3). Uridine and other unphosphorylated nucleosides cross cell membranes through **nucleoside transporters**, some of which offer facilitated passive diffusion, whereas others actively pump nucleosides. Peripheral cells then phosphorylate uridine to UMP, a process that is also called **salvage**. Apart from biosynthesis in the liver, uridine can also stem from the degradation of RNA in other cells (see Section 6 and Fig. 37.12).

A **deficiency of pyrimidine 5′-nucleotidase** is accompanied by hemolytic anemia. The deficiency is usually a consequence of the direct inhibition of the enzyme by $Pb^{2+}$ in **lead poisoning**; an inherited deficiency is rare. It is unclear how the deficiency is detrimental to erythrocytes.

**Chemotherapeutic and antiviral drugs** that are analogs of normal pyrimidine nucleosides enter cells through transporters for uridine or thymidine. Inside cells, kinases triphosphorylate these drugs. Examples of such chemotherapeutic drugs are **5-fluorouracil** and **gemcitabine** (2′,2′-difluoro-2′-deoxycytidine). 5-Fluorouracil is discussed in Section 5 and gemcitabine in Section 3. Examples of antiviral drugs taken up via nucleoside transporters are **zidovudine** (**AZT**; 3′-azido-2′,3′-dideoxythymidine) and **stavudine** (2′,3′-didehydro-2′,3′-dideoxythymidine).

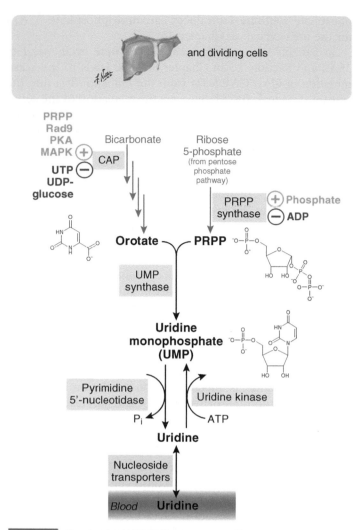

**Fig. 37.3** **Synthesis of UMP from orotate.** The liver exports uridine and other cells import it from the blood. ADP, adenosine diphosphate; CAP, carbamoyl phosphate; MAPK, mitogen-activated protein kinase; PKA, protein kinase A; PRPP, phosphoribosylpyrophosphate; UDP, uridine diphosphate; UTP, uridine triphosphate; Rad9 is a protein that plays a role in DNA repair and cell cycle control.

## 2. SYNTHESIS AND USES OF UTP AND CTP

*Cells phosphorylate uridine and UMP to UTP. UTP gives rise to CTP. UTP and CTP are used for the synthesis of RNA, phospholipids, and for UDP-glucose, which is used in a variety of processes.*

Uridine is phosphorylated to UTP, which can be converted to CTP (Fig 37.4; see also Fig. 37.3). Averaged over an entire cell (i.e., disregarding compartmentation), the concentration of UTP is on the order of 0.3 mM (i.e., about one-tenth the concentration of ATP). The concentration of CTP is about 0.1 mM.

The chemotherapeutic drugs gemcitabine (see Section 3) and 5-fluorouracil (see Section 5.1) are phosphorylated by the same enzymes as the uridine and cytidine nucleotides.

**UTP** gives rise to **UDP-glucose**, which is used for several different processes. UDP-glucose is used in **glycogen** synthesis (see Figs. 24.1 and 24.5); in the synthesis of **lactose** in the

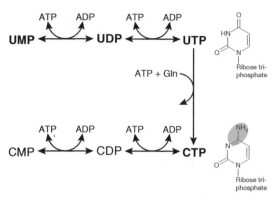

**Fig. 37.4** **The synthesis of uridine triphosphate (UTP) and cytidine triphosphate (CTP) from uridine monophosphate (UMP).** ATP, adenosine triphosphate; Gln, glutamine.

lactating mammary gland (see Fig. 20.11); in the synthesis of **glycosphingolipids** (see Fig. 11.1); for posttranslational **glycosylation** (see Chapters 7 and 13); in the synthesis of **UDP-glucuronate**, which is used for many detoxification reactions, including the conjugation of **bilirubin** in the liver (see Fig. 14.7); and in catalytic amounts for the degradation of **galactose** (see Fig. 20.9).

**CTP** is used in the synthesis of **phospholipids**, such as phosphatidylinositol, phosphatidylcholine, phosphatidylethanolamine, and phosphatidylserine (see Chapter 11; phospholipid synthesis is not covered in this book).

## 3. REDUCTION OF RIBONUCLEOTIDES TO DEOXYRIBONUCLEOTIDES

*Ribonucleotide reductase reduces certain pyrimidine and purine nucleotides to their respective deoxyribonucleotides for DNA replication and repair. Ribonucleoside diphosphate reductase is the target of the antineoplastic drugs hydroxyurea and gemcitabine.*

**Ribonucleoside-diphosphate reductase** (also called **ribonucleotide reductase**) catalyzes the reduction of ribonucleotides to deoxyribonucleotides in the **cytosol** (Fig. 37.5). This reduction physiologically occurs only with the nucleoside diphosphates UDP, CDP, ADP, and GDP. Ribonucleotide reductase activity is regulated allosterically by nucleotide binding to two distinct sites (activity sites and specificity sites), by transcription, and by regulatory proteins.

In **quiescent** cells, the concentration of deoxyribonucleotides is extremely low. During **DNA replication** or **repair**, the concentration of deoxyribonucleotides is relatively high but still lower than the concentration of ribonucleotides. Thanks to two different subunit compositions, the ribonucleotide reductase holoenzyme is active only during DNA replication or only during DNA repair.

Ribonucleotide reductase uses **thioredoxin** to reduce ribonucleotides to deoxyribonucleotides. **Thioredoxins** are proteins of about 100 amino acids that contain a Cys-X-X-Cys active-site sequence (X can be any amino acid). In *reduced* thioredoxin, the Cys side chains are free (i.e., –SH). In *oxidized* thioredoxin (i.e., thioredoxin disulfide), the two active-site

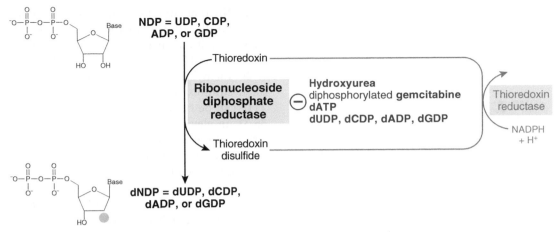

**Fig. 37.5** **The reduction of ribonucleotides to deoxyribonucleotides.** ATP, dTTP, dATP, and dGTP regulate the *substrate* specificity of ribonucleotide reductase (not shown). NDP, nucleoside diphosphate.

cysteine side chains form a disulfide bridge. Besides the reduction of ribonucleotides, thioredoxins also play a role in the reestablishment of –SH groups in proteins, antioxidant defense, immune defense, and apoptosis.

**Thioredoxin reductases** use NADPH to reduce thioredoxin disulfides to thioredoxins (see Fig. 37.5). Thioredoxin reductases contain **selenocysteine** in their active site (see Section 1.1 in Chapter 9). Thioredoxin reductase activity is increased in many cancer cells.

**Hydroxyurea** and **gemcitabine** are chemotherapeutic drugs that lead to a decreased rate of deoxyribonucleotide production (see Fig. 37.5). Hydroxyurea ($H_2N$–CO–NHOH) inhibits ribonucleotide reductase by reducing a protein tyrosyl radical that is crucial for enzyme activity. Hydroxyurea is used for patients who have **polycythemia vera** and are at high risk of thrombosis. Polycythemia vera is due to an abnormally increased red blood cell production. The disease is commonly treated with phlebotomy. Hydroxyurea also plays a role in the treatment of several other forms of cancer. Finally, hydroxyurea is used in patients with **sickle cell anemia** to decrease the incidence of vasoocclusive episodes. Hydroxyurea decreases sickling by leading to enhanced synthesis of hemoglobin F (attributed in part to nitric oxide that is released from hydroxyurea). Diphosphorylated gemcitabine (2′,2′-difluoro-deoxycytidine diphosphate) inhibits ribonucleotide reductase irreversibly. In addition, triphosphorylated gemcitabine is incorporated into DNA and thereby inhibits chain elongation. Gemcitabine is used in the treatment of metastatic **breast cancer**, certain stages of **non–small cell lung cancer**, advanced **ovarian cancer**, advanced **pancreatic cancer**, and a number of other tumors.

## 4. SYNTHESIS OF dTMP

*dUMP can form by various pathways. Thymidine synthase uses a one-carbon tetrahydrofolate to methylate dUMP to dTMP.*

Sometimes, dTMP, dTDP, and dTTP are abbreviated simply as TMP, TDP, and TTP, since only the thymidine deoxyribonucleotides play a known physiological role. Similarly, deoxythymidine is usually abbreviated to thymidine. For clarity, use of the prefixes "d" or "deoxy" is preferable.

dUDP, dUTP, or dCMP can give rise to **dUMP** (see Fig. 37.6), although little is known about the physiological relevance of these reactions.

**Thymidylate synthase** uses $N^5,N^{10}$-**methylene-THF** to reduce and methylate dUMP to **dTMP** (see Fig. 37.6). The reaction produces **DHF**. **DHF reductase** reduces DHF to THF (see Fig. 36.2), which is subsequently converted to $N^5,N^{10}$-methylene-THF. Control of dTTP synthesis most likely occurs via control of the production of dUMP.

## 5. CHEMOTHERAPEUTIC AGENTS THAT INTERFERE WITH dTMP SYNTHESIS

*The drug fluorouracil gives rise to fluoro-dUMP, which permanently inactivates thymidylate synthase and thus impairs the production of dTTP for DNA replication. Pemetrexed is also an inhibitor of thymidylate synthase. In contrast, methotrexate is a competitive inhibitor of dihydrofolate reductase. Methotrexate-induced accumulation of dihydrofolate and the depletion of methylene-tetrahydrofolate leads to decreased activity of thymidylate synthase, thus also impairing the production of dTTP for DNA replication.*

### 5.1. 5-Fluorouracil and Related Drugs

**Capecitabine, tegafur,** and **5-fluorouracil** all give rise to the same active metabolite, **5-fluoro-dUMP,** that impairs thymidylate synthase and hence DNA synthesis (Fig. 37.7). Capecitabine and tegafur are converted to 5-fluorouracil. 5-Fluorouracil gives rise to two toxic metabolites: 5-fluoro-UTP and 5-fluoro-dUMP. 5-Fluoro-UTP is incorporated into RNA. There is no proofreading mechanism for RNA synthesis,

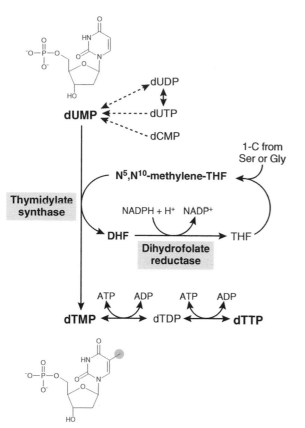

**Fig. 37.6** **Synthesis of deoxythymidine monophosphate (dTMP) from deoxyuridine monophosphate (dUMP).** The transfer of a one-carbon group to tetrahydrofolate (THF) to form $N^5,N^{10}$-methylene-THF is shown in Figs. 36.2 and 36.3.

and RNA that contains 5-fluorouracil is not fully functional. 5-Fluoro-dUMP is a **suicide substrate** for **thymidylate synthase** (i.e., it inactivates the enzyme irreversibly); it slows the synthesis of dTTP and thus inhibits DNA synthesis.

$N^5$-**formyl-THF** (also called **leucovorin**; see Chapter 36) is often administered together with 5-fluorouracil. $N^5$-formyl-THF can be converted into $N^5,N^{10}$-methylene-THF (see Fig. 36.3), an elevated concentration of which increases the substrate saturation of thymidylate synthase. Thus, $N^5$-formyl-THF increases the rate at which 5-fluorouracil incapacitates thymidylate synthase.

The effect of 5-fluorouracil on tumor cells also depends on the relative activities of **thymidylate synthase** and **dihydropyrimidine dehydrogenase**. The lower the thymidylate synthase activity is, the more tumor cells die from 5-fluorouracil treatment. Dihydropyrimidine dehydrogenase normally degrades 80% to 90% of administered 5-fluorouracil to dihydrofluorouracil (see Fig. 37.7). If a patient has decreased activity of this enzyme, 5-fluorouracil is unexpectedly toxic to the patient. Patients can be screened for dihydropyrimidine dehydrogenase deficiency. In patients who do not have this deficiency, the drug **gimeracil** is sometimes used to inhibit dihydropyrimidine dehydrogenase and thus boost the toxicity of 5-fluorouracil. Gimeracil is currently given together with tegafur.

5-Fluorouracil, capecitabine, and tegafur are used in the treatment of a wide variety of solid tumors, sometimes as part of a multidrug regimen. 5-Fluorouracil is also used topically for warts.

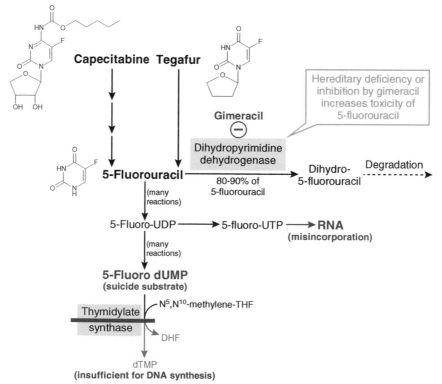

**Fig. 37.7** **Mechanism of action of 5-fluorouracil, capecitabine, and tegafur.** DHF, dihydrofolate; dTMP, deoxythymidine monophosphate; dUMP, deoxyuridine monophosphate; UDP, uridine diphosphate; UTP, uridine triphosphate.

## 5.2. Pemetrexed

Pemetrexed, like 5-fluouracil, inhibits **thymidylate synthase**, but it is not a suicide inhibitor. Pemetrexed also inhibits de novo synthesis of purine nucleotides, although this is of uncertain clinical relevance. Pemetrexed is used in the treatment of mesothelioma and nonsquamous non–small cell lung cancer.

## 5.3. Methotrexate

The antifolate drug methotrexate is a competitive inhibitor of **dihydrofolate reductase** and thus indirectly reduces thymidylate synthase activity (Fig. 37.8). Methotrexate is an analog of dihydrofolate. Methotrexate crosses the brush-border membrane via the reduced folate carrier (RFC; see Chapter 36). Inside cells, it is polyglutamylated and then stays in cells for many days. Methotrexate competes for the substrate binding site of dihydrofolate reductase and thereby inhibits binding of DHF. In the presence of methotrexate, the concentrations of THF and one-carbon-loaded THFs (e.g., $N^5,N^{10}$-methylene-THF) decrease. With a lower concentration of $N^5,N^{10}$-methylene-THF as a substrate, thymidylate kinase activity is decreased. Methotrexate also leads to an accumulation of DHF. DHF product inhibits thymidylate synthase. Hence, substrate deficiency and product inhibition both decrease thymidylate synthase activity.

Methotrexate has essentially two medical uses: one is related to the inhibition of DHF reductase, which is of use in treating malignancies, and the other is related to an immunosuppressive effect that is of use in the treatment of autoimmune diseases.

Methotrexate is used in the treatment of various leukemias (see Fig. 37.8) and solid tumors. The dose may be more than 0.5 g/m² of body surface. Neoplastic cells, normal cells in the bone marrow, normal fetal cells, and normal cells of the mucosa of the mouth, intestine, and bladder are especially sensitive to methotrexate.

Several **multidrug resistance proteins (MRPs)** pump methotrexate out of cells. These MRPs represent a subfamily of the **ATP-binding cassette (ABC) transporters**. ABC refers to a protein motif in these ATP-driven transporters; the genes for the MRPs contain the letters *ABCC*. Some of these transporters remove mono-, di-, and tri-glutamyl methotrexate from the cytosol. Methotrexate molecules with longer polyglutamate tails are less likely to be pumped out of cells, and they are more effective at inhibiting dTMP synthesis. The rare **Dubin-Johnson syndrome**, due to a heterozygous loss-of-function mutation in the *ABCC2* gene, is associated not only with an impaired excretion of conjugated bilirubin (see Section 5.2.2 in Chapter 14) but also with an impaired elimination of methotrexate. Hence, such patients need an unusually low dose of methotrexate.

**Resistance** to methotrexate can develop in several ways: reduced activity of folylpolyglutamate synthase leads to reduced retention of methotrexate inside cells and thus enhanced excretion of the drug. Active pumping of methotrexate by ABC transporters out of cells likewise diminishes the concentration of methotrexate inside cells. Gene amplification (insertion of many extra copies of the normal gene) of thymidylate synthase permits adequate dTMP synthesis despite the presence of methotrexate. Gene amplification of dihydrofolate reductase and mutations in the dihydrofolate reductase gene that decrease the methotrexate affinity of the enzyme facilitate reduction of DHF in the presence of methotrexate.

In some treatment protocols, methotrexate is infused at concentrations that would prove toxic were they not followed,

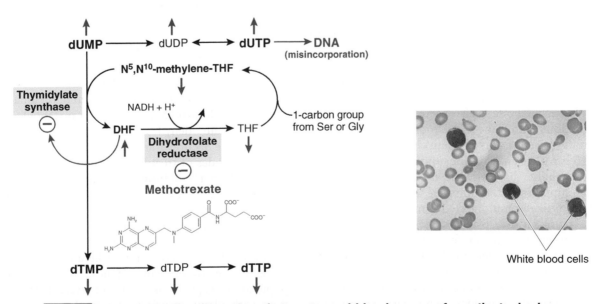

**Fig. 37.8 Mechanism of action of methotrexate, and blood smear of a patient who has acute lymphoblastic leukemia (ALL).** Red arrows indicate changes in concentration. Methotrexate is often part of the treatment regimen for ALL.

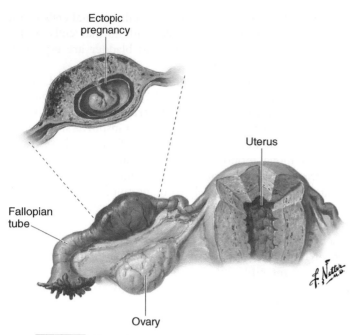

Fig. 37.9  **Ectopic pregnancy in the fallopian tube.**

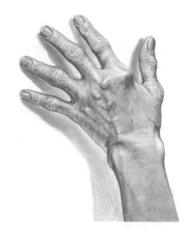

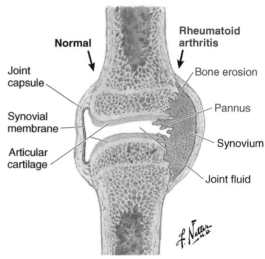

Fig. 37.10  **Rheumatoid arthritis.**

about a day later, by leucovorin ($N^5$-formyl-THF). This maneuver is sometimes called **leucovorin rescue**. With this protocol, more cancer cells are exposed to a therapeutic concentration of methotrexate and fewer cancer cells escape because of resistance to methotrexate.

Methotrexate is used in place of surgery to treat **ectopic pregnancies** (Fig. 37.9). An ectopic pregnancy is a pregnancy outside the uterus, usually in the fallopian tube. Methotrexate therapy preserves the affected fallopian tube, which would otherwise often be severed or removed during surgery. Methotrexate treatment is often reserved for patients who have amniotic sacs that are smaller than about 4 cm. Patients are commonly given a single dose of methotrexate (in the 0.15 g range) and a second or third dose if indicated. Resolution of the pregnancy is followed by measuring the concentration of chorionic gonadotropin in the serum. It usually takes about a month for the fetal tissue to resolve.

Sometimes, methotrexate is also used together with other drugs for **abortions** within the first 2 months of gestation.

Methotrexate is used weekly in relatively small doses (often at about 0.015 g/wk) as an **immunosuppressant** in the treatment of autoimmune diseases. The mechanisms by which methotrexate suppresses the immune system are poorly understood and likely multifaceted. Inhibition of purine nucleotide metabolism may play a role (see Section 2.1 and Chapter 38). Inhibition of dihydrofolate reductase likely plays only a minor role, and folic acid intake does not significantly diminish the effectiveness of methotrexate.

In the treatment of autoimmune diseases, methotrexate is most often prescribed to patients who have **rheumatoid arthritis** (Fig. 37.10), a disease that affects about 0.5% to 1% of the world's population. Affected patients often have joint

pain, joint swelling, and severe morning stiffness. The joints of the hands and wrists are most often involved early in the disease. The synovium is inflamed, and nearby cartilage and bone are destroyed. Therapy is aimed at preventing inflammation and destruction of the joint. Methotrexate, like leflunomide (see Section 1), is a **DMARD**.

Another drug used in the treatment of rheumatoid arthritis is **leflunomide**, which gives rise to a metabolite that inhibits dihydroorotate dehydrogenase in the orotate synthesis pathway (see Section 1 and Fig. 37.2).

Other modes of treatment of rheumatoid arthritis involve **biologicals** that bind **tumor necrosis factor-α (TNF-α)** or act as antagonists at the **interleukin-1 (IL-1)** or **interleukin-6 (IL-6)** receptor.

Methotrexate is sometimes used to treat **psoriasis** (Fig. 37.11) that covers more than 10% of the body. Psoriasis results in chronic hyperproliferation of keratinocytes that gives rise to scaly, sometimes itchy plaques. About 2% of the world population has psoriasis. There are several forms of the condition, with plaque psoriasis the most common. In place of methotrexate, patients can also be treated with a biological that binds TNF-α.

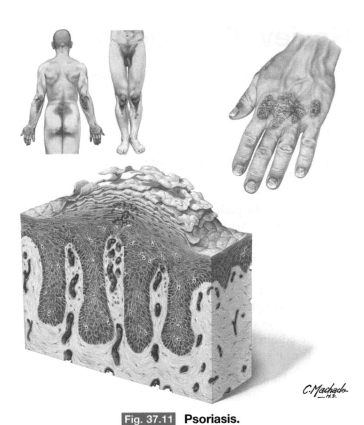

**Fig. 37.11** **Psoriasis.**

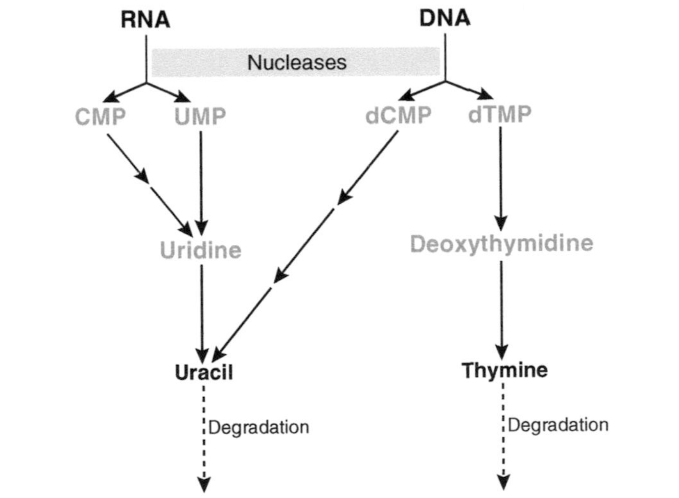

RNA      DNA

Nucleases

CMP   UMP     dCMP   dTMP

Uridine      Deoxythymidine

Uracil      Thymine

Degradation      Degradation

**Fig. 37.12** **Degradation of RNA, DNA, and pyrimidine nucleotides.** Compounds in green can be rephosphorylated and reused.

## 6. DEGRADATION OF PYRIMIDINE NUCLEOTIDES

*The degradation of RNA and DNA yields nucleosides, which can be rephosphorylated and reused.*

Degradation of RNA and DNA by nucleases yields pyrimidine mononucleotides (CMP, UMP, dCMP, and dTMP; Fig. 37.12) that can be rephosphorylated to pyrimidine trinucleotides and thus reused for the synthesis of RNA or the synthesis and repair of DNA. CMP and UMP can be degraded to uridine, which can also be rephosphorylated (see Fig. 37.3).

Similarly, dTMP can be degraded to deoxythymidine, which can be rephosphorylated.

## SUMMARY

■ Pyrimidine nucleotides are synthesized de novo mainly in the liver and in dividing cells. Synthesis involves the production of phosphoribosylpyrophosphate (PRPP) using ribose 5-phosphate from the pentose phosphate pathway. PRPP is produced only when the concentration of phosphate is adequate and the concentration of ADP is low (i.e., when a cell has normal ATP production). Pyrimidine nucleotide synthesis also involves the production of orotate, a pyrimidine base. Orotate is mostly synthesized when a cell performs DNA replication or repair. PRPP and orotate are joined to produce UMP.

■ The liver dephosphorylates UMP to uridine and releases uridine into the bloodstream. Peripheral cells salvage uridine and phosphorylate it to UMP. UMP is the starting point for the synthesis of all other pyrimidine nucleotides.

■ When carbamoylphosphate (CAP) accumulates in mitochondria due to a problem with the urea cycle, it leaks into the cytosol and enters the pathway for orotate synthesis. Measurement of orotate excretion in urine is useful in pinpointing the location of a urea cycle defect.

■ Leflunomide, used in the treatment of rheumatoid arthritis, inhibits the synthesis of orotate, which in turn impairs lymphocyte production.

■ UTP is aminated to CTP. Besides the synthesis of nucleic acids, UTP is used for the synthesis of UDP-glucose and UDP-galactose, whereas CTP is used for phospholipid synthesis.

■ Ribonucleotide reductase reduces UDP, CDP, ADP, and GDP to dUDP, dCDP, dADP, and dGDP, respectively. The protein thioredoxin is the reducing agent, and NADPH, in turn, reduces thioredoxins. The drugs hydroxyurea and gemcitabine inhibit ribonucleotide reductase. Hydroxyurea is used for instance in the treatment of polycythemia vera and sickle cell disease; gemcitabine is used against a diverse set of solid tumors.

■ Thymidylate synthase uses $N^5,N^{10}$-methylene-THF to methylate dUMP to dTMP; this reaction is unique in that it produces DHF. DHF reductase reduces DHF to THF. THF can then be loaded with another one-carbon group for further dTMP synthesis. dTMP synthesis is impaired in patients with a primary or secondary folate deficiency.

■ The antifolate methotrexate inhibits DHF reductase. As a result, DHF accumulates and feedback inhibits thymidylate synthase. In addition, $N^5,N^{10}$-methylene-THF becomes depleted, thus decreasing thymidylate synthase activity. This effect is useful in the treatment of certain leukemias, solid tumors, and ectopic pregnancies.

■ Patients with Dubin-Johnson syndrome are unusually sensitive to methotrexate because they have an inadequate activity of a transporter that removes methotrexate.

Cells can become resistant to methotrexate by reduced polyglutamylation of methotrexate, by amplification of the dihydrofolate reductase or thymidylate synthase gene, or by point mutation of the dihydrofolate reductase gene.

- Low-dose methotrexate has an immunosuppressive effect that is useful in the treatment of rheumatoid arthritis and psoriasis. The immunosuppressive effect seems to be independent of folates.
- Metabolism of the chemotherapeutic drugs capecitabine and tegafur yields 5-fluorouracil. 5-Fluorouracil can also be administered directly. The drug gimeracil inhibits an enzyme that degrades 5-fluorouracil. 5-Fluorouracil gives rise to 5-fluoro-dUTP, which is incorporated into RNA, making the RNA nonfunctional; it also gives rise to 5-fluoro-dUMP, which is a suicide substrate for thymidylate synthase. Without adequate thymidylate synthase activity, DNA replication and repair are impaired. Capecitabine, tegafur, and 5-fluorouracil are mainly used in the treatment of solid tumors.
- The drug pemetrexed also inhibits thymidylate synthase and is used in the treatment of mesothelioma and nonsquamous non–small-cell lung cancer.
- Degradation of RNA gives rise to CMP, UMP, and uridine, all of which can be reused.
- Degradation of DNA yields dTMP and deoxythymidine, which can be reused; dCMP is also formed but cannot be reused.

## FURTHER READING

- Capmas P, Bouyer J, Fernandez H. Treatment of ectopic pregnancies in 2014: new answers to some old questions. *Fertil Steril.* 2014;101:615-620.
- How Renoir coped with rheumatoid arthritis. *BMJ.* 1997;315:1704-1708. This paper is written by experts in rheumatoid arthritis. It nicely illustrates the natural history of untreated rheumatoid arthritis and dramatically describes the effect of the disease on the daily life of the famous painter.

# Review Questions

1. De novo pyrimidine biosynthesis is stimulated by which of the following?

    A. 5-Fluorouracil
    B. N-acetyl-glutamate
    C. Ornithine
    D. Phosphoribosylpyrophosphate
    E. UTP

2. An 85-year-old patient was taking methotrexate for his rheumatoid arthritis. When he moved into an assisted living community, the dose of methotrexate was accidentally changed from 15 mg once a week to 15 mg daily. After 9 days, the patient became very ill. He had labored breathing, nausea, fever, and chills. The patient was hospitalized. A blood sample revealed a low number of red and white blood cells as well as platelets. Which one of the following can be administered to the patient to counteract the toxic effects of methotrexate?

    A. Cobalamin
    B. Gemcitabine
    C. Gimeracil
    D. $N^5$-formyltetrahydrofolic acid
    E. S-adenosyl methionine
    F. Uridine

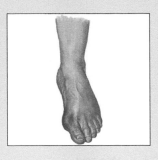

## SYNOPSIS

- The purine nucleotides contain the bases adenine or guanine. Adenosine triphosphate (ATP) is the predominant cellular purine nucleotide.
- Purine nucleotide metabolism is of clinical interest chiefly because of the high incidence of gout.
- Fig. 38.1 provides an overview of the relevant steps of adenine nucleotide metabolism. Guanine nucleotide metabolism is comparable but quantitatively less important.
- When needed, most cells can synthesize adenine and guanine nucleotides de novo.
- In cells with impaired energy production, the concentration of adenosine monophosphate (AMP) is increased. Such cells rapidly degrade AMP to hypoxanthine, which they release into the blood.
- Other cells salvage most of the hypoxanthine in the blood and reuse it to produce purine nucleotides. The liver and the intestine degrade the remaining hypoxanthine to urate, which they release into the blood.
- Urate serves as an antioxidant. In men and postmenopausal women, urate is present in blood plasma near the limit of its solubility.
- Urate is actively excreted by the kidneys. Certain diuretics and organic acids impair the excretion of uric acid (the protonated form of urate). Excretion is also impaired in patients with kidney disease.
- If uric acid is present in urine beyond its solubility, it crystallizes and forms kidney stones.
- The concentration of urate in the blood depends on the rates of urate production and excretion. If the concentration of urate in blood is abnormally high, needle-like crystals of sodium urate tend to form in joints and soft tissues. Occasionally, the crystals in joints give rise to an inflammatory reaction that is extremely painful.
- Gout is characterized by one or both of the following during a patient's life: kidney stones made up of uric acid, and highly painful inflammatory reactions to crystals of sodium urate in peripheral joints. Joint pain can be lessened by treatment with an antiinflammatory drug.
- Drugs available to treat the cause of gout inhibit the formation of urate, promote the excretion of urate, or degrade urate.
- Tumor lysis syndrome can develop in patients who receive cytolytic therapy. Damage to kidney tubules by uric acid crystals can be prevented with an enzyme that degrades urate.

## LEARNING OBJECTIVES

*For mastery of this topic, you should be able to do the following:*
- Explain how the pathways of de novo synthesis, degradation, and salvage of purine nucleotides fit together and how they are regulated.
- List the factors that influence the concentration of urate in the blood, considering urate overproduction and underexcretion.

- For the population at large, describe the effect of gender and age on the concentration of urate in the blood.
- Explain why patients with preeclampsia or eclampsia have hyperuricemia.
- Describe the cause of tumor lysis syndrome, the major risk for patients who have this syndrome, and the role of blood urate–lowering drugs in preventing kidney damage.
- Explain the pathogenesis of an acute attack of gout, starting with hyperuricemia.
- Describe the gold standard for the diagnosis of gout and describe how gout can be differentiated from pseudogout.
- Describe the natural history of an untreated acute attack of gout, as well as the long-term consequences of untreated or treatment-resistant gout.
- Explain the options for acute and long-term treatment of gout with lifestyle intervention and drugs, paying attention to the mechanisms of action.
- Describe the mechanisms by which the following contribute to hyperuricemia and gout: ethanol consumption, fructose consumption, hypoxia, psoriasis, hemolytic anemias, lead poisoning, lactic acidemia, and Lesch-Nyhan disease and its variants.
- Explain the pathogenesis of uric acid nephrolithiasis and list appropriate treatment options.

## 1. DE NOVO SYNTHESIS OF PURINE NUCLEOTIDES

*Adenine and guanine are purines. ATP and adenosine diphosphate (ADP) in mitochondria and the cytoplasm constitute the majority of all purine nucleotides. Adenine and guanine nucleotides can be synthesized de novo, starting with a 5-carbon sugar from the pentose phosphate shunt pathway.*

In biochemistry, the term **purines** entails a large collection of compounds that can be derived chemically from purine (Fig. 38.2) by substitution, such as adenine, adenosine, guanine, guanosine, inosine, hypoxanthine, xanthine, uric acid, the purine nucleotides inosine monophosphate (IMP), AMP, ADP, ATP, guanosine monophosphate (GMP), guanosine diphosphate (GDP), guanosine triphosphate (GTP), and the deoxyribose analogs of these nucleotides.

The concentration of some purine nucleotides in cells is as follows (tissues differ appreciably): ~4 mM ATP, ~1 mM ADP (only ~30 μM free ADP), ~0.1 mM AMP (<1 μM free AMP), and ~0.5 mM GTP. Fig. 38.2 provides a more detailed visual summary. ATP, ADP, and AMP in the mitochondria and the cytoplasm are involved in energy transfer. Almost all of the ADP and AMP is bound to proteins. The GTP/GDP/GMP ratio resembles the ATP/ADP/AMP ratio. The purine nucleotides contained in DNA and RNA make up only about one-tenth of a cell's purine nucleotide content.

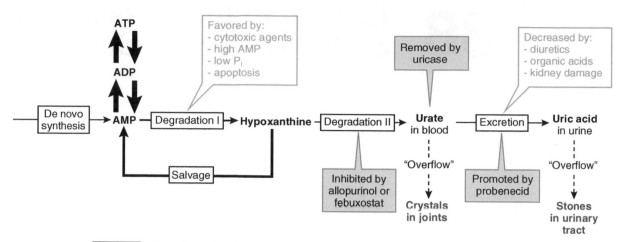

**Fig. 38.1** Overview of adenine nucleotide metabolism as it pertains to gout.

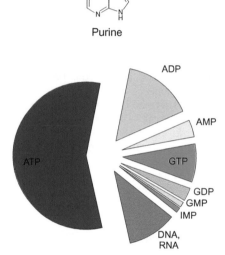

**Fig. 38.2** **Structure of purine and the approximate purine nucleotide content of cells.** The concentration of ATP is usually several mmol/L cell water. Structures of AMP and GMP are shown in Fig. 38.3. (Data from Traut TW. Physiological concentrations of purines and pyrimidines. *Mol Cell Biochem.* 1994;140:1-22.)

Almost all cells can synthesize AMP and GMP both by de novo synthesis and by salvage (see Section 2.4). In the entire human body, de novo synthesis constitutes only about 3% of all AMP synthesis; the rest occurs via salvage. In the de novo synthesis of AMP or GMP, IMP—a precursor purine nucleotide—is built from the ribose phosphoribosylpyrophosphate (PRPP) in many steps. IMP is then converted to AMP or GMP. Fig. 38.3 summarizes these reactions.

Details of purine nucleotide synthesis are as follows. **Well-energized cells** with an adequate concentration of phosphate synthesize **PRPP** from ribose 5-phosphate, an intermediate of the pentose phosphate shunt pathway (see Fig. 38.3; see also Chapter 21). PRPP synthetase is chiefly activated by **phosphate** and inhibited by **ADP**. As will be shown in Section 2.4, PRPP is also used for the salvage of hypoxanthine and guanine. As detailed in Chapter 37, PRPP is also used for the de novo synthesis of pyrimidine nucleotides.

The purine base is built up stepwise on the ribose of PRPP to form **IMP** (which contains the hypoxanthine ring structure; compare to Fig. 38.5). The first of these reactions is irreversible and catalyzed by **glutamine PRPP amidotransferase** (also termed **amido phosphoribosyl transferase**). The activity of this enzyme limits the rate of de novo synthesis. Glutamine PRPP amidotransferase shows cooperativity toward PRPP. As shown in Section 2.5, when IMP cannot be produced from salvage of hypoxanthine, the concentration of PRPP rises and activates the glutamine PRPP amidotransferase. AMP and GMP feedback inhibit this enzyme.

The immunosuppressant drug **mycophenolic acid** inhibits the conversion of IMP to GMP. This drug selectively decreases the concentration of GMP in lymphocytes because these cells have insufficient salvage to produce GMP from guanine and PRPP (see Section 2.4).

Controls on the conversions of IMP to **AMP** and **GMP** are such that appropriate amounts of AMP and GMP are produced.

Even though two of the reactions in purine nucleotide de novo synthesis require $N^{10}$-**formyltetrahydrofolate**, a **folate deficiency** in a patient does not diminish purine synthesis to a clinically significant extent (see Chapter 36).

Under normal circumstances, most ADP is phosphorylated to ATP by **oxidative phosphorylation**, whereby the creatine kinase–catalyzed reaction ADP + **phosphocreatine** + $H^+$ ↔ ATP + creatine plays a major accessory role in muscle and the central nervous system (see Chapter 23). About one-tenth as much ATP is derived from substrate-level phosphorylation in glycolysis (see Chapter 19). **Adenylate kinase** catalyzes the reversible reaction AMP + ATP ↔ 2 ADP. Because of this reaction, the physiological concentration of AMP is tied to that of ADP (i.e., when the concentration of ADP is high, that of AMP is also high). Furthermore, the concentration of AMP changes with the square of the concentration of ADP, making AMP particularly suitable as an indicator of a cell's phosphorylation state.

The concentrations of free GMP, GDP, and GTP are related to those of AMP, ADP, and ATP. **Guanylate kinase** uses ATP to phosphorylate GMP reversibly to GDP. **Nucleoside**

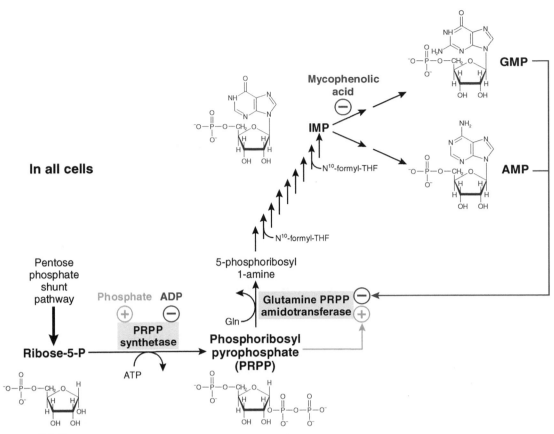

**Fig. 38.3** **De novo synthesis of adenine and guanine nucleotides.** Only well-energized cells (i.e., cells with an adequate concentration of phosphate and a low concentration of free ADP) synthesize PRPP. The de novo synthesis pathway is primarily active when the concentration of PRPP is elevated and the concentration of nucleoside mono- and diphosphates is low.

diphosphokinase uses ATP to phosphorylate reversibly GDP to GTP. Succinyl-coenzyme A (succinyl-CoA) synthetase in the citric acid cycle also phosphorylates GDP to GTP. As a consequence of the prevalence of these enzymes, the degree of phosphorylation of guanine nucleotides generally resembles the degree of phosphorylation of adenine nucleotides.

A large number of reactions dephosphorylate either ATP to ADP or AMP, or GTP to GDP or GMP.

## 2. DEGRADATION AND SALVAGE OF PURINE NUCLEOTIDES

*Whenever the concentrations of AMP and ADP in a cell rise substantially, or whenever the concentration of phosphate in a cell drops substantially, AMP is degraded. During intense exercise, skeletal muscle degrades AMP mostly to IMP and then resynthesizes AMP as part of a purine nucleotide cycle. Nonmuscle cells degrade AMP to hypoxanthine, which they release into the blood. The liver and the intestine oxidize excess hypoxanthine into urate. Most hypoxanthine is salvaged by cells that need more adenine nucleotides. Salvage is always preferred over de novo synthesis.*

*GMP is degraded to guanine under the same conditions as AMP. Cells can salvage guanine and produce GMP.*

*Guanine deaminase in the blood degrades guanine to xanthine, which is taken up mostly by the liver and oxidized to urate.*

*The kidneys excrete about 7% to 10% of the urate that is present in the glomerular filtrate. Organic acids such as ketone bodies, lactic acid, and thiazide diuretics lower this percentage, whereas uricosuric drugs (e.g., probenecid) increase it.*

### 2.1. Degradation of AMP and GMP to Hypoxanthine and Guanine

Almost all of a cell's AMP is bound to proteins, and **free AMP** is present only in **nanomolar** concentrations.

If the concentration of free **AMP** in a cell is abnormally high, or if the cytosol contains an abnormally low concentration of **phosphate**, AMP is rapidly degraded. The concentration of AMP may be high because certain reactions produce AMP at an increased rate (e.g., muscle contraction, metabolism of ethanol, phagocytic degradation of dying cells, pathologic futile cycling in glycolysis and gluconeogenesis), or because mitochondrial ATP production is impaired (e.g., due to hypoxia, poisoning of the electron transport chain, low intracellular free phosphate, or substrate limitation).

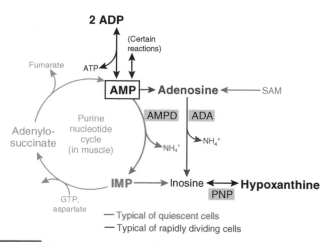

**Fig. 38.4** **Degradation of ADP and AMP to hypoxanthine.** Adenosine deaminase (ADA) and purine nucleoside phosphorylase (PNP) also handle deoxyadenosine and deoxyinosine, respectively. AMPD, AMP deaminase; SAM, S-adenosyl homocysteine, an intermediate in the activated methyl group cycle (see Chapter 36).

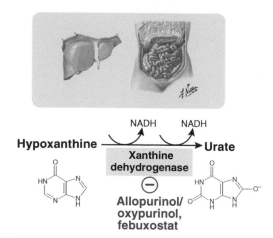

**Fig. 38.5** **Degradation of hypoxanthine to urate and inhibition by allopurinol and febuxostat.** Xanthine dehydrogenase oxidizes allopurinol to oxypurinol, a virtually irreversible inhibitor of xanthine dehydrogenase.

In skeletal muscle, **AMP deaminase** degrades AMP to IMP, which can be reaminated in two reactions to reform AMP (Fig. 38.4). This cycle is called the **purine nucleotide cycle.** No agreement exists yet on the perceived role of this cycle. AMP deaminase is most active when the concentration of ATP is low and that of ADP is high.

In the United States, about 2% of the population has **no active type 1 AMP deaminase**, the predominant AMP deaminase in muscle (other tissues express type 2 or type 3 AMP deaminase). The majority of type 1 AMP deaminase–deficient patients remain asymptomatic, but a minority experience early **exercise fatigue** and **muscle cramps**. In these affected patients, exercise may also lead to an abnormal increase in serum urate (see Section 2.2). For yet unclear reasons, partial and complete AMP deaminase deficiency is associated with improved **recovery from ischemic heart disease.**

While **nondividing cells** resemble skeletal muscle cells in that they degrade AMP via IMP, **rapidly dividing cells** usually degrade AMP via adenosine (see Fig. 38.4). Most tissues must release their hypoxanthine into the blood while the liver and the intestine can convert hypoxanthine all the way to urate (see Section 2.2)

Near-complete **adenosine deaminase (ADA) deficiency** leads to **severe combined immunodeficiency (SCID)** that develops over the first few months of life. ADA deficiency (see Fig. 38.4) leads to increased concentrations of the ADA substrates adenosine and deoxyadenosine, which in turn are phosphorylated to ATP and dATP. Deoxyadenosine and dATP are toxic to lymphocytes. The loss of B-, T-, and NK-lymphocytes can be followed as the disease develops. Patients who have on the order of 5% of the normal ADA activity experience later disease onset, sometimes only in adulthood. In North America, SCID develops in about 1 in 50,000 newborns, and ADA deficiency is responsible for about 20% of all SCID.

The immunosuppressive effect of the antifolate drug **methotrexate** is thought to involve inhibition of both adenosine deaminase and AMP deaminase, thereby leading to the accumulation of adenosine, which binds to adenosine receptors that inhibit neutrophils, monocytes, and macrophages.

**Purine nucleoside phosphorylase (PNP) deficiency** (see Fig. 38.4) also leads to SCID via increased, lymphotoxic concentrations of deoxyguanosine and dGTP. PNP deficiency is a very rare disease.

Most cells degrade **GMP** to **guanine**, which they release into the blood. Other cells that are in need of guanine nucleotides take up guanine and salvage it (see Section 2.4). Since the phosphorylation states of adenine nucleotides and guanine nucleotides are coupled, GMP and AMP are degraded in parallel.

Blood contains the enzyme **guanine deaminase** (also called **guanase**), which degrades guanine to xanthine. The liver takes up xanthine and oxidizes it to **urate** (see Section 2.2 below).

## 2.2. Degradation of Hypoxanthine to Xanthine and Urate

Hypoxanthine and xanthine are degraded to urate chiefly in the **liver**, and to some degree in the **intestine**. **Xanthine dehydrogenase** catalyzes the sequential oxidation of hypoxanthine to xanthine and xanthine to urate (Fig. 38.5). The intestine converts about one-third of the **adenine nucleotides in the diet** to urate. Both the liver and the intestine release urate into the blood.

In the bloodstream, urate functions as an **antioxidant** that reacts preferentially with **peroxynitrite** (O=N–O–O⁻). Peroxynitrite results from the reaction of superoxide anion (•O$_2^-$) and nitric oxide (•NO). If not removed by urate, peroxynitrite directly reacts with or gives rise to compounds that damage DNA and proteins. In contrast to its antioxidant effect, uric acid is also a **prooxidant** that favors lipid peroxidation.

The drugs **allopurinol** and **febuxostat** inhibit xanthine dehydrogenase (see Fig. 38.5). Xanthine dehydrogenase oxidizes allopurinol (an analog of hypoxanthine) to **oxypurinol** (alloxanthine). Oxypurinol then inhibits xanthine dehydrogenase virtually irreversibly. Febuxostat inhibits the molybdenum pterin catalytic center of xanthine dehydrogenase. As shown below, allopurinol and febuxostat are used to decrease urate production in certain patients who have gout (see Section 4; hypoxanthine is then excreted as such, or as its metabolite xanthine). Since xanthine dehydrogenase also metabolizes certain drugs, allopurinol and febuxostat also inhibit the degradation of drugs such as **azathioprine** and **6-mercaptopurine** (see Section 5 and Fig. 38.19).

Oxidation or proteolysis, for instance during **ischemia-reperfusion injury,** turns xanthine dehydrogenase into a **xanthine oxidase** that uses $O_2$ in place of $NAD^+$ and then produces $H_2O_2$ (hydrogen peroxide) in place of $NADH + H^+$. Ischemia-reperfusion injury occurs when tissues experience inadequate perfusion or hypoxia, followed by adequate perfusion and oxygenation. This happens, for instance, in the course of a **myocardial infarction** or a **stroke**. Injury leads to the activation of proteases, which convert xanthine dehydrogenase to xanthine oxidase. The $H_2O_2$ from hypoxanthine oxidation by xanthine oxidase gives rise to reactive oxygen species that damage proteins, lipids, and nucleic acids (see Chapter 21).

Pharmacological information generally refers to allopurinol and febuxostat as inhibitors of **xanthine oxidase** even though the normal pharmacological target is xanthine dehydrogenase. In fact, these drugs inhibit both enzymes.

**Recombinant urate oxidase** (also called **uricase**), such as **rasburicase** or **pegloticase**, can be infused into patients to reduce the concentration of urate in the blood by converting uric acid into **allantoin**. Allantoin is excreted in the kidneys. Virtually all animals express urate oxidase, but humans do not. The recombinant uricases are somewhat immunogenic. Rasburicase has a short half-life in the blood and is used principally for the treatment of tumor lysis syndrome. Pegloticase has a longer half-life in blood and is used principally for the treatment of gout when every other treatment fails.

Recombinant uricases are contraindicated in patients who have **glucose 6-phosphate dehydrogenase (G6PD) deficiency**. As the uricases oxidize uric acid to allantoin, they produce $H_2O_2$. The $H_2O_2$ gives rise to reactive oxygen species (ROS) and oxidative damage (see Chapter 21). G6PD-deficient patients may have an insufficient capacity to generate NADPH in red blood cells to counter the ROS and the oxidative damage. As a result, G6PD-deficient patients injected with a uricase may develop acute hemolysis and sometimes even methemoglobinemia.

## 2.3. Excretion of Urate by the Kidneys

The kidneys function as follows (Fig. 38.6): Blood flow through the kidneys is quite independent of blood flow in the rest of the body. The **glomeruli** of the kidneys filter some of the blood that flows through them; cells and proteins are retained, whereas about one-fifth of water and small molecules in blood plasma end up in the filtrate. The filtrate enters the **proximal tubule**, which actively reabsorbs small molecules such as glucose, amino acids, and ions; about 70% of the filtered water

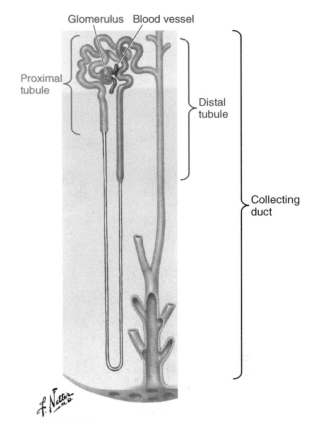

**Fig. 38.6** **Architecture of the kidneys.**

is passively reabsorbed through osmosis. The proximal tubules also secrete organic ions that are destined for excretion. The remaining liquid in the proximal tubule enters the **loop of Henle**, which also removes inorganic ions and water. In the **distal tubule** and the **collecting duct**, the further reabsorption of salt and water is regulated by hormones depending on the needs of the body to secrete either small amounts of hyperosmolar urine or large amounts of hypoosmolar urine. The distal tubules can also acidify the urine.

About **7% to 10%** of the urate in the glomerular filtrate ends up in the **urine**, and organic acids lower this fraction (Fig. 38.7). The excretion of urate by the kidneys is an area of active research. Our understanding of the physiological function and relevance of transporters is therefore preliminary. As a small molecule, urate passes through the glomerular filter. The proximal convoluted tubules take up about 99% of the urate in the filtrate. A subsequent portion of the tubules secretes about half of this urate via the transporters ABCG2 and NPT4. These transporters also secrete lactic acid, ketone bodies, and aspirin. Through competition for the transporter, an elevated concentration of these organic acids decreases the rate of urate excretion. About 40% of the secreted urate is then reabsorbed from the proximal tubules by several **urate transporters**. URAT1 among these transporters is inhibited by the uricosuric drug **probenecid**, and, as a side effect, by other drugs (see Section 4.2).

The urine is often supersaturated with uric acid. In some patients, **stones of uric acid** may form in the kidneys (see Section 4.3).

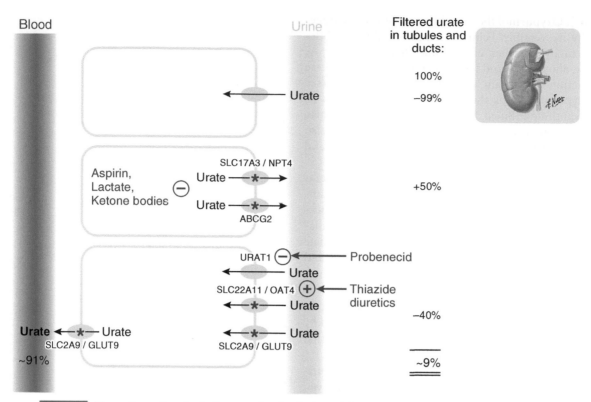

**Fig. 38.7** **Excretion of urate in the proximal tubules of the kidneys.** Only about 9% of the filtered urate ends up in the urine. Asterisks denote a genetic locus in or near the transporter gene associated with a person's genetic risk for gout.

About 25% of all urate is excreted via the **feces**. ABCG2, which also transports urate into the urine, is thought to play a significant role in urate excretion into the intestine. There are no established means of influencing fecal urate excretion.

## 2.4. Salvage of Hypoxanthine and Guanine

Cells that need to increase their adenine nucleotide content may take up the purine base **hypoxanthine** from the blood and react it with the ribose **PRPP** to make the nucleotide **IMP**, a precursor of **AMP** and **GMP** (Fig. 38.8). Cells synthesize PRPP only when they have an adequate concentration of phosphate and when the concentration of free ADP is low. The salvage reaction is catalyzed by **hypoxanthine guanine phosphoribosyl transferase** (commonly abbreviated **HGPRT** or **HPRT**). As indicated by the name of this enzyme, HGPRT can also salvage **guanine**, thereby producing GMP.

Patients who have **classic Lesch-Nyhan disease** have less than 2% of the normal **HGPRT** activity. The deficiency leads to mental retardation, profound motor disability, and a strong inclination toward self-mutilation. HGPRT is encoded on the X chromosome; hence boys are affected more often than girls. Female heterozygote carriers are usually normal. Patients with classic Lesch-Nyhan disease recycle almost no hypoxanthine. As a result, de novo synthesis and urate production are about 30-fold increased. The neurologic problems are likely due to an inadequate synthesis of purine nucleotides, especially in

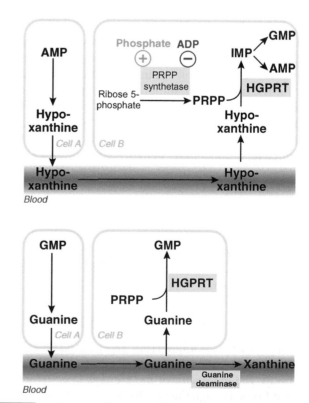

**Fig. 38.8** **Salvage of hypoxanthine and guanine.** Control over the salvage pathway rests with the production of PRPP. The liver degrades hypoxanthine and xanthine that have not been salvaged.

the basal ganglia. Urate overproduction leads to gout (see Section 4.1). Classic Lesch-Nyhan disease is very rare, and it represents one extreme of a spectrum of HGPRT deficiencies.

**Variant Lesch-Nyhan disease** is caused by milder deficiencies of HGPRT activity than classic Lesch-Nyhan disease. The mildest phenotype is associated only with hyperuricemia, but this seems to be uncommon. A more severe deficiency of HGPRT also causes motor handicaps and cognitive problems.

## 2.5. Balancing the Production of IMP From Salvage and De Novo Synthesis

For the production of IMP, **salvage** of hypoxanthine is **preferred over de novo synthesis**. In the human body overall, about **97%** of the production of purine nucleotides stems from the **salvage** of hypoxanthine, and about **3%** stems from **de novo** synthesis. The salvage enzyme, **HGPRT**, follows Michaelis-Menten type kinetics (Fig. 38.9). HGPRT has a

greater affinity for **PRPP** than does glutamine PRPP amidotransferase in the de novo synthesis pathway. In addition, in many tissues, maximal enzyme activity for HGPRT is larger than for glutamine PRPP amidotransferase. Hence, IMP is made mainly from hypoxanthine as long as sufficient hypoxanthine is available. **Glutamine PRPP amidotransferase**, the enzyme that limits the rate of de novo synthesis, shows cooperativity toward PRPP. Only when the concentration of PRPP is relatively high, usually because insufficient hypoxanthine is available for salvage, does glutamine PRPP amidotransferase become active.

Cells build up their adenine nucleotide content only relatively slowly. After losing adenine nucleotides, cells generally require many **hours** to several **days** to regain more than 95% of their normal adenine nucleotide content.

For the production of **GMP**, the same principles apply to balancing de novo synthesis and salvage from either guanine or hypoxanthine as for the production of AMP.

## 2.6. Daily Purine Turnover and Urate Excretion

There are two contributors to the daily purine load: the degradation of hypoxanthine and guanine to urate, and the conversion of dietary purines to urate (Fig. 38.10). About three-fourths of the daily purine load are excreted via the urine and one-fourth via the feces.

## 3. HYPERURICEMIA

*Men and postmenopausal women have the highest concentrations of urate in plasma. Whenever the body produces too much urate, the concentration of urate in the blood also rises, thereby giving rise to hyperuricemia. Likewise, whenever the kidneys inadequately filter blood or excrete a smaller fraction than the normal 7% to 10% of the filtered urate, hyperuricemia ensues. Pregnant women who have preeclampsia overproduce and underexcrete urate; serum urate therefore serves as one of several indicators of the severity of the disease. In persons who have chronic hyperuricemia, crystals of sodium urate tend to form in joints.*

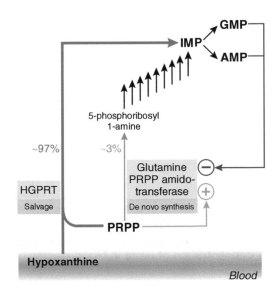

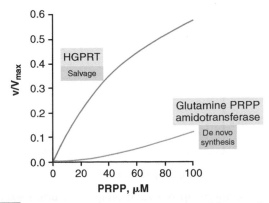

**Fig. 38.9** **Balancing salvage of hypoxanthine and de novo synthesis of IMP.**

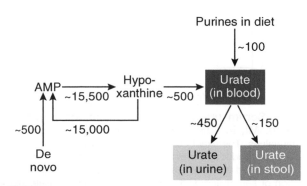

**Fig. 38.10** **Normal purine flux.** Numbers are approximate and given in milligrams per day.

## 3.1. Plasma Urate as a Function of Gender and Age

The concentration of urate in blood plasma is **age and gender dependent** (Fig. 38.11). In adults, estrogen increases uric acid clearance by the kidneys. Hence, premenopausal women excrete a greater percentage of filtered urate than men. Pregnancy normally further lowers the concentration of urate in women (this is also partly due to increased glomerular filtration). In transsexual persons, treatment with estrogens lowers serum urate, whereas treatment with testosterone increases it.

In population studies, the concentration of urate in blood is strongly **hereditary**. More than 25 different genetic loci are known to correlate with the serum urate concentration, although the individual contributions to the population variation are small. To date, about half of these loci could also be associated with protection from, or susceptibility to, gout.

## 3.2. Overproduction of Urate

The relationship between plasma urate concentration and the amount of urate the kidneys excrete per day is shown in Fig. 38.12. The kidneys of a patient who has a high urate production can excrete the larger amount of urate only under the condition of hyperuricemia. In other words, persons who overproduce urate have hyperuricemia. There is no physiological body store for urate. Any daily pathological deposition of urate as crystals of sodium urate in the joints is small compared with the daily urate production.

## 3.3. Underexcretion of Urate

If a patient has impaired perfusion of the kidneys, impaired glomerular filtration, decreased resecretion of uric acid into the proximal tubules of the kidneys, or increased reabsorption from the distal portion of the proximal tubules, the excretion of uric acid amounts to less than the normal 7% to 10%. The concentration of urate in the blood rises until daily uric acid excretion matches urate production (Fig. 38.13). This problem is commonly called urate **underexcretion**. However, this can be a misleading term because persons who produce a normal amount of urate and who "underexcrete" still excrete a normal total amount of urate per day. Underexcretion only refers to a low rate of urate excretion at a normal plasma urate concentration.

Hyperuricemia is thus present in both urate overproducers and urate underexcretors.

In patients who have hyperuricemia but are free of symptoms, possible causes of the hyperuricemia are usually explored, and diet, alcohol intake, and pharmacotherapy are adjusted, if possible. Drug therapy is usually not instituted.

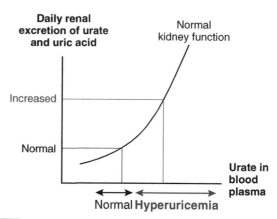

**Fig. 38.12** **Relationship between daily renal urate excretion and the concentration of urate in blood plasma.**

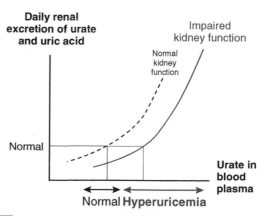

**Fig. 38.13** **Relationship between daily renal urate excretion and concentration of urate in blood plasma in patients who are urate underexcretors.**

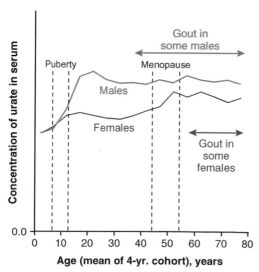

**Fig. 38.11** **Serum urate concentration in the population of Tecumseh, MI, in 1959–1960.** The data include both normal and abnormal values. The exact concentration of urate is omitted because current assays produce different numbers. The trends remain the same, however. (Modified from Mikkelsen WM, Dodge HJ, Valkenburg H. The distribution of serum uric acid values in a population unselected as to gout or hyperuricemia: Tecumsah, Michigan 1959-1960. *Am J Med.* 1965;39:242-251.)

## 3.4. Plasma Urate and Preeclampsia

Preeclampsia and eclampsia are a collection of life-threatening diseases that affect about **5% of pregnant women**, most often in their third trimester (Fig. 38.14). Vasospasms, diffuse intravascular coagulation, and the loss of fluid into the intravascular space (causing edema) decrease perfusion to almost all organs. Decreased renal perfusion and function lead to **underexcretion of urate**. Tissue hypoxia and necrosis, as well as degradation of red blood cells in clots, lead to **overproduction of urate**. Underexcretion and overproduction each increases the concentration of urate in serum. The concentration of total uric acid in blood plasma is a valuable predictor of preeclampsia and eclampsia, as well as an **indicator of the severity** and course of this disease. The principal treatment of preeclampsia and eclampsia is the delivery of the fetus. Seizures can be prevented with an infusion of magnesium sulfate.

## 3.5. Crystallization of Urate

Uric acid has a pK of 5.75; thus, above pH 5.75 (such as in blood), **urate** predominates, whereas below pH 5.75 (e.g., in acidic urine), **uric acid** predominates.

**Sodium urate** can form needle-like crystals. Sodium urate is present in blood near the limit of its solubility. This can be considered advantageous because of the antioxidant activity of urate. On the other hand, when plasma is **supersaturated** with sodium urate, sodium urate tends to crystallize on existing nuclei, preferentially in **joint synovia** and **soft cartilaginous tissues** (Fig. 38.15). This tendency is more pronounced at a lower temperature, which may explain why sodium urate crystals preferentially form in the **cooler** parts of the human body (e.g., limbs and auricles).

Depending on the pH of urine and the total concentrations of uric acid and sodium in it, crystals of either sodium urate or uric acid can form in the urinary tract (see Fig. 38.15). A **low daily urine volume** and a **high daily total uric acid production** both increase the chance of crystal formation. While a **low urine pH** favors the formation of **uric acid** crystals, a **high daily sodium excretion** and a **high urine pH** favor the formation of **sodium urate** crystals. The crystals can aggregate to form kidney stones.

## 3.6. Tumor Lysis Syndrome

Patients who undergo chemotherapy for certain neoplasms are at a particularly high risk of developing uric acid nephrolithiasis as part of tumor lysis syndrome. When tumor cells die, they liberate large amounts of hypoxanthine, potassium, and phosphate. The liver and intestine convert hypoxanthine to urate. This can lead to severe hyperuricemia and damage to kidney tubules by precipitation of calcium phosphate and/or the crystallization of uric acid. Tumor lysis syndrome can be fatal and is a feared complication of chemotherapy or radiotherapy, particularly in patients who have certain lymphomas or leukemias. Onset is usually 2 to 3 days after the start of therapy. In a current classification system, patients who have

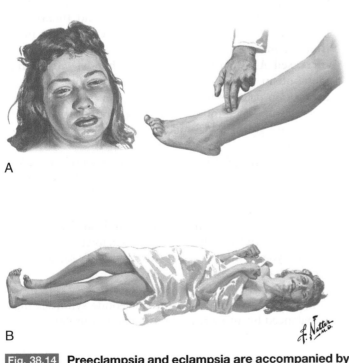

**Fig. 38.14** **Preeclampsia and eclampsia are accompanied by hyperuricemia.** (A) Preeclampsia is characterized by edema, high blood pressure, and proteinuria. (B) Eclampsia is accompanied by life-threatening seizures and internal hemorrhage.

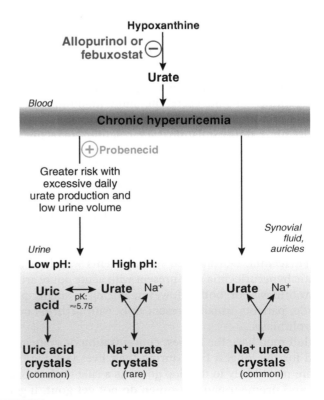

**Fig. 38.15** **Pathologic formation of crystals of sodium urate and uric acid.**

tumor lysis syndrome have two of the following abnormalities: increased $K^+$, increased phosphate, decreased $Ca^{2+}$ ($Ca^{2+}$ is low due to precipitation of calcium phosphate in the kidneys), and increased serum urate, or more than a 25% change in these values 7 days after starting chemotherapy.

Uric acid stone formation with tumor lysis can be minimized with a large fluid intake, oral bicarbonate or citrate, oral allopurinol, or intravenous recombinant urate oxidase (e.g., **rasburicase**). Compared with rasburicase, allopurinol has a slower onset, is not as effective in lowering blood urate, and may lead to the precipitation of xanthine in renal tubules. Hence, allopurinol is used in patients who are expected to produce only a moderate amount of extra urate. Hyperkalemia and hyperphosphatemia are addressed by the induction of diuresis and/or dialysis.

## 4. GOUT

*Patients who have chronic hyperuricemia may develop gout, which can manifest itself either as acute arthritis or kidney stones. Gout is a very common disease, particularly among elderly men. Acute gouty arthritis is due to joint inflammation in response to the presence of sodium urate. Kidney stones are usually due to aggregates of uric acid crystals. Urate-lowering therapy may involve inhibitors of xanthine dehydrogenase, drugs that increase the excretion of urate in the kidneys, and recombinant uric acid oxidase to destroy urate in the blood.*

### 4.1. General Comments About Gout

The term **gout** is sometimes used in reference to urate-dependent joint inflammation only, and sometimes in reference to both joint inflammation and formation of kidney stones. Both of these pathologies stem from aberrations in urate production and excretion. Joint inflammation stems from sodium urate crystals in joints that occasionally give rise to a highly painful inflammatory reaction, an **acute gouty arthritis**. **Nephrolithiasis** (presence of kidney stones) is due to the aggregation of crystals of uric acid or, rarely, sodium urate in the urine. Another form of **nephropathy**, although uncommon, results from crystallization of sodium urate in the hyperosmolar interstitial fluid of the renal medulla. Both nephropathy (related to uric acid or sodium urate) and arthritis are usually preceded by months to years of symptom-free **hyperuricemia**. During their lives, patients who have symptomatic hyperuricemia may present with acute gouty arthritis, nephrolithiasis, or both. However, during a single, painful episode, patients usually present only with arthritis or with nephrolithiasis.

Adult men have the highest concentration of urate in their blood for the longest time during their lives (see Fig. 38.11) and are most likely to develop gout. As a rule of thumb, **children and premenopausal women do not get gout**. If gout is present in a child or premenopausal woman, it may be due to a metabolic disease.

It is estimated that more than 95% of patients who have gout are urate **underexcretors** (see Section 3.3), often for unknown reasons. It is also not known why **hypertriglyceridemia** (see Chapter 28), **hypertension**, and the **metabolic syndrome** (see Chapter 39) are associated with impaired uric acid excretion. Chronic urate underexcretion is seen in the following circumstances:

- Decreased glomerular filtration in patients with advanced chronic **renal failure** and in patients who have **lead poisoning**.
- Inhibition of the excretion of uric acid into the kidney tubules by organic acids (see Fig. 38.7) in patients with chronic **lactic acidemia**, **ketoacidosis**, or **propionic acidosis**, as well as in patients who frequently metabolize large amounts of **ethanol**, and in patients who take certain diuretic drugs (especially **thiazides**, which are organic acids) or **aspirin** (acetylsalicylic acid) at a dose of 1 to 2 g/day.
- In chronically **dehydrated** persons, uric acid reabsorption by URAT1 is increased and excretion is decreased.

Perhaps as little as **1%** of all patients who have gout are urate **overproducers** (see Section 3.2), mostly for unknown reasons. Known causes of increased urate production are diseases and physiological states that lead to an **increased concentration of AMP** or **PRPP** or to decreased **salvage**. Urate production can be increased by the following:

- Metabolism of **ethanol** (see Chapter 30).
- Metabolism of **fructose** (see Chapter 20).
- Increased tissue turnover due to one of the following: **obesity, psoriasis** (see Chapter 37), **leukemia, lymphoma, hemolytic anemias, sickle cell** disease and **thalassemia** (see Chapter 17), **polycythemia vera, hemorrhage, infection, trauma,** or **cytolytic therapy.**
- **Increased AMP production** due to **hypoxia** or **ethanol metabolism.**
- Exercise in patients with a deficiency in muscle **glycogen** metabolism (e.g., muscle glycogen phosphorylase deficiency and glycogen debranching enzyme deficiency) (see Chapter 24).
- **ATP-consuming futile cycles** in patients who have a deficiency in the gluconeogenic pathway, such as glucose 6-phosphatase deficiency or fructose bisphosphatase deficiency (see Chapter 25).
- Exercise in patients with a **medium-chain acyl-CoA dehydrogenase (MCAD)** deficiency (see Chapter 27).
- **Lesch-Nyhan** disease (due to lack of salvage; see Section 2.4).
- Excessive activity of **PRPP synthetase** (a very rare mutation; increased de novo purine nucleotide synthesis must be balanced by an increased production of urate).

### 4.2. Acute Gouty Arthritis

Acute gouty arthritis is the most common presentation of symptomatic, long-term hyperuricemia. The higher

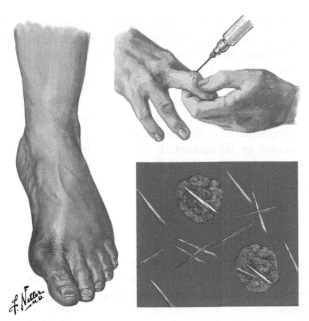

Fig. 38.16  **Acute gouty arthritis and its diagnosis.**

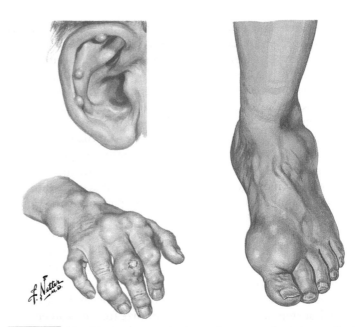

Fig. 38.17  **Tophaceous gout.** The sodium urate deposits are likely accompanied by repeated episodes of acute gouty arthritis and also by the erosion of nearby bone that can destroy a joint.

the concentration of urate in the blood, the greater is the chance that crystals of sodium urate form in the **synovial fluid**. Such crystals occasionally give rise to a very painful, acute inflammation called acute gouty arthritis. The inflammation typically affects a single joint, usually of the lower extremity, and most commonly the metatarsophalangeal joint (Fig. 38.16).

The **diagnosis** of an acute gouty attack often relies on aspirating fluid from the affected joint and finding negatively birefringent crystals under a polarizing microscope (see Fig. 38.16). If the compensator is oriented parallel to the crystals, the crystals appear yellow; if it is perpendicular to the crystals, they appear blue. The method allows crystals of sodium urate to be distinguished from crystals of calcium pyrophosphate, which are the cause of **pseudogout**.

The joint inflammation is self-limiting and, in the absence of treatment, resolves by itself within hours to weeks. The duration of the inflammation can be shortened with nonsteroidal antiinflammatory drugs (**NSAIDs;** e.g., indomethacin, naproxen, ibuprofen), **corticosteroids**, or **colchicine** (an inhibitor of leukocyte chemotaxis). None of these drugs appreciably affects the concentration of urate in the blood.

All patients with acute gouty arthritis should be informed about **lifestyle modification**. Obese patients should lose weight by using a combination of diet and exercise. Patients can reduce the dietary purine load by not eating **liver**, **kidney**, or **sweetbreads** (thymus) as well as limiting their consumption of **red meat** and **shellfish**. Patients can also limit their intake of **fructose** from sucrose, high-fructose corn syrup, and fruit juices. Finally, patients can limit their consumption of **ethanol**, particularly **beer** (because of its high purine content).

After one or more episodes of acute gouty arthritis, patients decide whether to start long-term **urate-lowering drug therapy**. In principle, the concentration of urate in the blood

can be lowered by decreasing urate production, increasing the efficiency of renal uric acid excretion, or a combination of these two processes. The major complication to be avoided is **nephrolithiasis**. Kidney stones with uric acid form most readily in patients with a low urine pH, a low urine volume, and an excessive production of urate.

The major urate-lowering drugs for long-term use are allopurinol, febuxostat, probenecid, and pegloticase. **Allopurinol**, an inhibitor of xanthine dehydrogenase (see Section 2.2), is currently preferred as long as patients do not have an HLA haplotype that is associated with allopurinol hypersensitivity syndrome, which in turn has about a 20% mortality rate. If allopurinol is contraindicated, **febuxostat**, another inhibitor of xanthine dehydrogenase, is used. **Probenecid** enhances renal urate excretion by inhibiting urate reuptake via the URAT1 transporter (see Section 2.3); it is thus a **uricosuric drug**. The use of probenecid is generally restricted to patients who are unlikely to form kidney stones. Patients can reduce their risk of uric acid stones by increasing their fluid intake and taking oral bicarbonate or citrate to alkalinize their urine. At times, patients are given both allopurinol and probenecid. If none of these drugs work, **pegloticase**, a uricase (see Section 2.2), can be used. The American College of Rheumatology recommends that the goal of urate-lowering therapy be a serum urate of 6 mg/dL or less.

**Fenofibrate, losartan,** and **amlodipine** have a uricosuric **side effect** that may be helpful in the treatment of gout. Like probenecid, these drugs inhibit the URAT1 transporter (see Section 2.3). Fenofibrate is used to treat hyperlipidemia. Losartan and amlodipine are both used to lower blood pressure.

If consecutive episodes of acute gouty arthritis are not, or cannot be, adequately treated, **tophi** (visible accumulations of sodium urate crystals; Fig. 38.17) form as a result of a **chronic** excess of urate production over urate excretion. The longer a patient is hyperuricemic, and the greater the hyperuricemia, the more likely a patient is to develop such tophi. Tophi are rarely present at the time of the first gouty attack. With current therapies, the formation of tophi can be prevented in almost all patients.

Patients who have gout due to **lead poisoning**, often referred to as **saturnine gout**, most commonly present with acute gouty arthritis in a **knee**. By contrast, patients who have the usual primary gout usually present with acute arthritis in the first metatarsophalangeal joint. Most patients in the United States with saturnine gout have absorbed too much lead from solder in equipment used for illegal alcohol distillation. Almost all of these patients have lead-induced kidney damage. Lead is stored in bone and stays in the body for decades (it has a half-life of ~20 years).

Treatment of saturnine gout is the same as for primary gout, but steps are also taken to minimize further lead poisoning and reduce lead in the body through **chelation** with $Ca^{2+}$-EDTA ($Pb^{2+}$ binds to EDTA in place of $Ca^{2+}$; $Ca^{2+}$ is present to prevent the hypocalcemia that EDTA would otherwise cause), dimercaprol, or succimer. Some of the lead-induced kidney damage is reversible.

### 4.3. Uric Acid and Sodium Urate in Nephrolithiasis

About 25% of patients who have symptomatic hyperuricemia first present with **uric acid nephrolithiasis** (uric acid **kidney stone**; Fig. 38.18). Most of these patients produce urine of a low pH and a high concentration of uric acid. **Sodium urate** is rarely found in stones.

The long-term prevention of uric acid nephrolithiasis is aimed at reducing the concentration of uric acid in urine.

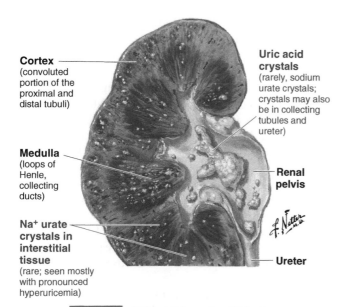

**Cortex** (convoluted portion of the proximal and distal tubuli)

**Medulla** (loops of Henle, collecting ducts)

**Na⁺ urate crystals in interstitial tissue** (rare; seen mostly with pronounced hyperuricemia)

**Uric acid crystals** (rarely, sodium urate crystals; crystals may also be in collecting tubules and ureter)

**Renal pelvis**

**Ureter**

**Fig. 38.18** Uric acid nephrolithiasis.

The patient can increase **urine volume** by increasing fluid intake, increase **urine pH** with oral **bicarbonate** or **citrate**, and decrease **urate production** with lifestyle changes (e.g., weight loss, decreased consumption of alcohol, fructose, and foods with high purine contents, such as organs or seafood). The physician should also treat any underlying disease that contributes to urate production (e.g., psoriasis or myeloproliferative disease). The patient can be prescribed **allopurinol** or **febuxostat**. If indicated by special circumstances, patients can be infused with recombinant **urate oxidase**.

## 5. THIOPURINES

*Thiopurines are purine analogs that have a mutagenic and immunosuppressive effect. They are used in the treatment of neoplasms, autoimmune diseases, and inflammatory diseases.*

The thiopurines have short-term anticancer and immunosuppression effects, yet their long-term use by transplant recipients is associated with an increased incidence of neoplasms, particularly skin cancer. Thiopurines are no longer used much in organ transplantation, but they are used for the treatment of acute lymphoblastic leukemia or inflammatory bowel disease (e.g., Crohn disease or ulcerative colitis).

While most cells can synthesize AMP either by the de novo synthesis pathway (see Fig. 38.3) or by salvage of hypoxanthine (see Fig. 38.8), activated lymphocytes synthesize most of their AMP by de novo synthesis. Therefore they are particularly susceptible to inhibitors of the purine de novo synthesis pathway.

The main clinically used thiopurines are **azathioprine**, **6-mercaptopurine**, and **6-thioguanine**. With the help of glutathione inside red blood cells, azathioprine is converted to 6-mercaptopurine (Fig. 38.19). In lymphocytes, HGPRT (see Section 2.4) acts on 6-mercaptopurine to form thio-IMP, some of which is methylated to methylthio-IMP, an inhibitor of glutamine PRPP amidotransferase, the first enzyme of de novo purine nucleotide synthesis. Both 6-mercaptopurine and 6-thioguanine are enzymatically converted to thio-dGTP, which is incorporated into DNA and may then be methylated. It seems likely that methylated thio-G presents a problem for DNA mismatch repair in a subsequent round of DNA replication, leading to cell cycle arrest and apoptosis.

About 0.3% of all patients are deficient in **thiopurine S-methyltransferase** (**TPMT**), degrade thiopurines abnormally slowly, and are therefore at substantial risk of a fatal adverse reaction. Before treatment, patients can be tested for erythrocyte TPMT activity if they have not recently received a blood transfusion.

Patients who take **allopurinol** or **febuxostat** need to be given a smaller dose of azathioprine or 6-mercaptopurine to account for decreased 6-mercaptopurine inactivation by xanthine dehydrogenase.

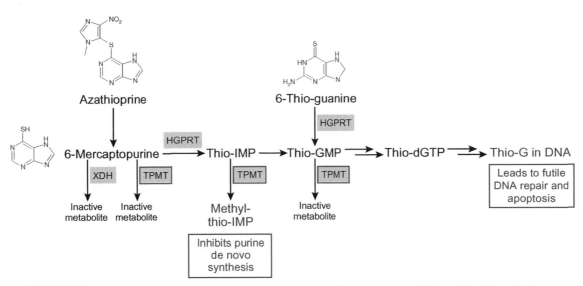

**Fig. 38.19** **Metabolism of the thiopurines azathioprine, 6-mercaptopurine, and 6-thioguanine.** TPMT-deficient persons are at risk for thiopurine toxicity. HGPRT, hypoxanthine guanine phosphoribosyl transferase; TPMT, thiopurine S-methyltransferase; XDH, xanthine dehydrogenase.

## SUMMARY

- When the concentration of phosphate is adequate, and that of ADP low, cells can synthesize phosphoribosylpyrophosphate (PRPP) from ribose 5-phosphate, an intermediate of the pentose phosphate pathway.

- De novo synthesis of AMP and GMP starts with PRPP and proceeds in many steps, two of which involve $N^{10}$-formyl-THF. However, a dietary folate deficiency does not impair purine de novo synthesis (it impairs only synthesis of dTMP).

- When cells accumulate purine nucleoside monophosphates, they rapidly degrade AMP to hypoxanthine and GMP to guanine, both of which they release into the blood. Other cells salvage ~97% of this hypoxanthine and guanine, thereby generating AMP and GMP.

- Cells that have a depleted nucleotide pool slowly reestablish the pool through salvage or de novo synthesis. Enzyme controls ensure that salvage is preferred over de novo synthesis.

- Only about 3% of the hypoxanthine is degraded to urate; this happens mostly in the liver and to a lesser extent in the intestine. The intestine also degrades some of the dietary purines to urate, which it releases into the blood.

- The intestine excretes about one-fourth of the daily amount of urate produced, and the kidneys excrete about three-fourths, mostly as uric acid.

- Men and postmenopausal women have the highest concentration of urate in the blood. In addition, the concentration of urate in the blood is strongly hereditary.

- Hyperuricemia can be the result of urate overproduction, urate underexcretion, or both overproduction and underexcretion. Chronic hyperuricemia leads to the formation of sodium urate crystals in the joints and can also lead to the formation of uric acid stones in the kidneys. In turn, these deposits can lead to acute gouty arthritis or nephrolithiasis, respectively.

- Further episodes of acute gouty arthritis can be prevented with urate-lowering therapy with the xanthine dehydrogenase inhibitors allopurinol or febuxostat, the uricosuric drug probenecid, or the recombinant uricase pegloticase. Further episodes of uric acid nephrolithiasis can be prevented with an increased volume and pH of the urine, allopurinol or febuxostat, or pegloticase. Patients with gout should also be counseled about weight loss as well as the dietary intake of purines, alcohol, and fructose.

- The thiopurines azathioprine, 6-mercaptopurine, and 6-thioguanine are converted to thio-GMP with the help of the salvage enzyme hypoxanthine guanine phosphoribosyl transferase (HGPRT). Thio-dGTP is incorporated into DNA and eventually leads to apoptosis. Thiopurines are used for their immunosuppressive and acutely antineoplastic effects, but they increase patients' long-term cancer risk.

## FURTHER READING

- Dalbeth N, Doyle AJ. Imaging of gout: an overview. *Best Pract Res Clin Rheumatol.* 2012;26:823-838.
- Merriman TR, Choi HK, Dalbeth N. The genetic basis of gout. *Rheum Dis Clin North Am.* 2014;40:279-290.
- Preston R. An error in the code. *New Yorker.* 2007;Aug 13:30-36. This is an account of Lesch and Nyhan's pioneering work on elucidating the cause of a syndrome that came to be called Lesch-Nyhan syndrome. Available at: <http://archives.newyorker.com/?i=2007-08-13#folio=004>.

# Review Questions

1. Patients with certain malignancies who undergo chemotherapy are at a particularly high risk of tumor lysis syndrome. When the concentration of urate in plasma is already high, uric acid nephrolithiasis can best be minimized by which of the following?

   A. Intravenous leucovorin
   B. Intravenous rasburicase
   C. Oral 6-mercaptopurine
   D. Oral probenecid
   E. Reduced fluid intake

2. The hyperuricemia of a 21-year-old male patient who has chronic gout and variant Lesch-Nyhan syndrome is best treated with which of the following?

   A. Intravenous lactic acid
   B. Intravenous rasburicase
   C. Oral allopurinol
   D. Oral probenecid

3. Most patients who have gout show which of the following?

   A. Excessive de novo synthesis of IMP
   B. Excessive degradation of AMP
   C. Insufficient salvage of hypoxanthine
   D. Overly active PRPP synthetase
   E. Overly active xanthine dehydrogenase
   F. Urate underexcretion in the intestine
   G. Urate underexcretion in the kidneys

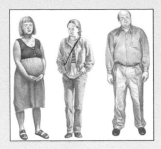

# Chapter
# 39

# Diabetes

## SYNOPSIS

- Type 1 diabetes is characterized by autoimmune destruction of pancreatic β-cells. When the remaining β-cells no longer secrete enough insulin, the concentration of glucose and fatty acids in the blood rises; eventually, diabetic ketoacidosis develops.
- The development of type 1 diabetes depends on both genetic predisposition and the environment.
- Patients with type 1 diabetes treat themselves with insulin, the amount of which they estimate based on carbohydrate intake, prevailing blood glucose concentration, and insulin sensitivity. Almost all currently used insulins are recombinant insulins.
- In type 2 diabetic patients, insulin secretion from pancreatic β-cells is inadequate to maintain the concentration of blood glucose within a normal range. The majority of patients with type 2 diabetes are overweight and have low sensitivity to insulin.
- Treatments for patients with type 2 diabetes include exercise, weight loss, and insulin as well as drugs that stimulate insulin secretion, increase insulin sensitivity, inhibit gluconeogenesis, slow glucose absorption in the intestine, or promote loss of glucose into the urine.
- Gestational diabetes is diabetes that becomes evident during pregnancy, a time of low insulin sensitivity caused by hormones from the placenta. During the postpartum period, most patients with this form of diabetes regain control of the concentration of glucose in the blood. However, they often develop type 2 diabetes years later.

## LEARNING OBJECTIVES

*For mastery of this topic, you should be able to do the following:*
- Describe the pathogenesis of type 1 diabetes and explain the major predisposing factor for this form of diabetes.
- Explain the procedure for diagnosing type 1 diabetes.
- Compare and contrast type 1 diabetes and neonatal diabetes.
- Explain the biochemistry of diabetic ketoacidosis, paying special attention to the role of pancreatic hormones.
- Describe the effects of an overdose of injected insulin on the metabolism of glucose, fatty acids, and ketone bodies.
- Describe the defense against insulin-induced hypoglycemia in healthy and in type 1 diabetic patients.
- Create a procedure for the screening and diagnosis of type 2 diabetes.
- Explain the changes in insulin sensitivity and insulin secretion that typically concur with the development of type 2 diabetes in obese patients.
- Describe the abnormalities that occur in glycogen metabolism and gluconeogenesis in patients who have type 2 diabetes.
- Describe the mechanisms by which weight loss and exercise can improve blood glucose control in type 2 diabetic patients.
- Compare and contrast the mechanisms of action of drugs that are used to treat type 2 diabetes, such as metformin, insulin sensitizers, α-glucosidase inhibitors, glucagon-like peptide 1

receptor agonists, dipeptidyl peptidase-4 inhibitors, sodium-glucose cotransporter-2 inhibitors, inhibitors of adenosine triphosphate–sensitive $K^+$ channels, and insulin.
- Compare and contrast the pathogenesis, blood chemistry, and treatment of hyperosmolar hyperglycemic state and diabetic ketoacidosis.
- Describe testing and treatment for gestational diabetes and estimate the likelihood that a patient with gestational diabetes will develop type 2 diabetes later on.
- Explain the acronym MODY, describe the inheritance pattern and prevalence of MODY, and discuss how a mutation in glucokinase can lead to diabetes.

## 1. OVERVIEW OF THE CLASSIFICATION OF DIABETES

*Diabetes is characterized by a blood glucose concentration that is frequently above a predetermined range. Patients with diabetes have a relative or absolute deficiency in insulin secretion, and they may not properly respond to insulin. Patients who lose most of their pancreatic β-cells to autoimmune attack have type 1 diabetes. Patients whose tissues have an abnormally low response to insulin and who no longer secrete an adequate amount of insulin have type 2 diabetes. Patients who develop diabetes during pregnancy have gestational diabetes. Patients who develop severe diabetes during the first 6 months of life and some patients who develop a milder form of diabetes as children or young adults have mutations in genes, the products of which affect pancreatic β-cell development or function. Patients with maturity-onset diabetes of the young (MODY) carry mutations that mostly lead to impaired insulin secretion.*

Diabetes is characterized by an abnormally high concentration of *glucose* in blood plasma. At a very early, preclinical stage of the disease, hyperglycemia occurs mostly after a meal; later, hyperglycemia is also present in the fasting state. When diabetes is recognized, most patients have hyperglycemia in both the fed and the fasting state.

Many different pathological processes can give rise to diabetes, and our understanding of these processes influences the way different forms of diabetes are categorized. Table 39.1 provides an overview of major, currently accepted types of diabetes.

In the Western world, most patients with diabetes have type 2 diabetes. Only about 5% to 10% of all diabetic patients have type 1 diabetes, about 1% to 5% have MODY, and about 1% to 2% have mitochondrial diabetes. Gestational diabetes affects about 5% of all pregnant women. Neonatal diabetes is

**Table 39.1    Common Classification of Types of Diabetes**

| Type | Description |
|---|---|
| Type 1 diabetes | Autoimmune destruction of pancreatic β-cells. Without treatment with insulin, patients develop life-threatening diabetic ketoacidosis. |
| Type 2 diabetes | Some reduction in volume of β-cells. Insufficient and somewhat altered insulin secretion, often coupled with insulin resistance. About 85% of patients are obese. |
| Gestational diabetes | Diabetes that is recognized for the first time during pregnancy. Years later, most patients develop type 2 diabetes. |
| Neonatal diabetes | Diabetes onset during the first 6 months of life. |
| Transient form | Intrauterine growth retardation. Hyperglycemia often around the fourth day of life. Remission often around 3 months of age. Most patients have excessive transcription of the imprinted genes for the protein PLAGL1 and the noncoding RNA HYMAI. |
| Permanent form | Caused by mutations in the genes encoding the inward rectifying K-channel 6.2, the sulfonylurea receptor type 1 (these two proteins give rise to $K_{ATP}$-channels), insulin, insulin promoter factor-1, or glucokinase, which lead to impaired insulin secretion. Some patients instead show altered imprinting of chromosome 6q. |
| Maturity-onset diabetes of the young (MODY) | Onset of diabetes is typically before 25 years of age. Many causes, but most patients have a mutation in the gene for HNF-4α, glucokinase, HNF-1α, or HNF-1β. Some forms can present as neonatal diabetes or increase the risk for gestational diabetes. |
| Latent autoimmune diabetes in adults (LADA) | Clinical picture is intermediate between type 1 and type 2 diabetes. Patients are adult and have autoantibodies to islet proteins, but they do not have ketoacidosis and initially do not require insulin. |
| Mitochondrial diabetes | In some patients who have a mitochondrial disease that impairs ATP production, often due to mutant mitochondrial DNA. |
| Diabetes due to a disease of the exocrine pancreas | In patients who do not have functional β-cells due to pancreatectomy, chronic pancreatitis, severe cystic fibrosis, or severe hemochromatosis. |

rare. The prevalence of latent autoimmune diabetes in adults (LADA) is difficult to judge because the disease is poorly defined and patients often receive a diagnosis of type 1 or type 2 diabetes. By some estimates, ~5% of type 2 diabetic patients have LADA, and LADA is up to twice as prevalent as type 1 diabetes.

## 2. METABOLISM DURING SEVERE INSULIN DEFICIENCY

*A severe deficiency of insulin gives rise to diabetic ketoacidosis, which is characterized by high concentrations of glucose and ketone bodies in the blood. Patients who have a somewhat less severe deficiency of insulin may instead develop the hyperosmolar hyperglycemic state, which is characterized by severe hyperglycemia and severe dehydration. Diabetic ketoacidosis is principally seen in type 1 diabetic and hyperosmolar hyperglycemic state in type 2 diabetic patients.*

### 2.1. Diabetic Ketoacidosis

As insulin deficiency develops due to autoimmune destruction of pancreatic β-cells, there is first diminished use of glucose, then excessive endogenous glucose production, and finally, excessive lipolysis and ketone body production. This sequence of events is explained by the insulin sensitivity of metabolism, as shown in Fig. 39.1. Glucose uptake requires the highest concentration of insulin; inhibition of glucose production by the liver and kidneys requires an intermediate concentration of insulin, and inhibition of lipolysis requires the lowest concentration of insulin.

**Diabetic ketoacidosis** is commonly defined as a condition during which the concentration of glucose is exceedingly high (>250 to 300 mg/dL, or >14 to 17 mM), the concentration of bicarbonate is low (≤18 mEq/L), the pH is low (≤7.30), and the serum osmolality is only modestly elevated (~290 to 320 mOsm/kg; Table 39.2). In addition, calculation of serum "anion gap" ($Na^+$ minus $Cl^-$ minus bicarbonate) yields a value greater than 10 mEq/L. Diabetic ketoacidosis develops only when the insulin deficiency is very severe. Hence, diabetic ketoacidosis is commonly seen in patients who have type 1 diabetes, and it is uncommon in patients who have type 2 diabetes.

During diabetic ketoacidosis, glucose production is near maximal, glucose consumption is minimal, lipolysis is excessive, and ketone body production far exceeds consumption (Fig. 39.2).

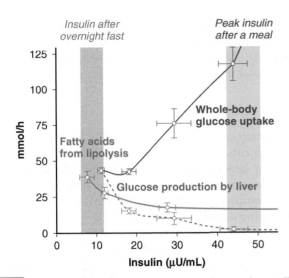

**Fig. 39.1** **Relative insulin sensitivity of adipose tissue lipolysis, glucose production by the liver, and whole-body glucose uptake.** Fifty millimoles of glucose are equal to 9 g of glucose (~36 kcal), and 50 mmol of fatty acids is equal to ~14 g of fatty acids (~120 kcal). 100 mM insulin equals ~14 µU/mL. (Data from Bonadonna RC, Groop L, Kraemer N, Ferrannini E, Del Prato S, DeFronzo RA. Obesity and insulin resistance in humans: a dose-response study. *Metabolism.* 1990;39:452–459; and Campbell PJ, Carlson MG, Hill JO, Nurjhan N. Regulation of free fatty acid metabolism by insulin in humans: role of lipolysis and reesterification. *Am J Physiol.* 1992;263:E1063–E1069.)

**Table 39.2** **Typical Laboratory Values for Patients With Hyperosmolar Hyperglycemic State and Patients With Diabetic Ketoacidosis**

| Analyte in Serum or Blood | Pure Diabetic Ketoacidosis | Pure Hyperosmolar Hyperglycemic State |
|---|---|---|
| Glucose | | |
| mg/dL | ≥250 | ≥600 |
| mM | ≥14 | ≥33 |
| Ketone bodies | Moderate to high | None or low |
| Bicarbonate (mEq/L) | ≤18 | ≥18 |
| pH | ≤7.30 | ≥7.30 |
| Osmolality (mOsm/kg) | variable | ≥320 |

Modified from Kitabchi AE, Umpierrez GE, Miles JM, Fisher JN. Hyperglycemic crises in adult patients with diabetes. *Diab Care.* 2009;32:1335–1343.

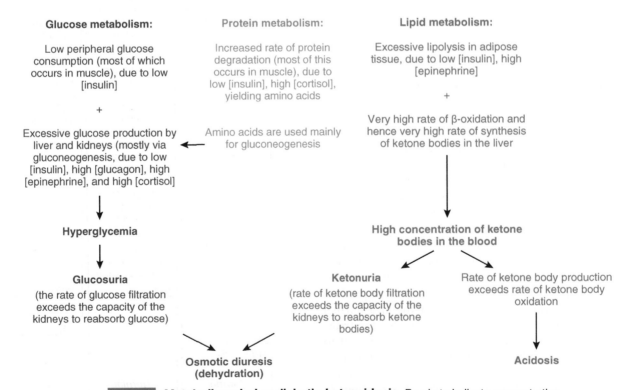

**Fig. 39.2** **Metabolism during diabetic ketoacidosis.** Brackets indicate concentration.

**Treatment** of patients who have diabetic ketoacidosis involves infusing saline solution, insulin, potassium, and glucose. The saline solution helps rehydrate the patient. Insulin stops the lipolysis and hence the production of ketone bodies. Acidosis, dehydration, diuresis, and insulin deficiency all alter potassium homeostasis. During acidosis, cells absorb H⁺ (and buffer it) in exchange for losing K⁺ thus causing hyperkalemia. When insulin is administered, K⁺ flows back into cells, potentially causing hypokalemia. Hence, potassium (as KCl) is given as needed. Hypokalemia can cause cardiac arrhythmia and respiratory arrest, whereas hyperkalemia can cause cardiac arrest. Glucose can also be infused so as to lower the concentration of glucose in the blood only gradually, which may lower the incidence of brain swelling that accompanies some episodes of severe diabetic ketoacidosis.

## 2.2. Hyperosmolar Hyperglycemic State

The hyperosmolar hyperglycemic state develops in diabetic patients who secrete too little insulin to inhibit gluconeogenesis, yet enough insulin to inhibit lipolysis. The syndrome is chiefly seen in a minority of *type 2 diabetic* patients, and it takes days to develop. During this time, the concentration of glucose in the blood climbs steadily. The concentration of insulin in the blood is too low to stimulate insulin-induced glucose uptake (this is the process that requires the highest concentration of insulin; see Fig. 39.1). Hyperglycemia induces somnolence, but per se it is not acutely toxic. When the concentration of glucose in the blood exceeds about 10 mM (180 mg/dL), the kidneys no longer reclaim all glucose from the glomerular filtrate, and glucose appears in the urine. The osmotic activity of glucose induces loss of extra water, which favors dehydration. With drinking, affected patients do not replace all of the water they lose. The osmolarity of serum increases. After several days, the dehydration and consequent decrease in blood volume impair oxygen delivery to the brain, causing mental impairment and then coma.

Hyperosmolar hyperglycemic state is often defined by laboratory values of the concentration of glucose in excess of about 600 mg/dL (33 mM), an osmolarity equal to or greater than 320 mOsm/kg, a pH equal to or greater than 7.3, and bicarbonate ($HCO_3^-$) in plasma equal to or greater than 15 mEq/L (see also Table 39.2). Comparison with the lab values of patients who have pure diabetic ketoacidosis shows differences in the concentrations of glucose, ketone bodies, and bicarbonate as well as in the osmolality.

In practice, the metabolic derangement of diabetic patients is frequently intermediate between diabetic ketoacidosis and hyperosmolar hyperglycemic state, reflecting a spectrum of insulin secretion and insulin sensitivity.

The **treatment** of patients who have hyperosmolar hyperglycemic state involves infusions of saline solution, insulin, potassium, and glucose. Saline solution is infused for rehydration. Insulin is infused to curb endogenous glucose production. Potassium is infused as needed to maintain a normal concentration of potassium in the blood (see also the treatment of diabetic ketoacidosis above). Glucose is infused to lower the concentration of glucose in blood plasma only gradually. In response to the prevailing high osmolarity, the brain of an affected patient has produced sizable concentrations of osmolytes (such as myo-inositol, N-acetyl-aspartate, taurine, creatine, and phosphocreatine). These osmolytes are degraded only slowly. Lethal swelling of the brain may occur during treatment of hyperosmolar hyperglycemic state, and there is concern that this may be due to water flowing into the brain due to the high concentration of intracellular osmolytes. For this reason, many algorithms call for a gradual reduction in blood glucose. However, while the above theory is plausible, a thorough understanding of the cause of the brain edema is still lacking. About 20% of patients who present with the hyperosmolar hyperglycemic state do not survive the episode.

## 3. DIAGNOSIS OF DIABETES

*The diagnosis of diabetes is based on the finding of an abnormally high concentration of glucose or an abnormally high fraction of hemoglobin $A_{1c}$ in the blood. The testing procedures yield groups of patients who have either frank diabetes or abnormalities that are associated with an increased risk of developing diabetes in the future.*

Diabetes is defined in the following ways: (1) as an abnormally high concentration of **glucose** in blood plasma after an overnight fast, at any time during the day, or 2 hours into an oral glucose tolerance test (described below); or (2) as an elevated fraction of **hemoglobin $A_{1c}$** (**$HbA_{1c}$**). Criteria for glucose testing of nonpregnant adults are shown in Fig. 39.3. $HbA_{1c}$ is described in Table 16.1. Blood for an $HbA_{1c}$ test can be collected at any time. This test should not be used in pregnant patients, those with hemolysis, or patients who receive a

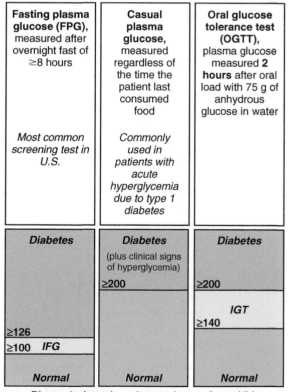

**Test:**

| Fasting plasma glucose (FPG), measured after overnight fast of ≥8 hours | Casual plasma glucose, measured regardless of the time the patient last consumed food | Oral glucose tolerance test (OGTT), plasma glucose measured **2 hours** after oral load with 75 g of anhydrous glucose in water |
|---|---|---|
| *Most common screening test in U.S.* | *Commonly used in patients with acute hyperglycemia due to type 1 diabetes* | |
| **Diabetes** | **Diabetes** (plus clinical signs of hyperglycemia) ≥200 | **Diabetes** ≥200 |
| ≥126 | | *IGT* ≥140 |
| ≥100 *IFG* | | |
| *Normal* | *Normal* | *Normal* |

Diagnosis, based on plasma glucose (in mg/dL)

**Fig. 39.3** **Tests for screening and diagnosis of diabetes.** Cutoff numbers are those of the American Diabetes Association. The World Health Organization and the International Diabetes Federation mostly use the same values. Conversion of glucose concentrations: 100 mg/dL = 5.56 mM, 110 mg/dL = 6.11 mM, 126 mg/dL = 7.00 mM, 140 mg/dL = 7.78 mM, 200 mg/dL = 11.11 mM. IFG, impaired fasting glucose; IGT, impaired fasting glucose tolerance.

blood transfusion or erythropoietin therapy. It is also inappropriate to perform this test in patients with certain hemoglobinopathies. An HbA$_{1c}$ value (standardized to the Diabetes Control and Complications Trial in the United States) of 6.5% or more is positive for diabetes.

There is incomplete concordance between tests for diabetes. The oral glucose tolerance test with determination of plasma glucose after 2 hours is the most sensitive test. This is largely attributable to the fact that most patients lose control over blood glucose after a meal before they lose control in the fasting state.

For a **definitive diagnosis** of diabetes, there must be clear clinical evidence of diabetes, a different test that also shows diabetes, or an immediate repeat test with a new blood sample that also shows diabetes. Similar principles apply to the testing of children and pregnant women.

**Prediabetes** is a popular term for impaired fasting plasma glucose, impaired glucose tolerance (Fig. 39.3), or an HbA$_{1c}$ of 5.7% to 6.4%, all of which are risk factors for diabetes. These patients can lower their risk of developing diabetes by exercising regularly and maintaining or achieving a normal body weight.

A **glucose tolerance test** measures the body's ability to clear glucose from the blood without excessive hyperglycemia. A patient is given a standardized amount of glucose, usually by mouth, and the concentration of glucose in the patient's blood is determined at two or more time points (Fig. 39.4). Pancreatic insulin secretion and the body's response to insulin both affect glucose clearance. In the absence of diabetes, the β-cells secrete sufficient insulin to compensate for any deficit in the body's response to insulin. Currently, tests with oral glucose are clinically limited mostly to the detection of gestational diabetes in pregnant women and to their follow-up. The oral glucose test is also frequently used in diabetes research.

Infants who develop diabetes before the age of 6 months have **neonatal diabetes** or MODY and should undergo DNA testing for mutations in genes that have been linked to these forms of diabetes. In the 6- to 12-month age cohort, type 1 diabetes is more likely than neonatal diabetes, and genetic testing can be limited to those who do not have antibodies against islets. The incidence of neonatal diabetes is at least ~1 in 400,000. The major causes of neonatal diabetes are listed in Table 39.1.

## 4. PATHOGENESIS, DIAGNOSIS, AND TREATMENT OF TYPE 1 DIABETES

*The likelihood that a person develops type 1 diabetes depends on the person's makeup of antigen-presenting proteins, other heritable factors, and the environment. Over a period of months or years, the pancreatic β-cells are destroyed by an autoimmune attack. Patients who develop type 1 diabetes present with pronounced hyperglycemia and frequently also with ketoacidosis. Type 1 diabetic patients need to be treated with insulin. The carbohydrate content of meals as well as other factors are used to estimate insulin needs. There are*

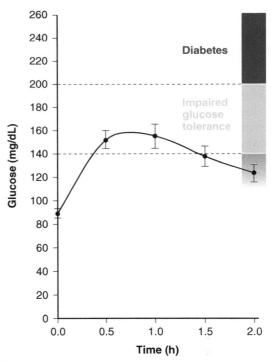

**Fig. 39.4** **The 75-g oral glucose tolerance test and its interpretation according to the American Diabetes Association.** The time course of the concentration of glucose represents the mean of ~150 nondiabetic individuals. (Data from Man C, Campioni M, Polonsky KS, et al. Two-hour seven-sample oral glucose tolerance test and meal protocol: minimal model assessment of beta-cell responsivity and insulin sensitivity in nondiabetic individuals. *Diabetes.* 2005;54:3265-3273; and Gerich J, Van Haeften T. Insulin resistance versus impaired insulin secretion as the genetic basic for type 2 diabetes. *Curr Opin Endocrinol Diabetes.* 1998;5:144-148.)

*long- and short-acting insulins, which are best suited to cover the body's needs between and after meals, respectively.*

### 4.1. Definitions

Type 1 diabetes is sometimes subdivided into type 1A and type 1B diabetes. At the time of diagnosis, type 1A diabetes is accompanied by autoantibodies to islet proteins. In contrast, patients with type 1B diabetes do not have islet autoantibodies. Among patients with type 1 diabetes, most have type 1A diabetes. The term type 1 diabetes in this text refers to type 1A diabetes.

### 4.2. Pathogenesis, Heredity, and Diagnosis

The development of type 1 diabetes depends on a person's genotype and environment.

Type 1 diabetes shows a polygenic pattern of inheritance. Certain alleles for class II **human leukocyte antigens** (**HLAs**) are the most common predisposing factor, and alleles for the **insulin promoter** are second most important. Other genes have a comparatively small influence.

Pancreatic β-cells die due to a direct attack by cytotoxic T cells, a bystander effect, or a combination of these. HLA proteins are located in the membrane of antigen-presenting cells, such as dendritic cells, activated macrophages, and activated B cells (i.e., lymphocytes, not pancreatic β-cells); on the surface of those cells, HLA proteins present short peptides to T cells. If T cells consider these peptides foreign, they might attack β-cells directly. Alternatively, β-cells might sustain damage due to the release of free radicals, NO, interleukin-1, and enzymes from nearby macrophages and neutrophils. Patients who have had clinically recognized type 1 diabetes for several years have only about 2% of the normal number of β-cells left. Most type 1 diabetic patients produce β-cells at a low rate throughout their lives; however, autoimmune killing keeps the total number of β-cells very low.

**Antibodies to islet cell antigens** are detectable years before onset of glucose intolerance due to type 1 diabetes and can be used to predict who will develop type 1 diabetes. These antibodies are typically directed against one or more of the following: insulin, glutamic acid decarboxylase (GAD), IA-2 (protein tyrosine phosphatase 2), and ZnT8 (also called SLC30A8, a zinc transporter in islet β-cells). The number of nucleotide repeats in a region 5′ to the insulin gene determines the expression of (a tiny amount of) insulin in the thymus. Insufficient insulin synthesis in the thymus might give rise to inadequate central tolerance.

Years after islet cell antibodies are first apparent, impaired glucose tolerance and glucose intolerance usually set in over a period of many months. As β-cells die and insulin secretion diminishes, there is first diminished use of glucose, then excessive endogenous glucose production, and finally excessive lipolysis and ketone body production (see Fig. 39.1; further details are provided in Chapters 24, 25, 27, and 28). Accordingly, patients who develop type 1 diabetes first have postprandial hyperglycemia and then fasting hyperglycemia. Typically, the concentration of glucose 2 hours after an oral glucose tolerance test rises markedly (by ~2 mM or ~35 mg/dL per month) only during the few months before onset of diabetes. With marked hyperglycemia, glucosuria (glucose in the urine) and polyuria (excessive urination due to the osmotic effect of glucose in the urine) set in. The affected person commonly does not recognize the gradual loss of glucose tolerance. Sometimes, glucose intolerance is accompanied by candidiasis, a yeast infection. Excessive lipolysis develops at a later stage, which gives rise to diabetic ketoacidosis. Patients with yet undiagnosed type 1 diabetes typically present with a history of polydipsia, polyuria, weight loss, and malaise and, in ~25% of cases, diabetic ketoacidosis. Ketoacidotic patients breathe deeply and rapidly, and their breath smells of acetone (acetone is spontaneously formed from acetoacetate, a ketone body; see Sections 5.1 and 7.3 in Chapter 27).

Once a patient is diagnosed with type 1 diabetes and receives treatment, **diabetic ketoacidosis** sets in whenever the concentration of insulin is extremely low compared with needs (see Section 2.1). In the absence of insulin, a type 1 diabetic patient develops diabetic ketoacidosis within hours to a day (depending on the half-life of the insulin that was last administered). Sometimes, a patient has the misperception that no insulin is needed when no food is consumed during

an acute illness. In truth, ill patients may have to increase their insulin dose beyond their normal baseline dose because illness causes the body to secrete relatively large amounts of glucagon, epinephrine, and cortisol.

In patients with type 1 diabetes, **diagnosis** is usually urgent and straightforward. The diagnosis of diabetes typically rests on finding a plasma glucose concentration of 200 mg/dL or higher (≥11.1 mM; see Fig. 39.3) as well as polyuria, polydipsia, and unexplained weight loss. An elevated concentration of ketone bodies in serum, a reduced concentration of bicarbonate, and a low blood pH can provide further support for a diagnosis of type 1 diabetes. In special cases, a test for islet cell antibodies may help distinguish type 1 from type 2 diabetes.

## 4.3. Treatment of Type 1 Diabetes

Type 1 diabetic patients depend on exogenous **insulin** for immediate survival. Current chief regimens are either a minimum of three to four injections per day with short- and long-acting analogs of human insulin (see below) or continuous and bolus infusion of short-acting insulin by a pump. Patients measure their blood glucose concentration by finger prick multiple times per day and adjust their insulin dose accordingly. A continuous glucose monitor with a sensor under the skin can provide additional data on interstitial glucose. The U.S. Food and Drug Administration has recently approved a wearable artificial pancreas, which consists of a glucose sensor, algorithms, and an insulin pump.

A few weeks after diagnosis, type 1 diabetic patients sometimes experience a **honeymoon** phase during which they require a reduced amount of exogenous insulin.

Type 1 diabetic patients need a **basal** concentration of insulin in the blood at all times and **boluses** of insulin to accommodate meals. Figs. 26.5, 26.8, 28.9, and 39.6 show that there is a basal concentration of insulin in nondiabetic volunteers. The basal concentration of insulin suppresses lipolysis (see Section 5.1 in Chapter 28) and endogenous glucose production (glycogenolysis and gluconeogenesis; see Section 2.2 in Chapter 24 and Section 3 in Chapter 25). A bolus of insulin covers the diet-derived spike in blood glucose by activating glucose consumption (see Fig. 39.1).

Patients who receive multiple insulin **injections** per day use a **rapid-acting insulin** to cover meal-related needs for insulin and a **long-acting insulin** to cover the baseline need for insulin. A rapid-acting insulin peaks 0.5 to 2 hours after injection, whereas a long-acting insulin does not have a clearly identifiable peak action and is effective for a half-day to a full day. Typically, patients inject about 50% of their daily insulin as a long-acting insulin (toddlers need only about 30% of the daily total). Insulin cannot be given orally because the digestive tract would degrade most of it before it reaches the bloodstream.

Patients who wear an insulin **pump** use only rapid-acting insulin. The pump delivers a bolus of programmable duration to cover meals and an ongoing infusion to provide for baseline needs.

Rapid-acting, intermediate-acting, and long-acting insulins are the result of applying knowledge of protein chemistry to a clinical problem and producing modified proteins with methods of molecular biology. The majority of insulin is now purified from transformed bacteria that synthesize a normal or mutated human preproinsulin, proinsulin, and insulin. Insulin is purified from an extract of such bacteria. This purified insulin does not contain C-peptide. The insulin is sometimes crystallized with $Zn^{2+}$; however, it can instead also be complexed with **protamine**, a DNA-binding protein that contains many positive charges.

A challenge in producing rapid- and long-acting mutant insulins is to produce molecules that do not lead to excessive activation of insulin-like growth factor-1 (IGF-1) receptors. Excessive activation of IGF-1 receptors leads to an increased rate of cell division and may give rise to a **neoplasm**.

The commonly used **rapid-acting insulins** are insulin lispro, aspart, and glulisine. Insulin **lispro** differs from normal human insulin in that it has a Pro28Lys and a Lys29Pro mutation. Insulin **aspart** has a Pro28Asp mutation. **Glulisine** has Asn3Lys and Lys29Gln mutations. These sequence changes impede dimerization of insulin and formation of hexamers around a zinc atom. Hence, in the subcutaneous space, these insulin analogs are mainly present as monomers and they therefore diffuse into the bloodstream at a higher rate than do insulins that form hexamers with Zn and then crystallize. The appearance of short-acting insulins in the bloodstream resembles the food-induced appearance of insulin in nondiabetic individuals.

The main currently used **intermediate-acting insulin** is insulin **NPH**. NPH stands for neutral protamine Hagedorn (Dr. Hagedorn in Denmark was one of the inventors of this technology). When insulin is complexed to protamine, the subcutaneous depot releases insulin into the bloodstream more gradually.

The main currently used **long-acting insulins** are insulin detemir, insulin glargine, and insulin degludec. Insulin **detemir** has a β-chain without Thr30, but with the fatty acid myristic acid (14 carbons) covalently linked to Lys29. As supplied, insulin detemir forms hexamers around a zinc atom. After injection, solute (phenol and cresol) is lost from the subcutaneous depot, and the hexamers pair up. Because large molecules diffuse only slowly, this dihexamer complex diffuses into the bloodstream only slowly. Insulin **glargine** has decreased solubility at physiological pH but it is soluble at low pH. Accordingly, insulin glargine is injected in a solution that has a pH of about 4. In the tissue, where the pH is above 7, insulin glargine precipitates and then dissolves relatively slowly. Insulin **degludec** misses ThrB30 and has LysB29 linked to glutamate and then two fatty acids. It dissolves in phenol and cresol, precipitates after injection, and forms dihexamers. The half-life is longer than 24 hours.

The control a diabetic patient has over the concentration of glucose in the blood is limited by multiple factors, including the accuracy with which the patient predicts his or her body's need for insulin, the patient's counterregulatory responses to hypoglycemia, stress, and the level of exercise. Most patients estimate their insulin needs for a meal based on meal carbohydrate content, insulin sensitivity, and current blood glucose concentration (Fig. 39.5). Consistently accurate prediction of insulin needs is impossible because the body's daily responses differ too much. If a patient injects too much insulin, a so-called **insulin reaction** can occur, which is characterized by a period of transient **hypoglycemia**, during which glucose consumption is excessive and endogenous glucose production is minimal. Hypoglycemia is dangerous because—depending on severity—it can lead to poor judgment, loss of consciousness, permanent vegetative state, or death.

Patients typically treat **hypoglycemia** with rapidly absorbed carbohydrate or, if severe, with glucagon. The carbohydrate can be consumed as glucose in solid or liquid form or as a regular food from which carbohydrate is readily available (e.g., sugar-containing liquids, such as fruit juice or soft drinks). **Glucagon** liberates glucose from liver glycogen stores and must be injected. Although a typical pharmacological dose of glucagon cannot stimulate lipolysis, it can always stimulate breakdown of liver glycogen. Glucagon is commonly used in children who are unconscious or who cannot swallow; however, it frequently elicits nausea or vomiting.

At the time of diagnosis, type 1 diabetic patients usually secrete a normal amount of **glucagon** and **epinephrine**, but these responses are lost after many years of the disease. Glucagon and epinephrine are the chief hormones that help counteract insulin-induced hypoglycemia. Without either hormone, a patient's body is defenseless against an overdose of insulin. Hence, patients with long-term type 1 diabetes are at increased risk of insulin-induced hypoglycemia.

Recurrent hypoglycemia leads to **hypoglycemia unawareness** and reduced secretion of counterregulatory hormones during hypoglycemia, components of the hypoglycemia-associated autonomic failure (HAAF) syndrome. About one-fourth of adults who have type 1 diabetes also have hypoglycemia unawareness. The molecular pathogenesis of HAAF is poorly understood. After several weeks without

| Carbohydrate intake: | Blood glucose correction: |
|---|---|
| **Amount Per Serving** | Finger stick: 150 mg/dL |
| Total Carbohydrate: 26 g<br>Dietary Fiber:          3 g | Target:         120 mg/dL |
| **Digestible Carbohydrate:**<br>26 g – 3 g = 23 g | Excess blood glucose:<br>150 – 120 = 30 mg/dL |
| **Insulin: 1 unit / 14 g CHO** | Insulin: 1 unit / 25 mg/dL |
| **Insulin dose for carbohydrate:**<br>23 / 14 = **1.64 units** | Insulin dose for blood glucose:<br>30 / 25 = **1.20 units** |

**Total insulin dose:  1.64 + 1.20 = 2.84 units**

**Fig. 39.5** **Calculation of insulin dose for one serving of a packaged food.** The person's insulin sensitivity determines how much carbohydrate 1 U insulin "covers" and by how much it lowers a high concentration of blood glucose. CHO, carbohydrate.

hypoglycemia, patients can become aware of hypoglycemia once again.

The **diet** of a type 1 diabetic patient is essentially that of a healthy person, except for an avoidance of rapidly absorbed sugars. Current insulins do not reach the bloodstream quickly enough to cover a large and rapid increase in blood glucose.

Treating physicians assess diabetic patients' control of their diabetes every 3 months by measuring the fraction of $HbA_{1c}$. This value reflects the plasma glucose concentration over a period of ~2 months (red blood cells are typically 0 to 4 months old). Two methods for the determination of $HbA_{1c}$ are currently in use. The United States uses a traditional method that is traced to a standard that contains several glycated hemoglobins and was used during a large diabetes treatment trial. European countries use a newer method that refers to a single glycated hemoglobin species and yields lower values than those yielded by the traditional method. In an attempt to minimize confusion, results from the old method are reported as a percentage, and results from the new method as mmol/mol. A patient with type 1 diabetes, on average, always has some hyperglycemia, which typically leads to an elevated $HbA_{1c}$. An $HbA_{1c}$ value less than 6.5% to 7.0% is considered acceptable (the $HbA_{1c}$ of a nondiabetic person is ≤5.6%), whereas a larger value should be a call to improved control of plasma glucose.

The $HbA_{1c}$ is misleadingly low in patients who have a shortened lifetime of red blood cells or certain other conditions (see Section 3).

Continuous glucose monitors measure the concentration of glucose in the interstitial fluid continuously and can often provide helpful information about daily excursions of the concentration of glucose. This information can be used to improve control of blood glucose.

# 5. PATHOGENESIS, DIAGNOSIS, AND TREATMENT OF TYPE 2 DIABETES

*Type 2 diabetes is usually diagnosed after a screening procedure or when a patient has a typical complication of type 2 diabetes, such as a stroke or myocardial infarction. Almost all type 2 diabetic patients take up an abnormally small amount of glucose in response to insulin, and all type 2 diabetic patients secrete an inadequate amount of insulin to maintain a normal concentration of glucose in the blood. A person's chance for developing type 2 diabetes depends on genetic factors, body weight, and age. Available treatments for type 2 diabetes can be well rationalized based on knowledge of glucose homeostasis. Treatments decrease the rate of influx of glucose into the blood, increase insulin secretion, increase the effect of insulin on metabolism, attenuate glucose production by liver and kidneys, or induce a significant loss of glucose into the urine.*

## 5.1. Pathogenesis

Type 2 diabetes is largely a result of the interplay of a patient's **genotype**, **diet**, **exercise**, and **age**.

More than 60 genetic loci are known to affect the risk of developing type 2 diabetes, and many more loci remain to be discovered to account for the contribution of genetics to a person's risk for type 2 diabetes. The genetic predisposition to type 2 diabetes is somewhat smaller than the genetic predisposition to type 1 diabetes. There is little overlap between genetic loci that predispose to type 1 and type 2 diabetes.

The locus that confers the highest risk for type 2 diabetes is in the *TCF7L2* gene (which encodes a transcription factor), and it increases risk only by a factor of ~1.4. Therefore the genetic risk for diabetes is an aggregate of many small risks. Surprisingly, diabetic persons and matched nondiabetic persons have about the same number of risk factors. As a result, testing of patients for diabetes-related loci does not yet provide useful clinical information.

**Age**, **family history**, and **obesity** are the major risk factors for diabetes that are used clinically. For instance, compared with a 25-year-old person, the diabetes risk of a 50-year-old is ~13 times and that of a 70-year-old is ~26 times higher. Also, the ~8% of the U.S. population with the highest familial risk for diabetes has 5 times the risk of the ~70% of the population with only an average familial risk. **Obesity** in **adults** is commonly assessed using **body mass index (BMI)**. The BMI is a useful measure of body fat in populations, not individuals, yet in clinical practice BMI is widely used with individual patients. The formula for calculating the BMI is as follows:

$$BMI = (\text{weight in kg})/(\text{height in m})^2$$

According to the widely used World Health Organization (WHO) definition, the term **overweight** is used for BMIs from 25 kg/m² to less than 30 kg/m² and the term **obese** for BMIs of 30 kg/m² or higher. **Morbid** or **extreme obesity** is sometimes defined as a BMI of 40 kg/m² or higher. Compared with a person with a BMI of 25 kg/m², a person with a BMI of 30 kg/m² is ~3 times more likely to develop diabetes and a person with a BMI of 40 kg/m² ~9 times more likely. About 80% to 90% of patients who have type 2 diabetes are obese. Obesity in **children** is assessed using special tables that take age into account, such as those published by the U.S. Centers for Disease Control and Prevention (see Kuczmarski et al. under the Further Reading section). **Insulin resistance** is a state in which the body, at a normal concentration of insulin, does not remove a normal amount of glucose from the blood. As a result, the pancreatic β-cells need to secrete more insulin to maintain a normal concentration of glucose in the blood. Hence, insulin resistance is accompanied by **hyperinsulinemia**. **Insulin sensitivity** is the opposite of insulin resistance.

In a research setting, insulin resistance can be assessed by infusing a patient with insulin to obtain a stable concentration of circulating insulin and by infusing glucose to maintain plasma glucose near a predetermined concentration. The less glucose that has to be infused, the more insulin resistant a patient is. An infusion of labeled glucose is commonly used to correct the data for endogenous glucose production by the liver and by the kidneys.

A decreased secretion of adiponectin, as in obesity, thus renders the body more insulin resistant. Obese patients with moderate insulin resistance typically have two to five times the concentration of insulin in the blood that is found in a lean, insulin-sensitive person (see Fig. 39.6).

Among patients with insulin resistance, the insulin desensitization is only partial, so that even markedly insulin-resistant patients always maintain a metabolic response to an increased concentration of insulin. Furthermore, the insulin resistance does not affect all organs and metabolic pathways to the same extent. Indeed, the hyperinsulinemia that accompanies insulin resistance can lead to a seemingly paradoxical effect of increased activity in an insulin signaling pathway in a particular organ even though whole-body glucose uptake in response to insulin is decreased.

A longitudinal study of Pima Indians showed that the following changes occurred as volunteers progressed from normal glucose tolerance to diabetes: increase in body weight, decline in insulin-stimulated glucose removal from the blood (i.e., increasing insulin resistance), decline in insulin secretion in response to an intravenous bolus of glucose, and finally, an increase in the body's endogenous glucose production (this glucose comes mostly from the liver and the kidneys; see Chapter 25). The concentration of glucose in the fasting state increases only late in the pathogenic process, and it appears to be due mostly to excessive endogenous glucose production. The immediate causes of the decline in insulin secretion are not known; however, chronically elevated concentrations of glucose and fatty acids, changes in the concentrations of adipose tissue–derived hormones, and decreased insulin sensitivity of the β-cells themselves have been blamed.

Most type 2 diabetic patients who are **lean** are insulin resistant like their obese counterparts. These lean patients presumably develop diabetes in the same way as some obese patients. A minority of lean type 2 diabetic patients have normal insulin sensitivity but secrete insulin at a reduced rate. The causes of impaired insulin secretion and signaling in these lean patients are unknown.

Type 2 diabetic patients still secrete insulin, but not enough to control the concentration of glucose in the blood. Autopsies of type 2 diabetic patients show that the pancreas contains ~50% of the normal volume of β-cells, which show signs of inflammation.

### 5.2. Diagnosis

Type 2 diabetes is usually discovered either on the basis of routine clinical vigilance and screening or after a patient has had a heart attack or stroke. Heart attack and stroke are often a consequence of protracted, unrecognized hyperglycemia. The American Diabetes Association recommends that screens involve only a fasting plasma glucose concentration (see Section 3). The WHO recommends that patients who have "impaired fasting glucose" also undergo an oral glucose tolerance test. For patients who have had a heart attack or stroke, the diagnostic test is performed following recovery from the acute illness; that is, at a time when the concentration of stress

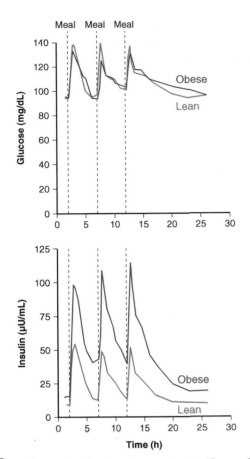

**Fig. 39.6** **Effect of obesity on the concentrations of glucose and insulin.** Mean of two studies with a total of ~20 volunteers in each group. Meals contained about 50% carbohydrate and were approximately appropriate for maintaining weight. (Data from Polonsky KS, Given BD, Van Cauter E. Twenty-four-hour profiles and pulsatile patterns of insulin secretion in normal and obese subjects. *J Clin Invest.* 1988;81:442-448; and McQuaid SE, Hodson L, Neville MJ, et al. Downregulation of adipose tissue fatty acid trafficking in obesity: a driver for ectopic fat deposition? *Diabetes.* 2011;60:47-55.)

Clinically, insulin resistance is apparent from a high plasma concentration of insulin in the fasting state or from a high daily amount of insulin needed to control blood glucose.

**Obesity** renders people **insulin resistant**. As a result, β-cells need to secrete more insulin to maintain normoglycemia (Fig. 39.6). Insulin resistance can be lessened by physical activity and weight loss.

Obese patients show insulin resistance of their skeletal muscles and adipose tissue. In response to insulin, the skeletal muscles thus take up an abnormally small amount of glucose. The skeletal muscles normally account for most of the insulin-induced whole-body glucose uptake. The adipose tissue of obese patients releases fatty acids at an abnormally high rate, and other tissues also oxidize fatty acids at an elevated rate so that the change in the concentration of circulating fatty acids is very small. Whether this contributes to insulin resistance in skeletal muscle is unclear. Furthermore, triglyceride-laden adipocytes alter their secretion of adipokines (hormones that stem from adipocytes). For instance, they secrete less **adiponectin**. Adiponectin makes tissues more sensitive to insulin.

hormones (also called counterregulatory hormones, including glucagon, epinephrine, and cortisol) is no longer markedly elevated. However, an immediate determination of an $HbA_{1c}$ value allows the degree of the patient's hyperglycemia in the ~2 months before the acute illness to be assessed.

As a rough rule of thumb, type 2 diabetic patients are older than 40 years. However, as obesity increases in the developed world, this limit is shifting; a remarkable fraction of obese teenagers currently have type 2 diabetes.

About 7% of the U.S. population has type 2 diabetes. In other developed countries, the incidence of type 2 diabetes is moving toward a similar value.

**Hyperosmolar hyperglycemic state** is more often seen in patients previously diagnosed with diabetes than on first presentation. This state (see Section 2.2) develops only in a small number of patients who have type 2 diabetes. Patients who are most susceptible to developing the syndrome are those who have had diabetes for a long time and therefore have poor secretion of insulin from β-cells, patients who forget to take their antidiabetic medication (e.g., due to dementia), and patients who live alone and without a care provider.

Type 2 diabetic patients develop **ketoacidosis** only very rarely. Patients with type 2 diabetes usually secrete enough insulin to have normal inhibition of lipolysis and hence do not develop ketoacidosis.

The **distinction between type 1 and type 2 diabetes** is often made on clinical grounds. A young, lean child with ketoacidosis is exceedingly more likely to have type 1 rather than type 2 diabetes. Conversely, an overweight, 70-year-old person is much more likely to have type 2 rather than type 1 diabetes. Nonetheless, autoimmune destruction of pancreatic β-cells is thought to be possible at any age. Testing of a patient's serum for antibodies to islet cells is possible; however, this test is only rarely performed because its outcome would not change the management of the patient's diabetes.

Some patients with diabetes have characteristics that are intermediate between type 1 and type 2 diabetes; this type of diabetes is called **latent autoimmune diabetes in adults** (**LADA**; Table 39.1). In Europe and the United States, about 4% of patients who have a diagnosis of type 2 diabetes have antibodies to glutamic acid dehydrogenase (an enzyme that produces the neurotransmitter γ-aminobutyric acid), a finding that is typical (but not diagnostic) of type 1 diabetes. For the first half year after diagnosis, patients with LADA generally do not need insulin; however, they need exogenous insulin sooner than other patients who have type 2 diabetes. In clinical care, no distinction is made between patients who have type 2 diabetes and patients who have LADA.

## 5.3. Treatment

Available treatments for type 2 diabetes can be well rationalized based on our knowledge of glucose homeostasis. Treatments decrease the rate of influx of glucose from the intestine into the blood, increase insulin secretion, increase the effect of insulin on metabolism, attenuate glucose production by liver and kidneys, or lead to a loss of glucose into the urine.

The American Diabetes Association recommends that patients who receive a diagnosis of type 2 diabetes first try a regimen of **diet, exercise**, and **metformin**. Weight loss and exercise are accompanied by increased insulin sensitivity, though they do not mend the defect in insulin secretion. Still, the increase in insulin sensitivity may allow the pancreatic β-cells to regain control of the concentration of glucose in the blood. Metformin decreases glucose production by the liver (see below). Additional drugs are recommended only if these measures fail to lower the $HbA_{1c}$ below 7% (according to the traditional method of measurement; see Section 4.3).

Type 2 diabetes is thought of as a slowly progressive disease. It may be controlled early on with diet, exercise, and perhaps one oral drug; however, it will eventually require further oral drugs or injected drugs. In the opinion of most physicians, type 2 diabetes does not vanish when a patient achieves normal glucose homeostasis with weight loss and exercise alone; it is then called controlled diabetes.

Patients who have type 2 diabetes do best when consuming a **diet** from which glucose enters the bloodstream only slowly. A steady, low flux of glucose from the intestine into the bloodstream requires secretion of less insulin than does a sudden, high influx of the same amount of glucose. In general, foods that contain **soluble fiber** are digested more slowly than foods that contain no fiber (see Section 1 in Chapter 18). Foods that release glucose only slowly are said to have a low glycemic index. **Fat** in a meal also slows gastric emptying and intestinal digestion of a meal. Although this effect is beneficial, most patients with type 2 diabetes also have lipid abnormalities, and they should therefore consume saturated fats and trans-fats only sparingly. A **low-carbohydrate, high-fat diet** (an Atkins type diet) requires considerably less insulin secretion than a high-carbohydrate diet. Multiple small meals also require less insulin to be secreted than do one or two large meals.

The drugs **acarbose** and **miglitol** competitively inhibit **α-glucosidases** and thus inhibit the production of glucose from dietary carbohydrates in the intestine. α-Glucosidases in the intestine are amylase, sucrase-isomaltase, and maltase-glucoamylase (see Section 2.2 in Chapter 18). Partial inhibition of α-glucosidases slows the degradation of starch and sucrose and thus allows for a more steady and lower flux of glucose into the blood; this glucose flux can often still be handled by insulin secretion from the failing β-cells. Side effects of these drugs are bloating and borborygmi, which are caused by bacteria that get to degrade an unusually large amount of carbohydrates (see Section 4 in Chapter 18).

Inhibitors of **ATP-sensitive K+ channels** ($K_{ATP}$-channels)**, glucagon-like peptide 1 (GLP-1) receptor agonists**, and inhibitors of the degradation of GLP-1 are used to boost insulin secretion from pancreatic β-cells as follows:

**Sulfonylurea** drugs and "**glinide**" drugs inhibit $K_{ATP}$-channels; this leads to increased insulin secretion (see Chapter 26). The different classes of drugs differ mainly in their chemical structure. Some of the inhibitors of $K_{ATP}$, such as *repaglinide* and *nateglinide* are short acting and can be taken before each meal; others, such as the sulfonylurea *glyburide* (also called *glibenclamide*), are long acting (several days) and are taken only once a day. Since the secretagogue effect of all $K_{ATP}$-channel inhibitors shows only a mild dependence on the concentration of glucose, all of these inhibitors can cause **hypoglycemia** (which may be life threatening). $K_{ATP}$-channel inhibitors cause mild weight gain because the increased amount of insulin secretion leads to increased synthesis of triglycerides and their deposition in adipose tissue.

**GLP-1 receptor agonists** enhance glucose-induced insulin secretion via GLP-1 receptors, which signal via cyclic adenosine monophosphate (cAMP; see Chapter 26). GLP-1 itself has too short of a half-life in the blood to be of pharmacological use. The currently approved drugs in this class are **exenatide**, which is a synthetic recombinant form of the Gila monster toxin **exendin-4**, a 39–amino acid peptide that is ~50% homologous to human GLP-1; **liraglutide**, an analog of human GLP-1 that is acylated with palmitic acid; **albiglutide**, a recombinant peptide consisting of two copies of modified human GLP-1 and one copy of albumin; and **dulaglutide**, a recombinant fusion protein of modified human GLP-1 and a fragment of a modified human immunoglobulin. All of these peptides must be injected because, if taken orally, they would be degraded in the intestine. GLP-1 receptor agonists reduce postprandial hyperglycemia (Fig. 39.7) by slowing gastric emptying, inhibiting glucagon secretion, and stimulating insulin secretion. GLP-1 and its analogs enhance insulin secretion only at a concentration of glucose above ~90 mg/dL (~5 mM). Hence, if taken alone, analogs of GLP-1 should not cause hypoglycemia. (Nevertheless, these drugs do carry a warning of hypoglycemia because hypoglycemia is possible in conjunction with drugs that produce hypoglycemia, such as

insulin and inhibitors of $K_{ATP}$-channels). GLP-1 normally has an appetite-suppressing effect; perhaps because of this, a side effect of GLP-1 receptor agonists is decreased appetite and nausea. A decrease in appetite obviously helps with weight loss.

The "**gliptins**" inhibit the degradation of the patients' own GLP-1 and thus lead to an elevated concentration of GLP-1. Gliptins currently approved in the United States are **sitagliptin**, **saxagliptin**, **linagliptin**, and **alogliptin**. The gliptins inhibit **dipeptidyl peptidase-4** (**DPP-4**), which degrades GLP-1 as well as other hormones, such as gastric inhibitory peptide (an incretin-like GLP-1; see Section 3.3.2 in Chapter 26). Gliptins are low-molecular-weight, nonpeptide compounds, and they can be taken by mouth. Like GLP-1 receptor agonists (see above), the gliptins by themselves do not cause hypoglycemia. An advantage of gliptins over GLP-1 receptor agonists is that they do not cause nausea; a disadvantage is that they are less effective in lowering $HbA_{1c}$.

**Pramlintide,** an analog of the peptide amylin (see Section 8.4 in Chapter 9 and Section 2.2 in Chapter 26), decreases food intake, slows gastric emptying, and inhibits glucagon secretion. These effects require that patients approximately halve their dose of short-acting insulin. Pramlintide is best suited for patients who cannot control their blood glucose concentration with insulin alone or with insulin plus oral antidiabetic drugs. Amylin is normally contained in secretory vesicles in pancreatic β-cells. Type 1 diabetic patients secrete virtually no amylin, whereas type 2 diabetic patients secrete progressively less amylin as they age. Amylin irreversibly aggregates when present at elevated concentrations (see Section 8.4 in Chapter 9). Pramlintide differs from amylin in three amino acid residues; this change renders pramlintide much more soluble than amylin.

The use of **sodium-glucose cotransporter-2 (SGLT2) inhibitors** in the treatment of type 2 diabetes is discussed in Section 6 of Chapter 18. SGLT2 is a $Na^+$-dependent glucose transporter located in the kidney tubules that normally recovers most of the glucose from the glomerular filtrate. Treatment with an SGLT2 inhibitor leads to glucosuria (glucose in the urine). Urinary tract infection is one of the most common side effects of SGLT2 inhibition and can be dangerous.

**Metformin** chiefly attenuates endogenous glucose production. Most patients with type 2 diabetes produce too much glucose, mostly from gluconeogenesis and especially during the overnight fast. In addition, type 2 diabetic patients also have an elevated concentration of free fatty acids in their blood and therefore have an abnormally low need for endogenously produced glucose. The mechanism of action of metformin is poorly understood. In the liver, metformin decreases flux in gluconeogenesis, perhaps by activating AMP-activated protein kinase (AMPK; see Fig. 25.7 and Sections 3 and 4.2.2 in Chapter 25). In muscle, metformin leads to the insertion of glucose transporters into the plasma membrane and to activation of glycogen phosphorylase; this increases glucose uptake and the production of glucose 6-phosphate from glycogen. In muscle and in liver, metformin increases β-oxidation of fatty acids (see Section 4 in Chapter 27). Predominantly in patients

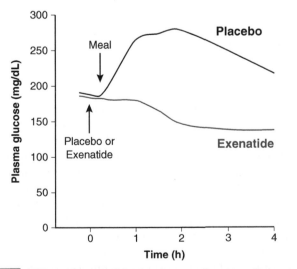

**Fig. 39.7** **Effect of exenatide on plasma glucose after a meal.** Volunteers with type 2 diabetes received an injection of exenatide (~0.09 μg/kg body weight) or placebo 15 minutes before a standardized breakfast. (Data from Fineman MS, Bicsak TA, Shen LZ, et al. Effect on glycemic control of exenatide (synthetic exendin-4) additive to existing metformin and/or sulfonylurea treatment in patients with type 2 diabetes. *Diabetes Care.* 2003;26:2370-2377; and Kolterman OG, Buse JB, Fineman MS, et al. Synthetic exendin-4 (exenatide) significantly reduces postprandial and fasting plasma glucose in subjects with type 2 diabetes. *J Clin Endocrinol Metab.* 2003;88:3082-3089.)

who have compromised function of the heart, lungs, liver, or kidneys, metformin may cause lactic acidosis. The lactic acidosis may be caused by inhibition of complex I of oxidative phosphorylation (see Sections 1.3 and 2 in Chapter 23). Metformin slightly decreases appetite.

The **thiazolidinediones** increase insulin sensitivity by increasing the activity of **peroxisome proliferator-activated receptor γ** (**PPAR-γ**). Currently, the thiazolidinediones **rosiglitazone** and **pioglitazone** are approved for use in the United States; however, there are major concerns that these drugs may damage the heart and its vasculature as well as have other adverse effects. Thiazolidinediones greatly increase insulin-stimulated glucose removal from the blood. The mechanism of action is only partially understood. PPAR-γ are nuclear receptors that heterodimerize with retinoid X receptors to form a functional transcription factor. This complex regulates transcription of genes that play a role in the metabolism of glucose and lipids. PPAR-γ is especially abundant in adipose tissue. There, activation by thiazolidinediones gives rise to more, younger, more insulin-sensitive adipocytes in the subcutaneous adipose tissue as well as increased activity of lipoprotein lipase and increased secretion of adiponectin from fat cells. Adiponectin, in turn, increases the insulin sensitivity of muscle and liver. In muscle, thiazolidinedione use is associated with increased AMPK activity (similar to metformin, see above). If used by themselves, thiazolidinediones do not cause hypoglycemia.

After about 3 to 5 years of use, monotherapy with one of the aforementioned oral agents generally fails to be sufficiently effective, most likely because of a further decline in function of pancreatic β-cells. At this point, agents with a different, noninterfering mechanism of action can be added, or **insulin** injections can be instituted. Indeed, insulin injections are used in all patients whose blood glucose cannot be controlled with oral medications.

**Short-acting insulins** are needed for patients whose β-cells secrete little or no insulin in response to meals, whereas **long-acting "baseline" insulins** can be used in patients who still have appreciable β-cell function. Because most patients with type 2 diabetes are insulin resistant, they need to inject much more insulin than do the typical type 1 diabetic patients.

Patients who have type 2 diabetes who start a new drug or take a drug that can cause hypoglycemia (particularly insulin) commonly measure their blood glucose concentration using a **glucose meter**.

## 6. MODY

*Maturity-onset diabetes of the young (MODY) is a collection of diseases that are caused by mutations in individual proteins that are essential for the normal function of β-cells.*

The term MODY dates from a time when type 2 diabetes was referred to as "maturity onset" and when the causes of MODY were still unknown. Patients with MODY are often misdiagnosed as having type 1 or type 2 diabetes.

All known types of MODY are due to mutations in proteins that are important for normal development and function of pancreatic β-cells; often, these proteins also affect the function of the liver. For the most common types of MODY, numerous mutations are known, and there is therefore an appreciable diversity of phenotypes.

The overall prevalence of MODY is likely ~1 in 1,000, though many persons are undiagnosed, especially if they have MODY-2 (see below).

A diagnosis of MODY is commonly entertained if a patient is lean, develops diabetes before 30 years of age, has a family member who also developed diabetes at such a young age, has no signs of insulin resistance (e.g., acanthosis nigricans), and either does not require insulin or has a significant plasma concentration of C-peptide (an indicator of endogenous insulin secretion; see Chapter 26). In the original working definition of MODY, patients also had to be free of diabetic ketoacidosis and islet cell autoantibodies. Among teenagers who do not have type 1 diabetes, one can expect the leaner patients to have MODY and the more obese to have type 2 diabetes. A calculator to estimate the probability that a patient has MODY is available at http://diabetesgenes.org/content/mody-probability-calculator.

The most common forms of MODY are MODY-2 and MODY-3. Both are inherited in an autosomal dominant fashion.

**MODY-2** is caused by a heterozygous loss-of-function mutation in the *GCK* gene, which encodes **glucokinase**. In Europe, the prevalence of MODY-2 is ~1 in 1,000. Glucokinase is the glucose sensor of the pancreatic β-cell (see Fig. 26.7). In the liver, in the fed state, glucokinase helps direct glucose into glycolysis and glycogen synthesis (see Section 5.6 in Chapter 19 and Sections 1.3 and 3.1 in Chapter 24). Affected patients have a higher set point for glucose-induced insulin secretion and therefore have mild hyperglycemia even in the fasting state. Hyperglycemia is recognizable at birth and increases slightly with age. Patients with MODY-2 do not seem to have a noticeably increased risk for diabetic complications. Treatment is usually not necessary, except during pregnancy. Oral antidiabetic agents are ineffective.

**MODY-3** is caused by a mutation in the *HNF1A* gene, which encodes HNF1 homeobox A (**HNF1A**). HNF1A is a transcription factor that stimulates the transcription of genes, the products of which are involved in the metabolism of glucose or fatty acids. At birth, patients have a normal concentration of blood glucose. However, they have a severe defect in insulin secretion that worsens with age. Typical onset of diabetes is at ~20 years of age. Some patients present with pronounced hyperglycemia and are misdiagnosed as having type 1 diabetes. Patients are typically treated with diet and a sulfonylurea. When endogenous insulin secretion has become insufficient, patients need to be switched to insulin therapy.

## 7. GESTATIONAL DIABETES

*Pregnancy is a time of marked insulin resistance and thus increased need for insulin secretion. Diabetes first shows up during pregnancy in about 5% of women. Patients who have gestational diabetes are treated with small modifications in diet and, if necessary, with insulin, glyburide, or metformin.*

Pregnancy requires a large increase in insulin secretion from the mother's pancreatic β-cells. After ~20 weeks of gestation, insulin resistance normally develops to the point that the pancreas has to secrete several times the usual amount of insulin, yet the β-cell mass increases only by a factor of ~1.4. Insulin resistance of the mother likely helps shunt glucose to the placenta to satisfy the fetus's large demand for glucose. The insulin resistance has been attributed in part to relatively high concentrations of placental growth hormone, placental lactogen, and progesterone. Age- and obesity-induced insulin resistance both increase a pregnant woman's chance of developing gestational diabetes. Approximately 5% of pregnant women do not secrete enough insulin during late pregnancy and thus have gestational diabetes.

When the fetus is exposed to chronic hyperglycemia, it synthesizes an inordinately large amount of fat. The fetal pancreas secretes insulin according to the prevailing concentration of glucose. The concentration of glucose in fetal blood is heavily dependent on the concentration of glucose in the mother's blood. The hyperinsulinemia in the fetus of a hyperglycemic mother stimulates the synthesis of fatty acids and triglycerides in the fetus. Excessive fetal lipid stores are the cause of **macrosomia** (weight in excess of 9 lb or 4.0 kg) and its attendant risks during delivery (e.g., shoulder dystocia; Fig. 39.8). Fetuses of hyperglycemic mothers also have relatively immature lungs.

In **newborns** of markedly hyperglycemic mothers, β-cells fail to properly reduce insulin secretion during normoglycemia or hypoglycemia. Accordingly, newborns of mothers with poorly controlled diabetes hypersecrete insulin and develop

**hypoglycemia**. This must be treated with glucose infusions. Over a period of days, provided the concentration of glucose is close to normal, the infant's β-cells adapt and eventually secrete the appropriate amount of insulin for normal glucose homeostasis.

Because untreated gestational diabetes can lead to the abovementioned serious complications, pregnant patients generally undergo **screening** for diabetes with a modified oral glucose tolerance test (see Section 3). This test is given at 24 to 28 weeks of gestation; that is, at a time when a woman's inability to secrete insulin in the face of mounting insulin resistance becomes apparent and when the fetus has not yet deposited a damaging amount of adipose tissue. In the United States, **glucose tolerance** during pregnancy is commonly tested as follows. Patients are given 50 g of glucose by mouth (without prior fasting), and a blood sample is taken 1 hour later. If the plasma glucose is above 135 to 140 mg/dL, the patient is tested further. In the second test, the patient fasts overnight and then undergoes a 100-g oral glucose tolerance test with samples taken at time points 0, 1, 2, and 3 hours. If plasma glucose values for two or more time points are above certain limits, the patient has gestational diabetes.

**Treatment** of patients who have gestational diabetes involves modest changes in **diet** and is augmented with drugs as needed. Even markedly overweight pregnant patients should not fast aggressively because pregnancy itself requires increased food intake for the health of both the mother and fetus. Only a few antidiabetic drugs are approved for use in pregnant women. Injected **insulin** to reduce baseline insulin secretion is usually adequate because the patient's β-cells can still take care of increased demand after meals. **Glyburide (glibenclamide)** is a long-acting oral sulfonylurea antidiabetic drug (see Section 5.3) that is used in place of insulin. **Metformin** (oral) mostly reduces endogenous glucose production (see Section 5.3).

Most women who have gestational diabetes become nondiabetic in the postpartum period. Unfortunately, gestational diabetes is a sign of future trouble. Within 10 years of being diagnosed with gestational diabetes, a majority of patients develop **type 2 diabetes.**

## 8. COMPLICATIONS OF DIABETES

*The main complications of diabetes lead to decreased vision, impaired peripheral nerve sensation, decreased kidney function, and dysfunction of the heart or large blood vessels. The main processes that cause these complications are thought to be spontaneous glycation of proteins and lipids; increased formation of damaging, oxygen-containing radicals; and insulin resistance.*

### 8.1. General Comments

Epidemiological studies have shown that diabetic patients who receive instructions to achieve good control of the concentration of **glucose** in plasma have fewer microvascular

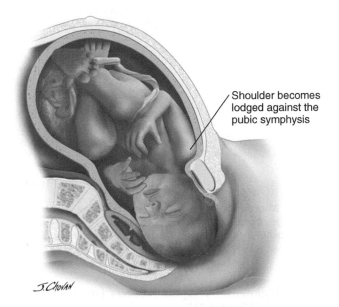

Shoulder becomes lodged against the pubic symphysis

**Fig. 39.8** **Shoulder dystocia.** Macrosomia from gestational diabetes can cause shoulder dystocia, a serious complication of a vaginal delivery. Shoulder dystocia may lead to permanent damage of the brachial plexus.

and macrovascular complications (see Section 8.2) of diabetes than patients who do not receive counseling and who have poor control. The difference in treatment results in a difference in the fraction of **HbA$_{1c}$**, which in turn correlates with the frequency of microvascular and macrovascular complications. Many of the complications of diabetes seem to result from chronic hyperglycemia, but there may be other causes as well. Complications of diabetes are also seen in patients who have forms of MODY that cause marked hyperglycemia. Patients who are obese or who have abnormalities of lipid metabolism are at risk of additional complications.

The current standard of care is a regimen of blood glucose testing and administration of drugs so that the concentration of glucose is fairly close to the normal concentration, yet not dangerously low.

## 8.2. Clinical Aspects of Complications of Diabetes

Diabetic complications are often divided into microvascular and macrovascular complications. **Microvascular complications** (Fig. 39.9) affect blood flow predominantly in the capillaries of the eyes, peripheral nerves, and kidneys. The capillaries have an abnormally small lumen, and the walls are leaky. This is associated with increased blood pressure, edema, and decreased blood flow to tissues (ischemia). For compensation, new blood vessels are produced. Major microvascular complications of diabetes are **retinopathy**, peripheral **neuropathy**, and **nephropathy**. **Macrovascular complications** include cardiovascular disease and peripheral vascular disease (arteries that supply the brain, heart, or lower extremities). Major macrovascular complications of diabetes are **heart disease**, **stroke**, **ulcers**, and **gangrene**.

**Retinopathy** may be accompanied by reduced blood flow to the retina due to vasoconstriction, local hypertension, leaky vessels, ischemia, proliferation of new blood vessels, and reduced visual acuity (see Fig. 20.4). Blindness can be the result of detachment of the retina, bleeding into the retina or vitreous, or ischemia of the macula (the region of the retina that provides vision of the highest acuity).

**Diabetic kidney disease** is accompanied by a decreased rate of filtration of blood (evident from serum creatinine), leakage of albumin into the urine (albuminuria), or both of these abnormalities. In patients with chronic hyperglycemia, capillaries to the glomeruli are lost and nearby cells fill the space with extracellular matrix (Fig. 39.10). In the glomerulus, the basement membrane and the foot processes of podocytes together form a size-exclusion filter. In patients with chronic hyperglycemia, a lack of adequate podocyte foot processes compromises this filter and allows albumin to pass into the filtrate.

Diabetic kidney disease is currently treated mainly with strict control of blood glucose and blood pressure. Blood pressure is reduced with angiotensin-converting enzyme inhibi-

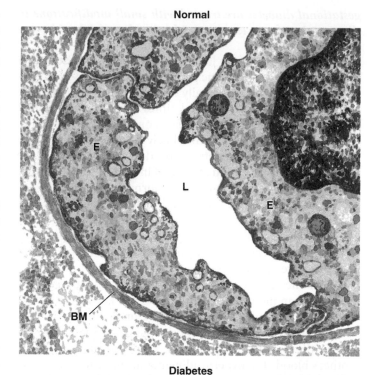

**Normal**

**Diabetes**

**Fig. 39.9** **Microvascular disease in diabetes.** Electron microscopic image of cross section of a skin capillary. BM, basement membrane; E, epithelial cell; L, lumen. The basement membrane is thickened and the lumen reduced.

tors and angiotensin receptor blockers (see Fig. 31.17 and Section 4.1 in Chapter 31).

**Peripheral neuropathy** is seen in almost half of all patients with diabetes. The neuropathy usually manifests itself with *numbness*. *Painful* neuropathy occurs in about 5% of all

**Normal**

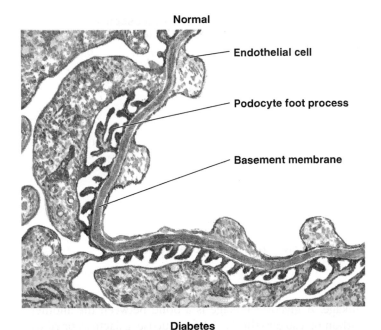

Endothelial cell

Podocyte foot process

Basement membrane

**Diabetes**

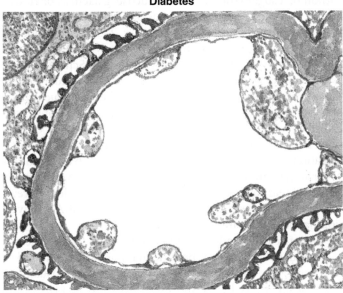

**Fig. 39.10** **Glomerulosclerosis as a consequence of long-term diabetes.** Based on transmission electron micrographs. Podocyte foot processes are damaged, the basement membrane is thickened, and the endothelium is compromised.

patients who have diabetes. The neuropathy is thought to derive from inadequate blood flow and damage to neurons.

Patients who have diabetes and peripheral neuropathy, macrovascular disease, and marked hyperglycemia are at an increased risk of developing diabetic **ulcers**, especially on their feet and lower legs; the ulcers may progress to **gangrene** (Fig. 39.11).

Diabetic patients who have insulin resistance (e.g., due to obesity) and dyslipidemia are at an increased risk for **vascular disease** (Fig. 39.12).

**Diabetic ulcer**

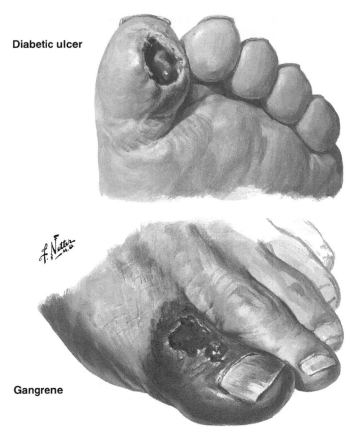

**Gangrene**

**Fig. 39.11** **Ulcer and gangrene as complications of diabetes.** Peripheral neuropathy impairs a patient's ready detection of lesions. Hyperglycemia and poor tissue perfusion favor infections. When gangrene develops, an amputation becomes necessary.

**Intermediate stage**

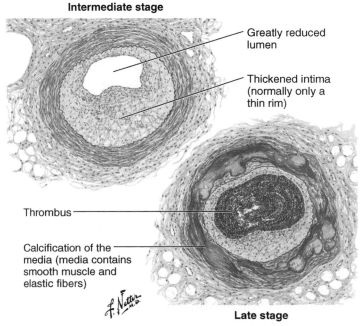

Greatly reduced lumen

Thickened intima (normally only a thin rim)

Thrombus

Calcification of the media (media contains smooth muscle and elastic fibers)

**Late stage**

**Fig. 39.12** **Atherosclerosis in patients who have diabetes.**

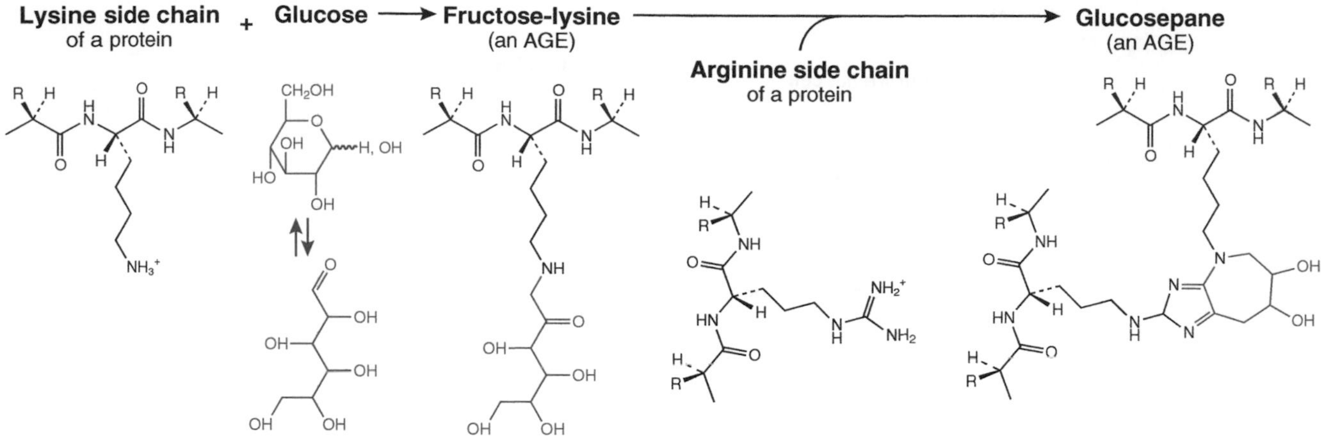

**Fig. 39.13** Nonenzymatic glycation of proteins by glucose gives rise to fructose-lysine and glucosepane. AGE, advanced glycation end product.

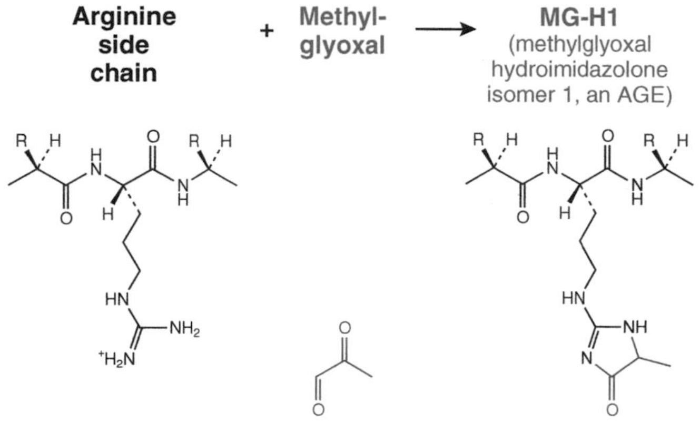

**Fig. 39.14** Methylglyoxal reacts with arginine side chains to form MG-H1, an advanced glycation end product.

## 8.3. Potential Biochemical Causes of Complications of Diabetes

### 8.3.1. Nonenzymatic Glycation

When a patient is hyperglycemic, the concentration of glucose is not only elevated in blood vessels, but also in the extracellular space and inside all cells that do not regulate glucose uptake.

Sugars in general are quite reactive. Glucose has relatively low reactivity; perhaps this is why it evolved to its current position in mammalian metabolism. Fructose and galactose are considerably more reactive than glucose. Several metabolites of glycolysis are also quite reactive. The 3-carbon sugar **dihydroxyacetone** is even reactive enough that it is used as a topical **tanning** agent (dihydroxyacetone readily reacts with amino groups in the epidermis to form a brown product, melanoidin). Dihydroxyacetone is used cosmetically for patients who have **vitiligo** (see Fig. 35.18 and Section 4.4 in Chapter 35).

The term nonenzymatic **glycation** refers to the spontaneous reaction between a sugar and a protein (or peptide, nucleic acid, or lipid) that results in a bond other than a glycosyl

linkage. A glycosyl linkage is a bond between the anomeric carbon of a sugar (this is C-1 for glucose, galactose, or ribose) and O, N, or S. In glycogen for instance, glucose residues are linked via O-glycosidic bonds (see Fig. 24.2). In ribonucleotides, a ribose is linked to a base via an N-glycosidic bond (see Fig. 1.1). In glycation, a sugar typically forms a Schiff base with a free amino group, and the Schiff base then undergoes an **Amadori rearrangement** that modifies the sugar such that it is no longer a glycosyl residue; that is, there is no longer a C linked to two O or one O and one N atom (Fig. 39.13; compare with Fig. 7.8). The formation of $HbA_{1c}$ is an example of a glycation reaction. Glucose forms a Schiff base with the N-terminal amino group of valine in β-globin. A subsequent Amadori rearrangement (see Fig. 39.13 for an analogous reaction) yields 1-deoxyfructosyl hemoglobin (i.e., $HbA_{1c}$). Glycation happens both inside and outside cells.

The term **advanced glycation end product** (**AGE**) refers to the product of a protein or peptide that was at one point linked to a sugar. In AGEs, the original sugar moiety is usually no longer a sugar (see below and Figs. 39.13 and 39.14).

Skin protein glycation parallels a type 1 diabetic patient's risk of microvascular and macrovascular complications. In skin, AGEs cross-link chiefly collagen. AGE content increases with age and with diabetes. The strongest associations between glycation products and risk of complications have been observed for **fructose-lysine, glucosepane,** and **methylglyoxal hydroimidazolone isomer 1** (**MG-H1**). Fructose-lysine is the product of glucose reacting with the free amino group of a lysine side chain (see Fig. 39.13). When fructose-lysine undergoes rearrangement and reacts with the side chain of an arginine residue, it gives rise to glucosepane. Methylglyoxal is thought to be chiefly formed from triose phosphates, such as dihydroxyacetone phosphate and glyceraldehyde 3-phosphate (see Fig. 19.2). A set of two ubiquitously expressed glyoxalases sequentially degrades methylglyoxal to lactate. Methylglyoxal readily reacts with the free guanidino group of an arginine side chain and thus gives rise to MG-H1 (see Fig. 39.14). There are many more AGEs, and the abundance of some of them also correlates with the risk for complications of diabetes.

Glycated proteins may have altered function, and they may activate AGE receptors (see below). Proteins of the extracellular matrix, such as collagens, elastin, and lens crystallins, have a relatively long lifetime and therefore accumulate an appreciable amount of AGEs. AGE–cross-linked collagens have altered physical properties and are also less susceptible to degradation. AGE-altered collagens especially affect the properties of blood vessels, basement membranes in the kidney glomeruli, and skin. When proteins that contain AGEs are degraded, they give rise to AGE-modified amino acids, which are excreted into the urine.

Besides amino groups on amino acids, amino groups on **phospholipids** are also susceptible to glycation reactions. In phospholipids, amino groups are present in phosphatidylethanolamine and phosphatidylserine (see Fig. 11.2).

In addition to AGEs produced in the body, AGEs from the **diet** and **tobacco smoke** contribute to a person's AGE load. When heated (as during cooking or baking), sugars react more readily with amino groups, forming AGEs. A fraction of dietary AGE is taken up via the intestine, and it has a highly appreciable effect on the amount of AGEs in blood. Tobacco leaves accumulate AGEs during curing. A person who smokes inhales some of these AGEs and absorbs them via the lungs.

Many different types of cells, especially endothelial cells, smooth muscle cells, and monocytes (which can become macrophages), have plasma membrane **receptors for advanced glycation end products; RAGE** is one such receptor. (RAGE also binds the Aβ-protein, as well as amyloid fibrils, which are rich in β-sheet structure; see Section 8 in Chapter 9). On binding an AGE, the RAGE signals across the membrane and, signaling via a variety of intracellular signaling pathways, alters the rate of transcription of certain genes. This change leads to increased production of reactive oxygen species (**ROS**; see Section 8.3.2) and evokes the secretion of **cytokines**, which in turn elicit **inflammation**. ROS stem, in part, from NAD(P)H oxidase and, in part, from the electron transport chain in mitochondria. Other AGE receptors facilitate the uptake and intracellular degradation of AGEs.

### 8.3.2. Damage by Reactive Oxygen Species

NADPH oxidase and the electron transport chain in mitochondria give rise to **superoxide radicals** ($\cdot O_2^-$), which in turn can give rise to **hydrogen peroxide** ($H_2O_2$), **hydroxyl radicals** ($\cdot OH$), **singlet oxygen**, or **peroxynitrite** ($ONOO^-$). NADPH oxidase is an enzyme that is present in phagocytic vacuoles and also on the cytoplasmic side of the plasma membrane, where it assembles in response to signaling from a variety of hormones, including cytokines. In the respiratory chain of mitochondria, it is mostly coenzyme Q interacting with complex III that gives rise to superoxide radicals (see Figs. 23.3 and 23.4). Radicals are discussed in Section 2.3 in Chapter 21. Singlet oxygen is a very reactive form of $O_2$ in which two electrons are in a high-energy electron configuration. Singlet oxygen is endogenously formed through various mechanisms. Peroxynitrite derives from the reaction of superoxide radicals ($\cdot O_2^-$) with the signaling molecule nitric oxide

(NO; see Section 5.2 in Chapter 16). Compounds such as singlet oxygen, hydrogen peroxide, and oxygen-containing radicals are lumped together under the term **ROS**.

Cells have several mechanisms to remove ROS, as detailed in Section 2.3 in Chapter 21. The extracellular space contains antioxidants that react spontaneously. The major extracellular antioxidants are –SH groups on proteins, urate, ascorbate (vitamin C), and vitamin E. Inside cells, enzymes remove most ROS that are precursors of more reactive ROS. For instance, superoxide dismutase converts $\cdot O_2^-$ to $H_2O_2$, and glutathione peroxidase or catalase minimizes the formation of $\cdot OH$ by reducing $H_2O_2$ to water (see Section 2.3 in Chapter 21 and Fig. 21.6).

In hyperglycemic patients, the rate of ROS production is abnormally high. Damage to **protein** and **lipids** occurs when a significant amount of radicals reacts with these molecules rather than antioxidants or radical scavengers. When ROS such as $\cdot OH$ react with lipids, they form lipid radicals, lipid peroxyl radicals, and lipid hydroperoxides. These radicals are removed by reaction with vitamin E and glutathione, whereas the hydroperoxides are reduced by glutathione (see Section 2.3 in Chapter 21).

Tissues of patients who have pronounced hyperglycemia and a markedly increased concentration of free fatty acids are most likely to show damage from ROS.

ROSs also damage **DNA** (see Section 2.3 in Chapter 21). In the presence of $Fe^{2+}$, $H_2O_2$ can give rise to $\cdot OH$, which is more reactive than either $\cdot O_2^-$ or $H_2O_2$. Hydroxyl radicals can react with deoxyguanosine and thereby damage DNA. Because a large amount of ROS is made in mitochondria, and because ROS react very rapidly, damage to mitochondrial DNA is presumably greater than damage to nuclear DNA. Both the nucleus and mitochondria have mechanisms to repair DNA. If damage to DNA is too extensive, apoptosis may be set into motion (see Chapters 2 and Chapter 8). Mitochondria can also be destroyed by autophagy (see Section 1.4 in Chapter 35).

Formation of ROSs potentiates the formation of **AGEs** (see Section 8.3.1) and vice versa. In fact, microvascular disease of the retinae, kidneys, and nerves appears to require both oxidative stress and hyperglycemia. An increased concentration of ROS leads to an increased rate of AGE formation. On the other hand, signaling by AGE receptors on the surface of cells induces the formation of ROS.

### 8.3.3. Deregulation of Metabolism

Most type 2 diabetic patients are **insulin resistant** and **hyperinsulinemic**. The molecular mechanisms that underlie the insulin resistance syndrome have yet to be elucidated. Insulin resistance is defined by the potency with which insulin stimulates glucose uptake. However, insulin receptors signal via several pathways and affect multiple pathways of metabolism. Analysis of tissues from diabetic patients shows that not all signaling pathways are similarly affected. The effects of altered insulin signaling on glucose and lipid metabolism in type 2 diabetic patients have yet to be elucidated.

Patients with type 2 diabetes typically have elevated concentrations of **glucose** and **fatty acids** in plasma. Uptake of glucose into muscle and adipose tissue is decreased. Endogenous glucose production, particularly gluconeogenesis, is excessive. Only a relatively small portion of glucose is stored as glycogen. The adipose tissue releases fatty acids at an abnormally high rate. In the liver, a high influx of fatty acids from the periphery and an elevated rate of fatty acid synthesis both contribute to increased production of triglycerides. This, together with insufficient clearance of very-low-density lipoprotein particles, leads to **hypertriglyceridemia**.

Many patients with type 2 diabetes have both altered metabolism and an increased risk of cardiovascular problems. The molecular links between these two pathologies are unclear; however, clinicians often use the term **metabolic syndrome** to define patients who are at risk of both diseases. A common definition of metabolic syndrome is the presence of three or more of the following five abnormalities: hypertension, hypertriglyceridemia, low high-density lipoprotein cholesterol, abdominal obesity, and impaired glucose homeostasis. In developed countries, ~10% to 30% of adults fulfill these criteria. The risk for cardiovascular disease seems to depend chiefly on the degree of a patient's hyperinsulinemia. By contrast, a patient's risk for retinopathy, nephropathy, and neuropathy mostly seems to parallel the degree of hyperglycemia.

During hyperglycemia, there is an appreciable increase in the synthesis of the sugar alcohol **sorbitol** from glucose. Sorbitol is synthesized via the **polyol pathway** (see Section 2 in Chapter 20 and Fig. 20.3). An overly active polyol pathway significantly reduces the availability of NADPH for the repair of oxidative damage (see Fig. 20.5). Hence, excessive sorbitol synthesis leads to impaired removal of **ROS** and increased damage of ROS to the lenses and to the microvasculature in the retinae, glomeruli, and peripheral nerves.

## SUMMARY

- The autoimmune disease that leads to the destruction of pancreatic islet β-cells, typically before about age 40, is called type 1 diabetes. Patients with this disease usually require treatment with insulin, lest they develop life-threatening diabetic ketoacidosis.

- In type 1 diabetic patients, injections of recombinant mutant human insulins, which quickly reach the bloodstream (e.g., lispro insulin, insulin aspart, insulin glulisine), are used to mimic the secretion of insulin from the pancreas of nondiabetic individuals. Similarly, recombinant insulins (e.g., insulin detemir, insulin glargine) that slowly reach the bloodstream are used to provide a basal amount of insulin throughout a 24-hour day. As an alternative to several injections per day, pumps can be used that infuse insulin into the subcutaneous space both continuously and in boluses for meals. For such a pump, patients typically use a short-acting insulin.

- Patients who have had type 1 diabetes for many years gradually lose their glucagon and epinephrine secretion in response to hypoglycemia. These patients are therefore highly susceptible to an excess dose of insulin. Since hypoglycemia can be life threatening, these patients need to manage their blood glucose concentration accordingly. For these and all other diabetic patients, hypoglycemia limits the use of insulin for normalizing the concentration of glucose in the blood.

- Patients who have type 1 diabetes on average have a higher concentration of glucose in plasma than do nondiabetic individuals. The higher the average concentration of glucose in plasma, the more likely type 1 diabetic patients develop complications, such as microvascular disease, retinopathy, nephropathy, and peripheral neuropathy.

- All type 2 diabetic patients have a defect in insulin secretion. All obese type 2 diabetic and most of the lean type 2 diabetic patients are insulin resistant. How insulin resistance eventually gives rise to deficient insulin secretion is unknown.

- Type 2 diabetes shows a multifactorial pattern of inheritance. For most patients who are genetically predisposed, obesity is necessary for type 2 diabetes to develop.

- Newly diagnosed type 2 diabetic patients are treated with diet and exercise, and often also with metformin. Diet and exercise lead to increased insulin sensitivity and thus help improve blood glucose homeostasis. Metformin chiefly reduces excessive endogenous glucose production.

- Other oral antidiabetic drugs used in the treatment of type 2 diabetes include: α-glucosidase inhibitors, such as acarbose, which slow the digestion of starch in the intestine; inhibitors of ATP-sensitive K-channels ($K_{ATP}$-channels), such as sulfonylureas and glinides, which induce insulin secretion from pancreatic β-cells; inhibitors of dipeptidyl peptidase-4 (DPP-4; gliptins), which slow the degradation of glucagon-like peptide-1 (GLP-1), which in turn potentiates glucose-induced insulin secretion; and insulin sensitizers, such as thiazolidinediones (glitazones).

- Injectable drugs that are used in the treatment of type 2 diabetes include exenatide, which is an analog of GLP-1 that boosts glucose-induced insulin secretion and pramlintide, which is an analog of amylin that decreases food intake, slows gastric emptying, and inhibits glucagon secretion; short- and long-acting insulins.

- Maturity-onset diabetes of the young (MODY) is due to one of several mutations, which are inherited in an autosomal dominant manner and lead to defective insulin secretion before about 25 years of age even in the absence of obesity. MODY is 20 to 100 times less common than pure type 2 diabetes.

- Gestational diabetes affects about 5% of pregnant women. If untreated, the fetus acquires extra fat, which complicates delivery. Most pregnant women undergo an oral glucose tolerance test at 24 to 28 weeks of gestation. Currently, insulin is the mainstay of treatment of gestational diabetes. Women who have gestational diabetes typically become normoglycemic soon after delivery. However, a majority of these women develop type 2 diabetes within the ensuing 10 years.

■ Complications of diabetes are thought to be due to hyperglycemia and hyperinsulinemia. Hyperglycemia increases the rate of spontaneous glycation of amino groups in proteins and phospholipids. Subsequent further reactions lead to advanced glycation end products (AGEs), such as glucosepane and fructose-lysine. AGEs damage the microvasculature and the renal glomeruli, leading to retinopathy, neuropathy, and nephropathy. Hyperglycemia also increases the production of reactive oxygen species (ROS) such as superoxide anion and hydroxyl radicals (•OH). AGE production increases ROS production and vice versa. AGEs and ROS together damage the microvasculature.

## FURTHER READING

■ American Diabetes Association. Classification and diagnosis of diabetes. *Diab Care.* 2016;39(suppl 1):S13-S22, This topic is updated annually in Supplement 1.

■ Atkinson MA, Eisenbarth GS, Michels AW. Type 1 diabetes. *Lancet.* 2014;383:69-82.

■ Chakera AJ, Steele AM, Gloyn AL, et al. Recognition and management of individuals with hyperglycemia because of a heterozygous glucokinase mutation. *Diabetes Care.* 2015;38:1383-1392.

■ Genuth S, Sun W, Cleary P, et al. Skin advanced glycation end products glucosepane and methylglyoxal hydroimidazolone are independently associated with long-term microvascular complication progression of type 1 diabetes. *Diabetes.* 2015;64:266-278.

■ Hanas R, John G, International $HbA_{1c}$ Consensus Committee. 2010 consensus statement on the worldwide standardization of the hemoglobin $A_{1C}$ measurement. *Diabetes Care.* 2010;33:1903-1904.

■ Kitabchi AE, Umpierrez GE, Miles JM, Fisher JN. Hyperglycemic crises in adult patients with diabetes. *Diab Care.* 2009;32:1335-1343.

■ Rizza RA. Pathogenesis of fasting and postprandial hyperglycemia in type 2 diabetes: implications for therapy. *Diabetes.* 2010;59:2697-2707. This is a comprehensive presentation of studies of endogenous glucose production and the fate of meal-derived glucose in human volunteers.

■ Rubio-Cabezas O, Hattersley AT, Njølstad PR, et al. ISPAD Clinical Practice Consensus Guidelines 2014. The diagnosis and management of monogenic diabetes in children and adolescents. *Pediatr Diabetes.* 2014;15(suppl 20): 47-64.

■ World Health Organization. Use of glycated haemoglobin ($HbA_{1c}$) in the diagnosis of diabetes mellitus. Available at <http://www.who.int/cardiovascular_diseases/report-hba1c_2011_edited.pdf>.

■ Kuczmarski RJ, Ogden CL, Guo SS, et al. *CDC Growth Charts for the United States: methods and development.* Atlanta, GA: National Center for Health Statistics; 2002.

■ World Health Organization. Definition and diagnosis of diabetes mellitus and intermediate hyperglycemia: a report of a WHO/IDF Consultation, Geneva, Switzerland, 2006. Available at <http://www.who.int/diabetes/publications/Definition%20and%20diagnosis%20of%20diabetes_new.pdf>.

# Review Questions

1. A 14-year-old boy was sent to a children's hospital in the afternoon because he was feeling unwell and was suspected of having diabetes. During the past 3 months, he had felt increasingly thirsty, urinated frequently, and lost weight, even though he seemed to eat a good amount of food. On the day of admission, the patient ate breakfast. The patient's height was 6 feet, 2 inches (1.88 m), and his weight was 143 lb (65 kg). Which of the following is most appropriate to test this patient for diabetes?

   A. Collect urine for 24 hours, then determine the amount of glucose lost via the urine during that time
   B. Fast the patient for at least 8 hours, give 75 g of glucose by mouth, and measure plasma glucose 2 hours later
   C. Fast the patient for at least 8 hours, then measure plasma glucose
   D. Give 75 g of glucose by mouth immediately, then measure plasma glucose 2 hours later
   E. Measure plasma glucose immediately

2. A 10-year-old boy who wrestles at school suddenly becomes disoriented, falls down, and becomes unresponsive. He wears a medical bracelet identifying him as having type 1 diabetes. This patient would most likely benefit from which of the following?

   A. Infusion of saline solution
   B. Injection of an antihypertensive drug
   C. Injection of glucagon
   D. Injection of insulin lispro
   E. Water (given orally)

3. During the past 10 years, a 60-year-old male patient has become progressively more obese. His BMI is now 35 kg/m². Which one of the following tests is most appropriate to test for diabetes?

   A. Fast overnight, then measure plasma glucose in the fasting state
   B. Measure acetoacetate or β-hydroxybutyrate in the blood
   C. Measure autoantibodies to γ-aminobutyric acid decarboxylase
   D. Measure the concentration of insulin or C-peptide in plasma

4. Which one of the following drugs can be expected to have a side effect of hypoglycemia when used as monotherapy in the treatment of type 2 diabetes?

   A. An α-glucosidase inhibitor
   B. An analog of glucagon-like peptide I
   C. An inhibitor of dipeptidyl peptidase IV
   D. An inhibitor of $K_{ATP}$-channels

5. A researcher wants to assess the function of β-cells in a group of patients who have had type 1 diabetes for several years and receive near-optimal treatment. Measurement of the concentration in blood of which one of the following is most promising?

   A. C-peptide
   B. Glucagon
   C. GLP-1
   D. Insulin
   E. Somatostatin

6. A 13-year-old lean boy is found to have diabetes. At the time of diagnosis, the boy is hyperglycemic but not keto-acidotic. He receives treatment with metformin at a usual dose. However, despite adherence to the prescribed drug for 4 weeks, the concentration of glucose in plasma is still unacceptably high. Which of the following would be the most appropriate next step?

   A. Double the dose of metformin
   B. Prescribe an α-glucosidase inhibitor
   C. Prescribe a thiazolidinedione (an insulin sensitizer)
   D. Prescribe injections of insulin
   E. Test for MODY

# Answers to Review Questions

## CHAPTER 1

1. **A.** See Fig. 1.5.
2. **B.** DNA contains negatively charged phosphate groups (see Fig. 1.2).
3. **D.** Irinotecan inhibits topoisomerase I.
4. **D.** C and G together form 3 H-bonds and are therefore thermally more stable than A and T, which form only 2 H-bonds. Furthermore, according to Chargaff's rule, A and T, as well as C and G, occur equally frequently due to base pairing.

## CHAPTER 2

1. **C.** MSH2 and MSH6 are both part of mismatch repair, and Lynch syndrome is a hereditary cancer predisposition due to an allele for a nonfunctional mismatch repair protein. *Incorrect:* A (caused by deficient NER), B (caused by a mutant *BRCA1* or *BRCA2* allele), and D (primarily a disease of the colon; it is not associated with a loss of MSH2).
2. **D.** See Section 3.
3. **A.** See Section 1.
4. **E.** Adducts of DNA with polycyclic compounds usually distort the DNA helix; see Section 3.
5. **B.** See Section 4.2.

## CHAPTER 3

1. **D.** See Fig. 3.3.
2. **B.** See Section 2.
3. **C.** See Fig. 3.10.

## CHAPTER 4

1. **D.** This is the only technique listed that can detect a point mutation.
2. **D.** The forward primer has the same sequence as the 5′ end of the sequence that is shown and is to be amplified; the reverse primer has a sequence that is complementary to the 3′ end of the sequence shown, but the primer sequence has to be read from its 5′ end.
3. **B.** This is the only technique listed that can detect a balanced translocation, and the translocation is large enough to be detected by this technique.
4. **B.** *Incorrect:* A (cannot detect inversions), C (inversion is too small to be recognized by G-banding), D (poorly suited to detecting chromosome rearrangements).

5. **B.** The daughter is homozygous for the mutant allele. *Incorrect:* A (the daughter's amplicons appear fully cleaved), C (the parents are heterozygotes, and the pathogenic allele gives rise to 2 bands), D (there is no evidence of this, and 310 is the uncleaved normal allele).

## CHAPTER 5

1. **E.** The same mutation leads to a variety of phenotypes. *Incorrect:* A-C (these refer to mutations, not phenotypes), D (this is not a question of individuals with the pathogenic genotype being positive for a disease).

## CHAPTER 6

1. **B.** The template strand is transcribed in the 3′→5′ direction, and the RNA is complementary to the template strand.
2. **E.** The TATA box is located at about nucleotide –30. *Incorrect:* A (located at about nucleotide +30), B (never in the region of the core promoter), C (near the start site of transcription, at about nucleotide +1), D (a nuclear receptor is a transcription factor, a protein).
3. **D.** Rett syndrome is due to a deficiency in MECP2, a protein that binds to methylated CpGs.
4. **A.** Almost all transcription factors bind to both DNA strands.
5. **A.** Acetylation of histone tails leads to a more open chromatin structure that is more conducive to transcription.
6. **C.** Exon 1 + exon 2 + poly(A) tail + cap. The UTRs are part of the exons; the intron is removed.

## CHAPTER 7

1. **A.** See Section 3.
2. **B.** The sequence from the coding strand can be used directly with the genetic code, except that U and T have to be exchanged.
3. **A.** Each codon is 3 nucleotides long, and only the exons minus the UTRs are translated (see Figs. 6.15 and 7.2).

## CHAPTER 8

1. **B.** An increased concentration of cyclin D1 leads to increased phosphorylation of RB, which then frees E2Fs (see Fig. 8.2). *Incorrect:* A, C-E (all of these alterations decrease the chance of a neoplasm).

2. **D.** Lynch syndrome is due to an inherited loss-of-function mutation of a mismatch repair protein that is present in all somatic cells, including lymphocytes. *Incorrect:* A and B (patients with these findings more often have sporadic colorectal cancer), C (the grandfather's colon cancer occurred at an age typical of sporadic colorectal cancer).
3. **C.** See Section 1.1.
4. **C.** This patient has polyposis, but the polyposis is not dominantly inherited as in FAP.

## CHAPTER 9

1. **D.** See Section 3.3.
2. **A.** See Section 2.1.
3. **D.** The amino group is definitely positively charged, and ALA has a net charge only if the carboxyl group is protonated.
4. **C.** See Section 4.2 and Fig. 9.8.

## CHAPTER 10

1. **D.** The enzyme from the cytoplasm most likely has lower activity at a pH of 5, and the protons act at a distance from the active site. *Incorrect:* A (there is most likely inhibition), B (there are no ionizable groups in the active site), C (the inhibition is most likely reversible), E (see B and C).
2. **C.** Half-maximal activity occurs at a higher concentration of DHF. *Incorrect:* A (the $K_m$ increases; see C), B (there is a ~20-fold shift in $K_m$, and the methotrexate curve will reach as high as the control curve only at about 2,000 μM DHF), D (there is no evidence for this).
3. **B.** The $K_m$ is identical (arrow) and the V (product formed) can be compared directly. *Incorrect:* A and C (the $K_m$ is identical [arrow], not different), D (the opposite is true).

## CHAPTER 11

1. **D.** Fig. 11.2 shows that it is negatively charged. *Incorrect:* A (both fatty acids are ester linked), B (a phospholipid does not contain isoprenes), C (it does not contain a sugar; it is a glycerophospholipid).
2. **C.** *Incorrect:* A (they flip phospholipids), B (it is a protein), D (it does not move aminophospholipids such as phosphatidylserine).

## CHAPTER 12

1. **A.** The parents both have thin basement membrane nephropathy due to heterozygosity for a mutation in the COL4A3 or COL4A4 gene, and each of their offspring has a 25% chance of being homozygous and thus having Alport syndrome.
2. **D.** Of the listed disorders, only Alport syndrome is associated with hematuria, and the father is asymptomatic.

## CHAPTER 13

1. **D.** See Section 1.2.
2. **A.** See Section 1.4.
3. **D.** This enzyme has insufficient activity in patients who have Hurler syndrome (see Section 2.4).

## CHAPTER 14

1. **A.** Acute intermittent porphyria shows autosomal dominant inheritance. *Incorrect:* B (X-linked), C and E (require that the mother is a carrier), D (most often acquired, though it can be inherited, but this is less common than A).
2. **B.** An example of such an autoimmune disease is primary biliary cholangitis. *Incorrect:* A would not give rise to an elevated concentration of bilirubin; C and E would give rise to a more modest increase in bilirubin, and the direct bilirubin would be less than 15% of the total bilirubin. If D gave rise to liver damage, the direct bilirubin would be less than 15% of the total bilirubin.
3. **B.** Infusion of lipids displaces bilirubin from albumin, which increases the chance that the infant develops kernicterus. Hence, lipid is infused at a rate that is low but sufficient to prevent a deficiency of essential fatty acids. *Incorrect:* A and C would not favorably affect bilirubin production, conjugation, or excretion.

## CHAPTER 15

1. **C.** Phlebotomy is the preferred treatment for HFE hemochromatosis. Iron chelators, such as desferrioxamine or deferasirox, can be used, but they are reserved for patients who do not tolerate phlebotomy. Treatment with iron would worsen iron overload that is apparent from the patient's serum ferritin.
2. **D.** The low hemoglobin, low MCV, low serum iron, somewhat high total iron binding capacity, low calculated transferrin saturation, and low serum ferritin all point to an iron deficiency (and thus speak against options A and C). The normal serum folate makes a folate deficiency (B) unlikely, and the normal serum cobalamin makes pernicious anemia (E) unlikely.
3. **B.** Chronic inflammation stimulates hepcidin secretion. Juvenile and HFE hemochromatosis, as well as iron-deficiency anemia, are associated with a low rate of hepcidin secretion.

## CHAPTER 16

1. **B.** This is due to an excessive rate of hematopoiesis. A, C, and D are incorrect because erythrocytes are normal.
2. **B.** Nitrites induce the formation of methemoglobin, which binds cyanide temporarily. *Incorrect:* A and C (treated with oxygen, not nitrite), D (treated with methylene blue, except in G6PD deficient patients).

3. **D.** Increases in the concentration of $H^+$, $CO_2$, and 2,3-BPG all increase the $P_{50}$ of hemoglobin for $O_2$.

4. **C.** The maximal saturation remains at 100%, but the $P_{50}$ shifts to a higher $pO_2$.

## CHAPTER 17

1. **C.** The woman's eggs have either no or one α-globin allele, and the man's sperm have either no or two α-globin alleles. The chance that an embryo has only one α-globin allele is $\frac{1}{2} \times \frac{1}{2} = \frac{1}{4}$.

2. **A.** An $HbA_2 + HbC + HbE$ of 5% can only indicate an elevated $HbA_2$; this, in turn, is a very strong indicator of β-thalassemia minor, to which a low hemoglobin and MCV fit well. *Incorrect:* B, C, and D ($HbA_2 + HbC + HbE$ is much less than 50%), D and E (HbS is 0%).

3. **D.** The patient has HbA and HbS as the major hemoglobins; in a patient with sickle cell trait, HbS is typically somewhat less abundant than HbA. *Incorrect:* A and E ($HbA_2 + HbC$ is normal), B (there is no indication of an abnormal $HbA_{1c}$), C and E (there is HbA).

4. **C.** The woman's eggs have either no or two α-globin alleles, and the man's sperm always have one α-globin allele, so the chance of the first-born having only one α-globin allele is $\frac{1}{2} \times 1 = \frac{1}{2}$.

5. **D.** The term sickle cell disease encompasses patients who have, for instance, hemoglobin SC disease or sickle cell/β-thalassemia. *Incorrect:* A is the genotype for β-thalassemia trait, B is for sickle cell trait, and C is for hemoglobin C disease.

6. **D.** The elevated bilirubin and LDH are indicative of a hemolytic anemia, and the low MCV can be due to a hemoglobinopathy. *Incorrect:* A (the fraction would be <15%), B (lab values are indicative of iron deficiency), C (lab values are indicative of polycythemia), E (MCHC is elevated, indicating a problem with DNA replication, not hemoglobin synthesis).

## CHAPTER 18

1. **E.** Lactulose is only digested by bacteria; if a significant amount of $H_2$ is produced in response to lactulose, the patient's lactose tolerance test is truly negative; if lactulose does not induce $H_2$ production, the patient's gut flora likely does not produce a significant amount of $H_2$, and the lactose tolerance test therefore cannot be interpreted. *Incorrect:* A could reduce the number of bacteria in the intestine and thus lower $H_2$ production, but the result would not be helpful in making a diagnosis. B, C, and D are most likely taken up normally and are therefore very unlikely to give rise to increased $H_2$ production.

2. **A.** Adipose tissue and muscle contain insulin-sensitive GLUT-4 transporters. *Incorrect:* B-E do not contain insulin-sensitive glucose transporters.

3. **B.** Lactase is not an α-glucosidase. *Incorrect:* A, C, and E are hydrolyzed by α-glucosidases. D is not hydrolyzed by human enzymes, only by bacteria, which do not produce glucose.

4. **D.** Protein malnutrition impairs the synthesis of disaccharidases. *Incorrect:* A, B, and C have no direct effect on lactase activity and play no role in the digestion of milk.

## CHAPTER 19

1. **F.** PFK1 is the rate-limiting enzyme and can be activated by fructose 2,6-bisphosphate in an insulin-dependent manner. *Incorrect:* A-E catalyze reversible reactions and can therefore not be effectively regulated. G, when activated, tends to decrease the concentration of intermediates between fructose 1,6-bisphosphate and phosphoenolpyruvate; this includes dihydroxyacetonephosphate.

2. **C.** The concentrations of all intermediates between fructose 1,6-bisphosphate and phosphoenolpyruvate are elevated, leading to an elevated concentration of 2,3-BPG. *Incorrect:* A is incorrect because a decrease in flux in one part of the pathway leads to a decrease in flux in the entire pathway; were it not for the 2,3-BPG bypass, both reactions would produce the same amount of ATP. B is incorrect because phosphoenolpyruvate cannot be transported across the plasma membrane. D is incorrect for the reason stated in A.

3. **C.** Hypophosphatemia inhibits the reaction from GAP to 1,3BPG. *Incorrect:* A and B are upstream of the deficiency and therefore would decrease; D and E are downstream of the deficiency and would increase.

## CHAPTER 20

1. **B.** Most cells form galactose 1-phosphate, which they can metabolize only slowly. The accompanying low concentration of free phosphate impairs ATP synthesis.

2. **C.** Fructose and galactose are both metabolized by the liver.

3. **E.** Aldolase B deficiency causes hereditary fructose intolerance, and sucrose gives rise to fructose.

## CHAPTER 21

1. **D.** The daughter of the affected male carries one G6PD-deficient X-chromosome, and there is a 50% chance that she will pass this on to her offspring. This applies to all X-linked disorders.

2. **B.** G6PD deficiency reduces the rate of NADPH production. *Incorrect:* A and D (primaquine is an oxidant), C (primaquine does not bind to G6PD), E (the sugar phosphate branch does not produce NADPH).

## CHAPTER 22

1. **C.**
2. **D.** Hypoxia incapacitates oxidative phosphorylation, which leads to an accumulation of NADH.

## CHAPTER 23

1. **B.** $O_2$ displaces CO. *Incorrect:* A, C, and D are ineffective.
2. **A.** Complex 1 deficiency is one cause of Leigh syndrome. *Incorrect:* B and C are associated with a deficiency of all complexes.

## CHAPTER 24

1. **A.** See Fig. 24.7.
2. **D.** Pompe disease only impairs the turnover of glycogen particles in lysosomes, leading to muscle weakness. *Incorrect:* A is associated with enlarged glycogen particles, B with glycogen particles of abnormal structure, and C with abnormally small glycogen particles.
3. **B.** See Section 3.3. *Incorrect:* A does not explain any abnormalities, C would not impair the formation of glucose from galactose via glucose 6-phosphatase, and D would not give rise to a high glycogen content.

## CHAPTER 25

1. **D.** Excess glucagon stimulates gluconeogenesis. *Incorrect:* A, B, C, and E are associated with a low rate of gluconeogenesis.
2. **D.** The deficiency leads to decreased use of lactic acid. *Incorrect:* In A-C, the opposite occurs.

## CHAPTER 26

1. **A.** See Section 3.3.2.
2. **C.** A mutant insulin can have normal immunoreactivity yet diminished biological activity (the receptor-binding region differs from the immunological epitope). *Incorrect:* A, B, D, and E (recombinant insulin had a normal effect).

## CHAPTER 27

1. **A.** See Figs. 27.3 and 27.9. *Incorrect:* B (the acyl carrier protein is part of fatty acid synthase in the cytosol, but fatty acid oxidation takes place inside mitochondria [or peroxisomes]), C (there is no such transporter in the inner mitochondrial membrane), D (the enzyme mentioned plays a role in ketone body oxidation, not in fatty acid oxidation).

2. **A.** The low bicarbonate is indicative of ketoacidosis, which is accompanied by ketonemia and ketonuria (see also Sections 5.4 and 7.3).
3. **B.** In the fasting state the liver synthesizes ketone bodies but not fatty acids, and it can never oxidize ketone bodies.

## CHAPTER 28

1. **E.** The liver synthesizes some fatty acids from glucose and receives others from the hydrolysis of infused triglycerides; the liver esterifies the fatty acids to triglycerides and exports them inside VLDL. *Incorrect:* A and B (without food, chylomicron production by the intestine is minuscule), C and D (IDL and LDL contain much less triglycerides than do VLDL).
2. **B.** *Incorrect:* A (de novo fatty acid synthesis occurs at only a low rate in the fed state, not the fasting state), C (VLDL give rise to LDL, not the reverse), D (the liver takes up chylomicron remnants, not chylomicrons; there are few chylomicrons in the fasting state; chylomicron remnants contain a relatively small fraction of triglycerides; and, in the fasting state, the triglycerides in the remnants are a minor source of triglycerides in VLDL).

## CHAPTER 29

1. Increased expression of LDL receptors mediates the cholesterol-lowering effect of statins. At least one functional allele of the LDL receptor (as in heterozygous familial hypercholesterolemia) is required for such an effect.
2. **A.** See Figs. 29.1 and 29.3.
3. **D.** Hypertriglyceridemia leads to delipidation and loss of HDL (see Fig. 29.7). *Incorrect:* A, C, and E would favor an increase in HDL cholesterol, and B would not have a significant effect.
4. **B.** This is a common cause of familial hypercholesterolemia (see Section 5.2). *Incorrect:* A and C-E do not cause high LDL cholesterol.

## CHAPTER 30

1. **A.** Hemodialysis is used in cases of severe ethanol poisoning. *Incorrect:* B (disulfiram would lead to an accumulation of toxic acetaldehyde), C (fomepizole would inhibit metabolism of ethanol), D (the hyperglycemia is mild and not dangerous), and E (there is no need for this).
2. **C.** Glucagon normally stimulates glycogenolysis, but due to a low rate of gluconeogenesis, glycogen stores are low in alcohol-abusing patients, particularly those who also have diabetes. *Incorrect:* A (there is no clinical precedent for this), B and D (per se, these can be true statements, but they are not the most direct answers to the question).
3. **B.** See Section 2.1.

## CHAPTER 31

1. **B.** See Fig. 31.17.
2. **B.** She produces too much aldosterone. *Incorrect:* A and C (the renin-angiotensin system is most likely functioning normally, and these drugs inhibit upstream signaling; aldosterone production in this patient is largely independent of the renin-angiotensin system), D and E (they do not reduce aldosterone synthesis or signaling).
3. **A.** Addison disease is due to destruction of the adrenal cortex; the low concentrations of cortisol and aldosterone lead to increased secretion of ACTH and renin. *Incorrect:* B (the opposite changes are occurring), C (these do not significantly affect cortisol and aldosterone synthesis), and D (the concentration of CRH is high).
4. **E.** This is the most likely reason the infant has a 46,XY disorder of sex development. *Incorrect:* A and D (would not cause development of female sex traits), B (would only affect the synthesis of estrogens), C (would accentuate male sex traits).

## CHAPTER 32

1. **B.** $PGE_3$ is made from EPA, and fish oil is the richest source of EPA. *Incorrect:* A (contains mostly DHA and very little EPA), C (contains mostly linolenic acid and virtually no EPA), D (is a poor source of ω-3 fatty acids).
2. **E.** Thromboxane $A_2$ stimulates platelet aggregation.
3. **E.** Zileuton inhibits 5-lipoxygenase (see Fig. 32.3). *Incorrect:* A (a $\beta_2$-adrenergic agonist that has no effect on eicosanoid synthesis), B (inhibits COXs, which are essential for the synthesis of prostanoids), C (prostaglandin $F_{2\alpha}$), D (a CYSLTR1 antagonist that has no effect on eicosanoid synthesis).
4. **B.** Misoprostol is a $PGE_1$ analog that increases bicarbonate and mucus secretion to protect the mucosa of the stomach and duodenum. *Incorrect:* A (it further inhibits prostaglandin synthesis; see Fig. 32.2), C (a $\beta_2$-adrenergic agonist that has no effect on prostanoid synthesis), D (a CYSLTR1 antagonist that has no effect on prostanoid synthesis), E (a 5-lipoxygenase inhibitor that has no effect on prostanoid synthesis).

## CHAPTER 33

1. **C.** See Section 2.
2. **C.** See Table 33.1.

## CHAPTER 34

1. **A.** G-cells in the antrum secrete gastrin, which leads to HCl secretion from parietal cells; see Figs. 34.1 and 34.2). *Incorrect:* B and C (histamine- and somatostatin-secreting cells are largely absent from the antrum; these options would increase HCl secretion). D and E (parietal cells and chief cells are largely absent from the antrum).
2. **B.** Pentagastrin stimulates histamine secretion, which in turn stimulates HCl secretion from parietal cells. *Incorrect:* A (acetylcholine stimulates gastrin secretion, not the other way around); C (somatostatin inhibits histamine secretion); D and E (no causal relationship).
3. **D.** Proton pump inhibitors reduce HCl secretion, which reduces somatostatin secretion, which reduces the inhibitory effect of somatostatin on gastrin secretion. *Incorrect:* A (somatostatin inhibits gastrin secretion); B and C (these lead to a high concentration of somatostatin, which inhibits gastrin secretion).

## CHAPTER 35

1. **E.** Ornithine carbamoyltransferase deficiency leads to an accumulation of ornithine and carbamoylphosphate that, in turn, leaks into the cytosol and gives rise to orotate. *Incorrect:* A and B lead to an elevated concentration of citrulline, and C and D do not give rise to a high excretion of orotate.
2. **B.** These drugs are commonly used to treat hyperammonemia in the hospital, and hemodialysis is indicated by the patient's state and the hyperammonemia. Incorrect: A (citrulline is only given for specific deficiencies of the urea cycle), C (essential amino acids would likely aggravate the hyperammonemia), D and E (neither addresses the life-threatening hyperammonemia).

## CHAPTER 36

1. **C.** *Incorrect:* The vitamins in A, B, D, and E play no role in the detoxification of methanol.
2. **D.** *Incorrect:* A and C are not specific for cobalamin deficiency, and B is not done (antibodies to intrinsic factor and/or parietal cells help in the diagnosis of pernicious anemia).
3. **C.** *Incorrect:* A is not specific for cobalamin deficiency, and B and D are not done.

## CHAPTER 37

1. **D.** PRPP is synthesized only when a cell's phosphorylation state is good, a prerequisite for pyrimidine nucleotide de novo synthesis. By contrast, UTP (E) exerts feedback inhibition. A-C have no effect on pyrimidine nucleotide de novo synthesis.
2. **D.** Methotrexate inhibits dihydrofolate reductase (DHFR) and thereby depletes the pool of one-carbon loaded THFs. $N^5$-formyltetrahydrofolic acid (leucovorin, folinic acid) can replenish this pool without requiring DHFR. None of the other options (A-C, E and F) replenish the pool of one-carbon THFs. Gemcitabine (C) inhibits ribonucleotide reductase, and gimeracil (D) inhibits the degradation of 5-fluorouracil; neither drug relieves methotrexate toxicity.

## CHAPTER 38

1. **B.** Rasburicase converts uric acid to allantoin. Allopurinol is also suitable to prevent tumor lysis syndrome, but rasburicase lowers existing hyperuricemia faster than allopurinol does. *Incorrect:* A and C have no hypouricemic effect. D and E would exacerbate the crystallization of uric acid in the kidneys.

2. **C.** Variant Lesch-Nyhan syndrome is due to reduced activity of HGPRT and therefore reduced salvage of hypoxanthine, resulting in increased urate production. Allopurinol inhibits urate production. *Incorrect:* A worsens the hyperuricemia by decreasing urate excretion. B is not a first-line treatment and is not sufficiently long-lived for the treatment of gout. D may cause uric acid nephrolithiasis.

3. **G.** The vast majority of patients who have gout are urate underexcretors. *Incorrect:* A-E all lead to urate overproduction, which is uncommon among patients who have gout. F is not thought to be common.

## CHAPTER 39

1. **E.** His blood glucose will likely be higher than 200 mg/dL (11.1 mM).

2. **C.** The boy is most likely hypoglycemic.

3. **A.** This is the standard approach for someone who is not in acute distress; see Section 3.

4. **D.** $K_{ATP}$ inhibitors stimulate insulin secretion even during hypoglycemia.

5. **A.** C-peptide is only secreted from the patient's own β-cells and parallels insulin secretion; injected insulin is free of C-peptide.

6. **E.** There is a good chance that he has MODY; a genetic diagnosis guides treatment.

# Index

Page numbers followed by "*f*" indicate figures, and "*t*" indicate tables.